CANCER PAIN

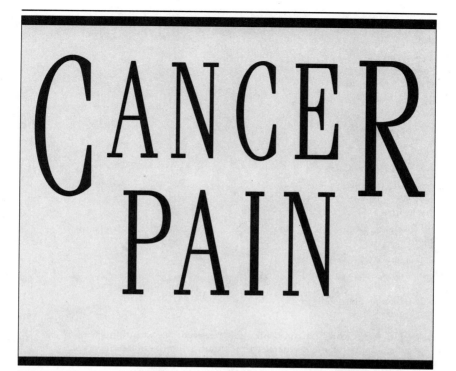

CANCER PAIN

RICHARD B. PATT, M.D.

Associate Professor of Anesthesiology, Psychiatry, and Oncology
Medical Director, Pain Treatment Center
Coordinator, Cancer Pain Programs
University of Rochester School of Medicine and Dentistry

with 38 contributors

J. B. LIPPINCOTT COMPANY
Philadelphia

Acquisitions Editor: Mary K. Smith
Developmental Editor: Anne Geyer
Project Editor: Amy P. Jirsa
Indexer: Sandra King
Designer: Doug Smock
Cover Designer: Cathy Cotter
Production Manager: Helen Ewan
Production Coordinator: Nannette Winski
Compositor: Bi-Comp
Printer/Binder: R. R. Donnelly Harrisonburg

6 5 4 3 2 1

Library of Congress Cataloging in Publications Data

Cancer pain / Richard B. Patt; with 38 contributors.
    p.   cm.
Includes bibliographical references and index.
ISBN 0-397-51138-8
1. Cancer pain. I. Patt, Richard B.
(DNLM: 1. Neoplasms—therapy. 2. Pain—therapy. 3. Palliative
Treatment—methods. QZ 266 C21621]
RC262.C291183 1993
616.99'406—dc20
DNLM/DLC
for Library of Congress   92-49630
                                         CIP

Foreword

The subject of cancer pain management has only recently been accorded sufficient attention and priority in the broad field of medicine. Indeed, many major specialty texts still devote only token amounts of space to the subject of cancer pain and its treatment. Recent major initiatives at a national and international level are rapidly changing the picture, however. In 1984, the World Health Organization identified cancer pain as a major world health problem. The International Association for the Study of Pain (IASP), initially concerned mainly with the subject of chronic pain, has increasingly focused also on cancer pain and the closely related subject of acute pain. IASP developed an official relationship with WHO for the specific purpose of participating in a global program aimed at making effective treatments available throughout the world by the year 2000. The development by IASP of undergraduate and postgraduate curricula has also provided an important framework on which to base a teaching initiative. Fortunately, in the past 5 years attention has now been given to the publication of comprehensive texts on the subject of cancer pain, but they are still very few in number. Thus this extensive and well-balanced text edited by Dr. Richard Patt fulfills an important need in this rapidly developing field.

The diagnosis and treatment of cancer pain now draws on knowledge and expertise from a very broad range of medical specialties. Thus Dr. Patt has appropriately drawn his authors from just such a cross-section of medical disciplines.

During the past 5 years that I have served as President and Past President of IASP, I have had an opportunity to visit many countries and to see first hand the work that is being done to improve the treatment of cancer pain. This has confirmed the estimates of WHO that currently only 50% of patients in developed countries receive effective pain relief and that this figure can vary to as low as 10% in some developing countries. In contrast, new knowledge and new methods are now capable of relieving in excess of 90% of cancer pain. Although the realization of this vast improvement is a complex task, dissemination of new knowledge does play an important part. Here again, Dr. Patt's book will make a valuable contribution, particularly because it is one of the first texts to deal comprehensively with this subject.

Michael J. Cousins, MD, FANZCA, Immediate Past President, International Association for the Study of Pain; Professor and Head, Department of Anesthesia and Pain Management, University of Sydney; Royal North Shore Hospital, St. Leonards, AUSTRALIA

Preface

In recent years the importance and value of effective management of cancer pain has achieved a high degree of recognition both in academic environments and with the lay public. Multiple specialties have assigned a high priority to cancer pain management in their programs of education, research, and clinical care. Patients and their families are articulating their concerns. Such changes are due in large part to the efforts of long-time workers in the field of pain management, including Bonica, Foley, Portenoy, Ventafridda, and Cousins. The factors responsible for this evolution are largely of a humane and ethical nature. The recognition that patients with cancer pain have historically been underserved, despite the availability of means for providing relief of pain, is coming to the fore. Cancer prevention and treatment, goals of inestimable importance, have historically been the subject of disproportionate funding and interest, almost to the exclusion of considerations of symptom control. That trend is undergoing slow reversal. The principles of cancer pain management described here work, and that is a corollary reason for enhanced interest: compassion breeds passion, especially when results are obtainable and measurable.

Part of health-care providers' attraction to cancer pain management is that symptoms are more amenable to treatment than are those in patients with nonmalignant pain—which are, in a sense, more responsive to management than treatment, per se. Working with patients who have nonmalignant pain involves rehabilitating and teaching patients to live with and accept residual pain. In contrast, symptoms are more often eliminated or significantly relieved in patients with oncologic pain. Issues of secondary gain and establishing disability rarely surface when pain is due to cancer. Opioid analgesics, of questionable and controversial value when administered chronically for nonmalignant pain, are considered effective and appropriate for use in patients with cancer pain.

Physicians are interventionists by nature, and cancer pain management allows for a wide range of intervention. Treatment with analgesics is the basis for the management of virtually all patients. The application of clinical pharmacology can be accomplished by the primary care provider or alternate specialists. Pharmacologic management is widely accessible because its underlying principles are based in common sense, and with motivation, careful observation, persistence, patience, and imagination, excellent results can be obtained in most patients. Despite their efficacy, the principles and techniques of pharmacologic management in current use are, to a large extent, still empirically based and provide a wealth of material for both the clinical researcher and basic scientist.

Some patients do not obtain adequate relief of pain despite aggressive efforts at pharmacologic management. A wide, sometimes dizzying array of choices of alternative therapeutic measures exists. Nerve blocks have an important historical and contemporary role in the management of pain. With only a few exceptions, the application of neural blockade in nonmalignant pain is limited to the injection of local anesthetic agents and corticosteroids. Treatment generally is of limited duration, and then usually in the context of a rehabilitation program. In contrast, neurolytic blocks are often appropriate choices in well-selected patients with cancer pain. Complications can be avoided by careful selection of the proper procedure and meticulous attention to technical detail.

Intraspinal opioid therapy, a relatively new but much-applied technique, promises to afford a reliable means for control of intractable pain of various types. Again, because therapy is likely to be of a finite duration, patients with cancer are superior candidates than are their counterparts with nonmalignant pain. Decision-making, however, can be problematic because of limited experience with alternative systems of implantation, drug delivery, and drug selection.

Our enthusiasm to provide relief of pain, no matter how great the need, must be tempered by a thorough evaluation of each patient's overall medical condition and an understanding of the importance of meticulous, frequent followup. Cancer is a multisymptomatic disease. Patients are best served when quality of life is regarded as the primary consideration guiding management. Relief of pain is best addressed in the context of control of other related symptoms such as confusion, nausea, vomiting, constipation, depression, and anorexia. Pain control is inadequate if it produces excessive sedation or intolerable nausea and vomiting. By the same token, most of these symptoms can be controlled, and should be addressed as aggressively as pain.

Finally, cancer is usually a multisystem disease, progressive and dynamic in character. Patients tend to be unwell but unlike the patients encountered in most medical and specialty practices, most care is provided in the setting of the patient's home. In most regions, systems exist to monitor patients' condition and to provide for their needs, in essence serving as the doctor's eyes, ears, and hands. Nevertheless, patients and their families need to be educated in how to handle their present circumstances and what to expect as illness progresses. Perhaps most of all, they require reassurance and reliable information.

Like the course of disease, requirements for symptom control do not remain static. Adequacy of pain control is affected by the development of tolerance, the evolution of metastatic lesions, and changes in the patient's medical and psychological condition. It is essential that in the course of monitoring the adequacy of symptom control, the practitioner recognize and understand the significance of related changes in patients' medical condition. Analgesic requirements and the patient's overall medical condition are often interdependent. It is not enough to apply the measures discussed here, but their implications vis-à-vis the patient's physiology and the pathophysiology of cancer need to be considered, particularly for the application of some of the more novel interventions. So, for example, although an epidural catheter may provide a means to modify symptoms dramatically, simply implementing therapy is insufficient; the clinician must also be able to problem-solve. He should, for example, be able to recognize catheter-related meningitis (and other problems), differentiate it from other processes, and provide alternate therapy if needed. Confusion and delirium may be related to treatment or alternatively may be a metabolic problem related to the disease, its treatment, or other factors. The onset of back pain and progressive neurologic symptoms may herald spinal cord compression, an oncologic emergency. Because of patients' limited access to hospitals and in virtue of the close followup ideally instituted by the pain control team, the symptom control specialist is often the first to be informed of this and like problems, and must possess resources to respond appropriately. This book supports the clinican in providing this valuable support to their patients.

ORGANIZATION

This text has intentionally adopted a broad scope in recognition of the evolving role of the practitioner managing oncologic pain and related symptoms. Treatment begins *prima facie* with assessment that must be broadly based and should include an understanding of the common cancer pain syndromes, including those due to treatment. These subjects, as well as the assessment and management of a long-neglected subject, pediatric pain, are included in the text's first section. The assessment of psychological problems is also covered initially, along with diagnosis, because these issues are likely to arise during assessment. As with medical management, an aggressive proactive approach to the behavioral determinants of suffering is preferred, and a sep-

arate section has been devoted to psychiatric issues that often arise in the course of illness: anxiety, depression, and delirium.

The section on treatment begins with an explication of the palliative roles of systemic chemotherapy and radiation therapy that should be of value to all specialists because, if justified by the risk that is entailed, eliminating the source of pain is beneficial whenever possible. Since oral drug therapy is the preferred initial treatment for most patients and usually remains an important adjunct, if not the mainstay of care, this subject has been given wide coverage, with particular attention devoted to issues of habituation versus legitimate and appropriate medical use, treatment aspects of persistent concern to patients, families, physicians, and healthcare administrators. The management of adverse drug effects, alternatives to opioids and alternative routes of administration are considered, with emphasis on the indications and limitations of these latter techniques. Although pain is the most common and often the most distressing symptom of advanced cancer, other important symptoms and their modification are addressed.

Considerable attention has been devoted to the role of nerve blocks. Areas covered include their indications, timing, selection, and avoidance and management of complications. The section on intraspinal opioids is particularly timely, endeavoring to correlate emerging concepts with selection of the proper patient, procedure, device, drug, and delivery system. The potential indications for neurosurgical intervention is covered as is orthopedic management. A wide range of oncologic emergencies are considered, mostly from the standpoint of early recognition and diagnosis. Finally, models for the organization of care are considered, including a section on the status of palliative care in developing nations, a most compelling issue. Regrettably, caring for patients with cancer often means ministering to dying patients and their families, an endeavor for which many of us are ill-prepared; hence a section of hospice care is featured. The management of patients with advanced malignancy requires a thorough and conscientious approach, and therefore an understanding of the systems required to facilitate assessment, followup, and emergency care is sensible and necessary. The appendices are a shorthand source of a variety of information intended to be of practical value to the clinician.

This text is intended to serve as a comprehensive reference for practitioners engaged in the management of cancer pain and related symptoms. It has been designed to be useful at both the resident and attending level, and for those for whom cancer pain management is a major focus, as well as those who are only occasionally involved in the treatment of these complex patients. As a reference, the text is expected to be extremely useful to practitioners from a variety of specialties who need to understand both the standard pharmacologic approaches to management as well as some of the more novel, sometimes invasive, approaches.

It has been emphasized throughout the text that although cancer pain management challenges even the most compassionate and tireless clinician, it is an endeavor that at the same time rewards involvement in unexpected, often very moving ways. Editing this text has been a like endeavor: I was encouraged by the enthusiasm and dedication of its authors, each world class experts in their respective fields, and also by their gentleness in dealing with my relentless efforts to complete this project. My department and its chairman, Ronald Gabel, were supportive as were my family who endured, proudly, special pains of their own. At times the book threatened to develop a life of its own and, for their understanding and professionalism, I thank the staff of J.B. Lippincott, especially Mary K. Smith, Anne Geyer, and Amy Jirsa. Like all wondrous things in life, the text has evolved in ways that could not have been predicted at the outset. I am pleased beyond all expectation with the quality of the text's constituent parts, as well as its final form, and I am hopeful that you will find its influence beneficial on your practice and your care of patients.

Acknowledgments

For secretarial assistance
Olga Welling

For design and artistic contribution
Anita Matthews

For assistance in production
Mary K. Smith
Anne Geyer
Amy P. Jirsa

For assistance in reviewing portions of the text

Robert Boas	Bertil Lofstrom
John Bonica	Richard Millard
Joseph A. Catania	Cyril Meyerowitz
J.E. Charlton	Russell Portenoy
Subhash Jain	Steven Rosen
Yashin Khan	Phillip Rubin
James Keller	Nancy Wells
Zachary Kramer	Tony Yaksh
Sampson Lipton	

For contribution of radiographs, questionnaires, and related materials

Steve Abrams	Russell Portenoy
Franz Boersma	Gabor Racz
Charles Cleeland	P. Prithvi Raj
Leonard F. Hirsch	Richard Rauck
Douglas M. Justins	Michael Stanton-Hicks
Dean Melnyk	C.P.N. Watson
Cyril Meyerowitz	

For invaluable personal support
My parents, Shirley and Howard Patt
Cheryl Kelley
Ronald Gabel
Richard Millard
Eileen Smith

Contributors

Steve Abram, MD
Professor of Anesthesiology
Medical Center of Wisconsin
Director, Milwaukee County Medical Complex Pain Clinic
Milwaukee, Wisconsin

Ina Cummings-Ajemian, MD, CM, CCFP
Associate Professor
Palliative Care Medicine Division
Department of Oncology
McGill University
Director, Palliative Care Service
Royal Victoria Hospital
Montreal, Quebec
CANADA

Michael Ashby, MBBS, MRCP(UK), FRCR
Clinical Senior Lecturer
Department of Medicine
University of Adelaide
Director of Palliative Medicine and Radiation Oncologist
Royal Adelaide Hospital
Medical Director, Mary Potter Hospice
North Adelaide, South Australia
AUSTRALIA

Judith E. Beyer, RN, PhD
Associate Professor
School of Nursing
University of Colorado Health Sciences Center
Denver, Colorado

William Breitbart, MD
Assistant Professor of Psychiatry
Cornell University Medical College
Assistant Attending Psychiatrist
Memorial Sloan-Kettering Cancer Center
New York, New York

Eduardo Bruera, MD
Associate Professor of Medicine
University of Alberta
Director, Palliative Care Program
Edmonton General Hospital
Edmonton, Alberta
CANADA

John A. Campa III, MD
Neuro-Oncology Pain Fellow
Department of Neurology
University of Cincinnati College of Medicine
Director, Neuro-Oncology Pain Service
Centennial Medical Center
Nashville, Tennessee

Joseph A. Catania, MD
Instructor in Anesthesiology
University of Rochester School of Medicine and
    Dentistry
Strong Memorial Hospital
Rochester, New York

Neil M. Ellison, MD
Clinical Professor of Medicine
Thomas Jefferson University
Associate, Medical Oncology
Geisinger Medical Center
Danville, Pennsylvania

Robin J. Hamill, MD
Assistant Professor of Anesthesiology and Critical
    Care Medicine
University of Virginia School of Medicine
Director of Preadmission Assessment Center
University of Virginia Health Science Center
Charlottesville, Virginia

C. Stratton Hill, Jr, MD
Professor of Medicine
Department of Neuro-Oncology
Director, Section of Pain and Symptom Management
University of Texas Medical School
MD Anderson Cancer Center Houston
Houston, Texas

Subhash Jain, MD
Director, Anesthesiology/Pain Management
Memorial Sloan-Kettering Cancer Center
Assistant Professor
Cornell University Medical Center
New York, New York

L. Douglas Kennedy, MD
Fellow, Pain Therapy Unit
Cleveland Clinic Foundation
Cleveland, Ohio

Michael R. Kurman, MD
Director of Oncology
Janssen Research Foundation
Janssen Pharmaceutica
Piscataway, New Jersey

W. David Leak, MD
Adjunct Staff
Department of Anesthesiology
The Cleveland Clinic Foundation
Medical Director
Pain Control Consultants, Inc.
Park Medical Center
Columbus, Ohio

Sampson Lipton, OBE, MD, FFA, RCS
Emeritus Consultant
Department of Medical and Surgical Neurology
Liverpool University
Medical Director, Pain Research Institute
Walton Hospital
Liverpool
UNITED KINGDOM

Richard W. Millard, PhD
Assistant Professor of Psychiatry (Psychology) and
    Anesthesiology
University of Rochester School of Medicine and
    Dentistry
Director, Pain Treatment Center
Strong Memorial Hospital
Rochester, New York

Richard Payne, MD
Associate Professor of Neurology
University of Cincinnati College of Medicine
Chief, Neurology Service
Veterans Administration Medical Center
Cincinnati, Ohio

Ricardo B. Plancarte, MD
Medical Director of Anesthesiology, Intensive Care,
    and Pain Clinic
Professor of Anesthesiology and Pain Clinic
Universidad Nacional Autonomo de Mexico
National Cancer Institute of Mexico
Mexico City
MEXICO

Russell K. Portenoy, MD
Associate Professor of Neurology
Cornell University Medical College
Associate Attending Neurologist
Memorial Sloan-Kettering Cancer Center
New York, New York

P. Prithvi Raj, MBBs, FCAnes
Professor of Anesthesiology
The Medical College of Georgia
Professor, Mercer University Southern School of
  Pharmacy
Executive Medical Director
Southeastern Pain Institute at Georgia Baptist Medi-
  cal Center
Atlanta, Georgia

Carla Ripamonti, MD
Palliative Care Service
National Cancer Institute
Milano
ITALY

John R. Roschuck
President, Preferred Medical Products
Thorold, Ontario
CANADA

Randy N. Rosier, PhD
Associate Professor of Orthopaedics, Oncology and
  Biophysics
University of Rochester School of Medicine and
  Dentistry
Strong Memorial Hospital
Rochester, New York

John C. Rowlingson, MD
Professor of Anesthesiology
Director, Pain Management Center
University of Virginia Health Sciences Center
Charlottesville, Virginia

Neil L. Schechter, MD
Professor of Pediatrics
Head, Division of Developmental and Behavioral
  Pediatrics
University of Connecticut School of Medicine
Director, Section of Developmental and Behavioral
  Pediatrics
Saint Francis Hospital and Medical Center
Hartford, Connecticut

Julia Ladd Smith, MD
Assistant Professor of Oncology in Medicine
University of Rochester/St. Mary's Hospital
Medical Director, Hospice of Rochester
Rochester, New York

John E. Stambaugh Jr., MD, PhD
Professor of Pharmacology
Jefferson Medical College
Division of Oncology Member, Cooper Medical
  Center
Attending Physician, Division of Oncology and
  Hematology
Underwood Hospital
Woodbury, New Jersey

Chad F. Swenson, RPh
Supervisor, Manufacturing Pharmacy Department
University of Rochester Medical Center
Rochester, New York

Mark Swerdlow, MD, MSc, FFARCS
Former Director
Northwest Regional Pain Relief Centre
Hope Hospital
University of Manchester School of Medicine
UNITED KINGDOM

James E. Szalados, MD
Fellow, Critical Care Medicine
University of Rochester School of Medicine and
  Dentistry
Rochester, New York

Ronald R. Tasker, MD
Professor
Department of Surgery
University of Toronto
Director of Neurosurgery
Toronto Hospital
Toronto, Ontario
CANADA

Rübén S. Velázquez, MD
Assistant Attending Physician, Department of
  Anesthesiology and Pain Clinic Service
Assistant Professor of Anesthesiology
Universidad Nacional Autonomo de Mexico
Assistant Professor of Anesthesiology
Spanish Hospital of Mexico
Mexico City
MEXICO

Steven D. Waldman, MD
Clinical Professor of Anesthesiology
University of Missouri, Kansas City
Medical Director, Pain Consortium of Greater Kansas
  City
Leawood, Kansas

Steven J. Weisman, MD
Associate Professor of Pediatrics
University of Connecticut School of Medicine
Co-Director, Children's Pain Service
University of Connecticut Health Center
Farmington, Connecticut

Nancy Wells, DNSc, RN
Assistant Professor of Clinical Nursing
University of Rochester School of Nursing
Clinical Nurse Research
Strong Memorial Hospital
Rochester, New York

Roberto Wenk, MD
Director, Palliative Care Programs of San Nicolás
Coordinator, World Health Organization Latin American Palliative Care Program, Argentina
San Nicolás, Argentina

Christopher L. Wu, MD
Chief Resident, Anesthesiology
Strong Memorial Hospital
University of Rochester School of Medicine and
  Dentistry
Rochester, New York

Contents

Section 1

Assessment

Chapter 1

Classification of Cancer Pain and Cancer Pain Syndromes

Richard B. Patt

CLASSIFICATION OF CANCER PAIN

A number of schemata for classifying cancer pain have been suggested (Table 1–1) that, when applied, have potential utility to aid in diagnosis and management.

CHRONICITY

One such classification is based on chronicity of symptoms (Table 1–2, Figs. 1–1 to 1–3). Acute pain is frequently associated with signs of sympathetic hyperactivity and heightened distress,[1] particularly when it is incident-related, as in the case of medical procedures like bone marrow biopsy or lumbar puncture.[2] Persistent (nonprocedural), acute pain has been characterized as a biologic "red flag," warning of ongoing tissue injury.[3] Indeed, it is often temporally associated with the onset or recrudescence of primary or metastatic disease, and its presence should motivate the clinician to seek its cause aggressively. Acute pain further signals the need for treatment with potent analgesics; this may resolve as antitumor therapy progresses (see Chapters 6–11, 14, and 15).[4]

In contrast, assessment and management of patients with chronic pain tend to be more complex.[5,6] Usually the source of pain has already been investigated, and is known or suspected. The continued presence

Table 1–1.
Methods for Classifying Cancer Pain

Chronicity
Severity
Pathophysiology/mechanism
Individual type and stage of disease
Pattern of pain
Syndrome

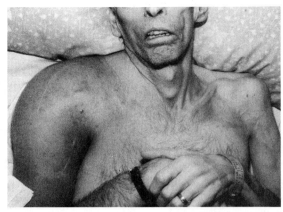

of symptoms implies that their cause cannot adequately be eliminated and suggests the need for some combination of palliation, adjustment, and acceptance. Having exceeded its value as a marker of injury, pain assumes the status of disease, and may, in itself, contribute markedly to a person's deterioration, both physiologic and psychological (see Chapters 5, 14, and 30).[5-8]

With time, biologic and behavioral adjustment to symptoms occurs and corroborating signs of tachycardia, hypertension, and diaphoresis are often absent. The patient may appear stoic with no outward signs of discomfort, or may display florid "pain behavior" (verbal signals, alterations in facial expression, gait, posture, and mood).[9] In either case, when physical signs are absent, care providers must guard against any tendency to minimize the importance of the patient's distress.

Chronic pain with superimposed episodes

Figure 1–1. Patient with lung cancer and chronic pain secondary to multiple bony metastases. As a result of radiation therapy and oral opioids, shoulder pain was reasonably well tolerated despite near-complete absorption of the scapula by tumor.

of acute pain (*ie*, breakthrough pain)[9a] is probably the most common pattern observed in patients with ongoing cancer pain.

INTENSITY

Classification of cancer pain based on its intensity is clinically relevant for several reasons. The consistent use of measurements of

Table 1–2.
Characteristics of Acute Versus Chronic Cancer Pain

Acute Pain	Associated with signs of sympathetic hyperactivity including tachycardia, hypertension, diaphoresis
	Associated with heightened distress
	Often temporally associated with the onset or recrudescence of primary or metastatic disease
	Signals need for treatment with potent analgesics, which may subside as antitumor therapy progresses
Chronic Pain	Signs of sympathetic hyperactivity often absent
	Pain behavior (groaning, alterations in facial expression, gait, and posture) often present
	Alterations in mood, depression and anxiety common
	Seek history of premorbid chronic nonmalignant pain

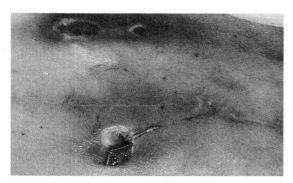

Figure 1–2. Same patient as in Figure 1 with an acute pain problem superimposed on chronic symptoms. Thoracolumbar spine had been surgically stabilized to forestall paraplegia. Severe, acute, low back pain ensued when the displaced rods began to protrude through skin of back, ultimately requiring a subarachnoid neurolytic block.

Dear Peggy,
Since I cant say when I will be able to see Dr. Patt, I'm hoping you get this any way.
My neck is much better but I developed problems with my back and couldnt walk straight. As a result I fell down a full flight of stairs & now have real problems. As soon as I can walk that far I will call to see Dr. Patt.
Happy Holidays
Ruth

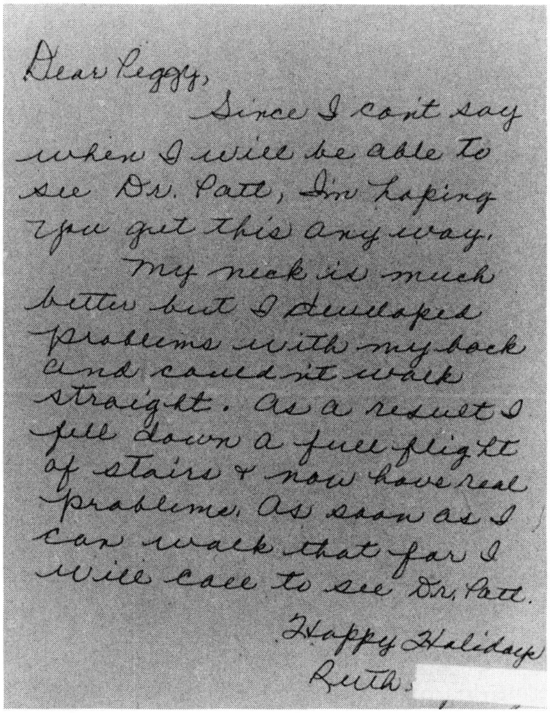

Figure 1–3. Letter from patient with chronic nonmalignant pain demonstrating the complex nature of this heterogeneous group of disorders.

pain intensity aids in reliable assessment of patients' progress, and may serve as a basis for interpatient comparison when data are being gathered for research purposes. Elevated pain scores should alert the clinician to the need for urgent or aggressive intervention. When drug treatment is being considered, the World Health Organization-advocated "analgesic ladder" model[10] is often applied (see Chapters 6 and 9). In this scenario, the severity of pain is the main determinant of the level at which the ladder is accessed, and helps decide if the patient should receive a nonopioid analgesic, a so-called "weak" opioid (*eg*, codeine, oxycodone), or a "more potent" opioid (*eg*, morphine, hydromorphone) as initial treatment.

PATHOPHYSIOLOGY

A general classification by pathophysiology distinguishes among nociceptive (somatic and visceral), neuropathic, and idiopathic or so-called "psychogenic" pain.[11] Shared characteristics and responsivity to various therapeutic interventions have been observed within each category, and hence this classification is useful when formulating an initial approach to treatment. However, despite similarities in mechanism and causation, each pain problem must still be regarded as a unique entity requiring an individualized plan that may need to be altered frequently. Factors that contribute to heterogeneity within a pathophysiologic group include the nature and severity of the insult, overall physical, emotional, and psychological condition, and interindividual differences in the response to drugs and other treatment (**threshold**). Further, in many patients the etiology of pain is the result of multiple, interacting mechanisms and components (sensory, affective, cognitive, and behavioral), the sum of which contributes to a complex pain syndrome that defies simple categorization.[12]

Somatic Pain

Somatic pain occurs as a result of activation of nociceptors in cutaneous and deep tissues.

Table 1–3.
Characteristics of Specialized Pain Conducting Fibers

Fiber Type	Diameter	Transmission	Type of Pain
A-delta	1–5 μm	6–30 m/sec	"Fast pain"; initial prick or sting-ing sensation after injury; well lo-calized
C	0.25–1.5 μm	0.25–1.5 m/sec	"Slow pain"; more lasting, gener-alized, dull ache

Nociceptors respond to a variety of events, including mechanical, thermal, and biochemical stimuli.[11] Biologic products of inflammation and tumor invasion, including serotonin, bradykinin, potassium, ATP, and prostaglandin E1 and E2 are postulated to act as algesic chemical mediators serving both to produce pain by direct activation of nociceptors and to lower the threshold of their activation (**sensitization**).[13–15] Activation of nociceptors results in the transmission of electrical impulses along thinly myelinated A-delta and unmyelinated C fiber afferents.[11,14,15] Known characteristics of A-delta and C fibers are listed in Table 1–3. Both elements enter the spinal cord through dorsal nerve roots and synapse in the dorsal horn, where impulses are modified and transmitted rostrally to the thalamus and cortex, primarily through the spinothalamic tracts, where the impulses are interpreted and appreciated as pain.

Somatic pain is typically constant and well localized, and is frequently characterized as aching, throbbing, or gnawing. Somatic pain tends to be opioid-sensitive, and amenable, at least temporarily to treat with interruption of proximal pathways by chemical blockade or surgery.

Visceral Pain

Visceral pain originates from injury to sympathetically innervated organs[16]. When pain is due to a lesion involving the abdominal or pelvic viscera, it is characteristically vague in distribution and quality, and is often described as deep, dull, aching, dragging, squeezing, or pressurelike. When acute it may be paroxysmal and colicky, and can be associated with nausea, vomiting, diaphoresis, and alterations in blood pressure and heart rate. Mechanisms of visceral pain include abnormal distention or contraction of smooth muscle walls (hollow viscera), rapid capsular stretch (solid viscera), ischemia of visceral muscle, serosal or mucosal irritation by algesic substances and other chemical stimuli, distention and traction or torsion on mesenteric attachments and vasculature, and necrosis.[17] The viscera are, however, insensitive to simple manipulation, cutting, and burning.[16]

Visceral involvement often produces **referred** or "transferred" pain,[17–19] a phenomenon of pain and hyperalgesia localized to superficial and/or deep tissues, often distant to the source of pathology. A number of mechanisms have been proposed to explain the occurrence of referred pain, including the presence of dual innervation of multiple structures, chemical irritation by tumor-mediated algesic substances, and central convergence of afferent impulses.[11] Examples include back pain of pancreatic or retroperitoneal origin, abdominal wall pain and allodynia from peritoneal irritation, upper extremity pain of anginal origin, phrenic nerve-mediated shoulder pain of hepatic origin, and knee pain from metastatic lesions of the hip.

Neuropathic Pain

Neuropathic pain refers to pain syndromes associated with aberrant somatosensory processes induced by injury to some element of

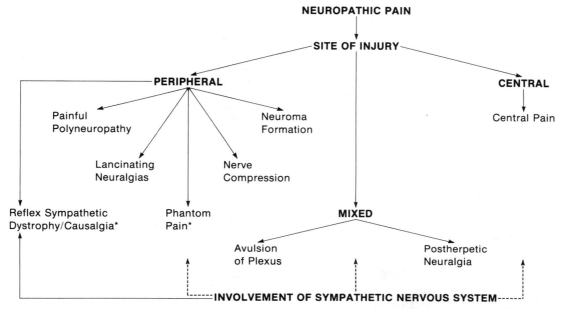

Figure 1–4. Classification of neuropathic pains by the site of neural injury. The dependence of the pain on sympathetic efferent activity has been reported for lesions at all locations, although it is far more prevalent with peripheral lesions and predominates in the sympathetically maintained pains, reflex sympathetic dystrophy, and causalgia. * Usually a peripheral lesion (reprinted with permission from Portenoy RK: Issues in the management of neuropathic pain. In Basbaum AI, Besson JM (eds): Towards a New Pharmacotherapy of Pain, p 393. New York: John Wiley and Sons, 1991

the nervous system (see Fig. 1–4 for proposed classification schema). The term "deafferentation pain" is used when the presumed site of aberrant processing is in the central nervous system; subtypes include central pain (injury to the central nervous system), avulsion of a nerve plexus, and phantom pain.[20] Sympathetically maintained pain is another subtype, exemplified in the cancer patient by tumor invasion or irritation of the sympathetic chain, producing a reflex sympathetic dystrophy. This entity may accompany Pancoast's syndrome or lumbosacral plexopathy, and is associated with causalgic, dysesthetic pain, often accompanied by typical vasomotor and dystrophic changes. These syndromes are amply discussed in Chapter 22. In the case of deafferentation, pain is usually localized to the area of sensory abnormality. When pain is of central origin, it tends to be located in the region that corresponds somatotopically to the lesion. Neuropathic pain is characteristically dysesthetic in nature. **Dysesthesia** refers to discomfort and altered sensations, distinct from the ordinary, familiar sensations of pain. Dysesthetic pain is variously described as burning, tingling, numbing, pressing, squeezing, and itching, and is typically described as extremely unpleasant, often even intolerable.

Neuropathic pain may be constant, steady, and spontaneously maintained (ie, present independent of external stimulus). In addition to continuous pain, there may be a component of superimposed, intermittent, shock-like pain, most often characterized as shooting, lancinating, electrical, or jolting in nature.

Associated findings, present in a variable proportion of patients, include, in roughly descending frequency, sensory loss, evoked pain, sympathetic dysfunction, and motor and reflex abnormalities.[20] Evoked pain implies an altered sensory threshold, and includes various similar phenomena recently defined by the International Association for the Study of Pain (IASP).[21] The term **dysesthesia** includes evoked as well as spontaneous abnormal sensation. **Hyperalgesia** refers to increased response to a stimulus that is normally painful, and **allodynia** refers to pain caused by a stimulus that does not normally provoke pain. Similar phenomena that may be present include **hyperesthesia**, an increased sensitivity to stimulation, and **hyperpathia**, which is a painful syndrome characterized by increased, often explosive reaction to a stimulus.

The development of neuropathic pain is idiosyncratic, and unpredictable even among patients with similar lesions. No consistent predisposing factors have been demonstrated with any certainty. Onset of pain may occur immediately after an injury or after a variable interval. When pain is delayed, as was the case in 61% of 168 consecutive patients with presumed deafferentation pain surveyed in one study,[20] it often follows a seemingly unrelated and sometimes trivial but stressful incident such as surgery, infection, or trauma.

Neuropathic pain is further characterized by persistence despite thorough applications of most standard analgesic therapies. In general, pain is relatively resistant to opioid therapy administered by standard or even neuroaxial routes, although this is not always the case.[22,22a] There is a tendency in some instances for favorable response to a heterogeneous group of centrally acting medications, sometimes referred to as **adjuvant** or **coanalgesic** drugs (see Chapter 10), agents developed for alternate purposes and only serendipitously observed to promote analgesia. These agents include the heterocyclic antidepressants, anticonvulsants, oral local anesthetics (sodium channel blockers), corticosteroids, and others. The dose–response relationship of these agents is unpredictable, and trials of 3 to 4 weeks in doses titrated upward to tolerance are recommended. Anecdotal re-

ports of successful treatment with topical agents, including capsaicin[23] and aspirin and chloroform,[24,25] are intriguing but of uncertain significance.

Neuropathic pain may be more resistant to further denervation than nociceptive pain, whether accomplished by ablative surgery or chemical neurolysis; both of these approaches warrant caution due to their potential for ultimately effecting increased pain. Ablative procedures may, however, result in short-term relief of pain, and in this regard have relatively greater merit in preterminal patients. Whenever possible, prognostic local anesthetic blockade should be performed before planned neuroablation, preferably repeatedly to exclude a placebo response.

Pain is often transiently relieved by proximal local anesthetic blockade, sometimes even for a duration in excess of the expected activity of the anesthetic drug. If this is the case, particularly for reflex sympathetic dystrophy, strong consideration should be given to repeating the blocks in a series in an effort to prolong periods of relief. Surgical sympathectomy often reliably reverses vasomotor changes, but long-term relief of pain is uncommon. Chronic electric stimulation of deep brain structures and the spinal cord has been reported to produce long-term relief of pain in selected cases (see Chapter 26).

Idiopathic or Psychogenic Pain

Great controversy surrounds labeling a pain syndrome as wholly psychogenic in origin. That a patient's psychological state contributes significantly to complaints of pain and suffering is well recognized,[26] and forms part of the basis for the **IASP's** definition of pain as ". . . an unpleasant sensory and emotional experience associated with actual or potential tissue damage or described in terms of such."[21]

It is often difficult to ascertain the degree to which psychological disturbances are secondary to pain versus the degree to which they are the cause of pain. Regardless, symptoms and their associated distress are real to the patient, independent of whether there are psychological factors involved in their maintenance. Pain is a subjective phenomena, and it is essential that the clinician maintain a willingness to believe the patient's report of pain and investigate its cause.

The presence of anxiety or depression and their relative contribution to complaints of pain should be carefully assessed so that appropriate supportive care and/or pharmacotherapy can be instituted (see Chapters 5, 13, 14, and 30). Attention to psychological needs and successful treatment of underlying depression have been shown to reduce complaints of pain.[27,28] Conversely, even aggressive therapy with morphine or surgery will not relieve pain that is psychologically based if these factors are overlooked.

Finally, as noted above, persistent pain may foster reactive depression: a higher incidence of depression has been demonstrated in cancer patients with pain than in matched cancer patients in whom pain is absent.[29] The observation that depression may be significantly reduced in cancer patients when pain is treated effectively[30,31] serves as a reminder that the combination of pain and disturbance of mood may be a signal to initiate more aggressive pain treatment.

STAGE OF DISEASE

Foley has devised a classification scheme (summarized in Table 1–4) based on patient type and stage of disease that she suggests is predictive of patients' response to therapy, and hence may be useful as a guide to clinicians.[32]

PATTERNS OF PAIN

Despite efforts at classification, pain in the cancer patient is still an individual phenomenon, and successful treatment requires that efforts at management be tailored to meet the needs of the individual patient.

Constant Pain

Pain may be constant and unremitting, in which case it is most amenable to drug therapy administered on an **around-the-clock** dosing schedule, contingent on time rather than symptoms. This approach to management endeavors to prevent pain rather than treat it retroactively, and is best accomplished by the proper use of long-acting analgesics or, in selected cases, infusions of analgesics.

Breakthrough and Incident Pain

Despite the establishment of an effective preventative schedule, breakthrough pain is still a common phenomenon that must be anticipated and addressed.[9a] **Breakthrough pain** refers to intermittent exacerbations of pain that can occur spontaneously or in relation to specific activity. Breakthrough pain that is related to specific activity, such as eating, defecation, socializing, or walking is referred to as **incident pain**. **End of dose failure** refers to exacerbations that occur predictably prior to the next scheduled dose of opioid. Breakthrough pain is best managed by supplementing the preventative regimen with analgesics with a rapid onset of action and a short duration. Once a pattern of incident pain is established, **"escape"** or **"rescue" doses** of analgesics can be administered in anticipation of the pain-provoking activity. End of dose failure is most amenable to increasing the dose of long-acting (basal) opioid or decreasing the interval between dosing. When treatment by infusion therapy (subcutaneous, intravenous, intraspinal) has been elected, the addition of patient-controlled analgesia (PCA), which permits patients to administer a preset amount of opioid at preset intervals, is an effective means to manage breakthrough and incident pain in selected patients (see Chapter 11).

Intermittent Pain

Pain that is intermittent and unpredictable in onset represents a further challenge to management. Around-the-clock dosing is likely to be unsatisfactory, as analgesia is often inadequate during painful episodes and sedation usually supervenes during pain-free intervals. Pain that occurs intermittently is usually best managed by the prn administration of an appropriately potent analgesic of rapid onset

Table 1–4.
Classification of Cancer Pain by Patient Type, Stage of Disease

Acute Cancer-Related Pain

Related to diagnosis or treatment	Patients tend to be hopeful
	Endure pain readily, often without seeking treatment
Recurrent pain	Identified with recrudescence of disease
	Psychological effects potentially devastating

Chronic Cancer-Related Pain — Psychological adaptation/maladaptation often established

Associated with treatment	Overriding concern is reestablishment of functional lifestyle
Associated with progression	Hopelessness, helplessness often predominate
Patients with preexisting chronic pain	Require intensive intervention and support
	Pain behavior established
	Accurate diagnosis essential
Patients with history of drug abuse	Difficult to evaluate and treat
	Risk of inadequate treatment
	Coordinate rehabilitation, social work
Dying patients	Adequacy of treatment has great impact on patient and family
	Assure comfort at all reasonable costs

Adapted from Foley KM: Treatment of cancer pain. N Engl J Med 1985;313:84.

and short duration, or, if an alternate route is being used, the addition of PCA. When intermittent pain is well localized there may be a role for nerve block therapy, as well.

CANCER PAIN SYNDROMES

Numerous distinct cancer pain syndromes have been recognized and described.[33] Syndromes related to cancer therapy are described in Chapter 3. Mechanisms of pain due to tumor invasion include obstruction of lymphatic and vascular channels, distention of a hollow viscus, edema, and tissue inflammation and necrosis. Severe symptoms are most often related to invasion of pain-sensitive structures by tumor mass.

OSSEOUS INVASION

Tumor infiltration of bone is cited as the most common cause of cancer pain,[34] and is most often secondary to primary disease in the prostate, breast, thyroid, lung, or kidney.[34,35] Skeletal metastases are clinically evident in one-third of patients with cancer, and are found in two-thirds of patients at autopsy.[36] Although the majority of skeletal metastases do not produce pain,[34,37] pain from bony metastases can produce a variety of symptoms. When present, pain is usually constant, but may be greatest at night and is often worse with movement or weight bearing. Patients may report a dull ache or deep, intense pain, and there may be referred pain, muscle spasm, or paroxysms of stabbing pain, particularly when bony lesions are accompanied by nerve compression.

Since up to 50% decalcification must be present before osseous lesions are visible on plain roentgenograms,[38] a bone scan (isotope scanning, scintigraphy) is preferred for detecting most bone metastases.[34] In certain settings (primary bone tumors, thyroid cancer, and multiple myeloma) plain films are considered to be more sensitive studies.[39] In addition, since radioisotope scanning reflects the current metabolic status of the bone and plain radiographs the net result of both new bone formation and old bone destruction, plain films may be valuable in patients with stabilized ("burned out") metastases.[40] Abnormal findings on scintigrams are not specific for malignant disease, and it is essential that they be interpreted together with other radiologic studies and in the context of clinical findings. Neoplastic involvement must be differentiated from changes related to infection, trauma, or degeneration because treatment differs, even in the patient with cancer. Scans may appear negative when lesions are predominantly osteoclastic, after radiotherapy, and when surrounding bone is diffusely involved with tumor, as is most likely to occur in patients with breast, lung, and prostate cancer.[40] Additionally, it has been pointed out that detection of osseous metastases in certain "hidden" sites[41] (T1 vertebral body, base of the skull, sacrum) may be difficult, particularly on plain films, because of overlying images of gas and normal bony structures.

Mechanisms of bone pain remain incompletely understood, but a biochemical explanation is attractive to explain how even small lesions can produce severe pain. Osseous metastases elaborate PGE_2, which is hypothesized to contribute to pain by sensitization of peripheral nociceptors (see Chapters 7, 10, and 25). Nonsteroidal anti-inflammatory agents and steroids are postulated to be effective in the treatment of painful bony metastases on the basis of their inhibition of the cyclooxygenase pathway of arachidonic acid breakdown, thus decreasing the formation of PGE_2 (see Chapters 7, 10, and 25). As deposits enlarge, stretching of the periosteum, pathologic fracture, and perineural invasion contribute to pain, and requirements for more potent analgesics increase. Palliative radiotherapy (see Chapter 15) is commonly successfully used to relieve pain emanating from bony metastases. Hormonal therapy (chemotherapy, orchiectomy, hypophysectomy) is often effective in reducing bony pain in patients with

hormonal-dependent disease (breast, prostate), although most of these agents, especially the estrogen agent tamoxifen, may increase pain transiently before it is relieved (tamoxifen flare) in a small proportion of patients.[42] This phenomenon has been observed in 3–9% of patients, may begin within a few hours or days, and typically subsides spontaneously within 1 month.[42]

Metastases to the Skull

Specific syndromes associated with metastatic spread of tumor to the base of the skull have been described by Greenberg et al[43] and Foley and colleagues (see Table 1–5).[44] Symptomatic metastases to the skull is usually, but not always, a late finding.[43] The presenting complaint is usually headache, which is often followed by the onset of neurologic abnormalities. Plain radiography and scintigraphy are often insufficient to make a reliable diagnosis. Supplementation with computed tomography (CT; thin slices and "bone windows") is desirable to diagnose bony disease, whereas magnetic resonance imaging (MRI) and lumbar puncture are useful to evaluate the soft tissues and to detect the presence of leptomeningeal disease, respectively.[44]

Vertebral Syndromes

The bony spinal column is a frequent site of metastases, especially from tumors of the lung, breast, and prostate. Tumor invasion restricted to the bone may result in severe, localized pain. Associated nerve compression tends to produce radiating pain and circumscribed neurologic changes. Vertebral involvement may be associated with epidural–spinal cord compression (see below and Chapter 29), which, if allowed to progress, is further associated with both pain and neurologic impairment (paraplegia and quadriplegia), and is a major cause of morbidity.

Focal back pain is usually the first sign of metastasis to the bony vertebral column, usually preceding neurologic changes by weeks. Cervical and lumbar involvement tend to produce unilateral symptoms, whereas tho-

Table 1–5.
Metastases to the Skull

Middle Fossa Syndrome

Often present with symptoms that are similar to trigeminal neuralgia, such as numbness, paresthesia and pain referred to the area subserved by the second or third divisions of the fifth nerve, except that objective signs of neuropathy (eg, corresponding sensory deficits and masseter) weakness may be present. Diplopia, dysarthria, headache, and dysphagia may develop as well.

Jugular Foramen Syndrome

Usually associated with occipital pain often radiating to the vertex and ipsilateral shoulder or neck, and may be accompanied by local tenderness and exacerbation with movement of the head. Neurologic signs consistent with dysfunction of cranial nerves IX through XII, and Horner's syndrome may be present. Lancinating throat pain (glossopharyngeal neuralgia) has been observed in association with the above symptoms or as the sole complaint.

Clivus Metastases

Associated with vertex headache exacerbated by neck flexion, and may be accompanied by either unilateral or bilateral cranial nerve dysfunction (VI through XII).

Orbital Metastases

Associated with retro-orbital or frontal headache, often with diplopia, visual loss, proptosis, and extraocular nerve palsies.

Parasellar Metastases

May invade the cavernous sinus and adjacent sphenoid bone, resulting in symptoms similar to orbital metastases.

Sphenoid Sinus Metastases

Suggested by bifrontal headache radiating to both temples with intermittent retro-orbital pain. There may be complaints of nasal stuffiness and diplopia, and a unilateral or bilateral VI cranial nerve palsy may be present.

Occipital Condyle Invasion

Associated with severe occipital pain that is exacerbated by movement and that may be accompanied by XII cranial nerve dysfunction.

Odontoid Fractures

Usually associated with erosion of the atlas. If accompanied by vertebral subluxation, progressive neurologic signs of spinal cord compression may develop.

Adapted from: Greenberg HS, Deck MDF, Vikram B et al: Metastases to the base of the skull: Clinical findings in 43 patients. Neurology 1981;31:530; and Elliot K, Foley KM: Neurologic pain syndromes in patients with cancer. Crit Care Clin 1990;6:393.

racic involvement is often bilateral. Periosteal invasion is responsible for the dull, steady, aching pain that is frequently observed. Pain is often exacerbated by recumbency, sitting, movement, and local pressure, and may be relieved by standing. Localized tenderness of the bony spinal column and radicular pain in the cervical, thoracic, or upper lumbar regions, findings that are uncommon in nonmalignant neuromusculoskeletal disorders, should alert the clinician to consider vertebral involvement by tumor. Although invasion of the upper lumbar vertebrae is usually heralded by dull backache and/or radicular signs, pain may be localized to the sacroiliac joints or iliac crests, and radiologic investigations of

the lumbar spine should be conducted when these symptoms are present. In addition, invasion of the second cervical vertebra may result in referred pain to the occiput, and C7–T1 invasion may produce interscapular pain.[45]

NEURAL INVASION

Invasion or compression of somatic nerves by tumor may be associated with constant, burning, dysesthetic pain, often with an intermittent lancinating component. Diffuse hyperesthesia and localized paresthesia are not uncommon, and muscle weakness and atrophy may be present if the affected structure is a mixed or motor nerve. Pain attributable to nerve compression by tumor was diagnosed in 40%, 20%, and 31% of patients referred to a tertiary care center, neurology service, and hospice, respectively.[46,47,48]

Spinal Cord Compression and Invasion

This syndrome is fully described in Chapter 29. Familiarity with the pertinent aspects of the clinical presentation and early diagnosis of spinal cord compression is warranted because the onset of this common disorder is heralded in almost all cases by pain, often independent of neurologic findings, and early intervention is essential to limit neurologic morbidity.

Cervical Plexopathy

Cervical plexopathy may result from local invasion by head and neck cancers or pressure from enlarged lymph nodes. Symptoms are primarily sensory in the distribution of the plexus, and are typically experienced as aching preauricular, postauricular, or neck pain.

Brachial Plexopathy
(Pancoast's or Superior Sulcus Syndrome)

Brachial plexopathy is associated most commonly with carcinoma of the lung (primary or metastatic) and breast, as well as lymphoma.[49] Pain occurs in up to 85% of patients with brachial plexus invasion, usually as an early symptom, often preceding other neurologic findings by up to 9 months.[50,51] The propensity for brachial plexus lesions to produce pain is highlighted by a study of 221 patients with pain due to lung cancer, in which Pancoast's syndrome comprised 31% of the cases, even though the incidence of Pancoast's tumor accounts for only 3% of lung cancers.[52] Early recognition with referral for radiotherapy, surgery, or chemotherapy is essential to limit neurologic morbidity, but unfortunately a diagnosis is often delayed. A number of reports of late diagnosis after prolonged symptomatic medical and chiropractic care emphasize the importance of maintaining a high index of clinical suspicion and considering early radio-

logic surveys in patients with unexplained shoulder and arm pain.[53,54] In one retrospective analysis of 58 patients with Pancoast's syndrome of pulmonary etiology, 54% of patients had pain that predated the diagnosis of cancer.[52] Median survival in this group was 11 months postdiagnosis.

The lower cord of the plexus (C8–T1) is affected most frequently, and pain is characteristically experienced as diffuse aching in the shoulder girdle with radiation down the arm, often to the elbow and medial (ulnar) aspect of the hand.[49,55] Dysesthesias, progressive atrophy, and neurologic impairment (weakness and numbness) usually occur. Horner's syndrome is a common concomitant finding. Although less common, invasion of the upper plexus (C5–6) may occur, usually with pain in the shoulder girdle and upper arm, radiating to the thumb and index finger.

Tumors may exhibit contiguous spread to the epidural space,[56,57,58] and brachial plexopathy associated with a paraspinal mass requires an evaluation of the adjacent epidural region with MRI or myelography. Differentiating between brachial plexus abnormalities due to radiation fibrosis and those due to tumor invasion can be difficult, as clinical findings are similar. In a large study comparing patients with radiation injury versus tumor involvement, Horner's syndrome and severe pain and weakness (C8–T1) were more common in the tumor group.[58] Patients with tumor typically complain of upper arm and elbow pain with radiating dysesthesias in the fourth and fifth fingers. The radiation group more commonly exhibited signs referable to dysfunction of the upper trunk (C5–C7 roots), including weakness of shoulder abduction and arm flexors (C5–C7). Pain is a less prominent finding after radiation injury, and is more likely to be characterized as aching in the shoulder and tightness and heaviness in the upper arm, accompanied by lymphedema.

Lumbosacral Plexopathy

Lumbosacral plexopathy due to invasion by tumor cells occurs most commonly in association with tumors of the rectum, cervix, breast, sarcoma, and lymphoma. That pain is a valuable diagnostic sign is emphasized by the findings in one large study[59] in which pain was the presenting symptom in 70% of patients, followed only weeks or months later by the development of significant weakness and numbness. Pain was the only symptom in 24% of patients studied. Reflex asymmetry, and mild sensory and motor changes, when present, were relatively early findings, and impotence and incontinence were relatively rare. In the same study, direct extension from local intra-abdominal disease was responsible for over two-thirds of cases, with metastatic disease accounting for a much smaller proportion. Pain may be local (85%), radicular (85%), or referred (44%), and is characteristically described as aching or pressure-like and only rarely as causalgic or dysesthetic.[59] Depending on the level involved, pain is referred to the low back, abdomen, buttock, or lower extremity.[59,60]

Several distinct patterns of symptoms have been identified.[51,59,60] The L1 or upper plexus syndrome may involve the ilioinguinal, iliohypogastric, and/or genitofemoral nerves, and is characterized by lower abdominal and groin pain, often accompanied by sensory loss but rarely motor loss. The so-called lumbosacral or lower plexus syndrome is associated with numbness of the foot, and flexor weakness of the ankle and knee. Involvement of the low sacral and coccygeal plexus is most often associated with severe, constant lower sacral pain that may be unilateral, bilateral, or midline, with or without rectal pain,[61] often with progression to perineal sensory loss and bowel or bladder dysfunction.[59] Suspected plexopathy must be differentiated from invasion of the spinal cord or cauda equina. Radiologic investigations of the pelvis and lumbar spine and diagnostic nerve blocks are helpful to corroborate clinical findings. For sacrococcygeal plexopathy, plain films, CT, and scintigrams may demonstrate bony invasion of the sacral plates and thereby suggest a coexistent lesion of the cauda equina. If symptoms are permitted to progress unchecked, patients are likely to become immobilized and depressed, and are subject to increased risks of venous thrombosis, decubitus, and infection.[59]

The differential diagnosis for patients with the above findings, as pointed out by Elliot et al,[44] includes psoas abscess and hemorrhage, abdominal aortic aneurysm, diabetic neuropathy, vasculitis, myofascial pain, and epidural spinal cord compression. Radiation fibrosis is more likely to be associated with edema and motor weakness than with pain as a prominent finding.[62] Weakness more often tends to be a bilateral phenomenon in patients with radiation plexopathy.[62] Rarely, lumbosacral plexopathy may exist without an apparent underlying cause.[63]

Other Neuropathic Syndromes

Meningeal carcinomatosis and cranial nerve invasion are considered under "Headache" (see below). Post-treatment neuralgias, such as those associated with mastectomy, thoracotomy, nephrectomy, radical neck dissection, radiotherapy, and chemotherapy are discussed in Chapter 3.

MUSCLE PAIN

It has only recently been well recognized that pain of muscular origin (cramps, myalgia, myofascial pain) is a much more common form of nonmalignant pain than previously thought,[64] and there is every reason to expect that it has been underdiagnosed in cancer patients as well.[65] Prior under-recognition is probably due in part to the inability of standard roentgenographic techniques to document muscle injury, as well as the varied, sometimes vague, and usually non-neurologic constellation of symptoms that is characteristically present. Muscle cramps in the cancer patient is the subject of a recent excellent review.[66]

Muscular pain or myalgia tends to be described as dull, aching, and sore in character, and is usually accompanied by stiffness and local tenderness.[67] The term "cramp" may be used synonymously, but is generally regarded as a condition that is more acute in onset and offset, more severe (but still dull), and often accompanied by muscle contraction. Spasm usually implies reflex contraction.[68] Myofascial pain (see below) refers to a chronic syndrome of regional muscle pain and dysfunction accompanied by trigger points (see below). In contrast, fibrositis or fibromyalgia (see below) is considered to be a systemic, multisymptomatic disorder accompanied by more generalized or widely distributed muscle pain with or without triggers.

Muscle pain may be due to a variety of etiologies. Pain may be secondary to an underlying disorder that irritates surrounding muscle in a reflex fashion or provokes splinting as a protective measure to immobilize the injury. Alternatively, muscle pain may be due to a systemic or metabolic cause, or may be a result of a self-perpetuating cycle of pain and spasm, such that an initial, often innocuous injury produces pain that is followed by localized reflex muscle spasm that in turn produces further pain, and so on, in an ever-widening spiral that may persist long after the original injury has resolved.[69]

Reversible causes of muscle pain should be sought, and, when possible, modified to eliminate the underlying source of pain. When no reversible causes are present or potentially reversible causes cannot be modified, efforts should turn to pharmacologic or procedural suppression of symptoms. Muscle pain tends to be poorly responsive to opioids, although a trial should not be summarily excluded. Traditional nonbenzodiazepine skeletal muscle relaxants are surprisingly ineffective, and have the disadvantage of being associated with a high incidence of sedation and dysphoria.[70] Well accepted pharmacologic measures include the administration of quinine (leg cramps), diazepam, baclofen, phenytoin, dantrolene, and carbamezapine.[66,67,70,71] Anecdotal reports of successful management with a variety of agents (procainamide, diphenhydramine, fluoride, riboflavin, vitamin E, verapamil, and nifedipine) require further investigation.[66]

Trigger points are small, tender areas of focal muscle spasm that often produce both localized and referred pain in response to the application of pressure.[72] They may be relatively isolated findings or a component of a more generalized fibromyalgia syndrome, in which case they tend to be associated with fatigue, sleep disturbances, morning stiffness, and depression.[73] Travell and Simons have described dozens of distinct pain patterns that they postulate arise when a given muscle is affected.[72] Although various devices have been developed to quantify soft tissue compliance and tenderness,[74] a diagnosis is usually made on a clinical basis.

The usual therapeutic approach to myofascial pain and trigger points is a rehabilitative one such as would be provided by a physical or occupational therapist,[75] although this modality may not be practical in many patients with advanced cancer. Useful measures include supervised exercise, gradual stretching, and a home exercise program combined with the application of local measures such as heat or ice, ultrasound, transcutaneous electrical nerve stimulation, and massage. The injection of local anesthetics and/or steroids into persistent trigger points is a well accepted intervention that can readily be applied by a variety of specialists or providers of primary care.[69] Performed in isolation, dramatic, often persistent relief may result; alternatively, these approaches are useful adjuncts to physical measures. Behaviorally based strategies that involve instructing patients in methods to reduce muscle tension and stress may play either a primary or adjunctive therapeutic role.

ABDOMINAL PAIN

Abdominal pain may arise from a variety of intra-abdominal and extra-abdominal sources (see "Visceral Pain" section).[19] Invasion or compression of a nerve root or peripheral somatic nerve characteristically gives rise to well localized, band-like abdominal wall pain that radiates in a characteristic dermatomal pattern and is often associated with hyperesthesia and other varieties of altered sensation. Alternatively, intra-abdominal disease and irrita-

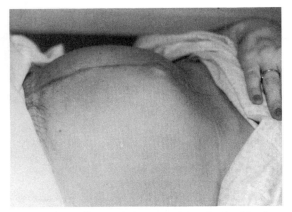

Figure 1–5. Thirty-eight-year-old patient with uterine malignancy and vague abdominal pain secondary to intrapelvic extension of tumor.

tion of the adjacent parietal peritoneum may result in nondermatomal pain referred to the abdominal wall (Fig. 1–5). Thoracic processes such as impingement of intercostal nerves by tumor or pleural disease may also result in pain referred to the abdomen and, alternatively, an intra-abdominal process may be accompanied by pain referred to a distant region (eg, shoulder pain secondary to diaphragmatic irritation). Muscle spasm may exceed its usual protective and warning function and evolve as an independent source of pain that is frequently overlooked (see "Muscle Pain" section).[18]

Intra-abdominal sources of pain include inflammation of the parietal peritoneum, obstruction of a hollow viscus, distention of the capsule of a solid viscus, chemical irritation, and acute ischemia. Intestinal obstruction is an important source of intra-abdominal pain resulting from extrinsic compression, invasion of the intestinal wall, and/or the presence of an intraluminal mass, all often superimposed on ileus or constipation. Symptoms vary depending on the level and grade of obstruction, but characteristically consist of intermittent, dull, crampy pain (colic) that is variable and often vague in distribution and that may be associated with nausea, vomiting, distention, a feeling of fullness, and altered bowel habit.[71,75] In contrast, biliary and ureteral colic tend to be more intense and are more often well localized to the right upper quadrant in the former case and flank, groin, or glans penis in the latter case, respectively.[76] The liver is a frequent site of tumor involvement. Hepatic metastases may be asymptomatic or may produce constant, dull pain localized to the epigastrium, accompanied by a feeling of fullness. Pain of hepatic origin may radiate to the midback, or, as a result of diaphragmatic irritation, to the right shoulder.

Pancreatic Cancer Pain

Pancreatic cancer pain has been well characterized.[77,78] Patients present most often with relentless, boring, midepigastric aching pain that radiates through to the midback, and that is often relieved by the assumption of the fetal position and worsened by recumbency. While this presentation is common, alternate symptomatology may be present in the patient with pancreatic cancer, perhaps due to related pathology, and it should be recognized that distinguishing among these heterogeneous syndromes is essential in order to select the most appropriate form of management. The classic presentation referred to above is most consistent with a likelihood of good outcome after celiac plexus block (see Chapter 22),[78a] whereas alternate symptoms suggest the need for alternate treatment and/or further diagnostic studies.

Multiple mechanisms have been proposed to explain pain observed in patients with pancreatic cancer. Local factors that contribute to pain include stretch of retroperitoneal nerves induced by bulky tumor mass (which may explain the increased comfort often observed with flexion of the trunk), direct invasion of autonomic nerves, ductal obstruction and distention, invasion of neighboring somatic nerves, and peripancreatic neuritis.[79] That back pain may be due to retroperitoneal invasion is supported by findings of a 21% incidence of back pain in a series of patients with testicular germ cell tumors, all of whom had periaortic nodal metastases.[80] Pancreatic cancer has a propensity for not only local but distant spread, and as a result, pain may originate from a variety of distant sites and mechanisms, including distention of the hepatic capsule, peritoneal invasion, portal vein obstruction, bowel obstruction, ascites, etc. Foley has appropriately stressed the need to identify other treatable causes of pain.[77] Careful proactive attention to a vigorous bowel cleansing regimen and proper antiemetic therapy (see Chapters 10, 12, 13, and 30) will reduce associated intestinal colic. The identification of obstructive lesions or infectious complications (cholangitis) may suggest a role for surgery or antibiotic therapy in selected patients. Pharmacotherapy and celiac plexus block are important therapeutic options, and are discussed elsewhere (see Chapters 6–11 and 22). In addition to standard pharmacologic and anesthetic measures, Levy suggests that steroids and diuretics may have a role in selected patients.[81]

Pelvic Pain

Pelvic pain syndromes are considered more fully in Chapter 22. In one series of 350 hospice patients, pelvic pain was present in 11% of patients, in whom it was associated with primary malignancies of the large bowel (21/40), gynecologic organs (9/40), and extra-abdominal disease (3/40).[82] Symptoms vary but often consist of a vague, poorly localized sensation of fullness, pressure, and discomfort that is characteristically bilateral. Alternatively, pain may be experienced as a fullness or intermittent shooting or red hot poker-like sensation in the rectum.[82]

Much of the above is also true for pain involving the perineum (see Chapter 22). One additional syndrome deserves mention, that of fungating tumor (malignant ulceration) associated with the local spread of rectal, anal, and vulvar carcinomas (see Fig. 1–6). Although early detection and intervention have reduced the incidence of these phenomena, when they occur they are usually associated with severe, intractable pain, local necrosis, odor, drainage, and, at times, fistula formation. Similar syndromes may occur in the head and neck, usually from squamous cell carci-

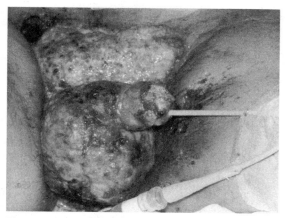

Figure 1–6. Locally invasive anal carcinoma in a 65-year-old man. Pain was ultimately unresponsive to all pharmacologic measures, including intraspinal opioids, as well as subarachnoid neurolysis. Pain ultimately controlled with midline myelotomy (commisurotomy).

noma, and are still occasionally reported in patients with breast carcinoma, especially in less developed nations.[83] The importance and effectiveness of local care have been stressed,[48,84] as well as a possible role for antibiotics. Bruera and MacDonald observed sudden increases of acute pain in seven patients that rapidly improved with antibiotic therapy.[85] Radiotherapy often slows tumor growth and relieves pain, but because disease may advance locally without significant distant organ involvement, patients may outlive the effects of such palliation.[86] We have had moderate success with midline commissurotomy (myelotomy) (see Chapter 26) in one patient who had failed trials of standard analgesics, neurolytic saddle block, and intravenous and intraspinal opioids. Recently, radical resection with flap rotation has been described as a successful means to achieve pain relief and extend survival.[87]

HEADACHE

Headache is a major but not invariable symptom of intracranial neoplasm,[88] present in 60% of patients in one survey, half of whom classified headache as their primary complaint.[89] Its pattern is undistinctive.[88,90] Patients typically describe pain that is steady, deep, dull, and aching, and that is rarely rhythmic or throbbing.[88] It is usually intermittent and may be worse in the morning and with coughing or straining. Characteristically, the intensity of pain is only moderate, rarely awakening patients from sleep and generally less than that which is typically described in so-called "benign" syndromes. Symptoms often respond to simple measures, including recumbency, the administration of aspirin or steroids,[91] and the application of cold packs. Symptoms often improve when radiotherapy is instituted to treat the underlying malignancy.[90,92]

The brain is not itself sensitive to noxious stimuli, although some, but not all, of its neighboring tissue is pain-sensitive,[93] and as a result, headache of neoplastic origin is nearly always referred, mediated by indirect mechanisms. Pain-sensitive structures include the venous sinuses and their tributaries, parts of the dura, especially at the base of the brain, the dural and cerebral arteries, the fifth, ninth, and tenth cranial nerves, and the upper three cervical nerves.[93] Mechanisms of headache are said to include traction, displacement and dilation of veins and arteries, inflammation near pain-sensitive structures, and direct pressure on cranial and cervical nerves. Reflex contraction of the cervical muscles is a common finding with headache in general, and may accompany headache of neoplastic origin or may even be the presenting symptom.[94]

Headache may be simply a manifestation of a chronic premorbid condition, unrelated to cancer except that it may be exacerbated by associated stress (see Chapters 5 and 14). Headache may occur with or without elevations of intracranial pressure (ICP), and although it is often regarded as a useful diagnostic sign (along with nausea, vomiting, mental status changes, and papilledema), raised ICP is not necessarily associated with headache, particularly when elevations in pressure are gradual or chronic.[95]

Leptomeningeal Metastases/Meningeal Carcinomatosis

Leptomeningeal metastases occur most commonly in patients with primary malignancies of the breast and lung, and lymphoma and leukemia. An 8–10% incidence was found in one autopsy study of patients with systemic cancer.[96] Diffuse infiltration of the meninges by tumor has the potential to produce protean signs and symptoms. About 40% of patients have headache or back pain, presumably due to traction on the pain-sensitive meninges, cranial and spinal nerves, and/or raised intracranial pressure.[97,98] Headache is the most common presenting complaint, is characteristically unrelenting, and may be associated with nausea, vomiting, nuchal rigidity, and mental status changes.[98] Other neurologic abnormalities include seizures, cranial nerve signs, papilledema, hemiparesis, ataxia, and cauda equina syndrome.

A diagnosis of leptomeningeal metastases is confirmed by analysis of cerebrospinal fluid that reveals the presence of malignant cells, and that may also be remarkable for an increased opening pressure, raised protein, and decreased glucose.[99] Computerized tomography, MRI, or myelography are recommended to evaluate the extent of disease.[44,100] The natural history of patients with leptomeningeal metastases is gradual decline and death over 4 to 6 weeks, although survival is regularly extended to 6 months or more when treatment with radiotherapy and/or intrathecal methotrexate is instituted.[101] Steroids are said to be useful in the management of headache.[44] We have seen the headache, neck, and back pain of one patient respond remarkably well to intraventricular morphine administered through an Ommaya reservoir.

Cervicofacial Pain

The head and neck are richly innervated by contributions from cranial nerves V, VII, IX, X, and the upper cervical nerves. Analgesia may be difficult to achieve because of the erosive, endophytic nature of many tumors and because physiologic splinting, ordinarily an important protective reflex, is often ineffective because pain is aggravated by relatively involuntary motion produced by swallowing, eating, coughing, talking, and other movements of the head. Pain may arise from a variety of mechanisms, and as such varies in character. Mechanisms include soft tissue ulceration, infection and compression from adenopathy or tumor, mucositis, bony erosion, and nerve invasion. When cranial nerves and their branches are affected, symptoms may be those of trigeminal or glossopharyngeal neuralgia (*eg*, sudden, severe lancinating pain radiating to the face, throat, or ear). Pain may be accompanied by altered sensation, trigger points, and impaired swallowing, breathing, and phonation.

Early consideration should be given to palliative radiotherapy (see Chapter 15). Depending on its underlying mechanism, pain may be responsive to treatment with nonsteroidal anti-inflammatory drugs, antibiotics, opioids, antidepressants, anticonvulsants, and/or oral local anesthetics. Neurolytic blocks, neurosurgery, and intraventricular opioids are often successful for pain that is otherwise intractable (see Chapters 17–26).

CONCLUSION

Careful assessment and frequent reevaluation are the hallmark of successful pain management. Although in each case the experience of pain is sufficiently personal and unique that an individualized treatment plan need be conceived, efforts to classify patients' complaints of pain may be rewarded by indications for the likelihood that a given strategy might be successful. Finally, it is important that the clinician be familiar with the range of known cancer pain syndromes.

REFERENCES

1. Sternbach RA: Pain: A Psychophysiological Analysis. New York, Academic Press, 1968.
2. Jay S, Elliot C, Ozolins M et al: Behavioral management of children's distress during painful medical procedures. Behav Res Ther 1985;23:513.
3. Sternbach RA: Acute versus chronic pain. In Wall PD, Melzack R (eds): Textbook of Pain, 2nd ed, p 242. Edinburgh, Churchill Livingstone, 1989.
4. Foley KM: Cancer pain syndromes. Journal of Pain and Symptom Management 1987;2:S13.
5. Sternbach RA: Pain Patients: Traits and Treatments. New York, Academic Press, 1974.
6. Black RG: The chronic pain syndromes. Surg Clin North Am 55:4, 1975.
7. Saunders C: The philosophy of terminal care. In Saunders C (ed): The Management of Terminal Malignant Disease. London, Edward Arnold, 1984, p 232.
8. Tunks E: Is there a chronic pain syndrome? In Lipton S et al (eds): Advances in Pain Research and Therapy, vol 13, p 257. New York, Raven Press, 1990.
9. Sanders S: Behavioral assessment and treatment of clinical pain: Appraisal and current status. In Hersen M, Eisler RM, Miller PM (eds): Progress in Behavior Modification, pp 249–291. New York, Academic Press, 1979.
9a. Portenoy R: Breakthrough pain: Definition, prevalence and characteristics. Pain 1990;41:273.
10. World Health Organization: Cancer Pain Relief. Geneva, World Health Organization, 1986.
11. Payne R: Cancer pain: Anatomy, physiology and pharmacology. Cancer (Suppl) 1989;63:2266.
12. Ahles TA, Blanchard EB, Ruckdeschel JC: The multidimensional nature of cancer pain. Pain 1983;17:277.
13. Perl ER: Characterization of nociceptors and their activation of neurons in the superficial dorsal horn: First steps for the sensation of pain. In Kruger L, Liebeskind JC (eds): Advances in Pain Research and Therapy, vol 6, p 23. New York, Raven Press, 1984.
14. Bonica JJ: Anatomic and physiologic basis of nociception and pain. In Bonica JJ: The Management of Pain, 2nd ed, p 28. Philadelphia, Lea and Febiger, 1990.
15. Bonica JJ, Yaksh T, Liebeskind JC et al: Biochemistry and modulation of nociception and pain. In Bonica JJ: The Management of Pain, 2nd ed, p 95. Philadelphia, Lea and Febiger, 1990.
16. Newman PP: Visceral Afferent Functions of the Nervous System. London, Arnold, 1974.
17. Procacci P, Maresca M: Pathophysiology of visceral pain. In Lipton S et al (eds): Advances in Pain Research and Therapy, vol 13, p 123. New York, Raven Press, 1990.
18. Kellgren JH: Somatic simulating visceral pain. Clin Sci 1939;4:303.
19. Cervero F: Visceral pain. In Dubner R, Gebhart GF,

Bond MR (eds): Proceedings of the VI World Congress on Pain, p 216. Amsterdam, Elsevier, 1988.

20. Tasker RR, Dostrovsky JO: Deafferentation and central pain. In Wall PD, Melzack R: Textbook of Pain, 2nd ed, p 154. Edinburgh, Churchill Livingstone, 1989.

21. Merskey H (ed): Classification of chronic pain: Description of chronic pain syndromes and definition of pain terms. Pain (Suppl) 1986;3:S1.

22. Jacobson L, Chabal C, Brody MC: Relief of persistent postamputation stump and phantom limb pain with intrathecal fentanyl. Pain 1989;37:317.

22a. Portenoy R: The nature of opioid responsiveness and its implications for neuropathic pain: New hypotheses derived from studies of opioid infusions. Pain 1990; 43:273.

23. Watson CP, Evans RJ, Watt VR: The post-mastectomy pain syndrome and the effect of topical capsaicin. Pain 1989;38:177.

24. King RB: Concerning the management of pain associated with herpes zoster and of postherpetic neuralgia. Pain 1988;33:73.

25. Kassirer M: King and Robert, Concerning the management of pain associated with herpes zoster and of postherpetic neuralgia, Pain 1988;33:73–78. Pain 1988;35:368.

26. Spiegel D, Bloom JR: Pain in metastatic breast cancer. Cancer 1983;52:341–345.

27. Wand NG, Bloom VL, Friedel RO: Effectiveness of tricyclic antidepressants in treatment of coexisting pain and depression. Pain 1979;7:331.

28. Spiegel D, Bloom JR: Group therapy and hypnosis reduce metastatic breast carcinoma pain. Psychosom Med 1983;45:333.

29. Bond MR, Pearson IB: Psychological aspects of pain in women with advanced cancer of the cervix. J Psychosom Res 1969;13:13.

30. Sternbach RA, Timmermans G: Personality changes associated with reduction of pain. Pain 1975;3;177.

31. Kissen DM: The influence of some environmental factors on personality inventory scores in psychosomatic research. J Psychosom Res 1964;8:145.

32. Foley KM: Treatment of cancer pain. N Engl J Med 1985;313:84.

33. Foley KM: Pain syndromes in patients with cancer. In Bonica JJ, Ventafridda V (eds): Advances in Pain Research and Therapy, vol 2, p 59. New York, Raven Press, 1979.

34. Galasko CSB: Skeletal Metastases, p 99. London, Butterworths, 1986

35. Enneking WF, Conrad EU III: Common bone tumors. Clin Symp 1989;41:1.

37. Pollen JJ, Schmidt JD: Bone pain in metastatic cancer of the prostate. Urology 1979;13:129.

38. Foley KM: Pain syndromes in patients with cancer. In Bonica JJ, Ventafridda V (eds): Advances in Pain Research and Therapy, vol 2, p 59. New York, Raven Press, 1979.

39. Edeiken J, Karasick D: Imaging in cancer. CA 1987;37:239.

40. Thrupkaew AK, Henkin RE, Quin JL III: False negative bone scans in disseminated metastatic disease. Radiology 1974;113:383.

41. Kanner R: Diagnosis and Management of Pain in Patients with Cancer. Basel, Karger, 1988.

42. DeVita VT Jr, Hellman S, Rosenberg SA (eds): Cancer: Principles and Practice of Oncology, 3rd ed, p 1252. Philadelphia, JB Lippincott, 1989.

43. Greenberg HS, Deck MDF, Vikram B et al: Metastases to the base of the skull: Clinical findings in 43 patients. Neurology 1981;31:530.

44. Elliot K, Foley KM: Neurologic pain syndromes in patients with cancer. Crit Care Clin 1990;6:393.

45. Payne R: Pharmacologic management of bone pain in the cancer patient. Clin J Pain (Suppl) 1989;5:S43.

46. Patchell RA, Posner JB: Neurologic complications of systemic cancer. Neurologic Clin 1985;3:729.

47. Gilbert MR, Grossman SA: Incidence and nature of neurologic problems in patients with solid tumors. Am J Med 1986;81:951.

48. Twycross RG, Lack SA: Symptom Control in Far Advanced Cancer: Pain Relief. London, Pitman, 1983.

49. Kori SH, Foley KM, Posner JB: Brachial plexus lesions in patients with cancer: 100 cases. Neurology 1981;31:45.

50. Foley KM: Brachial plexopathy in patients with breast cancer. In Harris JR, Hellman S, Henderson IC et al (eds): Breast Diseases. Philadelphia, JB Lippincott, 1987.

51. Scott JF: Carcinoma invading nerve. In Wall PD, Melzack R (eds): Textbook of Pain, 2nd ed, p 598. Edinburgh, Churchill Livingstone, 1989.

52. Watson PN, Evans RJ: Intractable pain with lung cancer. Pain 1987;29:163.

53. Yacoub M, Hupert C: Shoulder pain as an early symptom of Pancoast tumor. Journal of the Medical Society of New Jersey 1980;77:583.

54. Downs SE: Bronchogenic carcinoma presenting as neuromusculoskeletal pain. J Manipulative Physiol Ther 1990;13:221.

55. Batzdorf U, Brechner VL: Management of pain associated with the Pancoast syndrome. Am J Surg 1979;137:638.

56. Cascino TL, Kori S, Krol G et al: CT scan of the brachial plexus in patients with cancer. Neurology 1983;33:1553.

57. Kanner RM, Martini N, Foley KM: Epidural spinal cord compression in Pancoast syndrome (superior

pulmonary sulcus tumor): Clinical presentation and outcome. Ann Neurol 1981;10:77.

58. Foley KM: Overview of cancer pain and brachial and lumbosacral plexopathy. In Foley KM (ed): Management of Cancer Pain, p 25. New York, Memorial Sloan Kettering Cancer Center, 1985.

59. Jaekle KA, Young DF, Foley KM: The natural history of lumbosacral plexopathy in cancer. Neurology 1985;35:8.

60. Pettigrew LC, Glass JP, Maor M et al: Diagnosis and treatment of lumbosacral plexopathy in patients with cancer. Arch Neurol 1984;41:1282.

61. Twycross RG, Lack SA: Control of Alimentary Symptoms in Far Advanced Cancer. Edinburgh, Churchill Livingstone, 1986.

62. Thomas JE, Cascino TL, Earl JD et al: Differential diagnosis between radiation and tumor plexopathy of the pelvis. Neurology 1985;35:1.

63. Evans BA, Stevens JK, Dyck PJ: Lumbosacral plexus neuropathy. Neurology 1981;31:1327.

64. Travell J: Myofascial trigger points: Clinical view. In Bonica JJ, Albe-Fessard D (eds): Advances in Pain Research and Therapy, vol 1, p 919. New York, Raven Press, 1976.

65. Abrams SE: The role of non-neurolytic blocks in the management of cancer pain. In Abrams SE (ed): Cancer Pain, p 67. Boston, Kluwer Academic, 1989.

66. Siegal T: Muscle cramps in the cancer patient: Causes and treatment. Journal of Pain and Symptom Management 1991;6;84.

67. Mills KR, Newham DS, Edwards RHT: Muscle pain. In Wall PD, Melzack R (eds): Textbook of Pain, 2nd ed, p 420. Edinburgh, Churchill Livingstone, 1989.

68. Fisher AA, Chang CH: Electromyographic evidence of paraspinal muscle spasm during sleep in patients with low back pain. Clin J Pain 1985;1:147.

69. Raj PP: Prognostic and therapeutic local anesthetic blockade. In Cousins MJ, Bridenbaugh PO (eds): Neural Blockade, 2nd ed, p 899. Philadelphia, JB Lippincott, 1988.

70. Aronoff GM, Evans WO: Pharmacologic management of chronic pain. In Aronoff GM (ed): Evaluation and Treatment of Chronic Pain, p 435. Baltimore, Urban & Schwarzenberg, 1985.

71. Young RR, Delwaide PM: Spasticity: Parts I and II. N Engl J Med 1981;304:28,96.

72. Travell JG, Simons DG: Myofascial Pain and Dysfunction: The Trigger Point Manual. Baltimore, Williams and Wilkins, 1983.

73. Wolfe F, Smythe HA, Yunus MB, et al: The American College of Rheumatology 1990 criteria for the classification of fibromyalgia. Report of the Multicenter Criteria Committee. Arthritis Rheum 1990;33:160.

74. Fischer AA: Documentation of myofascial trigger points. Arch Phys Med Rehabil 1988;69:286.

75. Zohn DA, Mennell JM: Musculoskeletal Pain: Diagnosis and Physical Treatment. Boston, Little Brown, 1976.

76. Stillman M: Perineal pain. Adv Pain Res Ther 1991;16:359.

77. Foley KM: Pain syndromes and pharmacologic management of pancreatic cancer pain. Journal of Pain and Symptom Management 1988;3:176.

78. Reber HA, Foley KM (eds): Pancreatic cancer pain: Presentation, pathogenesis and management. Journal of Pain and Symptom Management 3:163, 1988.

78a. Jain S, Kestenbaum A, Shah N et al: Is celiac plexus block indicated for all upper abdominal cancer pain? Pain 1990;5(suppl):S-91.

79. Ihse I: Pancreatic pain. Br J Surg 1990;77:121.

80. Cantwell BMK, Mannix KA, Harris AL: Back pain: A presentation of metastatic testicular germ cell tumours. Lancet 1987;1:262.

81. Levy M: Pain management in advanced cancer. Semin Oncol 1985;12:394.

82. Baines M, Kirkham SR: Cancer pain. In Wall PD, Melzack R (eds): Textbook of Pain, 2nd ed, p 590. Edinburgh, Churchill Livingstone, 1989.

83. Ivetic O, Lyne PA: Fungating and ulcerating malignant lesions: A review of the literature. J Adv Nurs 1990;15:83.

84. Enck RE: The management of large fungating tumors (malignant ulceration). American Journal of Hospice and Palliative Care 1990;7:11.

85. Bruera E, MacDonald N: Intractable pain in patients with advanced head and neck tumors: A possible role of local infection. Cancer Treat Rep 1986;70:691.

86. Bates T: Radiotherapy, chemotherapy and hormone therapy in the relief of cancer pain. In Swerdlow M, Charlton JE (eds): Relief of Intractable Pain, 4th ed, p 329. Amsterdam, Elsevier, 1989.

87. Temple WJ, Ketcham AS: Surgical palliation for recurrent rectal cancers ulcerating in the perineum. Cancer 1990;65:1111.

88. Kunkle EC, Hernandez RR, Wolff HG: Studies on headache: The mechanisms and significance of headache associated with brain tumor. Bull NY Acad Med 1942;18:400.

89. Rushton JG, Rooke ED: Brain tumor headache. Headache 1962;2:147.

90. Zimm S, Wampler GL, Stablein D et al: Intracerebral metastases in solid tumor patients: Natural history and results of treatment. Cancer 1981;48:384.

91. Guitin PH: Corticosteroid therapy in patients with brain tumor. NCI Monogr 1977;46:151.

92. Black P: Brain metastasis: Current status and recommended guidelines for management. Neurosurgery 1979;5:617.

93. Ray BS, Wolff HG: Experimental studies on headache. Arch Surg 1940;41:813.

94. Simons DJ, Day E, Goodell H et al: Experimental studies on headache: Muscles of the scalp and neck as sources of pain. Association for Research in Nervous Mental Disease 1943;23:228.

95. Wolff HG: Headache and Other Head Pain, 2nd ed. New York, Oxford University Press, 1963.

96. Posner JB, Chernik NK: Intracranial metastases from systemic cancer. Adv Neurol 1978;19:579.

97. Olson ME, Chernik NL, Posner JB: Infiltration of the leptomeninges by systemic cancer: A clinical and pathologic study. Arch Neurol 1978;30:122.

98. Wasserstrom WR, Glass JP, Posner JB: Diagnosis and treatment of leptomeningeal metastases from solid tumor: Experience with 90 patients. Cancer 1982;49:759.

99. Schild SC, Wasserstrom WR, Fleischer M et al: Cerebrospinal fluid biochemical markers of central nervous system metastases. Ann Neurol 1980;8:597.

100. Lee YY, Glass JP, Geoffray A et al: Cranial computed tomographic abnormalities in leptomeningeal metastases. AJNR 1984;5:559.

101. Glass JP, Foley KM: Carcinomatous meningitis. In Harris JR, Hellman S, Henderson IC et al (eds): Breast Diseases, p 497. Philadelphia, JB Lippincott, 1987.

Chapter **2**

Comprehensive Assessment of the Patient with Cancer Pain

John C. Rowlingson

Robin J. Hamill

Richard B. Patt

PURPOSES

The evaluation of the patient presenting with cancer-related pain serves multiple purposes.[1,2] The initial encounter should be broadly based: rather than limiting inquiry to the pain syndrome per se, the process should encompass evaluation of the person, their feelings and attitudes about pain and disease, family concerns, and the patient's premorbid psychiatric history (*eg*, preexisting depressive or anxiety disorders, personality disorder, substance abuse). A compassionate but objective approach to assessment serves to instill confidence in the patient and family that will be of value throughout treatment. Thorough review of the patient's records and a detailed pain history serve both to help delineate the source of pain and to distinguish the degree to which the patient's complaints are related to nociceptive mechanisms versus psychological modulators. The primary care physician who has known the patient over time is a source of valuable information, and should be consulted personally. Psychological testing is of value, although in selected cases it must be abbreviated in consideration of poor physical or emotional condition.[3] That assessment must also be geared to the patient's cultural and educational background is highlighted by one Pakistani's comment that the questions were "eating her brain,"[4] and the development of a "fruit scale," that encourages patients to grade pain intensity by selecting a picture of the appropriate size fruit from a sequential scale ranging from a lemon to a watermelon.[5]

Ideally, consultation for the patient with cancer pain accomplishes more than simply rendering a diagnosis and treatment plan[6]; it should also orient the patient, family, and referring physician to what can realistically be accomplished, should serve an educational function, and should ultimately be reassuring to the patient. These goals are of practical value: patients with an improved understanding of their medical condition and confidence in their health care providers are more compliant, tend to have better outcomes, and are probably less likely to use emergency services inappropriately.[7,8,9] Table 2–1 summarizes the components of a comprehensive evaluation of the patient with cancer pain.

LOGISTICS AND UNDERLYING THEMES

WHY IS EXCELLENCE IN ASSESSMENT AN IMPERATIVE?

There is unanimous agreement among experts that careful assessment is an essential, indispensable precursor to the initiation of therapy for pain problems.[2,10–12] As a result, all the reasons that have been advanced as arguments for the importance of promoting excellence in the management of cancer pain[12–17] apply to striving for the same excellence in assessment. These include the high incidence of symptomatic cancer worldwide, the morbidity of uncontrolled pain (interference with functional status, rehabilitation, and compliance with antitumor strategies), and ethical and humanitarian rationales.[18]

WHAT SHOULD ASSESSMENT ENDEAVOR TO ACCOMPLISH?

Pain Control Versus Symptom Control

Although the purpose of consultation is ostensibly to promote improved pain control, our experience and that of others[19,20] has demonstrated that a broader view is frequently warranted. Pain control is desirable insofar as it fosters an improved quality of life, but it is apparent that this outcome is determined by multiple factors in addition to adequacy of pain control.[21,21a] For example, even independent of physical symptoms, coping with a diagnosis of cancer characteristically induces profound behavioral changes[22,23] that, if inadequately addressed, predictably detract from quality of life. Cancer is a multisymptomatic disorder[19,20,24] (Table 2–2), and attention to the other, equally distressing symptoms of cancer is essential if an enhanced quality of life is to be realized. A thorough review of systems and psychological as well as physical assessment will help identify other, potentially correctable symptoms that, if addressed, will improve the outcome of the consultation. Even when a consultant wishes to limit himself to pain control per se, the presence of other symptoms must be investigated, since clinical measures intended to reduce pain are often associated with side effects that may produce new symptoms or exacerbate preexisting symptoms (eg, constipation, fatigue, nausea, and vomiting).

This holistic approach to the care of patients with advanced irreversible disease (palliative care) has long been applied, but has only recently elicited widespread recognition as a legitimate activity for health care providers and an important part of educational curricula.[1,20,25] Subspecialty status in some quarters is only now forthcoming, and in others is completely lacking.[26–28] Palliative care is based on a combination of pragmatism and science. The former has parented numerous practices and guidelines for care, the efficacy of which have withstood the test of time. Well controlled clinical research is

Table 2–1.
Components of Comprehensive Assessment

Initial screening to determine appropriateness of referral and to plan resources

Review of medical record and radiologic studies

Review of patient responses to questionnaire

May wish to discuss with primary care provider and/or oncologist

Introduction of clinican or team, patient orientation to facility

Psychosocial history
  Marital and residential status
  Employment history and status
  Educational background
  Functional status, activities of daily living
  Recreational activities
  Support system
  Health and capabilities of spouse/significant other

Medical history independent of oncologic history
  Coexisting systemic disease
  Exercise tolerance
  Allergies to medications
  Medication use
  Prior illnesses and surgery

Thorough review of systems (see Table 2–2)

Oncologic history
  Prior malignancies
  Family history
  Diagnosis and evolution of disease
  Therapy and outcome (including side effects)
  Patient's understanding of disease process and prognosis

Pain history
  Premorbid chronic pain
  Premorbid drug or alcohol use
  Pain catalogue (number and locations)
  For each pain
    Onset and evolution
    Site and radiation
    Pattern (constant, intermittent, predictable, etc.)
    Intensity (best, worst, average, current)—0–10
    Quality
    Exacerbating factors
    Relieving factors
    How the pain interferes and with what
    Neurologic and motor abnormalities
    Vasomotor changes
    Other associated factors
    Current analgesics (use, efficacy, side effects)
    Prior analgesics (use, efficacy, side effects)

Physical examination (see text)

Team meeting, if applicable

Determination of need for further studies

Formulate clinical impression (diagnosis)

Formulate recommendations (plan) and alternates

Call oncologist and/or primary care provider, if applicable

Exit interview
  Explain probable cause of symptoms
  If appropriate, discuss nature of disease
  Discuss prognosis for symptom relief
  Discuss management options
  Discuss specific recommendations
  Arrange for follow-up
  Dictate summary to referring and consulting physicians

---

another necessary tool to further legitimize established practices, and is currently being applied more rigorously. One of the most profound lessons of the palliative care movement, "To cure sometimes, to relieve often and to comfort always,"[29] serves as a reminder to those in even the busiest of practices that we must be attentive to a whole person and not just a diseased organ or a pain syndrome.

WHEN SHOULD ASSESSMENT IDEALLY OCCUR?

Early Versus Late Consultation; the Expedient Consultation

Referral for chronic nonmalignant pain problems is frequently a lengthy process, much of which consists of gathering often extensive medical records, determining the suitability of the referral, and regrettably, at times, ascer-

Table 2–2.
Review of Systems (Symptom List)

Systemic/Constitutional	Gastrointestinal
Anorexia	Dysphagia
Weight loss	Nausea
Cachexia	Vomiting
Fatigue/weakness	Dehydration
Insomnia	Constipation
	Diarrhea
Neurologic	
Sedation	**Psychological**
Confusion	Irritability
Hallucinations	Anxiety
Headache	Depression
Motor weakness	Dementia
Altered sensation	
Incontinence	**Alterations in Urinary Function**
Respiratory	**Integument**
Dyspnea	Decubitus
Cough	Dry, sore mouth
Hiccough	

taining insurance status. If assessment is to take place in a multidisciplinary setting, a nurse manager, physician, or psychologist must evaluate which specialties should be involved, and then they must be scheduled. Standardized questionnaires (see below), often requiring input from the family, are usually mailed to the patient, and in addition the patient may be requested to complete additional work on site to assure validity (MMPI, Millon). Despite even high levels of distress, chronic nonmalignant pain, by definition, is rarely if ever an emergency, so the delay induced by these circumstances is rarely deleterious, and may even serve a therapeutic purpose by reinforcing the message that a beneficial outcome may be slow in coming.

Cancer pain is frequently characterized by features classically associated with acute pain, and as such a different model from that cited above should be adopted. Further, more expeditious and concise assessment is warranted in cases when a limited life expectancy serves as an impetus for maximizing the quality of remaining time.[13] Commonly, when a pain service is first establishing itself, a large pro-

portion of patients are referred in the late stages of disease when they are moribund and all other measures have failed. As the value of a service becomes more widely recognized, typically more timely referrals of patients in various stages of illness become more prevalent, a practice that should be encouraged.

In order to augment the confidence of referring sources, many pain centers have instituted a policy of scheduling the assessment of patients with cancer pain within 48 hours of referral, a practice that tends to be well received. It should be noted, however, that this type of policy, and, indeed, the high proportion of urgent referrals that is characteristic in this population, taxes resources immensely since the typically rigid daily schedule is easily interrupted.

WHERE SHOULD ASSESSMENT IDEALLY OCCUR?

The Consultative Environment

The setting where the assessment takes place should ideally be comfortable, spacious, and

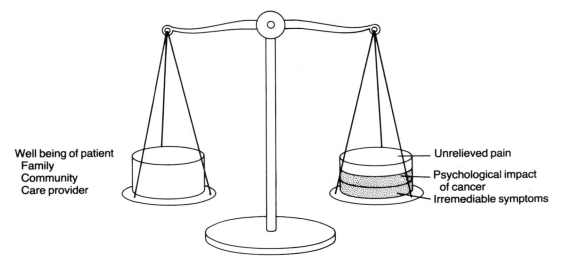

Figure 2–1.   Conceptualization of balance between well-being of patient, family, community, and care providers versus the sequelae of cancer. Shaded areas on right (psychological impact of diagnosis, irremediable symptoms) are difficult to modify. Effective management of unrelieved pain (clear area on right) may tip the "scale" back in favor of well-being for patient and cohorts.

nonthreatening.[30] Barrier-free access is essential since patients are frequently confined to a wheelchair or stretcher. Patients rarely present unattended, and ample space should be provided to accommodate family members and friends. Ideally, a family conference area is provided. Patients in whom cancer cure has failed may lack overall confidence in the health care system, and may also be apprehensive about exploring the unfamiliar idea of a pain consultation. Thus, a supportive staff, pleasant surroundings, and the presence of simple amenities like a water fountain and reading material will assist the patient and the family in feeling more at ease.

WHO SHOULD BE INCLUDED IN THE ASSESSMENT PROCESS?

The Companion

Although traditional medical models of assessment focus almost exclusively on the patient, cancer and cancer pain can readily be conceptualized as a disease with broader dele-terious effects, often affecting, in addition to the patient, the family unit, the community, and even health care providers (Fig. 2–1).[30–32] The nature of suffering that cancer patients typically experience has been well characterized,[33] and it is only logical to expect that the same feelings of helplessness, guilt, resentment, and sorrow are poignant issues for those close to the patient.

It is rare for a patient to present for consultation unaccompanied, and as a result the assessment process should adopt a policy that considers how to deal with the concerned spouse, parents, offspring, and others. There are significant advantages to including at least one pertinent relation in as much of the process as possible. The presence of a companion can help optimize the quality of the data collected by the clinician, particularly when the patient is stoic, unenthusiastic, or debilitated. The model of home-based hospice care that has developed in most countries usually requires that one family member be identified as being responsible for the patient's overall care, a guideline that is a U.S. Medicare requirement for eligibility.[34,35] Given the level of care that is often required, that individual may practically qualify as the patient's primary care provider, and his or her familiarity with the patient's routine, medical regimen, compliance, and complaints typically provides extremely valuable information.

The presence of a companion may also serve to influence compliance by helping optimize the quality of data collected by the patient, and this aspect of the consultation should not be discounted; it is of importance if the consultation is to be viewed, in part, as an educational endeavor.[36] Typically, even relatively well patients are poor consumers of health care, often seeming to invest more energy into the prospect of purchasing an automobile or appliance than into researching health care options. Whether due to the intimidating nature of the classic doctor–patient relationship[37,38] (authoritarian–deferential at its worst)[39] or denial of their disease process, patients often fail to ask important questions and may be reluctant to insist that doctors explain their condition in terms they understand. A friend or family member may assist the patient by prompting them to explore their concerns more completely. This concept is being explored by a pilot program initiated by Cancer Action, Inc. in Rochester, New York, that trains seasoned cancer patients to serve as advocates and companions for patients in active treatment.[40]

Finally, it is especially useful to involve a close companion in the decision-making process when validity of informed consent is an issue, especially if the patient is debilitated or his or her capacity is compromised by disease or treatment.

The Clinicians

There will always be debate as to in whose province properly falls the assessment and management of pain.[25,28,41,42] It is well accepted that a multidisciplinary or interdisciplinary approach to the management of the patient with pain is desirable, even optimal.[43–45] Nevertheless, multidisciplinary care is costly to administer in terms of time, effort, and expense, and as a result of this and other factors is not always readily available.[43] There

is every reason to expect that any of a variety of specialists can provide an adequate level of care, provided that they are knowledgeable, resourceful, and committed.[46] This is particularly true for cancer pain management, since the foundation of good care is pharmacologic management, which can readily be instituted by the well informed primary care provider. An astute clinician will ascertain the need for consultation from alternate specialists, and in this way the diverse needs of patients can be addressed even in the single-specialty practice.

When a treatment facility is staffed by multiple specialists, a prescreening process should determine which of these people should be involved in the initial assessment. As one of its goals, the assessment process should establish the need for further contact with alternate specialists. Residents, medical students, and specially trained nurses and other allied health professionals, can play an important role in gathering data, but a physician experienced in the assessment and management of patients with pain caused by cancer should always play a pivotal role throughout the consultation.

HOW SHOULD ASSESSMENT BE ACCOMPLISHED?

Preassessment

Some form of prescreening is essential to gain sufficient information to characterize the urgency of the referral, as well as to determine the nature of the resources that will need to be mobilized. This may be accomplished initially by the collection of basic demographic data by clerical personnel, supplemented by brief telephone contact between the referring source and clinician. While a detailed letter of referral and the full medical record are ideally reviewed well in advance of the evaluation, expediency frequently dictates that the patient be scheduled based on preliminary data or interphysician telephone contact, and that the patient's family or clerical staff collect pertinent records on the day of assessment. Referring physicians should still be encouraged to dictate a full letter of referral that summarizes the patient's clinical course, recent findings and impressions, and the questions they hope to have addressed by consultation. Nevertheless, every effort should be made to encourage referral by making the process as simple as possible.

Before meeting with the patient, all available data, including the medical record, radiologic studies, and pain questionnaires should be reviewed by members of the treatment team. When possible, contact with the primary care provider, treating oncologists, and other consultants will also help provide additional information.

Screening Instruments

Multiple, diverse instruments have been developed to obtain the variety of types of information that is of potential value in assessing patients with pain.[47,48] (See Appendix A.) Most centers select items from this plethora of tools to form their own unique questionnaire that is ideally completed by the patient before evaluation. The development and acceptance of a standard instrument would contribute to a better understanding of epidemiology and outcome, and is a highly desirable goal. All the instruments that will be discussed have some shortcomings, but of them the (Wisconsin) Brief Pain Inventory and the Memorial Brief Pain Assessment Card (see below) are becoming increasingly well accepted, and may emerge as standard tools for assessing cancer pain.

Ideally, the tools used for assessment will help characterize the quality of the pain experienced by the patient and will help quantify it as well. It is well accepted that pain cannot be directly correlated with tissue injury from as long ago as the time of Leriche, who said, "physical pain is not a simple affair of an impulse traveling at a fixed rate along the nerve. It is the result of a conflict between a stimulus and a whole individual."[49] When pain is conceived of as a highly personalized individual experience, it becomes obvious that it can be fully appreciated only by the person experiencing it, who must as a result be regarded as having a highly authoritative role in character-

izing the pain.[38] As such, it is almost universally recommended that some form(s) of self-report constitute the foundation for pain assessment.[50] Although these may be complemented by behavioral, psychometric, and observational instruments, these adjuncts should not be relied on exclusively. Several studies, mostly in burn patients, have demonstrated a relatively poor correlation between patients' and nurses' assessment of pain intensity,[51,52] and similar results have been obtained when cancer patients' self-reports have been compared with physician observations.[50,53] Similarly, a comparison of the responses of cancer patients and their next-of-kin was unable to demonstrate uniformly high correlations.[54]

Since pain is regarded as a subjective experience, quantitative measurement necessarily depends on subjective tools that endeavor to objectify self-report. The tool used most frequently is some variant of a unidimensional visual analogue scale (VAS),[47,55–57] that commonly consists of a horizontal or vertical line evenly "anchored" or divided into 10 segments numbered consecutively between 0 and 10 (Fig. 2–2). Patients may be instructed that 0 represents "total absence of pain" and 10 denotes the "most severe pain they can imagine." The patient is instructed simply to mark the number that best describes the level of pain they are experiencing at some given point in time. Technically for such a scale to be truly analogue in character, it should consist of only a line with anchors at each end and none in-between. Modified VASs for use with children substitute a continuum of smiling to crying faces for numbers, or may use colors or a pain "thermometer" (see Chapter 4 and Appendix B).[58] Frequently, a verbal version of the VAS proves easier to apply and may be more reliable in the presence of cognitive impairment.[59] A novel approach especially appropriate for rural and semiliterate patients is the Fruit Scale,[5] described above.

One of the most widely used instruments is the McGill Pain Questionnaire (MPQ),[60,61] a pen-and-paper instrument that, in addition to other components, instructs patients to make relevant selections from a list of 78 adjectives

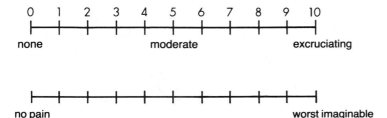

Figure 2–2. Examples of pain measurement scales, instruments used to assess pain, usually along a 100-mm continuum, with or without anchoring labels.

used to describe pain. The descriptors are organized into sets, and analysis of the types of words selected is intended to help evaluate the extent to which pain is predominantly sensory, affective, or evaluative in nature. Another feature of the MPQ is a schematic representation of the body that is shaded by the patient to indicate where pain is located. This component can be modified to provide additional information by instructing patients to inscribe a numeric value that signifies regional pain intensity in lieu of shading (Fig. 2–3). The use of the MPQ has been described in patients with cancer pain.[62,63]

That it is relevant to assess the patient's psychological status is illustrated in a well controlled study that determined that patients with a history of emotional problems were much more likely to report unmet emotional and social needs during the course of their illness, including perceptions that needs were inadequately addressed by their physicians.[64] Sophisticated tests assess psychological factors that often have an important bearing on pain, such as the patient's personal style, the presence of depression or anxiety, hypochondriasis, preoccupation with body image, etc. (see Chapter 5). While a comprehensive battery of psychological testing is usually considered to be an appropriate component of the assessment of the patient with chronic nonmalignant pain, it is essential that testing of the cancer pain patient be brief and not excessively demanding. Several practical, useful tools have recently been introduced that specifically target patients with cancer pain and that possess these attributes. These include the (Wisconsin) Brief Pain Inventory (BPI)[65,66]

and the Memorial Brief Pain Assessment Card.[67]

The (Wisconsin) Brief Pain Inventory (see Appendix A) requires on average 15 minutes for completion, and can be self-administered or used as an adjunct to the interview, apparently without affecting the reliability of results.[66] It includes several questions about the

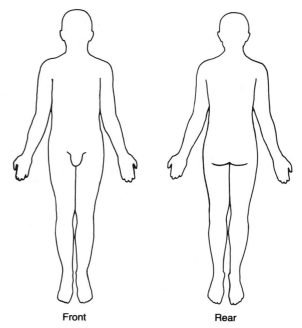

Front   Rear

Figure 2–3. Example of body outline used as an assessment tool for patients to generate a pain map. To obtain even more information, patients may be instructed to place a number between 0–10 over the shaded area to indicate the intensity of each pain.

characteristics of the pain problem, including its origin, and inquires into prior treatments and their efficacy. In addition, the BPI incorporates two valuable features of the MPQ, a graphic representation of the location of pain and groups of qualitative descriptors, which in this case were derived from a survey of a large number of cancer patients. Severity of pain is assessed by a series of visual analogue scales, tailored to the variable pain common with cancer by eliciting scores for pain at its best, worst, and on average. Finally, the perceived level of interference with normal function (enjoyment of life, work, mood, sleep, general activity, walking, relations with others) generated by the pain is quantified with visual analogue scales that are both numbered and labeled by the anchors "no interference" and "interferes completely." Preliminary evidence suggests that the BPI is cross-culturally valid[66] and is useful, particularly when patients are not fit to complete a more thorough or comprehensive questionnaire.

The Memorial Pain Assessment Card (see Appendix A) is a simple, efficient, and valid assessment instrument that can provide rapid evaluation, in clinical settings, of the major aspects of pain experienced by cancer patients.[67] It is easy to understand and use, and can be completed by experienced patients in less than 20 seconds. It consists of a two-sided, 8 1/2" × 11" card that is folded so that four separate measures are created. It features scales intended for the measurement of pain intensity, pain relief, and mood, and a set of descriptive adjectives. Its originators believe that it can be used to help distinguish among pain intensity, pain relief, and global suffering or psychological distress.[67]

One additional screening tool deserves mention because its intent and methodology are distinct from other available instruments. The Edmonton Staging System for Cancer Pain[68] is performed by the health care provider rather than the patient, and was developed to prognosticate the likelihood of providing effective relief of pain in cancer patients. Patients are staged with an alphanumeric code, similar to that used to characterize the clinico-histologic status of tumors.[69] The system's originators have provided preliminary validation that treatment outcome can be accurately predicted based on seven clinical features (mechanism of pain, the presence of incident pain, previous exposure to opioids, cognitive function, psychological distress, tolerance to opioids, a history of alcoholism or drug abuse).[68] Staging requires only 5 to 10 minutes to complete, and demands no special skills. Its value lies in identifying potentially problematic patients prospectively, further legitimizing clinical research on symptom control by introducing better standardization, and improving our ability to assess critically the results of different therapeutic interventions in large populations of patients.

COMPONENTS OF ASSESSMENT

HISTORY

The preliminary components of the assessment should be intentionally nonthreatening in their content, postponing the discussion of sensitive topics until the patient and his or her family have had an opportunity to "assess" the clinicians as compassionate and interested advocates. Initially, the patient is introduced to the team and oriented to the philosophy and protocols of the treatment facility, including the structure of the assessment process. A brief psychosocial history is obtained that should include such pertinent facts as the patient's marital and residential status, employment history and status, educational background, functional status, including ability to complete activities of daily living, recreational activities, and the nature of active networks of support. Other factors to be assessed include religious, cultural, and ethnic background. It is useful to determine the health and capabilities of the spouse or significant other as well as whether the patient or the spouse maintain the ability to drive. One of the authors had the experience of performing a neurolytic subarachnoid block in an unfortunate elderly man who subsequently developed mild unilateral lower extremity paresis, an occurrence that was even more distressing when it was learned that the patient was the only driver in the family.

A brief past medical history is obtained (exclusive of the oncologic history), focusing on the presence of coexisting systemic disease, exercise tolerance, allergies to medications, medication use, and prior surgery.

A thorough review of systems (ROS) is essential for the reasons previously cited; often the pain specialist can recommend interventions that will have potentially salutary effects on other symptoms that can be fully as distressing as pain. Constitutional changes associated with cancer (anorexia, weight change, and fatigue) should be sought, as well as evidence of central nervous system changes, which may range from mild sedation to lethargy, confusion, and even frank hallucinations. In addition, the history should assess the presence and degree of a variety of symptoms, including nausea, vomiting, dysphagia, dyspnea, constipation, diarrhea, alterations in urinary habit, visual acuity, and mood. As the ROS is being completed, efforts should be made to form differential diagnoses for symptoms and to correlate them with medication use.

One of the most sensitive areas of the interview relates to obtaining the oncologic history. Discussion of the status of the cancer should be prefaced with remarks that indicate an understanding of this fact. It is essential to gauge patients' reactions to this line of inquiry, which will range from a surprising level of willingness to engage in discussion to abrupt denial, and the interview approach must be altered accordingly. Whenever possible, it is useful to gain as much information as possible about the disease from the medical record. The patient's cognizance of the details and rationale of their treatment and prognosis reveals a great deal about the patient's styles of interaction and coping. Whatever the source, information should be obtained about any prior and family history of cancer, the evolution of the disease, antitumor treatment, and complications or side effects. Although usually an extremely delicate area of inquiry, it is useful to gain a sense of the patient's understanding of his or her prognosis, as this will affect how

treatment options are later framed. It may be useful to discuss these issues with a family member privately, as well as with the patient's oncologist.

Finally, a thorough pain history is obtained.[70,71] The pain history should include details of any premorbid chronic or acute pain problems and drug use. A quick overall survey should be obtained as to the number and locations of pain, since it is common for multiple sites of pain to be present, especially in patients with advanced disease.[72] In a prospective study of 100 new hospice patients, Twycross determined that 80% of patients had more than one pain, and 34% had four or more sites of pain.[73] Insofar as it is possible, separate pain histories should be obtained for each major complaint of pain, since their etiology may differ. Early on, a description of the chronologic evolution of the pain and its characteristics should be obtained to provide a context for more detailed questioning.

The site of pain and any radiation of pain should be determined, as well as its pattern (ie, constant, intermittent, breakthrough, or incident pain). The intensity of pain on average and at its best and worst should be assessed using a simple analogue scale. A certain amount of explanation is required to elicit optimal information about the quality and nature of the pain, since patients are often unaccustomed to thinking in this fashion. Factors that exacerbate and relieve the pain, even partially, should be sought, and might include movement, position changes, and the application of heat, cold, and massage. Total pain (see Chapters 1 and 30) should be assessed by determining the perceived effects of pain on sleep, appetite, posture, mood, sexuality, socialization, habits, recreation, etc.[13] Patients should be queried as to what they would choose to do differently if pain were not present.

PHYSICAL EXAMINATION

There is no definite agreement as to what constitutes the optimal extent of physical examination for the patient presenting for evaluation of cancer pain. Like careful history-taking, physical examination is a relatively noninvasive, cost-effective, time-conservative means of obtaining information.[70,74,75] Reports of previous examinations may provide useful information, but the temptation to rely on them exclusively should be avoided. Cancer is a dynamic and progressive disease, and as a result at least the essential components of the examination must be repeated, even if the patient is simply "referred for a procedure." Also, the recognition and interpretation of physical findings will differ among specialists. Ideally, every patient should receive a comprehensive examination, organized by region and/or system, although this is frequently abbreviated due to constraints of time, the patient's overall condition, and the urgency surrounding a specific problem.

The examination should be conducted with the patient in a hospital gown to facilitate access. Since this exchange of garments is depersonalizing and may be intimidating to the patient, meaningful exchange should be postponed until the patient is fully clothed. Whenever possible, the examination should follow a preset pattern to avoid omissions. Vital signs and weight should be obtained. Minimally, assessment should include a thorough examination of the site of pain, adjacent sites (to check for referred pain), sites of known tumor invasion, a complete musculoskeletal and neurologic examination, as well as auscultation of the heart and lungs. Signs of systemic disease may relate to the etiology of pain or other symptoms, may modify the patient's therapeutic options and be of value to other clinicians involved in the patient's care.[76]

The neurologic examination is geared to evaluate the extent of any neuromuscular deficits or altered sensation that may be present. It is critical that these findings be documented, particularly if a nerve block or neurosurgery are considerations. Findings may be present supporting a diagnosis of neuropathic pain that may have been overlooked by other specialists, and which would recommend other than standard treatment with opioid analgesics (see Chapters 1 and 10). Finally, since pain is an early, often overlooked sign, it is important to observe for signs consistent with spinal cord compression (see Chapter 29). Findings, particularly on examination of the neurologic and musculoskeletal systems, may be difficult to interpret when acute pain is present. Signs of simple nononcologic causes of pain such as trigger points (myofascial pain, muscle contraction headache) and positive straight leg raising (sciatica) should be sought as well.

Examining patients with advanced illness is challenging. When patients are debilitated there is a natural reluctance to subject them even to such relatively undemanding events as a thorough physical examination. In addition, the encounter may take place in a nonoffice setting such as the patient's home or a hospice. Nevertheless, because of their disease or self-imposed reclusivity, particularly after antitumor therapy has ceased, this population of patients is subject to reduced medical surveillance, and pertinent new findings may be noted. A recent survey, for example, found that of patients referred to a cancer pain service, 63% were determined to have previously unrecognized lesions discovered only through the assessment provided by the pain consultant.[76] In almost 20% of cases, this information provided an opportunity for primary antineoplastic or antibiotic therapy.

INTERVENTIONS

Diagnostic maneuvers are pursued to determine the underlying cause of pain so that, when possible, treatment can be directed at alleviating the source of pain in preference to relying on a purely symptomatic approach to treatment. Direction of treatment at the source of pain permits more focused, specific care, reducing the likelihood of complications from overtreatment of symptoms. Identification of psychological factors that may exacerbate and/or maintain the pain may suggest specific cognitive behavioral interventions or counseling directed at modifying these factors. Escalations of pain usually signal progressive injury to tissue and/or progressive disease, and anatomic localization of a painful lesion through radiologic studies or diagnostic nerve blocks may suggest additional treatment options. For example, the identification of spinal cord impingement or impending vertebral collapse may warrant mechanical or surgical stabilization to forestall paraplegia (see Chapter 29). Pain of unknown etiology may be an early symptom of recurrent disease or undiagnosed malignant neoplasm; this is particularly true for herpes zoster. Although diagnostic tests are not excluded because the patient has already been "worked up" or because antineoplastic treatment has been abandoned, a diagnosis is often possible on clinical grounds, and frequently only symptomatic treatment is warranted, particularly when expectancy of life is limited.

In an effort to determine the relative clinical utility of various diagnostic interventions, Rudy and colleagues[77] recently surveyed 80 pain specialists. Their results identified agreement for the relevance of 18 common biomedical procedures, but consistently demonstrated a strongly weighted reliance by experts on the results of physical examination to radiologic and other diagnostic studies. In descending order, the most highly clinician-weighted factors were the neurologic examination, observation of gait and posture, assessment of spinal mobility, and examination of muscular function, soft tissues, and the mobility of weight-bearing joints.

EXIT INTERVIEW

This portion of the assessment process is the one patients tend to value the most, and also represents an important opportunity to initiate patient education. It must be understood, however, that in spite of fatigue, denial, and passive styles of the patient and/or clinician, active participation by all parties must be encouraged. If multiple specialists have participated in the assessment, then the exit interview is preceded by a team conference intended to establish the issues to be discussed with the patient.

Insofar as it is possible, the basis for the patient's symptoms should be explained in simple terms[2] and in a tone sympathetic to the patient's understanding of the prognosis of his or her disease. Given the opportunity, many patients are surprisingly inclined to discuss their diagnosis and prognosis, would prefer that these topics be explained, and often express frustration that other clinicians have not addressed them more directly.[78–80] It is usually impossible to determine whether this phenomenon reflects a deliberate or unintentional omission by doctors to discuss these sensitive topics,[39,81,82] or denial on the part of the patient to really hear the doctor.[83,84] On the one hand, in one prospective study, 19% of patients who had clearly been told of a diagnosis of cancer repudiated the fact on subsequent interview.[79] On the other hand, the absence of a well-accepted, systematic, and reasoned strategy for discussing diagnosis and prognosis with patients is highlighted in a recent study by Lind and colleagues.[85] Of 55 patients interviewed retrospectively, over half of patients disclosed that they were alone when told they had cancer; 23% were told over the telephone, and 19% in the Recovery Room. This information was usually imparted by a surgeon; the primary care provider or oncologist first provided this information in only 11% and 8% of cases, respectively.

Since even palliative care experts are unable consistently to predict life expectancy with accuracy,[86,87] it is imprudent to answer questions of this type in overly exact terms. Depending on the consultant's relationship with the referring physician and on patient and family factors, the consultant may wish to either direct these questions back to the referring source, or, preferably, to respond truthfully and compassionately with general comments. These comments should be prefaced by a disclaimer that establishes medical science's inability to make such predictions accurately for a given individual. If indicated, the clinician could then suggest a range of survival, being careful to indicate possible exceptions, framing all explanations in a manner that erodes neither hope nor prayer.[2,30] Again, whereas discussion of these issues is often not indicated, in selected cases such dialogue establishes a basis for therapy that focuses on symptom control versus strategies intended to eradicate the tumor or prolong life. Specifically, the rationales for treatment with such measures as the administration of morphine or trials of invasive procedures are more readily understood in this context.

That the prognosis for cure of the underlying disease is often (but not always) dim is often well accepted, particularly in patients who are not newly diagnosed.[88] It is essential, however, that the prognosis for control of symptoms be clearly identified as an issue distinct from the outcome of disease, because, despite the fact that the prognosis for symptom control is often excellent,[89,90] patients typically harbor fears that their symptoms will progress without relief.[91] The likelihood of achieving control of symptoms should be communicated clearly, accurately, and, if warranted, enthusiastically, thus reassuring the patient and family. It should be emphasized that although symptoms usually can be managed, they are rarely eradicated, and that some trial and error and passage of time is usually required before a return to homeostasis is achieved.

Different styles of doctoring foster different approaches to outlining a treatment plan. Recognizing that patients are already suffering from loss of control,[92] our method and that of others[2] is to adopt an intentionally nonparental approach, consisting of outlining the potential relative benefits and risks of various therapeutic options. The simplest interventions that are most likely to yield beneficial effects without major alterations in routine or lifestyle are preferred, and more invasive approaches are outlined as alternatives. The discussion of treatment options is then concluded with a list of recommendations, thus satisfying patients who have a more passive style and who prefer to depend on the doctor to prescribe treatment more rigidly. Patients and family members should be encouraged to discuss these recommendations among themselves, and, if needed, with their other doctors. Depending on the urgency of the pain problem and the patient's inclinations, treatment may be initiated immediately or can be arranged for the near future. These practices further encourage the confidence of patients and reinforce their sense of autonomy. If treatment is prescribed, whenever possible it should be accompanied by a thorough explanation and the provision of teaching materials. Patients should be reassured that a complete dictated report will be promptly directed to the other clinicians who are involved in their care.

REASSESSMENT

Finally, the importance of frequent reassessment cannot be overemphasized. As has been stressed elsewhere in this text, cancer is a dynamic process that tends to be progressive and unpredictable. Whereas careful assessment establishes a foundation for a workable treatment plan, consistent follow-up is necessary to evaluate acute and chronic therapeutic responses and new or progressive problems.

Developing systems for providing follow-up care is challenging.[93,94] Among the distinguishing features of this patient population is that, at least over time, many patients become debilitated and disabled due to the presence of advanced symptomatic disease. Usually before the preterminal stage of illness there is a phase during which patients are able to make regular visits to the physician's office, in which case consistent and methodical outpatient care is provided. As illness progresses, these visits demand greater energy and resources from the patient and family, the doctor's office, and home care and transportation services. The potential negatives of an office visit begin to outweigh their potential benefit, particularly when the patient's condition has deteriorated but is stable.

Our medical training and standard models of care dictate that we provide care based on hands-on history and physical examination. In the setting of progressively debilitating disease, however, over time, the telephone becomes the conduit for much of our data acquisition and interventions. This is probably one of the most difficult adjustments a physician providing palliative care must make. In the best of all worlds, regular house calls would be common, but unfortunately they are not, although this trend may be reversing[95]; a recent survey of primary care physicians indicated that 53%–82% of clinicians engage in this practice.[96] Some of these difficulties can be reconciled by careful education and orientation of the family. They must be encouraged to keep accurate records, to be extremely observant, and to follow instructions; their access to the physician must be unimpeded by the demands of a busy practice. Fortunately, to bridge this gap, health care institutions have been developed to act as the physician's "eyes, ears, and hands" (*ie*, home care nursing, laboratory, and pharmacy services).[93,94] In order to be most effective, the physician must learn about the resources the community has to offer and make optimal use of them.

One of the most important community resources available to dying patients is hospice care (see Chapters 13 and 30).[35] To the uninitiated, hospice is often incorrectly regarded as a place where people go to die. Conceptually, hospice is probably best regarded as a philosophy of care; practically, it can be considered a context within which treatment occurs, indeed, almost as a treatment modality. The early part of hospice care's development occurred in the United Kingdom, where treatment was typically provided in an institutional setting resembling, in some ways, a hospital or nursing home. In the United States, hospice care has developed primarily as a home-based service, based partially on patients' preference to remain at home, but also on Medicare guidelines.[35] To be most effective, the physician providing palliative care must be familiar with the workings of local hospice care, and must help make it available and palatable to patients. Typically, a great deal of the doctor's education about what constitutes good home care may evolve from his or her contact with hospice.

SUMMARY

Assessment of the patient with symptomatic cancer is a complex, multifaceted, and challenging endeavor. As with management, assessment optimally includes input from not just the patient, but from their companions, other allied health care professionals, and community resources. Thorough and timely evaluations are conducted to preserve the patient's dignity and humanity, arrive at a definitive and broadly based set of diagnoses, and devise an individualized therapeutic program suitable to each patient's unique needs and goals. Frequent reassessment insures that comfort and quality of life, essential components of comprehensive cancer care, are optimized throughout the progress of the patient's disease.

REFERENCES

1. Buchanan J, Millership R, Zalcberg J et al: Medical education in palliative care. Med J Australia 1990; 152:27.
2. Twycross R: Palliative care: A compulsory issue. Adv Pain Res Ther 1990;13:297.
3. Copp LA, Anderson VC, Brown MJ et al: National Institutes of Health consensus panel: Integrated approach to the management of pain. Journal of Pain and Symptom Management 1987;2:35.
4. Sutton PM, Khan SM, Khan M: Cancer pain can be relieved. World Heath Forum 1990;11:210.
5. Romo JIR, Sanchez RP: Personal communication.
6. Portenoy R: Management of pain in patients with advanced cancer. Resident and Staff Physician 1987;33:59.
7. Lacroix JM: Low back pain factors of value in predicting outcomes. Spine 1990;15:495.
8. Cohrn RS, Ferrer-Brechner T, Pavlov A et al: Prospective evaluation of treatment outcome in patients referred to a cancer pain center. Adv Pain Res Ther 1985;9:655.
9. Tollison CD: Patient education influences pain recovery. Pain Management 1991;4:9.
10. Portenoy R: Practical aspects of pain control in patients with cancer. CA 1988;38:327.
11. Minton PJ: Evaluation and management of the patient with pain and metastatic cancer. In Lee JF (ed): Pain Management: Symposium on the Neurosurgical Treatment of Pain, p 166. Baltimore, Williams & Wilkins, 1976.
12. Benedetti C, Bonica JJ: Cancer pain: Basic considerations. In Benedetti C et al (eds): Advances in Pain Research and Therapy, vol 7, p 529. New York, Raven Press, 1984.
13. Saunders C: The philosophy of terminal care. In

Saunders C (ed): The Management of Terminal Malignant Disease, p 232. London, Edward Arnold, 1984.
14. Bonica JJ: Past and current status of pain research and therapy. Seminars in Anesthesia 1986;5:82.
15. Stjernsward J: Cancer pain relief: An important global public health issue. In Fields HL et al (eds): Advances in Pain Research and Therapy, vol 9, p 555. New York, Raven Press, 1985.
16. Stjernsward J, Teoh N: The scope of the cancer pain problem. In Foley KM, Bonica JJ, Ventafridda V (eds): Advances in Cancer Pain Research and Therapy, vol 16, p 7. New York, Raven Press, 1990.
17. Twycross RJ: Easing the pain of cancer. In Erdmann W, Oyama T, Pernack MJ (eds.): The Pain Clinic, vol 1, p 75. Amsterdam, VNU Science Press, 1986.
18. Wanzer SH, Federman DD, Adelstein SJ et al: The physician's responsibility toward hopelessly ill patients: A second look. N Engl J Med 1989;320:844.
19. Walsh TD: Symptom control in patients with advanced cancer. Am J Hospice Pall Care 1990;7:20.
20. Ventafridda V: Continuing care: A major issue in cancer pain management. Pain 1989;36:137.
21. Mor V: Cancer patients' quality of life over the disease course: Lessons from the real world. J Chronic Dis 1987;40:535.
21a. Ferrell BR: Quality of life as an outcome variable in management of cancer pain. Cancer 1987;63:2321.
22. Ahles TA, Blanchard EB, Ruckdeschel JC: Multidimensional nature of cancer pain. Pain 1983;17:277.
23. Derogatis LR, Morrow GR, Fetting J et al: The prevalence of psychiatric disorders among cancer patients. JAMA 1983;249:751.
24. Coyle N, Adelhardt J, Foley KM et al: Character of terminal illness in the advanced cancer patient: Pain and other symptoms in the last four weeks of life. Journal of Pain and Symptom Management 1990;5:83.
25. Maddocks I: The teaching of palliative care to medical students. Cancer Forum 1989;13:25.
26. Wodinsky HB: Palliative care in Canada: An overview. American Journal of Hospice Care 1989;6:44.
27. Odier C, Rapin CH, Carron JM et al: There is a palliative Europe to build. Journal of Palliative Care 1990;6:50.
28. Allbrook D: Who owns palliative care? Med J Australia 1990;152:170.
29. Twycross RG, Lack SA: Therapeutic in Terminal Cancer. Edinburgh, Churchill Livingstone, 1986.
30. Slaby AE: Cancer's impact on caregivers. Adv Psychosom Med 1988;18:135.
31. Carpenter PJ, Morrow GR: Clinical care of cancer patients: Close interpersonal encounters of the difficult kind. Journal of Psychosocial Oncology 1985;3:67.
32. Hall JE, Kirschling JM: A conceptual framework for caring for families of hospice patients. Hospice Journal 1990;6:1.
33. Kübler-Ross E: On Death and Dying. New York, MacMillan, 1970.
34. McDonald D: Nonadmissions: The other side of the hospice story. American Journal of Hospice Care 1989;6:17.
35. Rhymes J: Hospice care in America. JAMA 1990;264:369.
36. Weinstock E: Value of patient education in an outpatient cancer pain clinic. American Pain Society Abstracts, 1983.
37. Posner RB: Physician–patient communication. Am J Med 1984;77:59.
38. McCafferey M, Thorpe DM: Differences in perception of pain and the development of adversarial relationships among health care providers. In Hill CS, Fields WS (eds): Advances in Pain Research and Therapy, vol 11, p 113. New York, Raven Press, 1989.
39. Seelig MG: Should cancer victims be told the truth? J Miss State Med Assoc 1943;40:33.
40. Patt R: Personal communication.
41. Tammisto T: Intensive and terminal care: Unmanageable polarization or a fruitful combination of specialized anesthesiologic knowledge. Seminars in Anesthesia 1986;5:158.
42. Raj PP (ed): Practical Management of Pain, 1st ed. Chicago, Yearbook Medical Publishers, 1986.
43. Bonica JJ: Multidisciplinary/interdisciplinary pain programs. In Bonica JJ (ed): Management of Pain, 2nd ed, p 197. Philadelphia, Lea & Febiger, 1990.
44. Rowlingson JC, Toomey TC: Multidisciplinary approaches to the management of chronic pain. In Ghia JN (ed): The Multidisciplinary Pain Center, p 45. Boston, Kluwer Academic, 1988.
45. Gottlieb HJ: Multidisciplinary pain clinics, centers and programs. In Tollison CD, Kriegel ML (eds): Interdisciplinary Rehabilitation of Low Back Pain, p 259. Baltimore, Williams and Wilkins, 1989.
46. Lipton S: Pain relief. International Anesthesiology Clinics 1978;16:224.
47. Chapman CR, Casey KL, Dubner R et al: Pain measurement: An overview. Pain 1985;22:1.
48. Williams CR: Toward a set of reliable and valid measures for chronic pain assessment and outcome research. Pain 1988;35:239.
49. Ferrell B, Wisdom C, Wenzl C et al: Effects of controlled-release morphine on quality of life for cancer pain. Oncology Nursing Forum 1989;16:521.
50. Grossman SA, Sheidler VR, Swedeen K et al: Correlation of patient and caregiver ratings of cancer pain. Journal of Pain and Symptom Management 1991;6:53.
51. Van der Does AJW: Patients' and nurses' ratings of pain and anxiety during burn wound care. Pain 1989;39:95.

52. Choiniere M, Melzack R, Girard N et al: Comparisons between patients' and nurses' assessment of pain and medication efficacy in severe burn injuries. Pain 1990;40:143.

53. Peteet J, Tay V, Cohen G et al: Pain characteristics and treatment in an outpatient cancer population. Cancer 1986;57:1259.

54. O'Brien J, Francis A: The use of next-of-kin to estimate pain in cancer patients. Pain 1988;35:171.

55. Scott J, Huskisson EC: Graphic representation of pain. Pain 1976;2:175.

56. Wallenstein S: Measurement of pain and analgesia in cancer patients. Cancer 1984:53 (Suppl 10):2260.

57. Ahles AT, Ruckdeschel JC, Blanchard EB: Cancer-related pain: II. Assessment with visual analogue scales. J Psychosom Res 1984;28:121.

58. Miser AW: Assessment and treatment of children with pain. Anesthesia Progress 1987;34:116-118.

59. Banos JE, Bosch F, Canellas M et al: Acceptability of visual analogue scales in the clinical setting: A comparison with verbal rating scales in postoperative pain. Methods Find Exp Clin Pharmacol 1989;11:123.

60. Melzack R: The McGill pain questionnaire: Major properties and scoring methods. Pain 1975;1:357.

61. Melzack R, Torgerson WS: On the language of pain. Anesthesiology 1971;34:50.

62. Graham C, Bond SS, Gerkovich MM, et al: Use of the McGill pain questionnaire in the assessment of cancer pain: Replicability and consistency. Pain 1980;8:377.

63. Kremer EF, Atkinson JH, Ignelzi RJ: Pain measurement: Affective dimensional measure of the McGill pain questionnaire with a cancer pain population. Pain 1982;12:153.

64. Houts PS, Yasko JM, Kahn SB et al: Unmet psychological, social and economic needs of persons with cancer in Pennsylvania. Cancer 1986;58:2355.

65. Daut RL, Cleeland CS, Flanery RC: Development of the Wisconsin brief pain questionnaire to assess pain in cancer and other diseases. Pain 1983;17:197.

66. Cleeland CS: Assessment of pain in cancer. In Foley KM, Bonica JJ, Ventafridda V (eds): Advances in Pain Research and Therapy, vol 16, p 47. New York, Raven Press, 1990.

67. Fishman B, Pasternak S, Wallenstein S et al: The Memorial pain assessment card: A valid instrument for the evaluation of cancer pain. Cancer 1987;60:1151.

68. Bruera E, MacMillan K, Hanson J et al: The Edmonton staging system for cancer pain: Preliminary report. Pain 1989;37:203.

69. American Joint Committee for Cancer Staging and End Result Reporting: Manual for Staging of Cancer. Chicago, American Joint Committee, 1977.

70. Lipton S: Assessment of the patient with chronic pain. In Swerdlow M, Charlton JE (eds): Relief of Intractable Pain, 4th ed, p 79. Amsterdam, Elsevier, 1989.

71. Longmire D: The medical pain history. Pain Digest, 1991;1:28.

72. Twycross RG: Incidence of pain. Clin Oncol 1984; 3:5.

73. Twycross RG: Relief of pain. In Saunders CM (ed): The Management of Terminal Disease, p 65. Chicago, Yearbook Publishers, 1978.

74. Longmire D: The physical examination: Methods and application in the clinical evaluation of pain. Pain Digest, 1991;1:136.

75. Raj PP: Neurologic examination. In Raj PP (ed): Practical Management of Pain, 1st ed, p 78. Chicago, Yearbook Medical Publishers, 1986.

76. Gonzales GR, Elliott KJ, Portenoy RK, Foley KM: The impact of a comprehensive evaluation in the management of cancer pain. Pain 1991;47:141.

77. Rudy TE, Turk DC, Brena SF et al: Quantification of biomedical findings of chronic pain patients: Development of an index of pathology. Pain 1990;42:167.

78. Kelly WD, Freisen SR: Do cancer patients want to be told? Surgery 1950;27:822.

79. Aitken-Swan J, Easson EC: Reactions of cancer patients on being told their diagnosis. Br Med J 1959;1:779.

80. Gilbertsen VA, Wangensteen OH: Should the doctor tell the patient their disease is cancer? CA 1962;12:82.

81. Gilhooly MLM, Berkely JS, McCann K et al: Truth telling with dying cancer patients. Palliative Medicine 1988;2:64.

82. Bedell SE, Pelle D, Maher PL et al: Do-not-resuscitate orders for critically ill patients in the hospital: How are they used and what is their impact? JAMA 1986;256:233.

83. Wool MS: Understanding denial in cancer patients. Adv Psychosom Med 1988;18:37.

84. Davidson P: Facilitating coping with cancer pain. Palliative Medicine 1988;2:107.

85. Lind SE, Good DM, Seidel S et al: Telling the diagnosis of cancer. J Clin Oncol 1989;7:583.

86. Forster LE, Lynn J: Predicting life span for applicants to inpatient hospice. Arch Intern Med 1988;148:2540.

87. Enck RE: Prognostication of survival in hospice care. American Journal of Hospice and Palliative Care 1990;7:11.

88. Hinton J: Comparison of places and policies for terminal care. Lancet 1979;1:29.

89. Takeda F: Preliminary report from Japan on results of field testing of WHO draft interim guidelines for relief of cancer pain. Pain Clinics 1986;1:83.

90. Haram J: Facts and figures. In Saunders CM (ed):

The Management of Terminal Disease, p 12. London, Edward Arnold, 1978.

91. Angell M: The quality of mercy. N Engl J Med 1982;306:98.
92. Garland TN, Bass DM, Otto ME: The needs of hospice patients and primary caregivers: A comparison of primary caregivers' and hospice nurses' perceptions. American Journal of Hospice Care 1984;summer:40.
93. Vinciguerra V, Degnan TJ, Sciortino A et al: A comparative assessment of home versus hospital comprehensive treatment for advanced cancer patients. J Clin Oncol 1986;4:1521.
94. Council on Scientific Affairs: Home care in the 1990's. JAMA 1990;263:1241.
95. Cauthen DB: The house call in current medical practice. J Fam Pract 1981;13:209.
96. Siwek J: House calls: Current status and rationale. Am Fam Physician 1985;31:169.

Chapter 3

Pain Syndromes Due to Cancer Treatment

John A. Campa III

Richard Payne

INTRODUCTION

Pain is a common symptom in the patient with cancer. Estimates from the World Health Organization (WHO) suggest that 20%–50% of cancer patients will present with pain; 33% will have pain during treatment of their disease, and up to 75%–90% of patients with advanced cancer and terminal disease have pain[1]. Although the vast majority (about 70%) of patients with cancer will have pain directly related to neoplastic invasion into pain-sensitive bone and soft-tissue structures, as many as 20% of adults will have pain caused directly by *cancer therapy* (Table 3–1). This percentage is probably higher in the pediatric cancer population (see Chapters 4 and 28), especially given the frequency with which painful diagnostic procedures (*eg*, bone marrow biopsy, lumbar puncture, and venipuncture) are required for the evaluation and treatment of leukemia and central nervous system (CNS) neoplasms in this age group.[2]

This chapter reviews the most common pain syndromes related to cancer treatment (Table 3–1), and outlines approaches to evaluation and management. Treatment-related pain problems are important for several reasons: their appearance may be confused with more ominous pain syndromes associated with tumor recurrence or progression that may directly lead to death of the patient; when severe, compliance with recommendations for further therapy may be adversely affected; the incidence and prevalence of these syndromes appear to be increasing

Table 3–1.
Causes of Treatment-Related Pain

Chemotherapy-Related Pain

Oral mucositis
Peripheral neuropathy
Acute and chronic herpetic pain
Osteonecrosis secondary to steroids
Pseudorheumatism

Radiation-Related Pain

Osteoradionecrosis
Myelopathy
Brachial plexopathy
Lumbar plexopathy
Radiation-induced peripheral nerve tumors

Postsurgical Pain

Postmastectomy
Post-nephrectomy
Post-thoracotomy
Post radical neck dissection
Stump and phantom limb

Procedure-Related Pain

Bone marrow biopsy
Bone biopsy
Lumbar puncture and spinal headache
Venipuncture

in frequency; and, finally, they often pose particularly difficult management problems.

CHEMOTHERAPY-RELATED PAIN SYNDROMES

ORAL MUCOSITIS PAIN

This common complication of chemotherapy is usually seen within 1 to 2 weeks of the initiation of treatment, and is most common with the use of methotrexate, doxorubicin, daunorubicin, bleomycin, etoposide, 5-fluorouracil (5-FU), and dactinomycin.[3] Mucositis may be more severe when these agents are used in combination with radiotherapy, especially for bone marrow transplantation.[4] Inflammatory lesions (Fig. 3–1) typically peak in 2 to 3 weeks, and swallowing is usually impaired because of pain. Initially patients

may complain of increased sensitivity to solid or spicy foods. The lesions progress from erythema to ulcer formation and ultimately sloughing of tissue, phenomena that occur not only in the oral mucosa but also in the mucosa of the pharynx, esophagus, and anorectal region. Secondary hemorrhage and perforation may occur.

The diagnosis is almost always obvious, although occasionally these lesions may become superinfected by yeast or viral organisms, particularly *Candida albicans* and herpes virsus, respectively.

Treatment focuses on several issues. Adjustment of the diet is necessary to avoid foods that irritate the oral mucosa. In severe cases, parenteral nutrition may be required temporarily. Oral mouthwashes and rinses are the mainstay of therapy, and include chlorhexidine, diphenhydramine elixir, kaopectate, and viscous xylocaine.

Severe oral mucositis pain after bone marrow transplantation has been used as a model to evaluate the safety and efficacy of patient-controlled analgesia (PCA) drug delivery systems in cancer patients. In general, these studies have demonstrated that patients do not overuse morphine, and that the addiction liability of opioids is quite low in this setting.

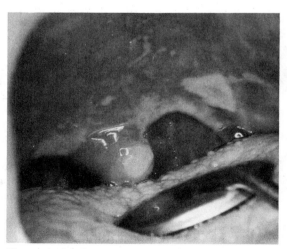

Figure 3–1. Painful oral mucositis in a cancer patient. Tongue is depressed with dental mirror to demonstrate lesions distributed over uvula and soft palate.

In fact, as is the case in postoperative pain management, patients generally use less morphine when it is administered by PCA as opposed to nurse or doctor-controlled intermittent intramuscular (IM) or intravenous (IV) administration.[5]

PAINFUL POLYNEUROPATHY

Vincristine and *cis*-platinum may produce sensory and motor neuropathy as a result of dose-related toxicity to the pons. This toxicity may be related to interference with fast axonal transport in peripheral nerves.[6,7]

Jaw pain or claudication may occur after a single large dose of vincristine. Dose reductions will usually eliminate the pain. Paresthesias are also common, and have been reported in 46%–57% of patients. Severe dysesthetic burning pain in the hands and feet, often accompanied by allodynia, is relatively common.

Cis-platinum neuropathy is mostly a sensory phenomenon, with little motor involvement.[8] Electrophysiologically, it is characterized by an absence of sensory nerve action potentials (SNAPS), normal motor nerve conduction velocity and compound muscle action potentials (CMAPS), and normal needle electromyography (EMG). The pathologic correlates include areas of demyelination and myelin degeneration seen in longitudinal sections at sural nerve biopsy.

In contrast, with vincristine neuropathy, motor involvement as well as sensory loss are prominent. Motor effects are remarkable in that there is a distinct predilection for the extensor muscles of the wrists and fingers in the upper extremity, and the presentation is usually as weakness in the distal muscle groups of the leg. Lower extremity weakness may be sufficiently severe to preclude the patient from walking or even standing without assistance, although this is rare. Findings on EMG studies are consistent with denervation; fibrillation and a reduced number of motor unit potentials in distal muscles, along with reduction in amplitude of SNAPS are observed. Sural nerve biopsy may demonstrate axonal degeneration. Clinically, vincristine neuropathy may be classified as an axonopathy.

Symptomatic management with adjuvant analgesics such as tricyclic antidepressants or anticonvulsants is usually of benefit, and improvement in the discomfort may be anticipated with the termination of treatment or a reduction in dosage. The roles of other recently investigated treatments for neuropathy such as topical capsaicin, oral mexilitine, and transdermal and oral clonidine, are unknown. However, these agents may be tried if pain is severe and more conventional treatments such as tricyclics and transcutaneous electrical nerve stimulation (TENS) have failed.

The diagnosis of chemotherapy-induced neuropathy is usually obvious, given the temporal relationship between the onset of symptoms and initiation of chemotherapy, and the usual reversal of symptoms when the specific offending drug is discontinued. However, in refractory or atypical cases, other causes of neuropathy should be considered, including diabetic neuropathy, tumor infiltration of peripheral nerves (especially in leukemia),[9] and tumors of peripheral nerves, especially in genetically susceptible individuals (*ie*, neurofibromatosis) who have been exposed to radiation[10] (see "Radiation Therapy," below).

STEROID-RELATED PAIN SYNDROMES

Corticosteroids are important components of cancer treatment, especially in leukemia and lymphoma chemotherapy regimens, as well as some chronic pain problems (see Chapters 10 and 13). In addition, they are essential for the management of neoplastic spinal cord compression and intracranial hypertension associated with brain tumor edema (see Chapters 1 and 29). In these settings it is often necessary for patients to take relatively high doses of corticosteroids for many weeks or months, and painful sequelae may ensue. These painful complications can occur by three mechanisms: 1) aseptic necrosis of the humeral and femoral joints[11]; 2) osteopenia and bone pain secondary to pathologic fractures; and 3) a "pseudorheumatoid" syndrome associated with rapid steroid withdrawal.

Aseptic necrosis of the femoral or humeral head (see Chapter 25) may occur after continuous or intermittent steroid therapy, and osteoporosis may appear in as few as 6 weeks after the initiation of therapy. Prednisone-related osteonecrosis may occur (rarely) with as little as 10 mg/day administered over many months. Symptoms are usually bilateral, but may occur unilaterally. This entity may present initially as pain over the knee, shoulder, or leg, exacerbated with motion and relieved with rest. This same pain characteristically predates radiologic changes by weeks to months. Bone scan and (especially) magnetic resonance imaging (MRI) scanning are the diagnostic imaging modalities of choice. Treatment involves the reduction, or, if possible, discontinuation of steroids, and, when needed, the use of nonsteroidal anti-inflammatory analgesics and opioid analgesics. Occasionally joint replacement is indicated if the underlying cancer is in remission.

"Rheumatic" complaints, including myalgias, arthralgias, tender muscles, and joint aches and pains may occur during the process of tapering and/or reduction in steroid doses ("pseudorheumatism"). Reinstitution of the steroid at a higher dose and then withdrawal over a more protracted period of time usually results in improvement.[12]

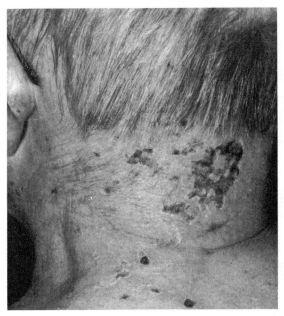

Figure 3–2. Painful, healing acute herpes zoster lesions distributed over the C3 dermatome; resolved with subcutaneous injection of local anesthetic and steroid mixture.

ZOSTER-RELATED PAIN SYNDROMES

Painful neuralgia may precede, follow, or occur concurrently with herpetic infection (Fig. 3–2).[13–15] Pain persisting 1 month or longer after healing of the rash occurs in 9%–14% of patients. Both sexes are affected equally. An anatomic predilection for the V1-ophthalmic division of the trigeminal nerve and the midthoracic dermatomes is characteristic. In cancer patients the infection commonly occurs over the site of tumor or at a previous radiation therapy port. Pain is burning, severe, localized over the area of sensory loss, and usually resolves with the disappearance of the rash.

Postherpetic neuralgia (PHN) is arbitrarily defined as pain persisting for more than 2 months after the disappearance of the rash. This problem is more common in patients past the age of 50 years, and may be associated with profound functional, personality, and mood effects comparable to those associated with other chronic pain syndromes. Many treatments have been proposed, but few have been tested in carefully controlled clinical trials. Recently, Rowbotham et al[16] reported a controlled trial that demonstrated the efficacy of codeine in PHN. This study is important because it is one of the few controlled trials that has demonstrated the efficacy of opioids in neuropathic pain. Controlled trials have also demonstrated that treatment with amitriptyline or desipramine, and carbamazepine are helpful for the burning and lancinating components of the pain (see Chapter 10). In a study of 33 patients with PHN, Watson et al concluded that topical capsaicin (0.025% concentration) may have a role in the management of PHN.[15] Capsaicin depletes substance P from afferent C-fibers. These fibers are thought to be important in mediating the burning pain associated with PHN, as substance P is thought to act as an algesic neurotransmitter agent at the central synapse of these fibers in the dorsal horn of the spinal cord. Watson et al found that 56% of the 23 patients completing the study had good or excellent pain relief after 4 weeks. Improvement in pain was reported by 78% of patients. Although this study demonstrates a potential role for the use of topical capsaicin in PHN, controlled clinical trials that would demonstrate true efficacy are still lacking. It is an attractive option for elderly patients, because one could potentially avoid the central nervous system side effects of systemically administered drugs such as the tricyclics and opioids. However, local burning on application of capsaicin, perhaps due to release of substance P, may be sufficiently severe to cause patients to discontinue treatment before a thorough trial has been completed.

Recent work by Rowbotham et al suggests that infrared thermography may be useful in identifying areas of pain and allodynia potentially responsive to local anesthetic infiltration.[17] Thermographic patterns of increased temperature were observed to correlate well with skin areas of maximal pain and allodynia. Curiously, sensory loss was minimal in thermographically determined "hot" regions, and was observed to be moderate to profound in the "cool" sites.

The pathology of herpes zoster infection is characterized by acute inflammation, necrosis, and hemorrhage in the dorsal root ganglia (DRG), with a mononeuritis extending out peripherally; both myelin and axonal degeneration ensue.[6] The pathophysiologic mechanisms underlying the pain of PHN are poorly understood; both central and peripheral mechanisms have been proposed as factors that contribute to pain. Ischemia and ultimate loss of large nerve fibers have been described

after herpes zoster infection. It has been suggested that a subsequent deficit in the pain-modulating effect of the large-fiber inhibitory system might permit increased nociceptive traffic through the dorsal horn of the spinal cord via small-diameter afferents. It has also been proposed that regeneration or damage to nociceptive afferents may contribute to painful dysesthesia.

Watson et al described findings in a single case studied at postmortem that support the above hypothesis.[18] They reported findings on a patient who had experienced severe pain in the right thoracic (T7–8) dermatomes during the final 5 years of his life, in whom the dorsal horn of the thoracic spinal cord of the affected side was atrophic from T4 to T8 at autopsy. Associated loss of both myelin and axons was noted, with fibrosis, cell loss, and nerve root involvement restricted to the T8 ganglion. Markers for unmyelinated afferents, substantia gelatinosa neurons, glial cells, and descending spinal projections were unchanged when the affected and nonaffected sides were compared, suggesting that unbridled unmyelinated nociceptive input may be a significant operative pain mechanism in PHN, as outlined above.

PAIN SYNDROMES ASSOCIATED WITH RADIATION THERAPY

Radiation-induced tissue changes may produce acute and chronic pain emanating from a variety of sources, including fibrosis, soft tissue ischemia, necrosis, and inflammation (see Chapter 15). Fibrosis may cause compression of contiguous neural tissue, leading to painful peripheral nerve dysfunction (eg, radiation-induced brachial plexopathy). Acute and chronic skin changes (Figs. 3–3, 3–4) may be associated with pain and impaired mobility, and are discussed in Chapter 15. Finally, radiation may directly injure large peripheral nerve plexus and spinal cord elements, or induce neurogenic tumors such as fibrosarcoma.

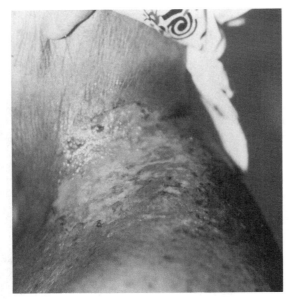

Figure 3–3. Acute skin injury after radiotherapy of a cervical epidural lesion in a patient with metastatic breast cancer. Initially painful, symptoms subsided as healing occurred over a 2-week period.

ORAL COMPLICATIONS OF RADIATION THERAPY

Oral complications of radiation therapy include mucositis, xerostomia, hypogeusia, dysphagia, infection, caries, trismus, and osteoradionecrosis. Mucositis has been discussed (see section on "Chemotherapy-Related Pain Syndromes"). The causes of oral complications of radiation therapy are multifactorial, and include the dose and type of radiation, its means of administration, the extent and type of disease, the age of the patient, concomitant surgery, and the pretreatment dental status. The incidence and severity of many of these problems can be reduced by pretreatment dental consultation and maintenance of careful oral hygiene, including fluoride prophylaxis.

TRISMUS

Trismus is most often related to radiation to the muscles of mastication and the temporo-mandibular joint, with resultant cell destruction and fibrosis. The onset of trismus is usually gradual and unpredictable, but it is most common when radiation is combined with surgery. Management consists of exercise performed during and after radiation treatment.[19,20]

OSTEORADIONECROSIS

Osteoradionecrosis is among the most serious and least readily reversible oral complications resulting from radiation therapy. The underlying pathophysiology involves loss of osteocytes; progressive, obliterative endarteritis; and hyalinization of blood vessels within the treatment field. The resultant hypoxic, hypocellular, and hypovascular tissue loses the ability to self-renew after injury (excessive precursor demand vis-a-vis supply). The mildest form (osteoradioatrophy) is asymptomatic, and is associated with only minimal radiographic changes. In cases of more severe injury (Fig. 3–5A,B) bone is devitalized, predisposed to infection, and healing is impaired. Septic osteoradionecrosis may be associated with pathologic fracture, necrosis, fistula formation with drainage, a fetid odor, and severe pain. Pain limits jaw mobility, and is exacerbated by talking and eating, predisposing to the insidious development of malnutrition.

Current estimates of the incidence of osteoradionecrosis (ORN) vary widely, with an average incidence reported at around 18% before 1971 and about 10% after 1971.[21–24] Factors implicated in the frequency of ORN are multiple and include the proximity of tumor to mandible, the quality and dose of radiation administered to the mandible, volume of mandible included in the field, external beam irradiation combined with interstitial brachytherapy, radiation combined with surgery, the patient's age, pre-radiation and postradiation dental care and hygiene, and the presence of dental prostheses. Most authorities agree that the replacement of orthovoltage (200–400 kV) by supervoltage and cobalt-60 radiation, with consequent reduction in dosage to bone and its blood supply, has de-

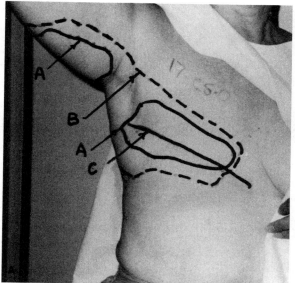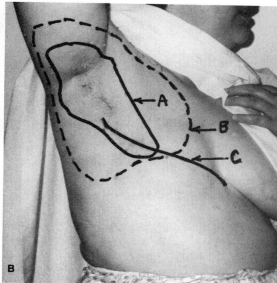

Figure 3–4.   A,B, These figures depict characteristic findings in two patients with postmastectomy pain syndrome. The solid line marked "A" represents the boundaries of sensory loss to pinprick, cold, and touch. The broken line marked "B" corresponds to the boundaries of allodynia, and the solid line marked "C" outlines the mastectomy scar. In both cases, pain and sensory changes correspond to the peripheral distribution of the intercostobrachial nerve. (Courtesy C. Peter N. Watson, MD, Smythe Pain Clinic, Toronto General Hospital.)

creased the frequency of ORN.[25] Doses greater than 4500 cGy and large doses per fraction have been implicated in increased risk for the development of ORN.[20] Osteoradionecrosis is more common in patients over the age of 50 years,[26] and in the presence of poor dental hygiene. The presence and early use of dental prostheses predisposes to ORN because of increased trauma. Access of organisms into irradiated tissue has been observed to be the single most consistent factor associated with ORN.[27,28]

Osteoradionecrosis is much more likely to occur in the mandible than maxilla, probably because the mandible depends on a single source of arterial blood, the inferior alveolar artery.[19–21,29] The onset of disease is most often within 6 months of treatment, but cases have been reported up to 25 years after therapy.[20,30] Post-radiation extractions should be performed only under the most extreme circumstances when all conservative measures have failed.

Prevention of Osteoradionecrosis

Prevention of ORN is facilitated by maintenance of good oral hygiene before, during, and after radiation treatment. A complete oral and dental evaluation with radiographs should be performed before treatment. Current recommendations include removal of decayed and impacted teeth with primary closure of incision sites. When periodontal disease is present, involved teeth should also be extracted. Antibiotics should be prescribed, and a minimum of 2 weeks should be permitted for healing before the initiation of radiation treatment.[20,24,27,31] Prophylaxis with daily, topical fluoride treatments, and the use of preradiation anti-inflammatory agents and topical anesthetics in combination with various irrigating solutions appear to be beneficial. Essential for prevention is a change in lifestyle, with the cessation of alcohol and tobacco use.[20,22,23]

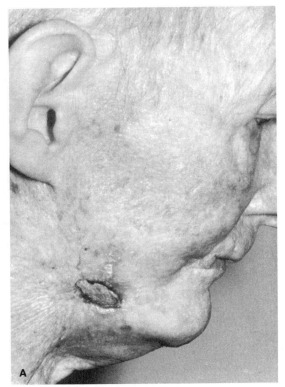

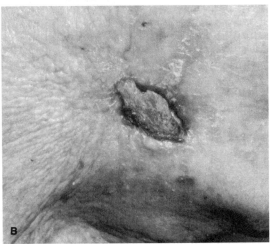

Figure 3–5. **A,** Painful osteoradionecrosis of mandible following curative radiotherapy for adenocarcinoma of a salivary gland in a 72-year-old-man; resistant to conservative management, pain was ultimately controlled with a series of alcohol injections of the mandibular nerve. **B,** Close-up view of necrotic, fractured bone.

Treatment of Osteoradionecrosis

Most aspects of conservative management for mild cases of ORN are identical to measures aimed at prevention: proper dental hygiene, oral rinses with antibiotics and fluoride, and systemic antibiotics. In addition, limited procedures intended to remove bone spicules while minimizing soft tissue trauma, with sequestrectomy and debridement, appear to be beneficial.[19,20,24]

Indications for more extensive surgery or the use of hyperbaric oxygen include intractable pain, trismus, deformity, fistula development, and nonhealing fractures persisting for more than 12 months.[24,32]

Hyperbaric Oxygen. The use of hyperbaric oxygen therapy in the management of ORN is based on the premise that injury is related to hypovascularity and tissue hypoxia. Healing depends on promoting neovascularization to supply the advancement of new tissue into necrotic spaces. Increasing oxygen concentration stimulates neovascularization, and also enhances the antibacterial activity of specialized leukocytes, increasing resistance to infection. Capillary budding, fibroblastic proliferation, collagen formation, and increased leukocyte microbial killing capacity have been observed when PO_2 is increased above 20 mm Hg in previously hypoxic areas.[33–36] This mechanism is supported by research demonstrating minimal effects on healing when hyperbaric oxygen is applied in the presence of adequate local circulation.[36]

Treatment is generally initiated at 3 to 36 months postirradiation, and usually consists of daily sessions of 1.5–2 hours' duration. Depending on clinical progress, 40 to 120 sessions are often administered, distributed over a 2- to 8-month time period. Treatment is with pressures averaging between 2-2.4 atmospheres. In wound areas with O_2 tensions of 5 to 15 mm Hg, treatment with 2.4 atmospheres has been observed to raise local oxygen tension to approximately 150 mm Hg.[35] Pain relief sometimes occurs after just 20 treatments. Treatment remains controversial because results are not consistently reproducible.

Therapy is contraindicated in patients with seizures, severe emphysema, asthma, and concurrent abuse of alcohol.[22,33,34] Potential complications of hyperbaric oxygen include pulmonary and cerebral oxygen toxicity, air embolism, decompression sickness, pneumothorax, and transient myopia.[32]

Surgery. In addition to its role as an initial intervention for oral cancer, surgery is often performed for the treatment of mild but persistent sequelae of ORN. Also, it is considered a definitive approach to eliminate the pain and deformity associated with more advanced ORN. Surgical options vary considerably, from simple sequestrectomy to hemimandibulectomy. Most techniques emphasize intraoral resection,[37] aiming to remove necrotic tissue and improve vascularity. Current emphasis includes the use of microvascular techniques and reconstruction with free osteocutaneous flaps.[23,27,37,38] The combination of hyperbaric oxygen and surgery appears to be beneficial for severe cases of established ORN.[35,37,39]

Nerve Blocks. A single case of ORN of the mandible treated with serial alcohol injections of the third division of the fifth cranial nerve, supplemented with phenol injections of the C2 root, has been reported.[40] This was a case of a patient who refused surgery due to fear of further disfigurement (see Fig. 5A,B). Nerve blocks resulted in improved speech, nutrition, and mood, but effects with each intervention tended to last only about 6 months. Serial treatment resulted in good symptom control until extrusion of necrotic bone and spontaneous healing were complete 3 years after treatment was initiated.

DELAYED RADIATION MYELOPATHY

This is an uncommon complication of radiation therapy delivered to the spine for palliation of bony or epidural metastasis, or to ports that overlap the spine, such as occurs with mediastinal radiation therapy for esophageal cancer and lymphoma. The differential diagnosis of suspected radiation-induced myelopathy includes epidural or intramedullary tumors, conditions that can almost always be excluded by MRI or myelogram-computed tomography (CT) imaging.

Four types of radiation myelopathy have been described.[41] The first type is an acute transient form, that usually presents 4–5 weeks after the administration of a range of radiation around 4,800 rads. Patients characteristically complain of numbness or paresthesias radiating from the neck to the spine and legs, and L'hermitte's sign (sudden electric-like shocks extending along the spine due to cervical flexion) is often present. Usually focal radicular or funicular motor or sensory loss cannot be demonstrated. Pathologic studies in animals reveal degeneration of paranodal myelin, and nodal widening.

The second type is rare and consists of a lower motor neuron syndrome that appears after a latency of 3–26 months and is manifest as diffuse lower extremity weakness.[41] Muscle atrophy, weakness, decreased deep tendon reflexes, and fasciculations appear as the process progresses. The cause of such selective anterior horn cell injury is unclear.

The third and rarest type (if it exists at all) is an acute and progressive form of radiation myelopathy that presents with the sudden appearance of acute paraplegia or quadriplegia, occurring within days of treatment.[41] The purported mechanism is acute arterial occlusion. Angiography demonstrated occlusion of the radiculomedullary and anterior spinal arteries in one patient after radiation-induced myelomalacia.[41]

Finally, the most common presentation of radiation-related myelopathy is a chronic progressive form. Although usually occurring in the first year after treatment, it may present from 4 months to 13 years after treatment. Symptoms are usually prominent in the lower extremities, and include numbness, burning paresthesias, and decreased sensation to pain and temperature.[41] Sphincter involvement is relatively common. Although motor weakness usually is not seen early in the clinical course, weakness and spasticity ultimately may supervene, and sensory levels may ascend as well as cross over. A Brown-Sequard syndrome may develop, that is, the patient may present with weakness and corticospinal tract signs (spasticity) in one extremity, and with pain and temperature deficits in the other. The syndrome is usually progressive, and the prognosis is grim.[41]

RADIATION-INDUCED BRACHIAL PLEXOPATHY

Brachial plexopathy (see Chapter 1) may be due to several different mechanisms. The most common etiologies in the patient with cancer are infiltration by tumor and radiation injury, but stretch injuries occurring during surgery, the development of a new primary tumor that infiltrates the plexus, and radiation-induced neurogenic tumors of the plexus have also been described.[42]

Radiation-associated syndromes may occur after treatment to the upper chest and mediastinum, such as is required for the primary therapy for lymphoma, and for adjuvant treatment of lung and breast cancer. In these clinical settings it is important to distinguish radiation-induced plexopathy from that produced by tumor infiltration of the plexus. This can often be achieved using clinical and radiographic criteria, although, rarely, exploration and biopsy of the brachial plexus region is required to establish a definitive diagnosis. A pattern of neurologic signs and symptoms referable to the upper plexus (C5–6) is common in radiation injury. It has been speculated that this distribution occurs because the lower trunk is partially shielded from radiation by the clavicle.[43] By contrast, the appearance of root signs and symptoms in the C8–T1 distribution, particularly when associated with a Horner's syndrome, strongly suggests involvement of the lower trunk of the plexus by tumor.

A typical presentation of radiation-induced plexopathy is numbness and paresthesias in the thumb and first finger of the hand, with concomitant weakness in the deltoid and biceps muscle groups and a diminished or absent biceps reflex, sometimes accompanied by edema. This constellation of signs is consistent with involvement of the C5–6 roots or upper trunk of the brachial plexus. In contrast, the typical presentation of tumor-associated plexopathy is the appearance of numbness and paresthesias in the fourth and fifth digits of the hand, and weakness in the triceps and intrinsic muscles of the hand, in association with an absent or diminished triceps reflex. This constellation of symptoms and signs denotes involvement of the C8–T1 nerve roots or lower trunk of the brachial plexus. Ptosis and miosis of the ipsilateral pupil (Horner's sign) is often present with metastatic plexopathy, because the tumor often invades the paraspinal ganglion as it grows in a medial direction. As such, the epidural space is usually also invaded (even in the absence of demonstrable vertebral body metastasis), and MRI or CT-myelographic imaging of the spinal cord is indicated in such cases.

Cervical spondylosis should be considered in the differential diagnosis, although the pattern of motor and sensory loss determined by a careful neurologic examination, EMG, and neuroradiologic imaging can usually distinguish cervical radiculopathy from brachial plexopathy. For example, weakness of *all* intrinsic muscles in the hand, including the opponens pollicis, denotes that not only are the C8–T1 nerve roots involved, but that there is involvement of the lower trunk of the brachial plexus as well (panplexopathy). It should be noted that the opponens pollicus muscle is innervated by the median nerve, whereas most of the other intrinsic muscles of the hand are subserved by the ulnar nerve. Both the median and ulnar nerves originate in the lower trunk of the plexus. Furthermore, electromyographic examination should demonstrate an absence of paraspinal fibrillations in brachial plexopathy, which, however, should be present in cervical polyradiculopathy.

In summary, several clinical findings help to distinguish plexopathy that is a result of radiation therapy from metastatic plexopathy. In the former, CT and/or MRI will usually not demonstrate a mass.[44] Radiation plexopathy is usually delayed in its appearance for up to 6 months (or as long as 20 years). Kori et al conclude that if the radiation therapy dose is less than 6,000 R, then radiation damage to the brachial plexus is unlikely, but if the dose is greater than 6,000 R and neurologic symptoms appear within a year, then radiation injury is the likely diagnosis.[43] Should the symptoms appear after 1 year, then the diagnosis may be either recurrent tumor or radiation injury.[42]

RADIATION-INDUCED LUMBOSACRAL PLEXOPATHY

This entity is less common than brachial plexopathy, a phenomenon with several possible explanations. Pelvic tumors for which radiation is indicated are generally associated with a poorer prognosis than breast cancer and lymphoma, likely tumors to affect the brachial plexus, and as a result many patients will not live sufficiently long to develop clinically significant radiation changes. Second, the lumbosacral plexus is embedded in the substance of the psoas muscle for much of its anatomic distribution, which, together with the bulk of the adjacent vertebral column, may partially shield it from direct radiation injury, although this factor is less likely to be operative with the use of current high energy techniques. Finally, doses below "nerve tolerance" are usually administered in this region out of respect for the vulnerability of adjacent bowel to injury.

The presenting symptoms of lumbosacral plexopathy (see Chapter 1) usually involve the appearance of an aching and pressure-like pain in the proximal lower limb (especially the quadriceps region in upper plexus involvement) or the perineum (in lower plexus involvement). The diagnosis of a postradiation syndrome is supported by prominent radiation changes involving the skin, lymphedema, and radiologic findings suggestive of radiation necrosis of the hip, pelvis, or sacrum. Pain is progressive, as is the development of lower extremity motor and sensory deficits, usually leading ultimately to monoparesis or paraplegia. When considering a diagnosis of radiation-induced lumbosacral plexopathy, every effort must be exerted to exclude a neoplastic etiology. In the former, as with brachial plexopathy, EMG studies typically reveal myokymic discharges (recurrent trains of motor unit potentials), findings that have not been reported with neoplastic plexopathy.[45] Since paraspinal fibrillation potentials are present in 50% of patients at EMG, a more appropriate designation of this entity would be "radiation lumbosacral radiculoplexopathy."

The differential diagnosis of lumbosacral plexopathy in the cancer patient includes inflammatory plexopathy, epidural spinal cord compression (especially cauda equina compression), and polyneuropathy of the lower extremities. Retroperitoneal and iliopsoas hemorrhage usually produce sudden onset of pain, with rapid progression to weakness in the lower extremities and associated flank, thigh, and lumbar paraspinal ecchymoses. Other causes of lumbosacral plexopathy to be considered that are usually suggested by the history include abdominal aortic aneurysm, diabetic plexopathy and "amyotrophy," and sciatic neuropathy caused by intragluteal injections. Painful inflammatory lumbosacral plexopathy was described by Bradley et al.[46] It is associated with an elevated sedimentation rate (range 56–123 mm/hr), and represents a treatable inflammatory syndrome that is not associated with vasculitis or neoplasia.

Jaeckle et al investigated the natural history of lumbosacral plexopathy in 85 patients with documented pelvic tumor.[47] Some useful generalizations are summarized below. The majority of patients (51%) presented as a lower (L4–S1) plexus process; 31% presented as an upper (L1–L4) plexus process, and 18% presented as a panplexopathy (L1–S3). In 70% of patients, pain occurred in the form of pelvic or radicular leg pain, and was the presenting complaint, followed by sensory symptoms and weakness weeks to months later. Weakness in a pattern that involved more than one nerve root was the most consistent clinical finding. Sensory loss and reflex asymmetry were present in the majority of patients. Only 9% had incontinence and 11% impotence, reflecting the rarity of autonomic involvement. The presence of metastatic lumbosacral plexopathy suggests advanced disease with a median survival of 5.5 months. Only 15% of patients studied had subjective improvement in pain or weakness at 1-month follow-up. Finally, Jaeckle et al's group concluded that epidural extension of tumor should be considered when 1) pain is severe, 2) in the presence of bilateral lower extremity weakness or sensory loss, and/or 3) in the presence of bowel or bladder incontinence.

Electromyography in patients with radiation-induced lumbosacral plexopathy shows the following abnormalities: fibrillation potentials, positive sharp waves, bizarre high-frequency discharges, and fasciculation. Myokymic discharges occur in about 30% of patients, along with bizarre low-frequency discharges, grouped discharges, and myoclonic discharges.

RADIATION-INDUCED NEUROGENIC TUMORS

These tumors may derive from local peripheral nerves or other surrounding soft tissues, and can present as either malignant peripheral nerve sheath tumors or as second primary tumors (sarcoma).[10,48] The presentation is usually that of an enlarging painful mass imaged over a previously irradiated site (brachial or lumbosacral plexus). Characteristically, their onset is associated with a long latency after irradiation (up to 4–41 years).[10] Factors that contribute to the generation of radiation-induced tumors include: high doses of radiation, long survival after radiation therapy, radiation damage to periaxonal extraneural tissues, and genetic factors associated with reduced host immune response or specific susceptibility to certain tumors.

POSTSURGICAL PAIN SYNDROMES

Surgery is often performed to promote cure, obtain tissue for pathologic diagnosis, and to "debulk" tumors to relieve obstructive symptoms or to provide an opportunity for adjuvant antitumor therapies (ie, radiation and chemotherapy) to be most effective. Postsur-

gical pain syndromes are defined as those persisting beyond the usual postoperative healing phase (usually 1–2 months), and are often associated with focal pain occurring as a consequence of nerve injury at a specific site due to surgical trauma. The following clinical syndromes are common in cancer patients, and are likely to be encountered in any oncology practice. Although they often are associated with substantial degrees of pain and impairment, recognition of these entities may relieve the patient of the concern that pain is secondary to recurrent tumor, although this must always be excluded.

POSTMASTECTOMY PAIN

This complication of cancer surgery is said to occur in up to 5% of women after mastectomy.[49] Although is has been described after simple mastectomy and even lumpectomy, it is apparently more common after radical mastectomy and axillary dissection. Axillary dissection may be associated with injury to the cutaneous branch of the intercostobrachial nerve (which originates from the T1 and T2 nerve roots). Pain is typically described as a burning numbness and dysesthetic squeezing sensation located along the anterior chest wall, axilla, and medial upper arm (see Figs. 3–4A,B). Hyperpathia and persistent spontaneous pain lead to guarding of the affected shoulder and upper extremity, often with the secondary development of frozen shoulder, contractures, and a reflex sympathetic dystrophy (RSD) syndrome. Pain may appear any time after surgery, but a latency of several weeks is common. It has been suggested that postmastectomy pain is more common after operative procedures that have been complicated by persistent drainage or infection around the surgical wound, although, as noted above, the most important correlate appears to be axillary dissection. Differential diagnosis includes brachial plexopathy and orthopedic abnormalities in the shoulder joint, such as torn rotator cuff.

Treatment options are limited and not usually satisfactory. The most commonly used therapies are those with an established role in the management of neuropathic pain. These include the use of tricyclic antidepressants, anticonvulsants, oral local anesthetics, as well as TENS units and physical therapy (see Chapters 1 and 10). When this syndrome is complicated by a frozen shoulder, suprascapular and/or stellate ganglion block combined with aggressive physical therapy are indicated. Injection of local anesthetic and steroids near a scar neuroma or trigger point may be helpful as well (see Chapter 19).

Watson et al recently treated 18 patients with postmastectomy pain using topical capsaicin (0.025%) with encouraging results.[50] After 4 weeks of treatment, 12 of the 14 patients demonstrated improvement, and 57% had good or excellent responses. At 6 months after completion of the study, 50% of patients reported sustained relief of pain.

Vecht et al have emphasized that differentiating between postmastectomy pain and a process involving the brachial plexus can be difficult.[51] Features favoring the presence of a lesion of the intercostobrachial nerve include a history of axillary lymph node dissection, an absence of lymphedema, no history of radiotherapy to the supraclavicular/axillary region, pain with a postoperative onset, pain in the axilla and/or shoulder as well as along the inner side of the upper arm, supraclavicular/axillary pain on palpation, and an absence of EMG and CT abnormalities.

POST-THORACOTOMY PAIN

Chest pain persisting past the usual postoperative healing time may be due to recurrent or progressive tumor growth, or may be a consequence of injury to chest wall structures during thoracotomy. Injury to the ribs and intercostal nerves may be due to the surgical incision, or may be related to retraction of the chest wall. Post-thoracotomy incisional neuralgia is typically burning in quality, and associated with hyperpathia. Chest wall pain that persists and worsens in intensity is always worrisome, and should prompt a thorough reassessment.[52] Chest CT, sputum cytology, bronchoscopy, and serum carcinoembryonic antigen (CEA) determinations are useful for excluding recurrent lung cancer.

The treatment of post-thoracotomy pain (see Chapters 10 and 19) depends on its etiology. Patients with intercostal neuralgia may be treated with TENS and tricyclics. Carbamazepine or other anticonvulsants may be helpful if lancinating pain is prominent. The results of recent uncontrolled experiences with topical capsaicin applied to the site of the thoracotomy scar have not been encouraging. For patients with recurrent or progressive pain related to tumor infiltration of the lung, bronchi, pleura, and chest wall structures, a variety of treatment options may be used. Opioid analgesics and adjuvants in combination with antitumor treatments such as radiation and chemotherapy may be employed. Pleural involvement with tumor may produce widespread and vaguely localized pain spreading diffusely throughout the chest wall. Anesthetic procedures with a potential therapeutic role include infiltration with local anesthetics and steroids, intercostal blocks (local anesthetic, neurolytics, or cryotherapy), subarachnoid or epidural neurolysis, or the placement of pleural catheters for the instillation of local anesthetics.

PAIN AFTER RADICAL NECK DISSECTION

Radical neck dissection for management of head and neck tumors may interrupt the cervical plexus and spinal accessory nerve, producing pain and weakness on this basis.[53] However, these tumors often recur and produce pain by locally infiltrating soft tissues of the neck, soft palate, and pharynx, and even the base of skull. In the latter instance, pain is often referred to the vertex of the skull and to the occiput. A recent report documented the role of low-grade infection as a cause of persistent pain in patients with radical neck dissection.[54]

In pain related to cervical plexus damage, the patient often describes an ongoing tightness or burning dysesthesia in the anterolateral neck, shoulder, jaw, and ear. Additionally, patients may experience painful lancinating paresthesias to the ear and angle of the jaw, as well as myofascial pain in the anterior chest, scapula, and shoulder. Management is similar to that described above.

PHANTOM AND STUMP PAIN

Phantom sensations are common after amputation, and should be distinguished from frank phantom pain and stump pain.[55] Stump pain is often due to neuroma formation, and is characterized by clearly identifiable trigger points and a positive Tinel's sign. Assessment ideally involves careful consultation with a physiatrist to assure that prosthetic devices fit properly. Treatment includes infiltration of trigger points with local anesthetic agents and the use of analgesics (see Chapter 19).

Phantom sensations occur in the vast majority of patients after amputation. The patient's experience is usually of a contorted and then shrunken limb. These perceptions are presumed to involve the expression of a learned "memory" represented in the central nervous system. Recent studies suggest that preamputation sensory blockade with anesthetic agents may prevent the occurrence of frankly painful chronic phantom sensation. The *post hoc* treatment of phantom pain is not satisfactory. Sherman has reviewed most of the available therapies.[55]

POSTNEPHRECTOMY PAIN

After operation in the region of the flank, injury to the L1 nerve may result in painful dysesthesias as well as a sensation of numbness, heaviness, and fullness in the flank, anterior abdomen, and groin.[56] Paraspinal tumor should be considered until proven otherwise by CT scan. An abdominal corset has been found to be helpful in providing better muscular support. The medical approach to treatment is similar to what has been outlined for other postsurgical syndromes.

PROCEDURE-RELATED PAIN IN CHILDREN

Children often experience significant pain and distress related to diagnostic procedures and therapy for cancer.[57,58] This previously neglected area of pain management has recently been the focus of considerable attention, and is well described in Chapters 4 and 28.

REFERENCES

1. World Health Organization: Technical Report Series. Cancer Pain Relief and Palliative Care. Geneva, World Health Organization, 1990.
2. Miser AW, Miser JS: The treatment of cancer pain in children. Pediatr Clin North Am 1989;36:979.
3. Shubert MM, Sullivan KM, Morten TH et al: Oral manifestations of chronic graft-versus-host disease. Arch Intern Med 1984;144:1591.
4. Carl W: Oral and dental care of patients receiving radiation therapy for tumors in and around the oral cavity. In Carl W, Saka K (eds): Cancer and the Oral Cavity, p. 167. Chicago, Quintessence, 1986.
5. Hill HF, Chapman CR, Karnell J et al: Self administration of morphine in bone marrow transplant patients reduced drug requirement. Pain 1990;40:121.
6. Green LS, Donoso A, Heller-Bettinger IE et al: Axonal disturbance in vincristine-induced peripheral neuropathy. Ann Neurol 1977;1:255.
7. Young DF, Posner JB: Nervous system toxicity of chemotherapeutic agents. In Vinken PJ, Bruyn GW (eds): Handbook of Clinical Neurology, Vol 9: Neurological Manifestations of Systemic Diseases, Part II, p 91. Amsterdam, North Holland Publishing Company, 1989.
8. Cowan JD, Kies MS, Roth JL et al: Nerve conduction studies in patients treated with cis-diamminedichloroplatinum (II) S: A preliminary report. Cancer Treat Rep 1980;64:1119.
9. Stillman MJ, Christensen W, Payne R et al: Leukemic relapse presenting a sciatic nerve involvement by chloroma (granulocytic sarcoma). Cancer 1988;62:2047.
10. Foley KM et al: Radiation-induction malignant and atypical peripheral nerve sheath tumors. Ann Neurol 1980;7:311.
11. Ihde DC, DeVita VT: Osteonecrosis of the femoral head in patients treated with intermittent combination chemotherapy (including corticosteroids). Cancer 1975;36:1585.

12. Rotstein J, Good RA: Steroid pseudorheumatism. Arch Intern Med 1957;99:545.

13. Watson PN, Evans RJ: Postherpetic neuralgia: A review. Arch Neurol 1986;43:836.

14. Portenoy RK, Duma C, Foley KM: Acute herpetic and postherpetic neuralgia: Clinical review and current management. Ann Neurol 1986;20:651.

15. Loester J: Herpes zoster and postherpetic neuralgia. In Bonica JJ (ed): The Management of Cancer Pain, 2nd ed, p 257. Philadelphia, Lea & Febiger, 1990.

16. Rowbotham MC, Reisner-Keller LA, Fields HL: Both intravenous lidocaine and morphine reduce the pain of postherpetic neuralgia. Neurology 1991;41:1024.

17. Rowbotham MC et al: Post-herpetic neuralgia: The relation of pain complaint, sensory disturbance and skin temperature. Pain 1989;39:129.

18. Watson CP et al: Post-herpetic neuralgia: Post-mortem analysis of a case. Pain 1988;34:129.

19. McClure D, Barker G, Barker B et al: Oral management of the cancer patient: Part II. Oral complications of radiation therapy. Compend Contin Educ Dent 1987;8:88.

20. Rothwell BR: Prevention and treatment of the orofacial complications of radiotherapy. J Am Dent Assoc 1987;114:316.

21. Ferguson BJ, Hudson WR, Farmer JC: Hyperbaric oxygen therapy for laryngeal radionecrosis. Ann Otol Rhinol Laryngol 1987;9:1.

22. Morton ME: Osteoradionecrosis: A study of the incidence in the northwest of England. Br J Oral Maxillofac Surg 1986;24:323.

23. Morton ME, Simpson W: The management of osteoradionecrosis of the jaws. Br J Oral Maxillofac Surg 1986;24:332.

24. Wang CC: Management and prognosis of squamous cell carcinoma of the tonsillar region. Radiology 1972;104:667.

25. Guttenberg SA: Osteoradionecrosis of the jaw. Am J Surg 1974;127:326.

26. Epstein JB, Wong FLW, Stevenson-Moore P: Osteoradionecrosis: Clinical experience and a proposal for classification. J Oral Maxillofac Surg 1987;45:104.

27. Dolezal RF, Baker SR, Krause CJ: Treatment of the patient with extensive osteoradionecrosis of the mandible. Arch Otolaryngol 1982;108:179.

28. Niebel HH, Neenan EW: Dental aspects of osteoradionecrosis. Oral Surg 1957;10:1011.

29. Yamashiro M, Amagasa T, Horiuchi J et al: Extensive osteoradionecrosis of the mandible associated with new bone formation. J Oral Maxillofac Surg 1987; 45:630.

30. MacDougall JA, Evans AM, Lindsay RK: Osteoradionecrosis of the mandible and its treatment. Am J Surg 1963;106:816.

31. Baker DG: The radiobiological basis for tissue reactions in the oral cavity following therapeutic x-irradiation. Arch Otolaryngol 1982;108:21.

32. Fattore L, Strauss RA: Hyperbaric oxygen in the treatment of osteoradionecrosis: A review of its use and efficacy. Oral Surg 1987;63:280.

33. Kivisaari J, Niinikoski J: Effects of hyperbaric oxygen and prolonged hypoxia on the healing of open wounds. Acta Chir Scand 1975;141:14.

34. Marchetta FC, Sato K, Holyoke ED: Treatment of osteoradionecrosis by intraoral excision of the mandible. Surg Gynecol Obstet 1967;125:1003.

35. Marx RE, Johnson RP: Problem wounds in oral and maxillofacial surgery: The role of hyperbaric oxygen. In Davis JC, Hunt TK (eds): Problem Wounds: The Role of Oxygen, p 65. New York, Elsevier, 1988.

36. Thom SR: Hyperbaric oxygen therapy. Journal of Intensive Care Medicine 1989;4:58.

37. Moran WJ, Panje WR: The free greater omental flap for treatment of mandibular osteoradionecrosis. Arch Otolaryngol Head Neck Surg 1987;113:425.

38. Panje WR: Mandible reconstruction with the trapezius osteomusculocutaneous flap. Arch Otolaryngol Head Neck Surg 1985;111:223.

39. Mansfield MJ, Sanders RW, Heimbach RD et al: Hyperbaric oxygen as an adjunct in the treatment of osteoradionecrosis of the mandible. J Oral Surg 1981; 39:585.

40. Patt R, Jain S: Management of a patient with osteoradionecrosis of the mandible with nerve blocks. Journal of Pain and Symptom Management 1990;5:59.

41. Berger PS: Neurological complications of radiotherapy. In Silberstein A (ed): Neurological Complications of Therapy: Selected Topics, p 137. Mount Kisco, NY: Futura, 1982.

42. Payne R, Foley KM: Exploration of the brachial plexus in patients with cancer. Neurology 1986;36:329.

43. Kori SH et al: Brachial plexus lesions in patients with cancer: 100 cases. Neurology 1981;31:45.

44. Cascino TL, Kori S, Krol G et al: CT scanning of the brachial plexus in patients with cancer. Neurology 1983;33:1553.

45. Chad DA et al: Lumbosacral plexopathy. Seminars in Neurology 1987;7:97.

46. Bradley WG et al: Painful lumbosacral plexopathy with elevated erythrocyte sedimentation rate: A treatable inflammatory syndrome. Ann Neurol 1984; 15:457.

47. Jaeckle KA et al: The natural history of lumbosacral plexopathy in cancer. Neurology 1985;35:8.

48. Ducatman BS et al: Malignant peripheral nerve sheath tumors: A clinicopathological study of 120 cases. Cancer 1986;57:2006.

49. Granek I, Ashikari R, Foley KM: Postmastectomy

pain syndrome: Clinical and anatomical correlates. Proc ASCO 1983;3:122.

50. Watson CP et al: The post-mastectomy pain syndrome and the effect of topical capsaicin. Pain 1989;38:177.

51. Vecht CJ et al: Post-axillary dissection in breast cancer due to lesion of the intercostobrachial nerve. Pain 1989;38:171.

52. Kanner RM, Martini N, Foley KM: Nature and incidence of post-thoracotomy pain. Proc ASCO 1982; 1:152.

53. Vecht CJ, Hoff AM, deBoer MF: Types and causes of pain in cancer of the head and neck. Pain 1990; (Suppl 5):S-354.

54. Bruera E, MacDonald N: Intractable pain in patients with advanced head and neck tumors: A possible role of local infection. Cancer Treat Rep 1986;70:691.

55. Sherman RA, Sherma CJ, Parker : Chronic phantom and stump pain among American veterans: Results of survey. Pain 1984:18:83.

56. Foley KM: Pain syndromes in patients with cancer. Med Clin North Am 1987;71:169.

57. Miser AW et al: The prevalence of pain in a pediatric and young adult cancer population. Pain 1987;29: 73.

58. Zeltzer LK et al: The management of pain associated with pediatric procedures. Pediatr Clin North Am 1989;36:941.

Chapter 4

Assessment of Cancer Pain in Children

Judith E. Beyer
Nancy Wells

INTRODUCTION

Dramatic advances have taken place in the scientific study of pediatric pain over the last decade.[1] Increased numbers of textbooks, journal articles, clinical, research, and consensus conferences addressing the topic of children's pain demonstrate the seriousness of clinicians and researchers in their search for new knowledge and improved assessment and management practices. The recent formation of a Special Interest Group on Pain in Childhood of the International Association for the Study of Pain (IASP) provides further evidence of the commitment of researchers and scholars to enhancing the scientific knowledge base for this previously neglected field of study. Research experts from around the world gathered for the first and second International Symposia on Pediatric Pain in 1988 (Seattle) and 1991 (Montreal), respectively. Nationally, the problems arising from pain in children with cancer have been examined in the Consensus Conference on the Management of Pain in Childhood Cancer,[2] and the Oncology Nursing Society (ONS) Position Paper on Cancer Pain.[3,4] Assessment of pediatric cancer pain using a variety of methods of measurement was emphasized in both forums as a necessary initial step in improving the management of cancer pain in children.

At least three recent developments can be expected to provide an impetus for needed changes in current practice in the assessment and management of pediatric cancer pain: 1) the global escalation of concern about the problems of cancer pain in children by health care clinicians and researchers; 2) the recognition of children's abilities to rate the intensity of their own pain; and 3) the development of more effective means to provide analgesia, such as the use of potent, rapid-acting analgesics and sedatives, the adoption of alternative routes for their administration, and the expansion of the use of anesthetics to reduce or eliminate cancer-related pain. To obtain optimal results from each of these developments, corresponding improvements in our ability to systematically measure pain in children are essential.

This chapter focuses on one aspect of childhood pain, the assessment of cancer pain. The purpose is to guide the clinician who provide care for children with cancer in understanding the importance, value, and process of using assessment instruments to examine the nature, intensity, and effects of pain experiences on children.

BACKGROUND AND RATIONALE

Systematic, accurate, and careful pain assessment is essential for all children experiencing pain, but it is especially important for children experiencing pain associated with the diagnosis and treatment of cancer. Pain is a common result of cancer and cancer therapy in children. In the United States, pain associated with neoplastic disease and therapy has been found in 48% of children hospitalized for cancer treatment, and 27% of children seen in outpatient settings.[5] The overall incidence of pain in Italian children with neoplastic diseases was estimated at 57%.[6] It seems reasonable to suggest that improvements in assessment and management of cancer-related pain would benefit a substantial number of children.

Accurate assessment is a prerequisite to and the cornerstone of good pain management, and in its absence pain management techniques cannot be effective. Numerous sources suggest that children are seriously undertreated for pain associated with a variety of conditions requiring surgery.[7-12] For children with cancer, disease-related pain is frequently both severe and persistent, and undertreatment with analgesics is common.[13-16] Simi-

larly, Zeltzer et al[17] indicated that efforts to control pain and anxiety during painful procedures tend to be instituted only as an afterthought, and often sedatives without analgesic properties are administered. At least part of the problem relates to inadequacies in the assessment of pain. For example, in 9 of 43 pediatric cancer patients referred for evaluation of psychiatric symptoms, consulting psychiatrists recommended increased attention to pain control.[18] In eight of the children in whom pain control was enhanced, psychiatric symptoms either diminished markedly or resolved completely. This outcome highlights the importance of both careful assessment and vigorous treatment of pain in the care of children with cancer.

For pain caused by cancer treatment, it is essential to monitor and relieve or prevent the child's pain in order to modify the negative experiences induced by pain. Otherwise, anticipatory nausea, vomiting, and fearfulness become a conditioned response, and to the child, the treatment becomes worse than the disease itself.[19] Children have reported that the pain related to bone marrow aspirations (BMAs) and lumbar punctures (LPs) is worse than the cancer,[19,20] thus highlighting the poor attention traditionally focused on control of pain during these procedures.

Accurate assessment of the child's experience of pain must be obtained before effective treatment can be identified. The person with the pain should always be considered the best judge and the final authority[21] on the intensity and quality of his or her own pain. This notion is well characterized by McCaffery's definition of pain, that ". . . pain is whatever the experiencing person says it is, occurring whenever he says it does."[22] Since there are no physiologic indicators that reliably provide objective information about the intensity or quality of pain, or diagnostic tests that provide useful information about the patient's pain experience, self-report remains the most valid and accepted indicator of pain in the verbal child. The assessment of pain in infants and toddlers continues to present a problem because of their inability to describe the nature of their experiences.

TYPES OF PEDIATRIC PAIN

In 1979, Beals[23] suggested it would be useful to categorize pain experienced by children with cancer as emanating from three sources: tumor invasion, therapy, and psychological. In 1990, Miser[24] further delineated five sources of pain associated with cancer in children: tumor invasion, therapy (*eg*, mucositis, infection, postsurgical, neuropathy, and radiation dermatitis), procedures (*eg*, venipuncture, BMA, and LP), debilitation (*eg*, decubitus ulcer and constipation), and incidental (*eg*, pain from unrelated medical conditions). Despite this heterogeneity, the bulk of the research on pediatric cancer pain focuses on procedure-related pain, particularly the pain induced by BMAs and LPs.[25] There is little written about the other types of pain associated with pediatric cancer, such as that due to the disease *per se*, and according to Jay et al, it is "nondata based."[25] In contrast to that on children, research on adults has focused on pain related to tumor invasion, almost to the exclusion of pain emanating from other sources. Miser and colleagues[5] are working to expand the knowledge base about the pain of cancer in children. They found that the majority of pain experienced by hospitalized children was related to tumor invasion (46%) or was a result of therapy (40%). These findings indicate that whereas a high incidence of pain is associated with the treatments instituted for either cure or palliation in children with neoplastic disease, pain due to tumor invasion should not be ignored.

ASSESSMENT OF PAIN IN CHILDREN WITH CANCER

Two recent documents address the needs of the pediatric oncology population and support the importance of and need for careful and systematic pain assessment in children. For the first time in history, health care providers have mobilized to work toward widespread improvements in the care of symptomatic pediatric patients with cancer. The first of these documents is the Report of the Consensus Conference on the Management of Pain in Childhood Cancer,[2] which was developed by a panel of 19 experts in pain and/or cancer from a variety of health care disciplines. Of the three papers contained in this report, one focused on assessment and methodologic issues,[26] one focused on the management of tumor-related pain,[27] and one focused on the management of procedure-related pain.[28] The second document is the ONS Position Paper on Cancer Pain.[3,4] Both of these documents adopted aggressive stands on the relief and elimination of cancer pain, and took equally strong positions on the role of systematic pain assessment as the foundation of effective pain management. The ONS paper focused on the nurse's role and responsibility in the assessment process, whereas the Consensus paper focused on specific guidelines for assessing pain in children by a variety of health care providers. These guidelines included recommendations to: 1) identify the factors that exacerbate pain; 2) believe the child's self-report of pain; 3) select and use validated instruments to measure pain; 4) identify behavioral clues that are highly suggestive of the presence of pain in infants and young children; 5) better characterize the importance of self-report, behavioral observation, and physiologic measures for various age groups; and 6) generate a Pain Problem List that identifies the multiple sources and dimensions of cancer-related pain. Both the ONS and Consensus papers recommend that pain intensity be monitored as a part of quality assurance programs. Both of these papers highlight the central importance of pain assessment and management in children with cancer.

The source of cancer-related pain, as well as the child's age and developmental level, serve as useful guides to the selection of appropriate pain assessment strategies. Recent research has focused on the validation of a variety of instruments designed to permit children to rate the intensity of their pain experiences. This work also has demonstrated that children, some as young as 3 years of age, are capable of indicating levels of pain in meaningful ways.[29-34] It was previously believed that because of limitations imposed by incomplete cognitive development, children were unable meaningfully to rate their pain in a reliable manner until they were 7 or 8 years old. These findings have served as a challenge to researchers to develop a variety of child-oriented assessment methods. Because most preschoolers are unable to quantify abstract phenomena, at least in a mature, adult fashion, new ways had to be developed to help them communicate the nature of their pain experiences to health care providers. Thus, over the past decade, research has made it possible to help children to communicate the nature of their hurt with the aid of pictures, poker chips, and other concrete objects (see below). As a result, researchers and clinicians have been able better to quantify the information children provide, to monitor the pain experience, and to design more effective individualized treatment plans.

Very few of these pain assessment instruments for children have been developed specifically for children with cancer; most have been developed for and tested more thoroughly in children recovering from surgery. Methods of measurement considered here include self-report, behavioral observation, and measurement of physiologic variables.

RELIABILITY AND VALIDITY

Consideration of the psychometric properties of testing instruments, particularly the concepts of reliability and validity, is a primary concern in any discussion of pain assessment. The application of these concepts to pediatric pain assessment instruments is discussed in general here, and is described in greater detail in a variety of other sources.[35–40]

In order for a clinician to feel confident that the assessment data obtained from patients are meaningful, the assessment device must possess an adequate level of validity. The **validity** of an instrument is essentially its ability to reflect the underlying concept it was designed to measure. Validity requires assessment at both conceptual and empirical levels, and, therefore, is more difficult to determine

than reliability. **Reliability** refers to the accuracy or consistency of an instrument, and may be assessed empirically within the instrument and/or over time.

For an instrument designed to measure pain intensity in children, there should be data that indicate it does in fact measure pain intensity. If, for example, a well controlled study shows that the pain scores obtained with a particular instrument decrease when a sample of children receives adequate doses of analgesics, these findings provide support for the validity of the assessment instrument. If, on the other hand, pain scores stay the same or increase after the administration of adequate doses of analgesics, then there is reason to doubt the instrument's validity. To establish validity, the instrument should be used in numerous studies conducted under a variety of conditions, and the results of these studies should substantiate that the instrument appropriately measures fluctuations in pain intensity. Because many of the pediatric pain instruments are new, very few have been tested extensively. However, there is sufficient evidence of adequate validity for a number of currently available instruments to support their use in clinical practice.

Validity can be assessed in many ways. **Content validity** refers to the degree to which the items that comprise the instrument are representative of the underlying concept. For example, a questionnaire's measure of the concept of anxiety should reflect the physiologic, emotional, and behavioral aspects of anxiety. Content validity is typically determined by a panel of experts who judge the relevance and importance of each item to the underlying concept.

Construct validity is the degree to which the instrument reflects the concept, and is usually determined by how the findings compare with expected hypotheses. One method used to determine construct validity is to apply the instrument to two groups that are known to differ on the concept being investigated. If the instrument demonstrates a measured difference between the two groups that is statistically significant, then the findings can be regarded as evidence of its construct validity. An example might be to apply an instrument to measure pain intensity to a group of children after surgery and to a group of children having preoperative physical examinations, with the expectation that pain scores should be higher in the group of postoperative children. Testing hypotheses based on theoretical notions about how the concept is related to and is different from other concepts also measure construct validity. For example, pain and fear are distinct concepts, but they tend to be related in children undergoing painful procedures. The distinction between concepts would be supported if two measures of pain were more highly correlated than measures of pain and fear in children undergoing painful procedures.

Criterion-related validity assesses the degree of correlation between the score of the instrument and an outside criterion variable. Unfortunately, for many of the psychologically based variables, such as pain and anxiety, there are few objective criteria available, particularly in children. An example of assessing criterion-related validity for pain in women in second-stage labor is to correlate their self-reported pain intensity with the amount of cervical dilatation present.

Reliability refers to the consistency and accuracy of an instrument, and is as important as validity when evaluating an instrument for clinical application. There are three types of reliability addressed here: inter-rater, internal consistency, and stability. The appropriateness of each type of reliability depends on the method of measurement and the nature of the underlying concept being measured. **Inter-rater reliability** reflects the consistency of measurement among two or more observers, and is an essential attribute for behavioral observation instruments. For example, two raters observing a child's pain behavior with the same instrument should produce similar scores if the instrument has good inter-rater reliability. Inter-rater reliability is typically described as the percent of agreement or degree of correlation between raters. **Internal consistency** is the degree to which the individual items on a multi-item scale reflect the underlying concept being measured. For example, if

the responses to 10 questions are summed to reflect a child's level of anxiety, the 10 items should be highly intercorrelated. **Cronbach's alpha coefficient** is the commonly used statistic to test the internal consistency of instruments. **Stability**, or **test-retest reliability**, reflects the consistency of a measure over time. To determine stability, the instrument is administered twice, and the correlation of measures between time intervals is examined. Stability is difficult, if not impossible, to assess in phenomena that are expected to change over time. Pain intensity, which characteristically fluctuates, is one such phenomenon. Variations in pain intensity might make an instrument appear to be unreliable when, in fact, the trait (pain) is unstable.

PAIN ASSESSMENT INSTRUMENTS FOR CHILDREN

The Report of the Consensus Conference on the Management of Pain in Childhood Cancer[26] recommended the use of multiple methods of measurement, including self-report, and behavioral and/or physiologic observation, when assessing pain in infants and children. Each of these types of measures will be discussed separately as they relate to the assessment of cancer pain in children.

SELF-REPORT

Numerous self-report techniques can be used to obtain data from children with cancer-related pain, including their verbal statements, verbal descriptors, pain diaries, pain drawings, pain maps, and pain intensity ratings. As an aid to gain more detailed information about children's experiences with cancer and associated pain, several books written by children have been published.[41,42] These sources provide rich data, from a qualitative perspective, on the thoughts, feelings, and perceptions of children with cancer (Figs. 4–1 and 4–2). Each method of assessment provides different types of information about the child's experience of pain, and each is useful

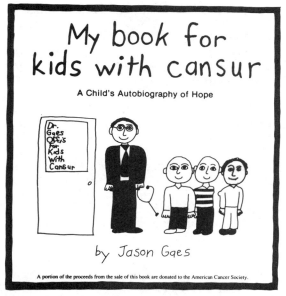

Figure 4–1. This is the title cover of the book written by 8-year-old Jason Gaes, intended as a resource for children with cancer and their families. In his book, Jason explained in detail his perceptions of the experience of having Burkitt's lymphoma and its successful treatment. (Melius Publishing Company, Inc. 515 Citizens Building, Aberdeen, SD 57401; 1-800-882-5171.)

in the assessment of children with symptomatic cancer. These methods are more thoroughly described elsewhere.[35–40] Briefly, verbal statements are the child's spontaneous explanation of his or her pain that may or may not be understandable to adults, but which usually have meaning within a developmental context. An example of this is when a child might report that the hurt was like "a lion's roar,"[35] in possible reference to Aesop's fable involving a lion with a thorn in its paw. Another example reflecting a young girl's headache was "Mommie, my barrettes are too tight" (verbal communication, Carolyn Aradine, 1985).

Over the past decade, investigators have developed instruments to assess the quality of pain experienced using **verbal descriptors**. This work was based on the McGill Pain Questionnaire,[43] which was developed to measure

pain quality and intensity in adults. Words that American children use to describe their pain have been studied by several groups of researchers.[44–50] The outcomes of these studies are instruments that consist of verbal descriptors of pain that children (school-age and older) use to describe the sensory, affective, and evaluative qualities of their pain experiences. Savedra, Tesler, Wilkie and colleagues[50] recently identified a set of 56 descriptors (as part of the Adolescent Pediatric Pain Tool; APPT) used by at least 50% of a large sample of school-age children and adolescents (Table 4–1). This level of agreement in a large, multiethnic sample provides evidence of content validity for the verbal descriptors identified by these researchers. Construct validity was established initially by a group of five clinical nurse specialists who agreed on the sensory, affective, and evaluative descriptor groups; this was confirmed sta-

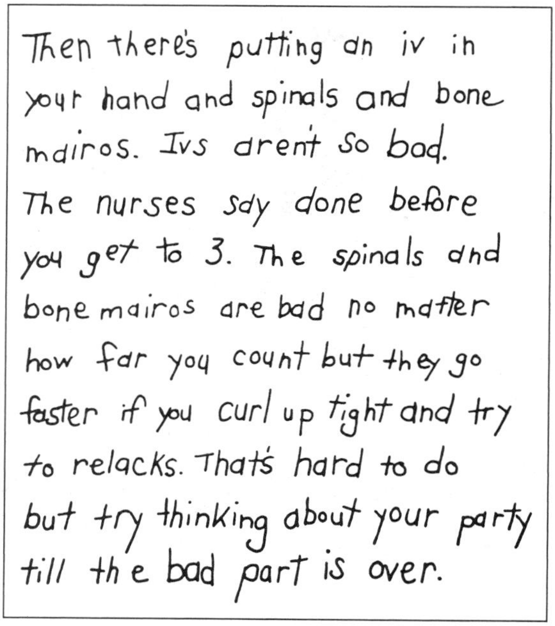

> Then there's putting an iv in your hand and spinals and bone mairos. Ivs aren't so bad. The nurses say done before you get to 3. The spinals and bone mairos are bad no matter how far you count but they go faster if you curl up tight and try to relacks. That's hard to do but try thinking about your party till the bad part is over.

Figure 4–2. A page from *My Book for Kids with Cansur* explaining Jason Gaes's view of lumbar punctures and bone marrow aspirations. (Gaes J: *My Book for Kids with Cansur.* Aberdeen, SD, Melius Publishing Co., Inc., 1987.)

Table 4–1.
Pain Word List for School-agers and Adolescents

Sensory

Aching	Like a sharp knife	Like a scratch
Hurting	Pinlike	Like a sting
Like an ache	Sharp	Scratching
Like a hurt	Stabbing	Stinging
Sore	Blistering	Shocking
Beating	Burning	Shooting
Hitting	Hot	Splitting
Pounding	Cramping	Numb
Punching	Crushing	Stiff
Throbbing	Like a pinch	Swollen
Biting	Pinching	Tight
Cutting	Pressure	
Like a pin	Itching	

Affective

Awful
Deadly
Dying
Killing
Crying
Frightening
Screaming
Terrifying
Dizzy
Sickening
Suffocating

Evaluative

Annoying
Bad
Horrible
Miserable
Terrible
Uncomfortable
Never goes away
Uncontrollable

Reprinted with permission of authors and publisher. From: Wilkie D, Holzemer W, Tesler M et al. Measuring pain quality: validity and reliability of children's and adolescent's pain language. Pain 1990;41:151.

tistically by factor analysis. In addition, the number of words selected by hospitalized children decreased over time, as would be expected as recovery occurs. Concurrent validity was supported by correlations between verbal descriptor scores, number of pain sites, and pain intensity scores. Test-retest reliability was supported by the high correlations between two measurement points in children whose pain intensity scores did not change.

Similarly, Abu-Saad[51] developed a 30-word verbal descriptor instrument for Dutch school-agers and adolescents. Internal consistency and content validity were shown to be adequate. Construct validity was examined through factor analysis, which showed three major factors: one affective/evaluative and two sensory. This instrument, which is in the early phase of its development, is currently being further examined for psychometric properties.

Abu-Saad examined the words used by

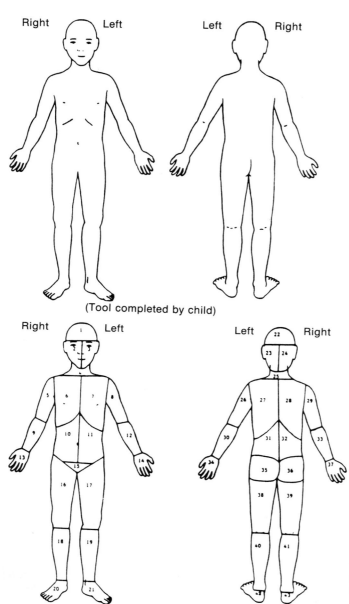

(Tool completed by child)

(Data analysis tool)

Figure 4–3. Body outlines for school-aged children and adolescents. Patients mark the body outlines to locate their pain. The segmented body outlines are used as templates to differentiate more finely 43 locations on the body. (Savedra M, Tesler M, Holzemer W, Wilkie D, Ward J: Testing a tool to assess postoperative pediatric and adolecent pain. In Tyler DC, Krane EJ (eds.): *Advances in Pain Research and Therapy*, vol 15, p 87. New York, Raven Press, 1990).

Arab–American, Asian–American, and Latin American children to describe pain.[52–54] Findings indicated that psychological causes of pain (*eg*, feeling unwanted or being yelled at) were identified by a larger group of Arab–American and Asian–American than Latin American children. Asian and Arab girls more frequently identified psychological causes, and used more affective and evaluative words for pain than boys. This supports gender role dif-

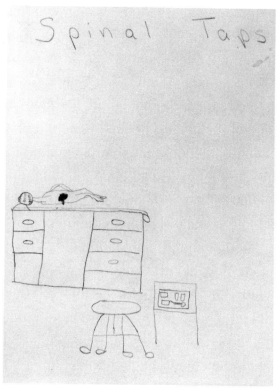

Figure 4–4. This is a drawing by Isaac, a 10-year-old with cancer. Note the vulnerability shown in the thin pencil lines and the position of the child on the table. The only color in this picture was the red paint carefully placed in the middle of the back at the site of the needle insertion for a lumbar puncture.

findings of Savedra et al,[44] no Asian children indicated that, when in pain, they felt brave or like hitting or kicking others. Abu-Saad explained that cultural expectations of obedience and self-control were higher in the Asian cultures than in Western cultures. These studies provide the first data available regarding cultural influences on pain experiences in children, and provide a rationale for cultural differences in response to pain.

Pain diaries are logs kept by children and adolescents to document their experiences of pain in the context of their daily lives. They are most often used in the treatment of children with chronic conditions, such as headache, recurrent abdominal pain, and juvenile rheumatoid arthritis.[55] Although pain diaries have not been used extensively in children with cancer pain, they have the potential to assist in identifying environmental and affective factors that influence the child's pain experiences.

Pain maps (Fig. 4–3) are body outlines on which children can locate and/or color the severity of their hurt. **Pain drawings** are simply children's artistic portrayals of their pain experiences (Figs. 4–4, 4–5). Because of the projective nature of children's drawings, specialized training is required for individuals who score the pictures. Pain drawings have been used extensively by health care providers to assist hospitalized children to express themselves about their pain experiences. Therefore, pain drawings may be more useful as a therapeutic intervention than as an assessment instrument.

Pain intensity ratings have been the main focus of self-report measures of children's pain. Research has shown that children can indicate the level of their pain when they are asked in developmentally appropriate ways. Self-report scales have taken many forms, and have emerged as useful, concrete ways for children to indicate how they feel. Researchers and clinicians can then quantify these pain indicators. Self-report of pain intensity provides a means to understand better children's experiences with pain, to monitor these experiences, and to evaluate the effects of interventions intended to relieve pain. As noted in

ferences, as Asian and Arab girls are expected to be more sensitive to emotional matters than boys.[52,53] In the Arab sample, boys were found to use words like "brave, angry, and feel like crying but don't" to describe how they felt when in pain. Girls used words like "embarrassed, sad, like running away." Again, this suggests gender role differentiation in the Arab culture, in which girls are considered docile, dependent, and emotional, whereas boys are considered assertive, brave, and strong.[52] There seemed to be little difference in the type of descriptors selected by the children to describe pain, except that the Asian children selected fewer sensory descriptors (*eg*, stinging, cutting, burning). Unlike in the

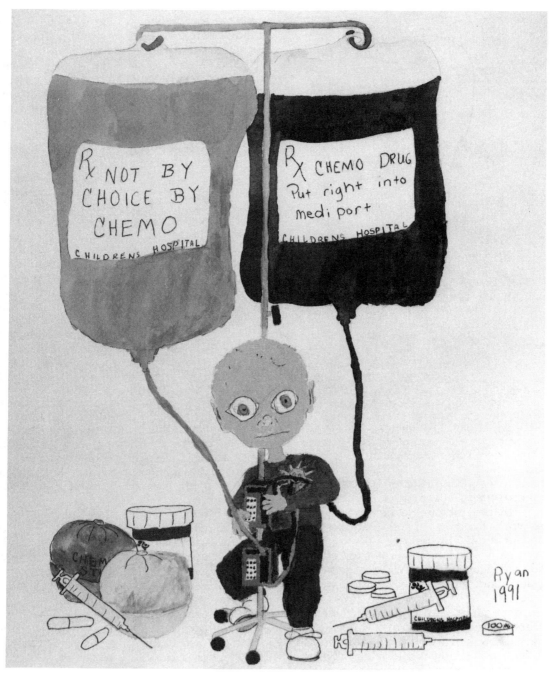

Figure 4–5. This is a drawing by Ryan, a 14-year-old with a brain tumor. Note the prominence of the medication in the foreground, the small size of the child, the wide-eyed look of fear and vulnerability on the face of the child, and the size of the bags of "chemo" looming above the child.

the report of the Consensus Conference on Pediatric Cancer Pain,[26] rather than asking children about improvement in pain relief, as is often done with adults, they should be asked systematically for their pain intensity scores. In this way, patterns in pain escalation and relief can be closely monitored.

The type of self-report that is most appropriate for a given use depends, in part, on the child's cognitive level. Between the ages of 1.5 and 2.5 years, toddlers are able to identify and communicate the presence or absence of hurting, but more refined quantifications of levels of intensity are not usually possible.[26] By the age of 3 years, a variety of instruments of a concrete nature can be used to measure pain intensity, with most involving pictures or objects with some relevance to pain or discomfort. By the age of 7 or 8 years, schoolagers are adequately adept at the use of numbers and more abstract words to rate the intensity of pain symbolically and numerically, such as with a 0–10 or 0–100 numerical scale or a verbal descriptor scale (Fig. 4–6). As children mature cognitively, they become able to use the scales developed for adults, such as the more abstract graphic rating scales, visual analogue scales (10 cm vertical or horizontal), and verbal rating scales (eg, mild, moderate, and severe). In summary, younger children are capable of indicating their level of hurt concretely, and the researcher or clinician then quantifies this indicator, whereas older children are able to quantify the level of their pain intensity by themselves. It should be noted that in the presence of illness, injury, or hospitalization, adolescents and children may regress[56], and more concrete tools may be necessary to obtain their pain intensity ratings during these periods.

Some of the most commonly used self-report measures include the following.

Eland's Color Scale/Body Outline[57]

Although validity has not been established for Eland's color scale, there appears to be clinical value in having children use the body outlines to indicate the location of pain and to color it according to the intensity experienced (Fig. 4–7, Table 4–2). In Eland's method, children first select four colors indicating four levels of hurt, from "no hurt" to "the worst hurt anybody could ever have."[58] They are then given these colors and asked to use them on body outlines (front and back views) to indicate the intensity for all pain experienced. Early work with the color scale and body outlines indicated that some children identified the presence of infection[9] and tumor metastases[59] before these disorders were diagnosed by the physician. Although the colors used by children could not be validated as a pain measurement device, the location of painful sites on body outlines has been supported by research. Of 172 4- to 10-year-old children studied by Eland, 168 correctly placed an "X" on a body outline.[9] Similarly, Savedra and Tesler[60] reported that in a study of 175 8- to 17-year-olds, 172 (98%) children correctly marked at least one pain site, and 140 (80%) marked all pain sites correctly. Correct location in both studies was evaluated by observation of the child's condition and review of the patients' records.

The Oucher

The Oucher (Fig. 4–8) is a self-report scale designed for use by 3- to 12-year-old children to measure pain intensity. It includes a 0–100 scale on the left for older children, and a six-picture photographic scale on the right for younger children. The six pictures are photographs of a 4-year old child after surgery in increasing levels of discomfort, from "no hurt" to the "biggest hurt you could ever have."

Content validity for the Oucher is supported by the findings of a study in which children were asked to sequence the photographs according to pain intensity.[61] Various forms of construct validity of the original (Caucasian) Oucher were supported when: 1) Oucher pain scores were found to vary in expected directions before and after surgery and analgesic administration;[29,30] 2) when pain scores were strongly and positively correlated[31] with pain scores on Hester's Poker Chip Tool;[32] and 3) when low to nonexistent correlations were found between Oucher pain scores and two measures of hospital fears.

No	Little	Medium	**Large**	**Worst**
Pain	Pain	Pain	**Pain**	**Possible**
				Pain

Figure 4–6. Word-graphic rating scale. The children are asked to make a mark on the line to indicate the intensity of their pain. The score is obtained by measuring with a metric ruler from the left side of the scale to the children's line. (Savedra M, Tesler M, Holzemer W, Wilkie D, Ward J: Testing a tool to assess postoperative pediatric and adolescent pain. In Tyler DC, Krane EJ (eds): *Advances in Pain Research and Therapy*, vol 15, p 87. New York, Raven Press, 1990).

Test-retest reliability was found to be adequate, using an indirect method (rating cartoon children in pain) of obtaining pain scores.[62] The difficulties of estimating reliability of actual pain on a single-item scale (like the Oucher) of a fluctuating variable (like pain) should be recognized.[63]

New Hispanic and African–American versions of the Oucher demonstrate adequate content validity in studies similar to those used with the original Oucher.[64,65] Content validity was further determined as adequate for the white, Hispanic, and African–American versions, using a coding method for facial expressions.[66] Studies of construct validity for the Hispanic and African–American versions are currently underway.

Hester's Poker Chip Tool

The Poker Chip Tool (PCT), first reported in 1979,[32] has been modified several times. Its final form includes the use of four red poker chips, each one representing "a piece of hurt," from "a little bit of hurt" to "the most hurt you could ever have."[33] Children are asked to indicate the intensity of their pain by selecting the number of poker chips that best represents "how many pieces of hurt you have."

Psychometric studies found PCT scores 1) varied in expected directions before and after surgery and analgesic administration;[29,30] 2) correlated strongly and positively with scores on the Oucher;[31] and 3) were unrelated to two measures of hospital fears.

Hester and colleagues[33] reported additional research that provides support for reliability obtained from a generalizability coefficient. This coefficient reflects the accuracy of generalizing from a score or observation to a universe of observations. Adequate support was also found for convergent validity, and partial support was obtained for discriminant validity. Validity was determined statistically based on criteria for the proportion of variance explained in pain ratings from subjects (children), parents, and nurses.

Facial Line Drawings

Several researchers have used line drawings of a series of faces as scales for the measurement of pain intensity in children.[49,67–69] The facial line-drawn scale of LeBaron and Zeltzer[67] included five faces, three of which were crying. As originally designed, the instrument was administered first, asking children how "scared" they were and then asking how much "hurting" they had. There were no findings to support the validity of the instrument as a measure of pain intensity, but it served to stimulate further the development of other instruments in an attempt to clarify the concept of pain intensity.

McGrath, de Veber, and Hearn,[34] and McGrath[40] (Fig. 4–9) developed a pain affect scale (nine facial drawings, including four positive, one neutral, and four negative) to be used in conjunction with a visual analogue scale to measure pain intensity. The faces scale was used to measure happiness and sadness associated with pain. The validity of this method of measurement is still under investigation.

Varni and colleagues[49] reported on a visual analogue scale for 5- to 15-year-olds with rheumatoid arthritis. This scale included a

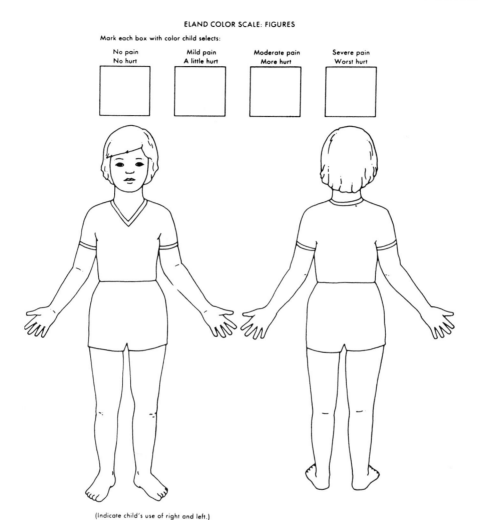

Figure 4–7. Eland's Color Scale. Instructions for use are in Table 4–2. (Cited in McCaffery M, Beebe A: *Pain: Clinical Manual for Nursing Practice*. St. Louis, The C.V. Mosby Company, 1989.)

happy face on the extreme left side and a sad face on the extreme right side of a 10-cm horizontal line positioned to imply a continuum. Children indicated the amount of their hurt by drawing a vertical line across the visual analogue scale; the child's pain score was obtained by measuring the distance in centimeters from the left side of the horizontal line. Construct validity was estimated as adequate

when positive correlations were found between pain scores and physicians' ratings of the activity of arthritic disease. Reliability was assessed as adequate when children could distinguish between present pain and the worst pain of the previous week.

Maunuksela and coworkers[68] introduced the use of two pediatric pain measurement devices in Finland. One was a five-face line

Table 4–2.
Eland Color Scale: Directions for Use

After discussing with the child several things that have hurt the child in the past:
1. Present eight crayons or markers to the child. Suggested colors are yellow, orange, red, green, blue, purple, brown, and black.
2. Ask the following questions, and after the child has answered, mark the appropriate square on the tool (*eg,* severe pain, worst hurt), and put that color away from the others. For convenience, the word "hurt" is used here, but whatever term the child uses should be substituted. Ask the child these questions:
   "Of these colors, which color is most like the worst hurt you have ever had, (using whatever example the child has given) or the worst hurt anybody could ever have?" Which phrase is chosen will depend on the child's experience and what the child is able to understand. Some children may be able to imagine much worse pain than they have ever had, whereas other children can understand only what they have experienced. Of course, some children may have experienced the worst pain they can imagine.
   "Which color is almost as much hurt as the worst hurt (or, use example given above, if any), but not quite as bad?"
   "Which color is like something that hurts just a little?"
   "Which color is like no hurt at all?"
3. Show the four colors (marked boxes, crayons, or markers) to the child in the order he or she has chosen them, from the color chosen for the worst hurt to the color chosen for no hurt.
4. Ask the child to color the body outlines where he or she hurts, using the colors chosen by the child to show how much it hurts.
5. When the child finishes, ask the child if this is a picture of how he or she hurts now or earlier. Be specific about what "earlier" means by relating the time to an event (*eg,* at lunch or in the playroom).

Reprinted with permission of JoAnn Eland, RN, PhD and publisher. From: McCaffery M, Beebe A. Pain: Clinical manual for nursing practice. St. Louis, C.V. Mosby Co., 1989.

drawing, and the other was a red wedge-shaped line on a white card (0–50 numeric scale); both were designed to represent increasing pain intensity. There were high correlations between these two self-report scales, thus suggesting their convergent validity. There were moderate correlations between behavioral pain assessment by the nurse and the self-report, thus suggesting construct validity. However, there was no report of the psychometric properties of the behavioral scale as a measure of pain.

A scale introduced by Bieri et al[69] includes nine line drawings of faces (Fig. 4–10). and is designed to measure pain intensity in children from 3 years of age and older. The authors reported a five-phase investigation designed to develop and examine the content validity, reliability, and scaling of the instrument in approximately 6- to 9-year-old children. In Phase I, 53 children drew faces according to their perceptions of changes that occur in expression from increasing levels of pain. Five adults with artistic abilities created five scales based on the children's drawings. In Phase II, 181 children ordered the five sets of faces from the most to the least painful. The final set of faces for the scale was determined from the set that received the most agreement for each position by the largest number of children. In Phase III, 240 children were given a 1-meter-long red wedge with the "no pain" and "most

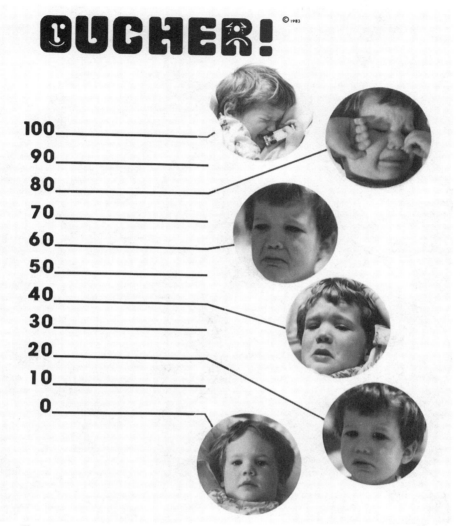

Figure 4–8. The Oucher, developed and copyrighted by Judith E. Beyer, RN, PhD, 1983. Children use either the numerical or photographic scale to indicate the intensity of their hurt.

pain" faces already mounted at the two ends. The children then positioned the remaining five faces on the wedge. The mean placement of pictures in centimeters was the interval between faces, and was compared with an "ideal" interval scale. Although these intervals were uneven, (from +2 to −7 cm "off" from an "ideal" interval scale), they were in the expected order, and, according to the au-

thors, the mean interval was a "good approximation to"[69] an interval scale. In Phase IV, the researchers had children reproduce a specific order of the nine pictures (half were in random order; half were in the correct order of increasing pain). Half and three-quarters of the sample were able to reproduce the pain order 2 hours after initial introduction and on the following day, respectively, as compared

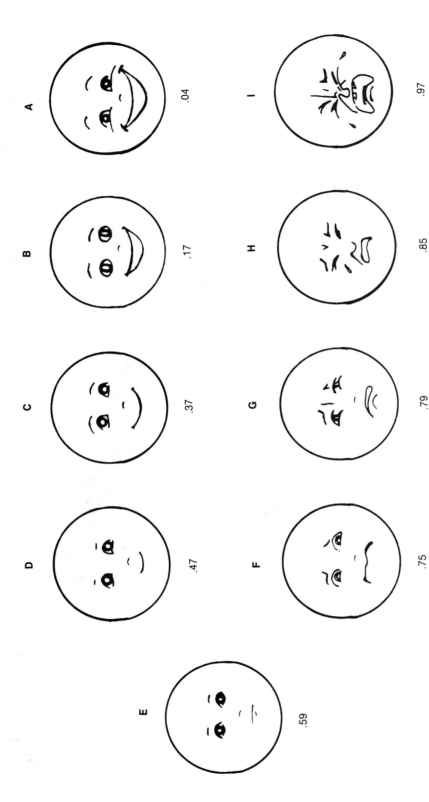

Figure 4–9. McGrath's faces scale of the affective dimension of pain in children. Children are presented with one of three different randomly ordered face sheets. They select the face that best represents how they feel in relation to their pain conditions, from "the happiest feeling possible" to the "saddest feeling possible." This figure is actually the scoring card used to quantify children's responses. The numbers represent the magnitude of pain affect (between 0 and 1) shown in each face based on previous research on children. (McGrath PA: *Pain in Children: Nature, Assessment, and Treatment.* New York, Guilford, 1990.)

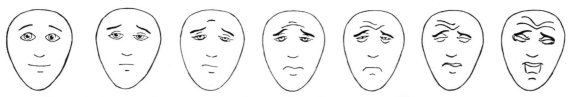

Figure 4–10. The Faces Pain Scale (Bieri D, Reeve R, Champion GD, Addicoat L, Ziegler J: The Faces Pain Scale for the self-assessment of the severity of pain experienced by children: Development, initial validation, and preliminary investigation for ratio scale properties. *Pain* 41:144, 1990).

with 16% and 0%, respectively, in the random order group. The authors concluded that subjects had a memory of the underlying theme of pain. This may be the case, or it may simply represent an ordering of intensity of any emotion. Fifty-eight percent of the subjects were able clearly to identify the expressions as physical or emotional pain/sickness. In Phase V, 35 6-year-olds were asked to rate the intensity of specific childhood pain experiences, using the faces scale twice (at a 2-week interval). The rank correlation coefficient (for test-retest reliability) was adequate, even when different investigators were involved in the data collection. The work to date is impressive, although construct validity studies to examine whether or not the scale actually measures pain intensity in children have yet to be reported. The authors suggest that it is questionable "whether the scale is specifically a measure of pain or pain affect, or whether it is a general measure of reaction to distress" (p. 146).[69] The authors contend that their scale does not confuse happiness and pain, like several of the other "smiley face" scales.

Other Pain Measures

Several other self-report scales have appeared recently that represent interesting, creative, and potentially useful methods to obtain children's self-reports of pain. Although promising, there is currently only limited empirical evidence to suggest that these instruments are valid measures of pain intensity. These include:

1. Molsberry's Hurt Thermometer[70]—Children are asked to move a red elastic strip on a vertical thermometer-like device to indicate 0–4 "degrees" of hurt.
2. The Ladder Scale[71,72]—Children are asked to rate the amount of their hurt by using a drawing of a nine-rung ladder.
3. The Squiggle Scale[73]—Children are asked to rate their pain (or fear) on the squiggle scale by selecting one of four different horizontally arranged lines (varying from a straight, flat line to a very wavy line).

In conclusion, a variety of methods has been used successfully with children to obtain their own descriptions and perceptions of their pain experience. These methods include verbal statements, verbal descriptors, pain diaries, pain maps, pain drawings, and pain intensity ratings.

BEHAVIORAL OBSERVATIONS

A variety of observational instruments has been developed to measure pain in children. These instruments include measures of behaviors indicative of pain and anxiety, based on the assumption that children experience a significant amount of anxiety in the presence of acute pain. The underlying concept has been labeled **behavioral distress**.[74,75] Three broad areas of behavior are typically included in the measurement of behavioral distress: communication (*ie*, vocalization and verbalization), facial expression, and motor movement. Because the method used in these instruments is observation, inter-rater reliability is essential to ensure consistency of measurement. Internal consistency is also relevant for behavioral distress scores that are derived from the sum of ratings on individual behavioral items. Construct validity has been determined primarily by examining the correlation between behavioral distress and self-reported pain and anxiety (described above), and between behavioral distress and observer-rated pain and anxiety (described below).

The age and developmental level of the child determine the type and magnitude of behaviors exhibited. As children develop, behavioral responses to aversive stimuli become more discreet, directed, and controlled. In infants, behavioral measures of pain include cry patterns[76-79] and reflex responses to inflicted pain.[80] Reliable changes in infant facial expression in response to aversive stimuli have been reported and appear to be the most valid indicator of pain/distress in this age group.[79,81-83] Infants learn to anticipate pain over the first year of life,[84] and with development, motor movements in response to nociception become more purposeful.[84,85] Verbal (as opposed to vocal) response to pain occurs around the 18th month.[85] The magnitude and variety of behaviors exhibited to aversive stimuli decrease between the ages of 6 and 7,[86,87] and the type of behaviors exhibited changes around the age of 10.[67] Adolescents, who have greater behavioral control, respond to pain in a more restrained, "adult-like" manner. Because of this, behavioral items used in scales to measure distress in adults may be applied to adolescent children.

Behavioral instruments have been developed for the purpose of assessing pain that arises from three sources: tumor invasion, therapy, and procedures. There is a considerable degree of overlap among these measures, particularly between measures to assess therapy- and procedure-related pain. Anxiety is a common response to both of these sources of acute pain. In addition, pain related to therapy and procedures may be perceived as beneficial, because cure or symptom relief is the goal. Tumor-related pain may be experienced for a longer duration with less expectation of

resolution. Therefore, tumor-related pain in terminal children tends to be associated more closely with depression,[88] and may be less willingly tolerated.[25]

Tumor-Related Pain

Pain arising from tumor invasion accounts for almost 50% of the pain experienced by hospitalized children with cancer.[5] Cancer is a heterogeneous disease, and as such, tumor-related pain can involve multiple organs, sites, and qualities of pain. Therefore, appropriate measures of this type of pain will necessarily be broad and general.

The Gustave–Roussy Child Pain Scale. Gauvin-Piquard and colleagues[88] have developed the only reported instrument that measures behavioral distress in children with tumors. Sixteen behaviors reflecting pain, anxiety, and depression were initially included in this scale. The final version of this scale includes 10 behaviorally defined items (Table 4–3), five reflecting pain, two reflecting anxiety, and three reflecting depression (written communication, Annie Gauvin-Piquard, 1991). The child is observed over a 4-hour interval using a five-point response format. This scale was initially tested on young children (2–6 years), and as a result, its applicability to older children has not been empirically demonstrated. Construct validity and internal consistency of this instrument were supported by the identification of three factors congruent with the underlying concepts of pain, anxiety, and depression. Inter-rater reliability was not reported. It is interesting to note that in their sample, pain and depression, but not anxiety, were highly intercorrelated. In contrast to acutely painful interventions (eg, BMA and LP), pain and anxiety were not correlated in this sample, suggesting that children with a life-threatening disease respond to pain in a distinct manner.

Therapy-Related Pain

A variety of instruments has been developed to measure postsurgical pain in children. These measures are readily adapted to chil-

Table 4–3.
The Gustave–Roussy Child Pain Scale*

Factor	Items†
Pain	Antalgic rest position
	Spontaneous protection of painful areas
	Anatalgic behavior during movement
	Control exerted by child when moved
	Reactions when painful areas are examined
Expression of Pain	Somatic complaints
	Child points out painful areas
Psychomotor Atonia	Lack of expressiveness
	Lack of interest in surroundings
	Slowness and infrequency of movements

* Written communication, Annie Gauvain-Piquard, 1991.
† Six items deleted from original scale.

dren with cancer who undergo surgery as part of their treatment. With some modification, behavioral items from these scales may be used to assess acute pain arising from other aspects of therapy, such as mucositis and radiation dermatitis.

Postoperative Infant Behavior. Attia and colleagues[89] described a nine-item observation scale, using a three-point response format, to measure postsurgical pain in infants (1–7 months). Behavioral items include the presence of sleep, quality of cry, and response to voice. Inter-rater reliability and internal consistency of this scale were not reported. Construct validity was supported in that infants who received fentanyl after surgery were rated as being more comfortable (ie, less pain observed) on the observation scale than infants who did not receive analgesics.

Infant–Toddler Behavior. Mills[85] described an instrument to measure acute pain behavior in infants (0–36 months). The types of behaviors identified included motor movement, communication, and facial expression, but varied according to the developmental level of the infant. Observations were made over a 30-minute period, and were coded in 1-minute segments. Inter-rater reliability of the instrument was adequate. Mills acknowledges

her work has not yet evolved into a well-developed and validated instrument. It is, however, promising in the context of behavioral pain measurement in infants and toddlers.

Children's Hospital of Eastern Ontario Pain Scale (CHEOPS). The CHEOPS was developed to measure postsurgical pain in children aged 1 to 7 years.[90] The six behaviors on the CHEOPS (Table 4–4) are rated using a four-point response format indicating increasing discomfort. Each level in the four-point response format is operationally defined, which increases consistency in scoring among observers. Inter-rater reliability ranged from 90% to 99% agreement between raters. Validity of the CHEOPS was supported by strong associations found between behavioral distress and independent observer rating of pain, and the significant reduction in behavioral scores following narcotic administration. More recently, Beyer, McGrath, and Berde[91] noted that children who reported moderate to high levels of postoperative pain inhibited their behavioral responses, thus producing "flat" CHEOPS scores. This reduction in behavior in the presence of moderate to severe pain raises questions about the sensitivity and validity of this scale during the early postoperative recovery period (within 36 hours after

Table 4–4.
Children's Hospital of Eastern Ontario Pain Scale (CHEOPS)*

Item	Score	Behavior†
Cry	1	No cry
	2	Moaning
	3	Crying
	4	Scream
Facial	0	Smiling
	1	Composed
	2	Grimace
Child verbal	1	None
	1	Other complaints
	2	Pain complaints
	2	Both complaints
Torso	1	Neutral
	2	Shifting
	2	Tense
	2	Shivering
	2	Upright
Touch	1	Not touching
	2	Reach
	2	Touch
	2	Grab
Legs	1	Neutral
	2	Squirming/kicking
	2	Drawn up/tense
	2	Standing
	2	Restrained

* McGrath PJ, Johnson G, Goodman J et al: CHEOPS: A behavioral scale for rating postoperative pain in children. In Fields H, Dubner R, Cervero F (eds): Advances in Pain Research and Therapy, vol 9, p 398. New York, Raven Press, 1985.
† Each level of behavior is operationally defined; see source.

discharge from the recovery room). It also supports the necessity of using multiple methods to measure pain in children to assess their pain experiences accurately.

Summary Scale of Distress Behavior. Maunuksela and colleagues[68] developed an instrument applicable to children aged 2 to 18 years. Subjects were globally rated on a 10-point scale, based on observation of behaviors such as movement or rigidity of limbs, irritability, and cardiovascular response. This behavioral instrument differs from those previously reviewed in that a single score is obtained that summarizes varying levels of behavior on all observation items. Inter-rater reliability was not reported. Construct validity was supported by the correlations found between the behavioral measure and various self-report measures of pain.

Observational Pain Scale (OPS). The OPS was developed to measure pain in adolescents.[92] This five-item scale uses a three-point response format. The OPS includes a physiologic item, blood pressure, in addition to behavioral items indicative of pain. No reliability data have been reported. The strength of the association between the OPS score and self-reported pain increased as the level of reported pain increased. Thus, in adolescents, behavioral distress is a better indicator of pain that occurs at moderate to severe levels. This is in contrast to the findings of Beyer et al,[91] using the CHEOPS in a younger population.

Procedure-Related Pain

The majority of instruments developed to measure procedure-related pain focus on responses to bone marrow aspiration (BMA), a common procedure in children undergoing cancer treatment. In addition, instruments that may be applicable to procedure-related pain in children with cancer have been described to measure behavioral distress in response to other aversive procedures, such as lumbar puncture (LP) and venipuncture.

Pain Behavior Rating Scale (PBRS). The PBRS was developed to measure responses to BMA in children from 8 months to 18 years.[74] This 13-item scale, with a binary (0,1 coding) response format, was used to record behaviors during four phases of the procedure: two anticipatory phases (called from waiting room, entering procedure room), an intraprocedural, and a recovery phase. Inter-rater reliability and internal consistency of the PBRS were found to be adequate.[74,93] In initial testing, the behavioral distress score obtained from the PBRS significantly correlated with an independent observer's rating of distress, indicating construct validity of the distress score.

Katz et al[74] reported age and gender differences on the PBRS. Young children (1–6.4 years) exhibited significantly greater behavioral distress at all four phases of the procedure when compared to the older children (10–18 years). The young school-aged children (6.6–9.1 years) exhibited distress similar to the older children during the anticipatory and recovery phases, but distress equal to the young children during the procedure. These age differences were replicated in a sample of Dutch children,[93] and in children undergoing venipuncture.[94] An analysis of gender differences revealed that girls expressed greater distress in the recovery phase than did boys. No gender differences were found in the anticipa-

tory or procedure phases.[74] Van Aken et al[93] found that boys exhibited less anticipatory distress at an earlier age than did girls. Jacobsen et al,[94] in a more restricted age sample (3–10 years), found no gender differences on the PBRS.

Observation Scale of Behavioral Distress (OSBD). Jay et al[86] modified the behavioral items and response format of the PBRS in their OSBD. The initial scale contained 11 items with a binary response format; in the revised scale 8 behaviorally defined items were retained[87] (Table 4–5). Jay et al retained the four observation phases, but used a time sampling technique of continuous 15-second segments within each phase to produce a frequency score for each behavior. The behaviors are weighted by their intensity to provide a more sensitive measure of behavioral distress. Inter-rater reliability and internal consistency of the OSBD were adequate.[87] Construct validity was supported by moderate to strong correlations between behavioral distress and self-reported pain,[86,87,95] parent ratings of their child's anxiety,[87] and nurse ratings of the child's distress.[87,95] Pulse also correlated with behavioral distress during the procedure, further supporting the construct validity of the instrument.[96] The age differences in behavioral distress reported by Katz et al[74] were replicated in this sample,[86] but no gender differences were found.

Procedure Behavior Checklist (PBCL). The PBCL was also developed to measure behavioral distress during BMA.[67] This is a nine-item scale that uses a five-point intensity rating format. The behavioral items on the PBCL are similar in content to the OSBD and PBRS. One rating is made for each of three phases: anticipatory, intraprocedural, and recovery. Inter-rater reliability was adequate; internal consistency was not reported. A moderate correlation was found between behavioral distress and self-reported anxiety in the anticipatory phase, and between self-reported pain and anxiety in the procedural phase of the BMA. Behavioral distress scores obtained on the PBCL also correlated with an independent

Table 4–5.
Observational Scale of Behavioral Distress—Revised (OSDB)*

Behavior	Definition
Information seeking	Any questions regarding medical procedure
Cry	Onset of tears and/or low-pitched nonword sounds of more than 1-second duration
Scream	Loud, nonword, shrill vocal expressions at high pitch intensity
Physical restraint	Child is physically restrained with noticeable pressure and/or child is exerting bodily force, and/or child is exerting bodily force and resistance in response to restraint
Verbal resistance	Any intelligible verbal expression of delay, termination, or resistance
Seeks emotional support	Verbal or nonverbal solicitation of hugs, physical or verbal comfort from parents or staff
Verbal pain	Any words, phrases, or statements in any tense that refer to pain or discomfort
Flail	Random gross movements of arms, legs, or whole body

* Elliott C, Jay S, Woody P: An observation scale for measuring children's distress during medical procedures. J Pediatr Psychol 1987;12:546.

observer's rating of pain and anxiety at all three phases of the procedure.

LeBaron and Zeltzer[67] found, consistent with previously reported studies, that older children (10–18 years) exhibited fewer distress behaviors during the BMA than younger children. There were no age-related differences in distress in the anticipatory and recovery phases, and there were no gender differences found in this sample.

Behavioral Distress During Venipuncture. Carpenter[73] developed an instrument to measure behavioral distress in children undergoing venipuncture. This instrument includes physiologic manifestations of pain/anxiety, in addition to communication, facial expression, and body movement. Responses are scored in a binary format over the course of the venipuncture. Reliability data were not reported for this instrument. Construct validity was supported by the correlations found between behavioral distress and an independent observer's rating of the child's fear. No age or gender differences were noted in this sample, which may be related to the narrow age range of the children (4–8 years).

CHEOPS Applied to Brief Pain. The CHEOPS was recently applied to children aged 3 to 17 years during venipuncture.[97] Children were observed using time sampling before and during venipuncture for the six behaviors included in the CHEOPS (see Table 4–5). Correlations among behavioral distress, nurse-rated distress, and self-reported pain provided support for the construct validity of the use of this instrument in this setting. Consistent with previous research, younger children (3–6 years) were more behaviorally distressed before and during the aversive procedure than older (7–17 years) children. Age was the most important predictor of both behavioral distress and self-reported pain in this sample of children. No gender differences were noted. This study indicates the applicability of the CHEOPS, an instrument originally developed for measurement of postoperative distress, to a brief procedure associated with moderate and momentary pain.

Modified Frankl Behavior Rating Scale. Frankl's behavior rating scale was developed to measure distress in children undergoing dental procedures.[98] This five-point scale has been modified[99] and tested in children receiving injections.[96,100] In Broome's modification,[100,101] each point on the scale is precisely

Table 4–6.
Modified Frankl Behavior Rating Scale*

Score	Behavioral Definition
1	Definitely positive: Good rapport with operator, no signs of fear, interest in procedures and appropriate verbal contact
2	Slightly positive: Cautious acceptance of treatment, but with some reluctance, questions, or delaying tactics; moderate willingness to comply with nurse, at times with reservation, but follows direction
3	Neutral: No expression on face, no physical sign of acceptance or resistance
4	Slightly negative: Minor negativism or resistance (accessible to treatment techniques), minimal to moderate reserve, fear, nervousness, or crying
5	Definitely negative: Refusal of treatment, overt resistance and hostility, extreme fear, forceful crying, massive withdrawal and/or isolation

* Broome R, Endsley R: Parent and child behavior during immunization. Pain 1989;37:85.

defined to reflect increasing levels of distress (Table 4–6). Inter-rater reliability was adequate for both modifications of the behavior rating scale.[96,100] Gonzalez et al[96] found a significant correlation between the scores of the modified Frankl scale and the OSBD, providing support for the construct validity of both scales. Construct validity was partially supported in that, in 4- to 8-year-olds, more distress was observed during injection when a parent was present than when parents were absent.[96] Broome and Endsley[100] found that maternal behavior and anxiety were not consistently related to the child's behavioral distress during the procedure. However, the lack of findings may be related to methodologic difficulties rather than a lack of construct validity of the modified scale. Further research is necessary to determine the construct validity of this behavioral scale.

PHYSIOLOGIC MEASURES

Although a variety of physiologic parameters has been measured in both clinical and research settings in an attempt to characterize better the experience of pain in children, none has been shown consistently to vary with fluctuations in self-reported pain intensity. Clinically, it has been assumed that vital signs, such as heart rate, respirations, and blood pressure would correlate positively with the level of pain the child experiences. This has not, however, been demonstrated in empirical studies. As noted by McGrath,[39] "As yet, there are no physiological responses that directly reflect the child's perception of pain." Clinically, it is useful to observe these variables in conjunction with others; however, changes in these parameters occur with other psychophysiologic events, such as fear, anxiety, apprehension, upset, and distress, as well as with physiologic events, such as fluid overload, hypoxia, and allergic reaction to medications. In addition to traditional vital signs, other parameters that have been measured in conjunction with infant/child pain, including serum beta endorphin levels, palmar sweat or skin conductance levels, skin temperature, transcutaneous oxygen levels, and plasma cortisol levels. Although the concept of searching for objective pain indicators is clinically and empirically interesting, consistency in methodology or findings has not been demonstrated, and as a result conclusions about physiologic concomitants of pain, at this point, remain tentative.

CONCLUSIONS

Recent advances in the study of pediatric pain measurement have enhanced the value of clinical pain assessment. Because of the frequent occurrence of pain in the child with cancer, potentially arising from a variety of sources, careful monitoring of the intensity of these experiences is essential. Health care professionals need to use the most appropriate methods of assessing children's pain, which includes selecting instruments that provide valid and reliable information. A variety of self-report and behavioral observation instruments is available for children of varying stages of cognitive development; those most developmentally appropriate for the particular child should be selected. Equipped with this knowledge, the health care professional can more appropriately prescribe and evaluate treatment for pain in children with cancer.

Because pediatric cancer pain is complex, multidisciplinary approaches to pain assessment and management are most productive. No single discipline alone can solve the many problems that arise as a result of cancer pain. The physician is in a key position to work toward the development of pain teams[102] on which a variety of health care professionals serve.

The use of self-report measures demonstrates that health providers value the child's explanation of his or her own experience. These data are necessary to evaluate the effects of pain-relieving interventions, and help guide therapeutic decision making. After adequate orientation and instruction, pain scores can be obtained in only a few seconds from the child.

Behavioral observations pose greater difficulty for clinical use because of the necessity of establishing inter-rater reliability and making repeated observations over a specific time period. Observations of pain behavior, however, are important adjuncts to the child's self-report. Observation instruments have been developed that measure behavioral distress in children with cancer pain. There is widespread agreement that the broad areas of behavior measured include communication, facial expression, and motor movement. Selection of a behavioral instrument for clinical use depends on multiple factors, such as the source of cancer pain, the age and developmental level of the child, and the degree of precision and accuracy desired.

The instruments themselves must be used properly, that is, in the way in which they were designed and for the intended age group. If self-report instruments are used, children need to be shown how to use them through careful and age-appropriate explanation, and need to be given an opportunity to practice. Parents should be encouraged to allow the child to provide their own scores without parental influence. If behavioral measures are used, attention must be paid to the reliability of those doing the ratings and to the specifics of time sampling procedures.

One of the most important aspects of assessing pediatric pain is the integrated use of multiple methods of measurement. In this way, a comprehensive profile of the child's pain is obtained, which facilitates more individualized and effective treatment. At the minimum, essential information includes obtaining self-report and behavioral data. Both McGrath[40] and Varni and colleagues[49,103] strongly urge the use of multidimensional pain assessment to thoroughly investigate the child's pain complaint. Although this may not always be feasible in the acute care setting, it is particularly relevant for the child with recurrent or chronic pain. Thus, in addition to the child's self-report and behavioral observations, these authors recommend taking extensive pain histories and carefully assessing the child's cognitive, affective, socioenvironmental, medical, and biologic milieu from interviews with both the child and his or her parents. Further, detailed evaluation information about the efficacy of the treatment for the child's pain is also obtained.

The variety of self-report and behavioral instruments available today for the assessment of pain reflects the degree of interest and activity in pediatric pain. Despite this intense activity and many recent advances in the field of pediatric pain, McGrath[1] reminds us that although we are off to a "good start," there is still much to accomplish before a solid scientific base is well established. It is our challenge to use this scientific base in our continuing efforts to enhance pain control for children with cancer.

REFERENCES

1. McGrath PJ: Paediatric pain: A good start. Pain 1990;41:253.
2. Schechter N, Altman A, Weisman S, eds: Report of the Consensus Conference on the Management of Pain in Childhood Cancer. Pediatrics 1990;86 (Suppl 5:2):813.
3. Spross J, McGuire D, Schmitt R: Oncology Nursing Society position paper on cancer pain: Part I. Oncology Nursing Forum 1990;17:595.
4. Spross J, McGuire D, Schmitt R: Oncology Nursing Society position paper on cancer pain: Part II. Oncology Nursing Forum 1990;17:751.
5. Miser A, Dothage J, Wesley R et al: The prevalence of pain in a pediatric and young adult cancer population. Pain 1987;29:73.
6. Cornaglia C, Massimo L, Haupt R et al: Incidence of pain in children with neoplastic diseases. Pain 1984;18 (Suppl 2):S28.
7. Beyer J, DeGood D, Ashley L et al: Patterns of postoperative analgesic use with adults and children following cardiac surgery. Pain 1983;17:71.
8. Burokas L: Factors affecting nurses' decisions to medicate pediatric patients after surgery. Heart Lung 1985;14:375.
9. Eland J, Anderson J: The experience of pain in children. In Jacox AJ (ed): Pain: A Sourcebook for Nurses and Other Health Professionals p 453. Boston, Little, Brown, 1977.
10. Mather L, Mackie J: The incidence of postoperative pain in children. Pain 1983;15:271.
11. Schechter N: The undertreatment of pain in children. Pediatr Clin North Am 1989;15:1.
12. Schechter N, Allen D, Hanson K: Status of pediatric pain control: A comparison of hospital analgesic usage in children and adults. Pediatrics 1986;17:11.
13. Eland J: The role of the nurse in children's pain. In Copp L (ed): Recent Advances in Nursing: Perspectives on Pain, p 29. London, Churchill Livingstone, 1985.
14. Miser A, Miser J: The treatment of cancer pain in children. Pediatr Clin North Am 1989;36:979
15. Zeltzer L, LeBaron S: Hypnosis and non-hypnotic techniques for reduction of pain and anxiety during painful procedures in children and adolescents with cancer. J Pediatr 1982;101:1032.
16. Zeltzer L, Zeltzer P: Clinical assessment and pharmacologic treatment of pain in children: Cancer as a model for the management of chronic or persistent pain. Pediatrician 1989;16:64.
17. Zeltzer L, Altman A, Cohen D et al: Report of the subcommittee on the management of pain associated with procedures in children with cancer. Pediatrics 1990;86 (Suppl):826.
18. Steif B, Heiligenstein E: Psychiatric symptoms of pediatric cancer pain. Journal of Pain and Symptom Management 1989;4:191.
19. Jay S, Elliott C, Ozolins M et al: Behavioral management of children's distress during painful medical procedures. Behav Res Ther 1985;23:513.
20. Kuttner L: Management of young children's acute pain and anxiety during invasive medical procedures. Pediatrician 1989;16:39.
21. Meinhart N, McCaffery M: Pain: A Nursing Approach to Assessment and Analysis, p 11. Norwalk, CT, Appleton-Century-Crofts, 1983.
22. McCaffery M: Nursing Management of the Patient in Pain, 2nd ed. Philadelphia, JB Lippincott, 1979.
23. Beals J: Pain in children with cancer. In Bonica J, Ventafridda V (eds): Advances in Pain Research and Therapy, vol 2, p 89. New York, Raven Press, 1979.
24. Miser AW: Evaluation and management of pain in children with cancer. In Tyler DC, Krane EJ (eds): Advances in Pain Research and Therapy, vol 15, p 345. New York, Raven Press, 1990.
25. Jay S, Elliott C, Varni J: Acute and chronic pain in adults and children with cancer. J Consult Clin Psychol 1986;54:601.
26. McGrath PJ, Beyer J, Cleeland C et al: Report of the subcommittee on assessment and methodologic issues in the management of pain in childhood cancer. In Schechter N, Altman A, Weisman S (eds): Report of the Consensus Conference on the Management of Pain in Childhood Cancer. Pediatrics 1990;86 (Suppl 5:2):814.
27. Berde C, Ablin A, Glazer J et al: Report of the subcommittee on disease-related pain in childhood cancer. In Schechter N, Altman A, Weisman S (eds): Report of the Consensus Conference on the Management of Pain in Childhood Cancer. Pediatrics 1990;86 (Suppl 5:2):818.
28. Zeltzer LK, Altman A, Cohen D et al: Report of the subcommittee on the management of pain associated with procedures in children with cancer. In Schechter N, Altman A, Weisman S (eds): Report of the Consensus Conference on the Management of

Pain in Childhood Cancer. Pediatrics 1990;86 (Suppl 5:2):826.

29. Aradine C, Beyer J, Tompkins J: Children's perceptions before and after analgesia: A study of instrument construct validity. Journal of Pediatric Nursing 1988;3:11.

30. Beyer J, Aradine C: Patterns of pediatric pain intensity: A methodological investigation of a self-report scale. Clinical Journal of Pain 1987;3:130.

31. Beyer J, Aradine C: Convergent and discriminant validity of a self-report measure of pain intensity for children. Children's Health Care 1988;16:274.

32. Hester N: The preoperational child's reaction to immunizations. Nurs Res 1979;28:250.

33. Hester N, Foster R, Kristensen K: Measurement of pain in children: Generalizability and validity of the Pain Ladder and the Poker Chip Tool. In Tyler D, Krane E (eds): Advances in Pain Research and Therapy: Pediatric Pain, vol 15, p 79. New York, Raven Press, 1990.

34. McGrath PA, de Veber LL, Hearn MT: Multidimensional pain assessment in children. In Field H, Dubner R, Cervero F (eds): Advances in Pain Research and Therapy: Proceedings of the Fourth World Congress on Pain, vol 9, p 387. New York, Raven Press, 1985.

35. Hester N, Foster R, Beyer J: Clinical judgment in assessing children's pain. In Watt-Watson J, Donovan M (eds): Pain Management: Nursing Perspective. St Louis, C.V. Mosby Co., 1992.

36. Lavigne J, Schulein M, Hahn Y: Psychological aspects of painful medical conditions in children: I. Developmental aspects and assessment. Pain 1986;27:133.

37. McGrath PJ, Unruh A: Pain in Children and Adolescents. Amsterdam, Elsevier, 1987.

38. Ross D, Ross S: Childhood Pain: Current Issues, Research and Management. Baltimore, Urban and Schwartzenberg, 1988.

39. McGrath PA: An assessment of children's pain: A review of behavioral, physiological and direct scaling techniques. Pain 1987;31:147.

40. McGrath PA: Pain in Children: Nature, Assessment, and Treatment. New York, Guilford, 1990.

41. Gaes J: My Book for Kids with Cansur. Aberdeen, SD, Melius Publishing, 1987.

42. Krementz J: How it Feels to Fight for Your Life. Boston, Little, Brown, 1989.

43. Melzack R: The McGill Pain Questionnaire: Major properties and scoring methods. Pain 1975;1:277.

44. Savedra M, Gibbons P, Ward J et al: How do children describe pain? A tentative assessment. Pain 1982;14:95.

45. Savedra M, Tesler M, Ward J et al: How do adolescents describe pain? J Adolesc Health Care 1988;9:315.

46. Savedra M, Tesler M, Holzemer W et al: Testing a tool to assess postoperative pediatric and adolescent pain. In Tyler DC, Krane EJ (eds): Advances in Pain Research and Therapy: Pediatric Pain, vol 15, p 85. New York, Raven Press, 1990.

47. Tesler M, Ward J, Savedra M et al: Developing an instrument for eliciting children's description of pain. Percept Mot Skills 1983;56:315.

48. Tesler M, Savedra M, Ward J et al: Children's words for pain. In Funk S, Tornquist E, Champagne M et al (eds): Key Aspects of Comfort: Management of Pain, Fatigue, and Nausea. New York, Springer, 1989.

49. Varni J, Thompson K, Hanson V: The Varni/Thompson Pediatric Pain Questionnaire: Chronic musculoskeletal pain in juvenile rheumatoid arthritis. Pain 1987;28:27.

50. Wilkie D, Holzemer W, Tesler M et al: Measuring pain quality: Validity and reliability of children's and adolescents' pain language. Pain 1990;41:151.

51. Abu-Saad H: Toward the development of an instrument to assess pain in children: Dutch study. In Tyler D, Krane E (eds): Advances in Pain Research and Therapy: Pediatric Pain, vol 15, p 101. New York, Raven Press, 1990.

52. Abu-Saad H: Cultural components of pain: The Arab–American child. Iss Comp Pediatr Nurs 1984;7:91.

53. Abu-Saad H: Cultural components of pain: The Asian–American child. Children's Health Care 1984;13:11.

54. Abu-Saad H: Cultural group indicators of pain in children. Matern Child Nurs J 1984;13:187.

55. Feuerstein M, Dobkin P: Recurrent abdominal pain syndrome. In Gross AM, Drabman RS (eds): Handbook of Clinical Behavioral Pediatrics, p. 291. New York, Plenum, 1990.

56. Thompson RH: Psychosocial Research on Pediatric Hospitalization and Health Care: A Review of the Literature. Springfield, IL, Charles C Thomas, 1985.

57. Eland J: Minimizing pain associate with prekindergarten intramuscular injections. Issues in Comprehensive Pediatric Nursing 1981;5:361.

58. McCaffery M, Beebe A: Pain: Clinical Manual for Nursing Practice. St. Louis, CV Mosby, 1989.

59. Eland J: Pain in children. Presented at the NIH Consensus Development Conference: The Integrated Approach to Management of Pain, May 19–21, 1986, Bethesda, MD.

60. Savedra M, Tesler M: Assessing children's and adolescents' pain. Pediatrician 1989;16:24.

61. Beyer J, Aradine C: Content validity of an instru-

ment to measure young children's perceptions of the intensity of their pain. Journal of Pediatric Nursing 1986;1:386.

62. Belter R, McIntosh J, Finch A et al: Preschoolers' ability to differentiate levels of pain: Relative efficacy of three self-report measures. Journal of Clinical Child Psychology 1988;17:329.

63. Beyer J, Knapp T: Methodological issues in the measurement of children's pain. Children's Health Care 1986;14:233.

64. Denyes M, Villarruel A: Measurement of pain in Afro-American and Hispanic children. Presented at the First International Symposium on Pediatric Pain, July 22–24, 1988, Seattle, WA.

65. Villarruel A, Denyes M: Pain assessment in children: Theoretical and empirical validity. Advances in Nursing Science 1991;14:32.

66. Neuman B, Denyes M, Stettner L et al: Facial expression as an emotional response to pain: A study of instrument content validity. Pain 1990; (Suppl 5):S25.

67. LeBaron S, Zeltzer L: Assessment of acute pain and anxiety in children and adolescents by self-reports, observer reports, and a behavioral checklist. J Consult Clin Psychol 1984;52:729.

68. Maunuksela E, Olkkola E, Korpela A: Measurement of pain in children with self-reporting and behavioral assessment. Clin Pharmacol Ther 1987;42:137.

69. Bieri D, Reeve R, Champion D et al: The Faces Pain Scale for the self-assessment of the severity of pain experienced by children: Development, initial validation, and preliminary investigation for ratio scale properties. Pain 1990;41:139.

70. Molsberry D: Young children's subjective quantification of pain following surgery. Unpublished Master's Thesis, The University of Iowa, Iowa City, 1979.

71. Hay H: The measurement of pain intensity in children and adults: A methodological approach. Unpublished Master's Research Report, McGill University, Montreal, Quebec, 1984.

72. Jeans ME, Hay H, O'Brien C: Pain assessment in children and adults: A methodological study. Manuscript in preparation, 1992.

73. Carpenter P: New method for measuring young children's self-report of fear and pain. Journal of Pain and Symptom Management 1990;5:233.

74. Katz E, Kellerman J, Siegel S: Behavioral distress in children with cancer undergoing medical procedures: Developmental considerations. J Consult Clin Psychol 1980;48:356.

75. Katz E, Kellerman J, Siegel S: Anxiety as an affective focus in the clinical study of acute behavioral distress: A reply to Shacham and Daut. J Consult Clin Psychol 1981;49:470.

76. Fuller B: Acoustic discrimination of three types of infant cries. Nurs Res 1991;40:156.

77. Fuller B, Horii Y: Differences in fundamental frequency, jitter and shimmer among four types of infant vocalizations. J Commun Dis 1986;19:111.

78. Fuller B, Horii Y: Spectral energy distribution in four types of infant vocalization. J Commun Dis 1988;20:111.

79. Grunau R, Johnston C, Craig K: Neonatal facial and cry responses to invasive and non-invasive procedures. Pain 1990;42:295.

80. Franck L: A new method to quantitatively describe pain behavior in infants. Nurs Res 1986;35:28.

81. Grunau R, Craig K: Pain expression in neonates: Facial action and cry. Pain 1987;28:395.

82. Izard C, Huebner R, Riser D et al: The young infant's ability to produce discrete emotion expressions. Dev Psychol 1980;19:132.

83. Johnston C, Strata M: Acute pain response in infants: A multidimensional description. Pain 1986;24:373.

84. Craig K, McMahon R, Morison J et al: Developmental changes in infant pain expression during immunization injections. Soc Sci Med 1984;19:1331.

85. Mills N: Pain behaviors in infants and toddlers. Journal of Pain and Symptom Management 1989;4:184.

86. Jay SM, Ozolins M, Elliott C et al: Assessment of children's distress during painful medical procedures. Health Psychol 1983;2:133.

87. Elliott C, Jay S, Woody P: An observation scale for measuring children's distress during medical procedures. J Pediatr Psychol 1987;12:543.

88. Gauvain-Piquard A, Rodary C, Rezvani A et al: Pain in children aged 2 -6 years: A new observational rating scale elaborated in a pediatric oncology unit: Preliminary report. Pain 1987;31:177.

89. Attia J, Amiel-Tison C, Mayer M-N et al: Measurement of postoperative pain and narcotic administration in infants using a new clinical scoring system. Anesthesiology 1987;A32(3A):A532.

90. McGrath PJ, Johnson G, Goodman J et al: CHEOPS: A behavioral scale for rating postoperative pain in children. In Fields H, Dubner R, Cervero F (eds): Advances in Pain Research and Therapy, vol 9, p 395. New York, Raven Press, 1985.

91. Beyer J, McGrath PJ, Berde C: Discordance between self-report and behavioral pain measures in children aged 3–7 years after surgery. Journal of Pain and Symptom Management 1990;5:350.

92. Broadman L, Rice L, Hannallah R: Evaluation of an objective pain scale for infants and children. Reg Anaesth 1988;13:45.

93. van Aken M, van Lieshout C, Katz E et al: Development of behavioral distress in reaction to acute pain in two cultures. J Pediatr Psychol 1989;14:421.

94. Jacobsen P, Manne S, Gorfinkle K et al: Analysis of child and parent behavior during painful medical procedures. Health Psychol 1990;9:559.

95. Jay SM, Elliott C: Behavioral observation scales for measuring children's distress: The effects of increased methodological rigor. J Consult Clin Psychol 1984;52:1106.

96. Gonzales J, Routh D, Saab P et al: Effects of parent presence on children's reactions to injection: Behavioral, physiological, and subjective aspects. J Pediatr Psychol 1989;14:449.

97. Fradet C, McGrath PJ, Kay J et al: A prospective survey of reactions to blood tests by children and adolescents. Pain 1990;40:53.

98. Frankl S, Shiere F, Fogels H: Should the parent remain with the child in the dental operatory? Journal of Dentistry for Child 1962;29:150.

99. Shaw E, Routh D: Effect of mother's presence on children's reaction to aversive procedures. J Pediatr Psychol 1982;7:33.

100. Broome M, Endsley R: Parent and child behavior during immunization. Pain 1989;37:85.

101. Broome M: Parental presence, childrearing practices, and child medical fears as predictors of young children's response to pain. Unpublished Doctoral Dissertation, University of Georgia, Athens, GA, 1984.

102. Berde C, Sethna N, Masek B et al: Pediatric pain clinics: Recommendations for their development. Pediatrician 1989;16:94.

103. Varni J: Behavioral management of pain in children. In Tyler DC, Krane EJ (eds): Advances in Pain Research and Therapy: Pediatric Pain, vol 15, p 215. New York, Raven Press, 1990.

Chapter 5

Behavioral Assessment of Pain and Behavioral Pain Management

Richard W. Millard

INTRODUCTION

The ideal armamentarium against cancer pain includes behavioral treatment methods. Such approaches have not been as widely implemented as pharmacologic or anesthetic/surgical treatment methods. This is in contrast to treatment for chronic nonmalignant pain, where behaviorally focused programs are commonly employed.[1] Although cancer pain has a clearer nociceptive basis, it is still a multidimensional process, and thus potentially mediated by behavioral factors.[2-4]

The primary goal of this chapter is to address this gap by reviewing programs of assessment and treatment that are influenced by findings from behavioral research. This frame of inquiry includes both cognitive (intellectual) and affective (emotional) processes that may be modified to potentially reduce pain and suffering. A secondary goal is to review obstacles that can arise in implementing effective behavioral pain management programs.

How different is cancer pain? Turk and Fernandez[2] challenge the assumption that reports of such pain are simply a direct manifestation of tissue damage, and suggest that expectancy, distress, placebo, and behavioral variables can each make important contributions. The relationship between distress and pain intensity is virtually the same for cancer pain and chronic nonmalignant pain.[5] Spiegel and Bloom[6] reported that a significant amount of pain in patients with metastatic breast cancer could be accounted for by mood and beliefs about pain.

This parallels findings derived from patients with nonmalignant pain, whose experience of pain and disability has been closely linked to psychological variables.[7] Collectively, these results form a cogent argument against the "putative uniqueness"[2] of cancer pain, and suggest that there is little merit in conceptualizing it as an entirely biomedical concern.

The distinction between acute and chronic pain, which is critical to treatment planning for nonmalignant conditions, becomes less clear for cancer pain. Features of both types of pain are present. Like in acute pain, there is an easily discernible sensory–physiologic process that produces nociception and helps to explain why pain occurs. Cancer pain frequently continues for more than a few months, however, and is thus accompanied by profound changes in mood and behavior.[8] This introduces a range of psychological factors that can contribute to the experience of pain. It is well known that patients exhibit varying responses to pharmacologic, anesthesiologic, or surgical interventions. Behavioral methods can contribute greatly to overall pain management by both serving to help explain variations in response to treatment, and by exerting a salutary effect when behavioral variables are major contributors to pain and suffering.

The behavioral interventions that have been devised for patients with symptomatic cancer more frequently seek to reduce procedure-related symptoms[9] than to improve overall adjustment to the course of the illness. This chapter will emphasize the latter strategies, highlighting those approaches that aim to maintain quality of life by reducing pain and associated suffering. Many of the interventions that are reviewed in this chapter have potential value in treating pediatric cancer pain (see Chapters 4 and 28). Unlike adults, children are less likely to have pain resulting from solid tumors, and this may change the nature of pain that is experienced.[8] In addition, children assign different meanings to pain,[10] and, depending on their verbal skills and prior experience, are likely to use different means to convey distress. The general framework of assessment and treatment, however, is similar for children and adults.

ASSESSMENT

Comprehensive assessment necessarily precedes any treatment, because it helps reveal the extent to which pain may be influenced by physiologic, behavioral, cognitive, or affective variables. These four areas serve as a useful framework for organizing information that is collected during the evaluation. This section will review assessment methods in each area; examples are shown in Table 5–1.

A standardized approach to assessment is preferred. This helps to achieve reliability by controlling for differences that may exist between interviewers, and aids in drawing accurate comparisons among patients. Unless noted to the contrary, each of the measures that are listed in this section have been shown to possess attributes of reliability and validity when used with medical populations. When possible, specific information about applications in patients with cancer pain are noted.

The accuracy of findings derived from conventional psychological assessment procedures may be confounded by the presence of illness. Any measure that is used must allow for the possible presence of other symptoms that can interfere with the assessment process. For instance, the Minnesota Multiphasic Personality Inventory (MMPI), which is widely used in evaluation of nonmalignant chronic pain, may not be appropriate for many patients with cancer. The presence of fatigue, active disease processes, and ongoing drug treatment may limit the patient's ability to complete testing, or may result in invalid findings.

Omnibus pain questionnaires such as the McGill Pain Questionnaire or the Multiaxial Pain Inventory are overly long for some patients with cancer pain. The Wisconsin Brief Pain Questionnaire (BPQ)[11] is a shorter questionnaire devised specifically to assess patients with cancer pain, and has been subjected to careful psychometric analysis. The BPQ obtains information concerning pain intensity, beliefs about pain, and levels of associated disability. It is recommended when using the BPQ that supplemental information about mood or situational influences on pain

Table 5–1.
Multimodal Assessment of Cancer Pain

Area	Suggested Methods	Major Content Areas
Physiology	Clinical interview Review of medical record	Pain site Pain intensity Disease variables Medication usage
Behavior	Clinical interview Companion interview Functional assessment Direct behavioral observation	Temporal pattern of pain Pain behavior Disability Family variables Social history
Cognition	Clinical interview Neuropsychological screening Measures of appraisal/coping	Brain function Beliefs, expectancies Perceived meaning, controllability of pain

Affect	Clinical interview
	Measures of distress,
	  affective constraint
		Mood
		Fear, anxiety
		Isolation
		Ability to experience emotional
		  concerns

may be collected during the interview process.

The Varni Thompson Pediatric Pain Questionnaire is available for children, and has been formulated in separate versions for children, adolescents, and parents.[12] As this questionnaire was not specifically developed to assess cancer pain, its content, in some instances, may require modification.

Considerable care is necessary when preparing the patient for assessment. Eliciting the patient's awareness of the illness process is an important first step in establishing a relationship conducive to treatment. Contact with a psychologist or other mental health figure can be easily misunderstood. It may be necessary to dispel a sense of stigma that accompanies such an encounter, and to convey the clear message that the patient's symptoms are not being minimized in any way. Some patients may need encouragement to speak candidly and to resist the desire to appear stoic.

PHYSIOLOGIC VARIABLES

This phase of assessment is used to specify physiologic variables that might affect pain or influence the provision of behavioral therapies. Some patients seem reassured by beginning with an account of physical problems, because it allays concerns that pain is implicitly depreciated by the involvement of mental health personnel. This encourages the development of rapport, predicated on acceptance of the symptoms as genuine and worthy of attention.

The clinical interview is a primary tool used to acquire information about physiologic status. Its accuracy may be enhanced when it is augmented by a questionnaire such as the BPQ.[11] At the outset, inquiries can address specific pain characteristics, including site, onset and duration, and intensity. The common analogue method of measuring pain intensity on a scale from 0 to 10 (10 denoting highest intensity) is useful in documenting average or present pain intensity, and provides an index against which to measure treatment outcome. The pattern of medication use is one potentially important physiologic determinant of pain intensity. Depending on the patient's analgesic regimen, some degree of pain may occur in relation to the dosing schedule of narcotic or sedative/hypnotic medication,[13] relating to combined physiologic and expectancy effects.

BEHAVIORAL VARIABLES

The concept of pain behavior is central to assessment of pain. Because pain is an inherently subjective phenomenon, direct observations are limited to what the patient tells or shows the examiner. These actions are summarized as pain behavior, and may include visible signs of distress as well as withdrawal from family, friends, or society at large. Behavioral approaches are based on the assumption that pain behavior can be occasioned by historical events, beliefs about disease, or personal distress. The behavior may serve to avoid something, or it may serve to obtain something.[14] This mode of analysis is applied frequently in programs designed to manage nonmalignant chronic pain, and is theoretically applicable to cancer pain as well.[2]

The interviewer will wish to document pain behavior and its situational correlates. Are there certain activities or events that produce increased pain? What usually is done as a result? Does the patient have any conception of how pain may influence the actions, thoughts, or feelings of other people?

Inquiries about the pattern of pain can reveal information that is important for planning behavioral interventions. It may become apparent that pain is severe in anticipation of treatment-related procedures.[9,15] Pain that seems to occur most often in the presence of family members would suggest that the family setting is an appropriate focus of treatment. The occurrence of pain over time as the day progresses suggests that pain accompanies fatigue, and could be ameliorated to some ex-

tent by efforts to reduce stress. Concurrent personal stressors, often direct effects of the disease, may also be revealed as significant concerns.

The scope of inquiry can be broadened by adopting a social-learning perspective (ie, by inquiry about historical events). These could be remote in time, especially in instances where developmental trauma or childhood experiences have affected the manner in which the patient establishes relationships with other people.[16] In other instances, pain behavior may have been vicariously modeled, for instance in the case of a patient who has seen a spouse or family member experience pain in association with cancer.[3] These developmental concerns are broadly important within the behavioral analysis.

Because it is essentially an environmental assessment, an integral part of any behavioral interview consists of speaking individually with a companion of the patient. The information that emerges from this meeting is frequently useful. How does the companion know that the patient has pain? How does he or she react in response? What kinds of changes have been observed over the course of the problem? This individual may be more willing to discuss salient issues than the patient, who may feel obliged to remain taciturn or stoic. The companion interview can help to create a working relationship with other family members, who may then become actively involved in aspects of a behavioral treatment program.

An appropriate questionnaire can complement the structured behavioral interview. The Biobehavioral Pain Profile (BPP)[17] is a 57-item measure constructed to assess both situational and cognitive/affective influences on cancer pain. Other measures have been developed for assessing the behavioral impact of illness. The Sickness Impact Profile (SIP) is an example of a comprehensive measure whose psychometric properties have been amply recorded among groups with chronic illness.[18] It assesses both physical and psychosocial aspects of disability. The SIP takes an average of about 40 minutes to complete, however, and a briefer screening checklist such as the

Functional Assessment Screening Questionnaire[19] or Pain Disability Index[20] may be preferred. Pain behavior can also be observed directly, using methods to code the occurrence of guarded movement, grimacing, rubbing, verbalization, or other actions. This approach has proven useful in documenting pain behavior in patients with head and neck cancer pain,[21] as well as other malignancies.[22]

COGNITIVE VARIABLES

A broad array of topics is included in this area, all concerning ways in which pain may be modified by how the patient thinks.

The integrity of cortical function is of primary concern, not because this will determine pain, but more because it may affect the patient's capacity to engage in treatment. Delirium or dementia (see Chapter 14) can emerge in association with disease processes.[23] If there is reason to suspect that neurologic or cognitive abilities have been compromised, practical screening devices are available to assess for the presence of deficits. The widely used Folstein Mini Mental State grades cognitive status, and can be administered in about 5 minutes[24]; it primarily samples verbal and memory functions. The Cognitive Status Examination[25] also evaluates reasoning, motor, and spatial skills, while still maintaining brevity. A psychologist may assist in selecting portions of larger standardized instruments such as the Wechsler Memory Scale or Wechsler Adult Intelligence Scale as alternatives to a comprehensive neuropsychological assessment. Whereas cognitive loss does not preclude participation in a behavioral management program, formal thought disorder (eg, hallucinations, delusions) that emerges in connection with disease processes may be problematic. The occurrence of such thinking can usually be discerned during a clinical interview.

The basic goal in the cognitive phase of the evaluation is to identify patient beliefs regarding pain. Various descriptive models have been applied toward this task,[26] and these may guide the interviewer in eliciting salient information. Yalom[27,28] has documented clinical experiences with cancer patients, emphasizing the importance of affective concerns related to existence and death. An increased awareness of mortality may engender a reordering of priorities in life, and a renewed desire to live more fully for present needs. Taylor[29] cites concerns about meaning, mastery, and self-esteem as critical issues in coping with cancer. A cognitive model of information processing used by Leventhal[30] suggests that patients ordinarily comprehend illness as if it were acute, and cope according to "schema" that determine emotional responses. Other explanations also emphasize the interaction between cognitive and affective processes in determining how physical symptoms[31,32] and cancer pain[33] are experienced.

Lazarus and Folkman[34] describe a practical model of coping that can help in classifying how patients appraise or think about pain.[35] The most upsetting appraisals of pain seem to involve fear or perceptions that it is uncontrollable. Coping responses can be classified as emotional (blaming self, avoidance, wishful thinking), or may be focused on identifying resolutions. The Ways of Coping Checklist has been used to specify coping responses among patients with cancer[17] and other medical problems.[36] Another model seeks to classify patients as being "repressors," who minimize distress and behave passively, or "sensitizers," who are prone to adopt a more expressive and proactive approach to diversity. This individual difference has been investigated using measures such as scales from the Millon Behavioral Health Inventory, to study progression of cancer,[37] or the Taylor Manifest Anxiety Scale and Marlowe Crowne Social Desirability Scale, to study biochemical correlates of pain.[38] Other short measures evaluating appraisal and/or coping include the Biobehavioral Pain Profile (BPP)[17] (factors assessing loss of control and fear of pain), the Pain-Related Control Scale and Pain-Related Self-Statement Scale (PRCS, PRSS),[39] and the Vanderbilt Pain Management Inventory.[40] Of these, only the BPP has been designed specifically for cancer patients, although the others are potentially appropriate.

AFFECTIVE VARIABLES

It is affective (or emotional) variables that often precipitate a psychological evaluation. As with other areas, a structured clinical interview can be supplemented by scales or questionnaires. Within the clinical interview, it is advisable to screen for specific criteria of affective disorder. Depression, as a response to perceived loss, is perhaps the most logical correlate of cancer. In addition, chronic pain is frequently linked to depression.[41] Psychiatric criteria (DSM-IIIR) can be used to characterize affective disturbances, although some items may be spuriously endorsed due to the presence of other symptoms of cancer (such as fatigue, loss of sleep/appetite, etc.), rather than affective disorder. This may occur with symptoms of anxiety as well. The coexistence of affective variables may result in a cycle of anxiety, depression, and anger.[33]

The Center for Epidemiologic Studies Depression Scale[42] provides a separate score for somatic items, making it possible to eliminate those symptoms of depression that might be confused with manifestations of the primary disease. The Profile of Mood States (POMS) has been used in a number of studies to evaluate affective concerns among cancer patients.[5,43,44] It has the advantage of providing scores for the presence of tension, anger, and a high level of energy, in addition to states other than depression. Alternatively, the Hamilton scale[45] is available as a clinician-rating scheme. Its content can be modified by eliminating potentially confounding somatic items.[46]

Alexythymia is a construct that has been cited as an important affective variable among patients with physical disorders.[47] Taken literally from the Greek, this term means an inability to read ("alex") feelings or emotions ("thymia"). Dalton and Feuerstein[17] assessed alexythymia in cancer patients using the Schalling–Sifneos Personality Scale,[48] and found that it was associated with increased intensity of cancer pain. This phenomenon may also be present among patients who exhibit somatization or who characteristically amplify body sensations.[31] Standardized assessment of this construct has not proven to be a straightforward task, although the Toronto Alexythymia Scale[49] has accrued the most secure psychometric support to date.

Other affective concerns are even less readily assessed by standard questionnaires. These include feelings of isolation or abandonment, feelings of loss, anger, frustration with therapeutic failures, resentment of sickness, and other powerful emotions produced by the circumstances of illness. A proper clinical interview should be sufficiently unstructured so that inferences may be derived to verify the occurrence of such themes.

INTERVENTION

EDUCATIONAL APPROACHES

It is essential to allocate sufficient time before beginning treatment to make certain that treatment goals are consensually accepted. The patient, family, and other caregivers may be expecting that pain will be the primary focus of a behavioral program. In fact, the goals of treatment could alternatively include reduced suffering, improved quality of life, improved mood, or acquisition of more efficient coping skills. These objectives need to be discussed and understood in relation to the experience of pain, so that false expectations are not promoted. It is similarly advisable to discuss any beliefs that participation in behaviorally focused treatment will alter the disease process or prolong life. There is no solid evidence that attention to psychological processes exerts a curative effect,[50] and any impact on duration of survival may well be indirect.[51]

Turk and Rennert[52] recommend a preparatory pretreatment phase. This provides an opportunity to orient the patient away from being a passive recipient of treatment, and instills the notion that personal efforts can be applied toward learning to control pain. Behavioral methods are organized around the assumption that the patient can play an active role in changing the way that he or she responds to events, including pain. Some patients will resist even the most articulate descriptions of this principle, and thus are unlikely to prosper by treatment.

The educational approach is an extension of the evaluation phase, and is ideally conceptualized as the clinician and patient mutually investigating the pain, its meaning, and its effects. The therapist's assuming the role of a teacher or coach may help in fostering this alliance.[53] As with other diseases, the amount and quality of information that the patient possesses regarding the disease and its symptoms may have a bearing on how effectively he or she manages it.[30, 52] To this end, a tutorial format is sometimes well received because it provides a way to reduce uncertainties.

During the educational phase, discussions may cover distinctions between nociception and pain, and ways that pain can be multiply determined. A program of self-monitoring often helps the patient spontaneously to identify salient behavioral factors. The patient may begin to describe his or her own internal thought processes and recognize ways in which these thoughts influence pain or distress.[52] This process forms a basis for the development of cognitive-behavioral techniques.

Over the course of two or three meetings, sufficient ground may be covered for the patient to acquire a more sophisticated understanding of pain. This alone may yield reductions in distress, although it more frequently serves to prepare the patient for some of the discrete methods that follow.

BIOFEEDBACK

The goal of biofeedback treatment is to train a patient to modify physiologic activity. Respiration, muscular activity, temperature, skin conductance, or other variables are measured, and this information is made available to the patient, who then attempts to change thoughts or behavior in a way that results in a more quiescent physiologic state. The utility of biofeedback has been challenged on the basis that the mechanical paraphernalia that it employs may actually divert attention away from salient psychological topics.[54] At its best, this method can help a patient to develop an increased awareness of his or her potential to exert personal control over physical symptoms. Biofeedback seems to assist in reducing nonmalignant headache and facial pain,[55] yet there has been little extension of these protocols to patients with cancer pain. Fotopoulos and coworkers[56] applied a biofeedback protocol among seven cancer patients and reported modest benefit, although gains were not well maintained. In the case of cancer pain, they recommended that treatment be individually tailored to the site or characteristics of the disease process. Such limitations may account for the lack of findings from controlled investigations. Biofeedback remains a conceivably beneficial yet largely untested adjunct for certain patients.

RELAXATION METHODS

Relaxation approaches comprise a variety of techniques that are used to achieve simultaneous alterations in behavior, cognition, and physiologic activity. Relaxation methods stem from ageless Asian traditions of meditation that have been more recently subjected to empirical scrutiny and classification.[57] Four general types of relaxation methods may be distinguished, as represented in Table 5–2.

Progressive Muscular Relaxation

Progressive muscular relaxation is a structured process in which the patient alternately contracts and releases several muscle groups of the body.[58] Its rationale is that by increasing awareness of voluntary muscular activity, a more sedate mental state might be achieved. The exact therapeutic mechanism is not well understood, although this method has been employed with good results for managing headache[54] and procedure-related symptoms of cancer.[59,60] Although there is relatively less information about its application for ongoing cancer pain, this is frequently the most practical relaxation method to use, because it is easy to conduct and it can be comprehended by

Table 5–2.
Excerpted Instructions for Relaxation Methods

Progressive Muscular Relaxation

"Hold your hands out in front of you, but not so hard that they hurt. Study the tension in your hands and forearms. And now let go quickly. Relax your hands and let them rest at your sides. Note the difference between the tension and the relaxation."

Meditation

"Each time you exhale, think clearly to yourself of the word 'calm.' Let yourself become as relaxed as possible as you allow your breath to flow easily and gently through your body until I ask you to end this exercise. . ."

Autogenic Techniques

"I feel quite quiet."
"My whole body is quite heavy, comfortable, and relaxed."
"Warmth is flowing into my hands."

Imagery/Visualization

"Imagine you are beside a stream in the forest. It is a sunny day in the middle of June. Feel the sun on your skin. Hear the rhythm of the water flowing by. The stream is full of trout. . ."

---

patients who desire a structured or concrete process.

Meditative Techniques

These techniques have been promoted as a part of contemporary medical practice by Benson,[61] who used the expression "relaxation response" to describe a calm and receptive mental state that is achieved by resting in a quiet environment and focusing on an object or word. The patient is given minimal instructions, apart from being told to breathe slowly and to adopt a quiet or passive attitude. This technique's lack of formal structure may appeal to some patients, much as the perceived structure of progressive muscular relaxation appeals to others. There has been scant evaluation of this method as an approach for managing cancer pain, although it may modify pain by reducing anxiety.[62] It is difficult specifically to evaluate meditation because its basic elements, rest and diversion of attention, are common to other relaxation methods as well.

Autogenic Training

This approach makes uses of mental phrases to reduce sympathetic activity. After achiev-

ing a comfortable and relaxed position, the patient is typically asked to concentrate on feelings of warmth, heaviness, or slowed respiration or heart rate.[63] Statements such as "my legs are heavy and warm" or "my heartbeat is calm and regular" are mentally repeated.[57] Autogenic training tends to be offered as an adjunct to relaxation methods, for example in efforts to modulate immune function.[64] There is little evidence documenting its exclusive application for the management of pain.

Imagery

Imagery is frequently used as a component of autogenic training, as well as in a separate procedure. The patient is asked to create a vivid mental picture of a pleasant setting, such as a meadow or beach. Other applications involve more specific suggestions, for example that the patient concentrate on an image that symbolizes the disease process, and its subsequent modification.[65] Turk and Rennert[52] recommend using vivid images that will distract, if not necessarily relax, such as imagining that a succulent lemon is being sliced on a white china plate. In general, imagery material does not include direct references to pain. Pain-specific images may, however, be invoked during hypnotic procedures, techniques that have received relatively more attention as means to modify cancer pain.

The relative merits of these different approaches are difficult to determine because they share common features, that is, they involve producing a quiescent state and divert attention. In clinical practice, the individual patient's personal preferences may influence the selection of a relaxation method. Disease variables such as fatigue or cognitive status may also interfere with the implementation of a relaxation training program.

HYPNOSIS

The state of hypnosis is characterized by constrained attention, reduced physiologic activity, and heightened suggestibility.[66] Both anecdotal evidence[67] and limited findings from controlled research[51] support its utility for managing cancer pain. In one study, a program of self-hypnosis and group therapy reportedly achieved more favorable results than either self-hypnosis or group therapy applied alone in the management of pain secondary to metastatic breast carcinoma.[51] As with relaxation methods, it is difficult to equate hypnotic procedures across settings. Hypnosis can share many of the same features as relaxation programs, such as imagery, breathing exercises, or deep concentration. In a study designed to investigate the importance of assigning labels to therapy, Hendler and Redd[68] compared responses to equivalent treatments that were labeled as either hypnosis or relaxation. The study sample consisted of patients undergoing treatment intended to reduce procedure-related symptoms. Patients were more resistant to participating in hypnosis, and felt that it would be less useful than relaxation training. These findings exemplify certain popular beliefs that potentially can detract from the value of hypnosis for managing cancer pain. In contrast to relaxation methods, hypnosis is a less self-regulated approach. A hypnotic induction generally, if not always,

implies the need for an external figure or authority to conduct treatment. It may not be perceived as scientifically based, or may carry a surplus meaning of mysticism that might be counterproductive in some patients. There are likely to be persistent individual differences affecting one's ability to become absorbed in the process of hypnosis,[69] so that some patients could be less appropriate for this treatment than others.

COGNITIVE THERAPY

The utility of cognitive therapy methods has been increasingly emphasized for pain management,[70] although there are few controlled investigations of their application in cancer pain management. The approach is potentially useful in modifying appraisals of pain (ie, as threatening or uncontrollable), and in achieving more effective cognitive or behavioral coping strategies. Cognitive therapy is used to counter thoughts that contribute to depressed mood,[71] and its application may assist in achieving reduced suffering.

Various techniques are used as components of this kind of treatment, including diversion of attention or substitution of healthier thoughts and images.[70] Turk and Rennert[52] describe how these techniques can be applied in a multimodal program devised to manage cancer pain. Their approach begins with pretreatment preparation, which emphasizes educating the patient about pain, and which is intended to increase the patient's awareness of internal thought processes. In doing so, it should become apparent how pain intensity or suffering are adversely influenced by certain thoughts. The patient is instructed in a program of self-monitoring to track such patterns. During therapy sessions, the patient and therapist work together closely to reinterpret thoughts that accompany or precede episodes of pain and distress. Relaxation methods are offered as an adjunct to help divert attention away from somatic concerns, and to rehearse ways that physiologic arousal can be diminished. The program requires active involvement of the patient at multiple stages:

at identifying thoughts, completing home-work assignments, role-playing, or participating in other structured exercises. A unifying theme and overall objective in all these procedures is the achievement of an increased sense of self-mastery.

In an empirical study, Nehemkis and co-workers[72] evaluated attributions of pain among 25 patients with various cancer diagnoses. Cognitive reappraisals of pain were apparent, but these did not seem to affect pain intensity. Perceived control was regarded to be an important mediating variable. Although treatment was not rendered in this study, it stands out as a rare example of a controlled investigation of the kinds of thought processes that might be modified by the application of cognitive therapy for cancer pain.

GROUP OR FAMILY THERAPY

Although they are not strictly behavioral approaches, group and family methods may modify pain behavior. Yalom[27,73] details the methodology involved in employing a group format to elicit emotional expression and to improve how patients cope with cancer. Controlled research extending this approach[44] has found that weekly supportive group psychotherapy combined with "self-hypnosis" for pain resulted in beneficial outcomes. These were mostly measured in terms of prolonged survival, a finding that may be more directly attributable to increased compliance or involvement with regular oncologic care. Pain, depression, and anxiety were reduced by this approach, and quality of life was improved. Although the mechanism of these changes needs to be further specified, the findings point toward the potential value of group psychotherapy that seeks to modify the stigma of death or improve social integration. A common ingredient to this and cognitive methods is that both approaches seek to enhance perceptions of self-control in the face of perceived threat.

Other studies have used group treatment for patients with cancer, but have focused mostly on outcome variables other than ongoing pain and suffering, such as survival time[65] or the severity of procedure-related symptoms.[74]

Multimodal formats feature combinations of various treatments. For example, Simonton et al[65] employed a 5- to 10-day psychotherapy program that included group and individual counseling, in addition to training in use of self-regulated mental exercises (ie, progressive muscular relaxation, breathing exercises, imagery, etc.). This type of design makes it difficult to draw conclusions about what components of treatment are most influential. Pain may not be distinguished as a primary outcome variable within multimodal treatment. Similarly, it is not possible to cite systematic intervention for cancer pain that has specifically used family therapy methods, although family contact often occurs within the context of behavioral methods during the initial, educational phase of treatment.

IMPLEMENTING BEHAVIORAL PAIN MANAGEMENT PROGRAMS

There are practical reasons that serve to explain the relative paucity of studies describing behavioral management of cancer pain. Too often, treatment is offered when other approaches have failed or when disease-related habits and beliefs are entrenched and thus less responsive to modification. Late application of these methods will suppress their potential therapeutic power, especially because most of the interventions need to be devised prospectively.[52] It is often impractical to establish sophisticated skills-training programs during later stages of illness (see above).

The prospect of a behavioral program should be broached at the outset of any discussion about pain stemming from cancer. In addition to affording adequate time for the patient to learn pain-management skills, this action will convey the message that such treatment is acceptable and available.

Ahles[75] cites other disease variables that impede behavioral programs. Cancer is rarely static, and is a heterogenous disease. It consists of many types, with or without metastases, and cancer or its treatment may or may not impair cognition. Prognosis is variable and often unpredictable, resulting in attrition of subjects. Biomedical treatments are intensive, and may produce side effects that also hamper the implementation of a regularly scheduled behavior therapy routine. Pharmacologic agents can modify sensitivity to treatment.[75] All of these variables may combine toward delaying the implementation of well developed treatment programs, such as might be more readily available for more homogenous disorders. It may be advisable to conduct clinical studies with smaller and more precisely defined samples, perhaps using single-subject designs.[76] The Edmonton staging system for cancer pain[77] suggests variables that can be matched in order to achieve more meaningful comparisons.

In most health care settings, office procedures or facilities for care are not readily conducive to the establishment of behavioral programs. Even if treatment is rendered on an outpatient basis, there is likely to be a host of other concerns that may be competing for more immediate attention. Private space can be at a premium, especially in an inpatient setting, where the commotion of adjacent hospital activities makes relaxation methods unusually difficult to conduct. The patient is in essence confirmed in a clearly defined "sick" role, as the victim or object of treatment. This is incongruent with guiding assumptions of behavioral and cognitive approaches, which emphasize that the patient must take important actions on his or her own. In addition, some patients will prefer simply not to make use of a treatment approach that seeks to achieve self-regulation of symptoms.

Bonica[78] explains how traditional medical practice does not favor multidisciplinary models of care. However, cancer pain is poorly addressed in unilateral treatment. Unless all members of a treatment team have an understanding and commitment toward psychologically focused methods, the patient could simply perceive it as a treatment of exclusion or "last resort."[75] This undermines treatment efforts, and emphasizes the importance of achieving a consensual philosophy of care pervading the actions of everyone who is part of the multidisciplinary team. It is necessary to revise conceptions that cancer pain is somehow unique, or unworthy of psychological management.[2] The integrative model of Melzack and Wall[79] has emphasized that pain is an emotional, as well as sensory phenomenon.

CONCLUSION

The aim of this chapter has been to describe behavioral approaches that are potentially useful in the management of patients with cancer pain. Given the prevalence of such methods for other types of pain, this area seems to have been unjustifiably overlooked. In devising behavioral treatment, the assessment process necessarily includes careful analysis of physiologic, cognitive, and affective variables. It ordinarily consists of a structured interview, accompanied by carefully selected standardized questionnaires or tests. Interventions need to be devised prospectively, and are not limited to programs that seek to relieve pain. These may alternatively seek to modify beliefs or emotion, instill alternative coping strategies, or generally improve quality of life. The successful application of these approaches requires a supportive interdisciplinary context, as well as a curious and committed outlook by the patient.

REFERENCES

1. Turner JA, Clancy S, McQuade KJ et al: Effectiveness of behavioral therapy for chronic low back pain: A component analysis. J Consult Clin Psychol 1990; 58:573.
2. Turk DC, Fernandez E: On the putative uniqueness of cancer pain: Do psychological principles apply? Behav Res Ther 1990;28:1.
3. Dalton JA, Feuerstein M: Biobehavioral factors in cancer pain. Pain 1988;33:137.
4. Ahles TA, Blanchard EB, Ruckdeschel JC: Multidimensional nature of cancer pain. Pain 1983;17:277.
5. Schaham S, Reinhardt LC, Raubertas RF et al: Emotional states and pain: Intraindividual and interindividual measures of association. J Behav Med 1983; 6:405.

6. Spiegel D, Bloom JR: Group therapy and hypnosis reduce metastatic breast carcinoma pain. Psychosom Med 1983;45:333.
7. Smith TW, Follick, MJ, Ahern DK et al: Cognitive distortion and disability in chronic low back pain. Cognitive Therapy and Research 1986;10:201.
8. Jay SM, Elliott C, Varni JW: Acute and chronic pain in children with cancer. J Consult Clin Psychol 1986;54:601.
9. Morrow GR, Dobkin PL: Anticipatory nausea and vomiting in cancer patients undergoing chemotherapy treatment: Prevalence, etiology, and behavioral interventions. Clinical Psychology Review 1988; 8:517.
10. Thompson KL, Varni JW: A developmental cognitive-behavioral approach to pediatric pain assessment. Pain 1986;25:283.
11. Daut RL, Cleeland CS, Flanery RC: Development of the Wisconsin Brief Pain Questionnaire to assess pain in cancer and other diseases. Pain 1983;17:197.
12. Varni JW, Thompson KL: The Varni/Thompson pediatric pain questionnaire. Unpublished manuscript, 1985.
13. Portenoy R, Foley K: Management of cancer pain. In Holland JC, Rowland JH (eds): Handbook of Psychooncology, pp. 369–382. New York, Oxford, 1989.
14. Fordyce WE: Pain and suffering: A reappraisal. Am Psychol 1988;43:276.
15. Patterson KL, Ware LL: Coping skills for children undergoing painful medical procedures. Issues in Comprehensive Pediatric Nursing 1988;11:113.
16. Rowland JH: Developmental stage and adaptation: Adult model. In Holland JC, Rowland JH (eds): Handbook of Psychooncology, pp. 519–543. New York, Oxford, 1989.
17. Dalton JA, Feuerstein M: Fear, alexythymia and cancer pain. Pain 1989;38:159.
18. Bergner M, Bobbitt RA, Carter W et al: The Sickness Impact Profile: Development and final revision of a health status measure. Med Care 1981;19:787.
19. Millard RW: The functional assessment screening questionnaire: Application for evaluating pain-related disability. Arch Phys Med Rehabil 1989;70:303.
20. Tait RC, Pollard CA, Margolis RB et al: The Pain Disability Index: Psychometric and validity data. Arch Phys Med Rehabil 1988;68:438.
21. Keefe FJ, Brantley A, Manual G et al: Behavioral assessment of head and neck cancer pain. Pain 1985;23:327.
22. Ahles TA, Coombs DW, Jensen L et al: Development of a behavioral observation technique for the assessment of pain behaviors in cancer patients. Behavior Therapy 1990;21:449.
23. Fleishman S, Lesko SM: Delirium and dementia. In Holland JC, Rowland JH (eds): Handbook of Psychooncology. New York, Oxford, 1989.
24. Folstein MF, Fetting JH, Lobo A et al: Cognitive assessment of cancer patients. Cancer 1984;53:2250.
25. Barrett ET, Gleser GC: Development and validation of the cognitive status examination. J Consult Clin Psychol 1987;55:877.
26. Rowland JH: Intrapersonal resources: Coping. In Holland JC, Rowland JH (eds): Handbook of Psychooncology, pp. 25–43. New York, Oxford, 1989.
27. Yalom I. Existential Psychotherapy. New York, Basic Books, 1980.
28. Yalom I: Love's Executioner. New York, Basic Books, 1989.
29. Taylor SE: Adjustment to threatening events: A theory of cognitive adaptation. Am Psychol 1983;38: 1161.
30. Leventhal H, Nerenz DR: A model of stress research with some implications for the control of stress disorders. In Meichenbaum D, Jaremko ME (eds): Stress Reduction and Prevention, pp. 219–251. New York, Plenum, 1983.
31. Barsky AJ, Klerman GL: Overview: Hypochondriasis, bodily complaints, and somatic styles. Am J Psychiatry 1983;140:273.
32. Watson D, Pennebaker JW: Health complaints, stress, and distress: Exploring the central role of negative affectivity. Psychol Rev 1989;96:234.
33. Chapman CR: Psychologic and behavioral aspects of cancer pain. In Bonica JJ, Ventafridda V (eds): Advances in Pain Research and Therapy, vol 2, pp. 655–662. New York, Raven Press, 1979.
34. Lazarus RS, Folkman S: Stress, Appraisal, and Coping. New York, Springer, 1984.
35. Turner JA, Clancy S, Vitaliano PP: Relationship of stress, appraisal, and coping to chronic low back pain. Behav Res Ther 1987;25:281.
36. Vitaliano PP, Maiuro RD, Russo J et al: Raw versus relative scores in the assessment of coping strategies. J Behav Med 1987;10,1.
37. Goldstein DA, Antoni MH: The distribution of repressive coping styles among non-metastatic and metastatic breast cancer patients as compared to non-cancer patients. Psychology and Health 1989;3:245.
38. Jamner L, Schwartz GE, Leigh H: The relationship between repressive and defensive coping styles and monocyte, eosinophile, and serum glucose levels: Support for the opioid peptide hypothesis of repression. Psychosom Med 1988;50:567.
39. Flor H, Turk DC: Chronic back pain and rheumatoid arthritis: Predicting pain and disability from cognitive variables. J Behav Med 1987;11:251.
40. Brown GK, Nicassio PM: Development of a questionnaire for the assessment of active and passive coping strategies in chronic pain patients. Pain 1987;31:53.
41. Romano JH, Turner JA: Depression and chronic pain: Does the evidence support the relationship? Psychol Bull 1985;97:18.

42. Frerichs RR, Aneshensel CS, Yokopenic PA et al: Physical health and depression: An epidemiologic survey. Prev Med 1982;11:639.
43. Johnson JE, Lauver DR, Nail LM: Process of coping with radiation therapy. J Consult Clin Psychol 1989;57:358.
44. Spiegel D, Bloom JR, Kraemer HC et al: Effect of psychosocial treatment on survival of patients with metastatic breast cancer. Lancet 1989;ii;888.
45. Hamilton M: A rating scale for depression. J Neurol Neurosurg Psychiatry 1960;23:56.
46. Reding M, Orto L, Willensky P et al: The dexamethasone suppression test: An indicator of depression in stroke but not a predictor of rehabilitation outcome. Arch Neurol 1985;42:209.
47. Papciak AS, Feuerstein M, Belar CD et al: Alexythymia and pain in an outpatient behavioral medicine clinic. Int J Psychiatry Med 1987;16:347.
48. Apfel RJ, Sifneos PE: Alexythymia: Concept and measurement. Psychother Psychosom 1979;32:189.
49. Taylor GJ, Bagby RM, Ryan DP et al: Validation of the alexythymia construct: A measurement-based approach. Can J Psychiatry 1990;35:290.
50. Jamison RN, Burish TG, Wallston KA: Psychogenic factors in predicting survival of breast cancer patients. J Clin Oncol 1987;5:768.
51. Speigel D, Bloom JR, Yalom I: Group support for patients with metastatic breast cancer. Arch Gen Psychiatry 1981;38:527.
52. Turk DC: Rennert Pain and the terminally ill cancer patient: A cognitive-social learning perspective. In Sobel H (ed): Behavior Therapy in Terminal Care, pp. 95–123. Cambridge, Ballinger, 1981.
53. Loscalzo M, Jacobsen PB: Practical behavioral approaches to the effective management of pain and distress. Journal of Psychosocial Oncology 1990; 8:139.
54. Turner JA, Chapman CR: Psychological interventions for chronic pain: A critical review. I. Relaxation training and biofeedback. Pain 1982;12:1.
55. Blanchard EB: Management of Chronic Headaches: A Psychological Approach. New York, Pergamon, 1985.
56. Fotopoulos SS, Graham C, Cook MR: Psychophysiologic control of cancer pain. In Bonica JJ, Ventafridda V (eds): Advances in Pain Research and Therapy, vol 2, p 231. New York, Raven Press, 1979.
57. Lichstein KL: Clinical Relaxation Strategies. New York, Wiley, 1988.
58. Jacobson E: The origins and development of progressive relaxation. Behavior Journal of Therapy and Experimental Psychiatry 1977;8:119.
59. Morrow GR, Morrell C: Behavioral treatment for the anticipatory nausea and vomiting induced by cancer chemotherapy. N Engl J Med 1982;307:1476.
60. Redd W, Andrykowski MA: Behavioral intervention in cancer treatment: Controlling aversion reactions to chemotherapy. J Consult Clin Psychol 1982;50:1018.
61. Benson H: The Relaxation Response. New York, Morrow, 1975.
62. Mastrovito R: Behavioral techniques: Progressive relaxation and self-regulatory therapies. In Holland JC, Rowland JH (eds): Handbook of Psychooncology, pp. 492–501. New York, Oxford, 1989.
63. Pikoff H: A critical review of autogenic training in America. Clinical Psychology Review 1984;4:619.
64. Kiecolt-Glaser JK, Glaser R, Strain EC et al: Modulation of cellular immunity in medical students. J Behav Med 1985;9:5.
65. Simonton OC, Matthews-Simonton S, Sparks TF: Psychological intervention in the treatment of cancer. Psychosomatics 1980;21:226.
66. Kroger WS: Clinical and Experimental Hypnosis. Philadelphia, JB Lippincott, 1977.
67. Hilgard ER: Hypnosis in the Relief of Pain. Los Altos, CA, William Kaufmann, 1975.
68. Hendler CS, Redd WH: Fear of hypnosis: The role of labeling in patients acceptance in behavioral intervention. Behavior Therapy. 1986;17:2.
69. Roche SM, McConkey KM: Absorption: Nature, assessment, and correlates. J Pers Soc Psychol 1990;59:91.
70. Fernandez E, Turk DC: The utility of cognitive coping strategies for altering pain perception: A meta-analysis. Pain 1989;38:123.
71. Beck AT: Cognitive Therapy and the Emotional Disorders. New York, International Universities Press, 1976.
72. Nehemkis AM, Charter RA, Stampp MS et al: Reattribution of cancer pain. Int J Psychiatry Med 1982–83;12:213.
73. Yalom I, Greaves C: Group therapy with the terminally ill. Am J Psychiatry 1977;134:396.
74. Forester B, Kornfeld DS, Fleiss JL: Psychotherapy during radiotherapy: Effects on emotional and physical distress. Am J Psychiatry 1985;142:22.
75. Ahles TA, Cohen RA, Blanchard EB: Difficulties inherent in conducting behavioral research with cancer patients. The Behavior Therapist 1984;7:69.
76. Bonica JJ: Multidisciplinary/interdisciplinary pain programs. In Bonica JJ, Loeser JD, Chapman CR et al (eds): The Management of Pain, 2nd ed. Philadelphia, Lea and Febiger, 1990.
77. Hersen M, Barlow DH: Single Case Experimental Designs. Elmsford, NY, Pergamon, 1976.
78. Bruera E, MacMillan K, Hanson J et al: The Edmonton staging system for cancer pain: Preliminary report. Pain 1989;37:203.
79. Melzack R, Wall PD: The Challenge of Pain. New York, Basic Books, 1982.

42. Frerichs RR, Aneshensel CS, Yokopenic PA et al: Physical health and depression: An epidemiologic survey. Prev Med 1982;11:639.

43. Johnson JE, Lauver DR, Nail LM: Process of coping with radiation therapy. J Consult Clin Psychol 1989;57:358.

44. Spiegel D, Bloom JR, Kraemer HC et al: Effect of psychosocial treatment on survival of patients with metastatic breast cancer. Lancet 1989;ii;888.

45. Hamilton M: A rating scale for depression. J Neurol Neurosurg Psychiatry 1960;23:56.

46. Reding M, Orto L, Willensky P et al: The dexamethasone suppression test: An indicator of depression in stroke but not a predictor of rehabilitation outcome. Arch Neurol 1985;42:209.

47. Papciak AS, Feuerstein M, Belar CD et al: Alexythymia and pain in an outpatient behavioral medicine clinic. Int J Psychiatry Med 1987;16:347.

48. Apfel RJ, Sifneos PE: Alexythymia: Concept and measurement. Psychother Psychosom 1979;32:189.

49. Taylor GJ, Bagby RM, Ryan DP et al: Validation of the alexythymia construct: A measurement-based approach. Can J Psychiatry 1990;35:290.

50. Jamison RN, Burish TG, Wallston KA: Psychogenic factors in predicting survival of breast cancer patients. J Clin Oncol 1987;5:768.

51. Speigel D, Bloom JR, Yalom I: Group support for patients with metastatic breast cancer. Arch Gen Psychiatry 1981;38:527.

52. Turk DC: Rennert Pain and the terminally ill cancer patient: A cognitive-social learning perspective. In Sobel H (ed): Behavior Therapy in Terminal Care, pp. 95–123. Cambridge, Ballinger, 1981.

53. Loscalzo M, Jacobsen PB: Practical behavioral approaches to the effective management of pain and distress. Journal of Psychosocial Oncology 1990; 8:139.

54. Turner JA, Chapman CR: Psychological interventions for chronic pain: A critical review. I. Relaxation training and biofeedback. Pain 1982;12:1.

55. Blanchard EB: Management of Chronic Headaches: A Psychological Approach. New York, Pergamon, 1985.

56. Fotopoulos SS, Graham C, Cook MR: Psychophysiologic control of cancer pain. In Bonica JJ, Ventafridda V (eds): Advances in Pain Research and Therapy, vol 2, p 231. New York, Raven Press, 1979.

57. Lichstein KL: Clinical Relaxation Strategies. New York, Wiley, 1988.

58. Jacobson E: The origins and development of progressive relaxation. Behavior Journal of Therapy and Experimental Psychiatry 1977;8:119.

59. Morrow GR, Morrell C: Behavioral treatment for the anticipatory nausea and vomiting induced by cancer chemotherapy. N Engl J Med 1982;307:1476.

60. Redd W, Andrykowski MA: Behavioral intervention in cancer treatment: Controlling aversion reactions to chemotherapy. J Consult Clin Psychol 1982;50:1018.

61. Benson H: The Relaxation Response. New York, Morrow, 1975.

62. Mastrovito R: Behavioral techniques: Progressive relaxation and self-regulatory therapies. In Holland JC, Rowland JH (eds): Handbook of Psychooncology, pp. 492–501. New York, Oxford, 1989.

63. Pikoff H: A critical review of autogenic training in America. Clinical Psychology Review 1984;4:619.

64. Kiecolt-Glaser JK, Glaser R, Strain EC et al: Modulation of cellular immunity in medical students. J Behav Med 1985;9:5.

65. Simonton OC, Matthews-Simonton S, Sparks TF: Psychological intervention in the treatment of cancer. Psychosomatics 1980;21:226.

66. Kroger WS: Clinical and Experimental Hypnosis. Philadelphia, JB Lippincott, 1977.

67. Hilgard ER: Hypnosis in the Relief of Pain. Los Altos, CA, William Kaufmann, 1975.

68. Hendler CS, Redd WH: Fear of hypnosis: The role of labeling in patients acceptance in behavioral intervention. Behavior Therapy. 1986;17:2.

69. Roche SM, McConkey KM: Absorption: Nature, assessment, and correlates. J Pers Soc Psychol 1990;59:91.

70. Fernandez E, Turk DC: The utility of cognitive coping strategies for altering pain perception: A meta-analysis. Pain 1989;38:123.

71. Beck AT: Cognitive Therapy and the Emotional Disorders. New York, International Universities Press, 1976.

72. Nehemkis AM, Charter RA, Stampp MS et al: Reattribution of cancer pain. Int J Psychiatry Med 1982–83;12:213.

73. Yalom I, Greaves C: Group therapy with the terminally ill. Am J Psychiatry 1977;134:396.

74. Forester B, Kornfeld DS, Fleiss JL: Psychotherapy during radiotherapy: Effects on emotional and physical distress. Am J Psychiatry 1985;142:22.

75. Ahles TA, Cohen RA, Blanchard EB: Difficulties inherent in conducting behavioral research with cancer patients. The Behavior Therapist 1984;7:69.

76. Bonica JJ: Multidisciplinary/interdisciplinary pain programs. In Bonica JJ, Loeser JD, Chapman CR et al (eds): The Management of Pain, 2nd ed. Philadelphia, Lea and Febiger, 1990.

77. Hersen M, Barlow DH: Single Case Experimental Designs. Elmsford, NY, Pergamon, 1976.

78. Bruera E, MacMillan K, Hanson J et al: The Edmonton staging system for cancer pain: Preliminary report. Pain 1989;37:203.

79. Melzack R, Wall PD: The Challenge of Pain. New York, Basic Books, 1982.

Section 2

Pharmacologic Treatment

Chapter 6

General Principles of Pharmacotherapy

Richard B. Patt

ASSESSMENT

As has been emphasized throughout the introductory section of this text, all management efforts and interventions begin, *prima facie*, with careful assessment. Ideally, the scope of assessment extends to include biologic determinants (the pain syndrome, the neoplastic process, associated symptoms, intercurrent medical conditions) and psychosocial determinants (beliefs, cultural milieu, economic status, family interactions). Whether assessment is accomplished by a multidisciplinary team, a cadre of consultants, or a sole practitioner, these factors must be integrated, and, together, form the basis for a cogent treatment plan. To confound the process further, 1) problems are often of an urgent nature, and 2) each determinant is potentially dynamic, a factor that necessitates frequent reassessment and revision of the treatment plan.

INTERINDIVIDUAL VARIABILITY

Cancer pain, and indeed pain in general, is characterized by interindividual variability that manifests itself in multiple ways. For example, not all bone metastases result in pain. When present, reports of pain vary dramatically, as do responses to therapy. The regular administration of an aspirin-like drug may suffice for some patients, whereas others will require morphine. In the latter group, even patients with similar disease characteristics will vary dramatically in their analgesic requirements, to the extent that daily doses of morphine may need to be dispensed in milligrams for some patients and grams for others.

Even in the same patient, one standard opioid analgesic may produce dose-limiting side effects, whereas a similar drug may be tolerated without difficulty. If the experience of cancer pain and patients' therapeutic response were uniform or even predictable, then management would be a simple technical task, and this textbook would be unnecessary, or at least much more brief. It is this interindividual variability that makes cancer pain management a challenging and demanding endeavor.

PHARMACOLOGIC MANAGEMENT

Throughout this text and other excellent reviews of cancer pain management, the primacy of pharmacologic management is emphasized. This modality has been proven to be effective in adults and children and across different cultures. Treatment is titratable, and is suitable for pain that is multifocal and/or progressive. Effects and side effects are reversible, and widespread implementation does not depend on sophisticated technology or scarce resources.

OPIOIDS

Treatment with opioids is widely acknowledged as the mainstay of pharmacologic management. More liberal, thoughtful prescribing of opioids is warranted, and would reduce global suffering; interestingly, the successful results of opioid therapy are more limited by our reluctance to implement treatment than by the intrinsic properties of these drugs.

OPIOID ALTERNATIVES

Despite the central role of opioid therapy, careful polypharmacy is usually indicated; patients benefit from a balanced selection from a multitude of potentially useful drugs. The nonsteroidal anti-inflammatory agents have an important role in the management of osseous metastases and other syndromes, but are often ignored in favor of opioids. An entire new heterogenous class of drugs, the analgesic adjuvants or coanalgesics (antidepressants, corticosteroids, anticonvulsants, sodium channel blockers, amphetamines) are being explored for their potential to control neuropathic and other pain syndromes. Further controlled research is essential to characterize better the role of these and more standard analgesics.

ROUTE OF ADMINISTRATION

Ideally, analgesics are administered orally because of simplicity and cost-effectiveness, and to promote independence. Even when pain is severe and multifocal, good control can usually be achieved by oral administration through careful application of pharmacokinetic and pharmacodynamic principles.

Alimentary dysfunction, a relatively common event in patients with advanced cancer, is the most common and appropriate indication for using alternative routes for drug administration. The limits of accepted alternative routes have been expanded (rectal and subcutaneous administration). Some novel routes are becoming more widely accepted (intraspinal, transdermal administration), and others are the focus of ongoing research (inhaled and transmucosal administration). Further controlled research is needed to determine the relative merits of drug administration by these and other routes.

NONPHARMACOLOGIC MANAGEMENT

Pharmacotherapy provides sufficient relief for most patients with cancer pain. The judicious application of nonpharmacologic methods promises to control pain in the 10%–30% of patients whose symptoms persist despite aggressive pharmacotherapy, or in whom dose-limiting side effects prevent adequate control. Various nonpharmacologic measures of controlling pain have enjoyed enduring acceptance, whereas the endorsement of others has lapsed. Unfortunately, the same rigorous methodology that characterizes many drug trials has not often been applied to determine the potential benefits, risks, and relative indications for many of these procedures. Nevertheless, these measures should be considered as important adjuncts and alternatives for pa-tients with intractable pain. Neurolytic nerve blocks and selected neurosurgical procedures are effective in many patients with well localized pain. Intraspinal opioids are effective for patients with more generalized or multifocal pain, particularly when opioid side effects have resulted in a prominence of dose-limiting side effects.

Chapter 7

Role of Nonsteroidal Anti-Inflammatory Drugs in the Management of Cancer Pain

John E. Stambaugh, Jr.

INTRODUCTION

Pain due to cancer may arise from a variety of sources (see Chapter 1). Identifying the specific etiology of cancer pain in each case serves as an important guide to management,[1,2] and will become increasingly important as new, more specific therapeutic interventions are developed. Acute cancer pain may be attributable to a cause that is either treatable (*eg*, focal metastases) or self-limited (*eg*, sprain, muscle spasm), and is an indication for short-term analgesic use until the primary source is either effectively treated (*eg*, radiotherapy), or until the pain resolves with the passage of time and provision of supportive care. In chronic cancer pain, careful efforts should be made to determine the etiology of pain, since, over time, cancer pain, like chronic nonmalignant pain, may take on multifactorial attributes that can amplify or modulate symptoms.

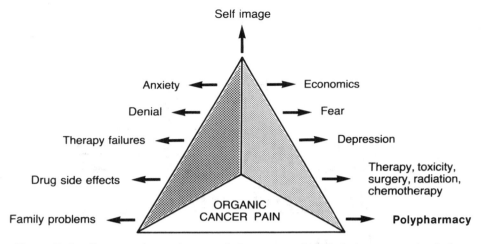

Figure 7–1. Cancer pain can be regarded as a pyramid with its base comprised of organic pain, compounded by treatment, social, economic, and emotional factors. Each of these components contributes a different degree of significance for each patient with the final result interpreted as pain.

As shown in Figure 7–1, chronic cancer pain can be viewed as a composite of the organic component of the neoplasm plus factors related to treatment, socioeconomic, and emotional aspects.[3–7] Cancer pain results primarily from nociceptive stimuli originating with tissue injury produced by tumor growth. With time, reported pain may ultimately emanate from a small organic component combined with relatively greater contributions from the other listed factors. In such cases, despite a reduction in the organic component of the syndrome, pain intensity may persist or actually increase due to the influence of these associated factors. In some cases, chronic cancer pain may wholly result from the described associated factors, including distortion of self-image, treatment, depression, and anxiety.

Chronic cancer pain serves no biologic purpose, and patients with long-term pain syndromes represent difficult management problems to the clinician. It is important that all facets of the pain problem be addressed by the treatment plan. In addition to trials of escalating doses of standard analgesics, effective pain management often involves the ap-propriate use of antidepressants, anxiolytics, and psychosocial intervention.

The purpose of this chapter is to describe the optimal use of NSAIDs in the management of cancer pain. Properly applied, such methods may contribute to more balanced analgesia and more effective pain control in patients with cancer pain, both early in the course of disease and in advanced or terminal malignancy.

MECHANISMS OF ACTION OF THE NSAIDS IN CANCER PAIN

Pain due to cancer results from bone metastases in 75% of cases, presumably as a result of expanding cancer within the bone.[1,16] That even small metastases may produce severe pain argues for an underlying biochemical mechanism. Metastatic bone pain appears to result from the release of arachidonic acid from damaged cell membranes, with the consequent production of prostaglandins and leukotrienes, as illustrated in Figure 7–2. Both of these substances are substrates for the formation of other chemical mediators that con-

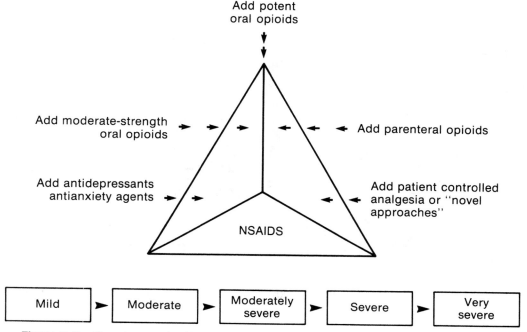

Figure 7–3.   The pharmacologic management of cancer pain is most effectively achieved by carefully individualized combination therapy. In most cases, the NSAIDs form the basis for such an analgesic regimen.

Later, the oral opioids in short-acting and/or controlled-release preparations should be added as the intensity of pain progresses to moderate or severe levels. The doses of these agents are serially adjusted, with the analgesic dose titrated according to pain intensity. A similar strategy is adopted when treatment with parenteral opioids is indicated. Even in the presence of severe pain, efforts should be made to continue NSAID therapy to take advantage of potentially additive or synergistic analgesia.

Whether used initially or added to an opioid regimen, the NSAIDs may reduce the daily dosage of opioid needed to control pain adequately. Such combination analgesia has been postulated to result from an additive mechanism.[26,45–47] The existence of an additive mechanism is supported by a recent study designed to determine the effects of ibuprofen on oxycodone analgesia in patients with moderate to severe cancer pain.[29] In this study, adequate pain control was first achieved with an opioid analgesic (oxycodone), and then either placebo or ibuprofen was added to the analgesic regimen. As shown in Figure 7–4, ibuprofen but not placebo significantly reduced the amount of oxycodone required to manage pain. The effect of the addition of ibuprofen was highly significant, evidenced by significant reductions in oxycodone use over the 2–3 days after the introduction of the NSAID. In sharp contrast, oxycodone use actually increased in the placebo-treated group, perhaps as a result of the development of tolerance. This clinical trial clearly demonstrates that, when used as a part of the treatment regimen for moderate to severe cancer pain, the NSAIDs may significantly reduce opioid requirements, probably as a result of an additive mechanism. Although additional clinical research is needed to better define the

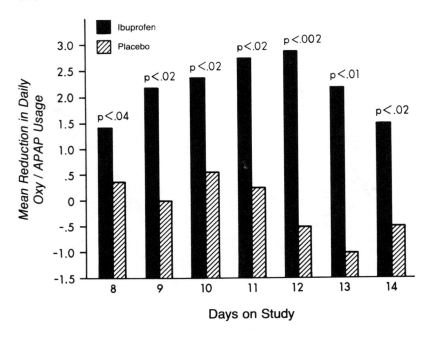

Figure 7-4. In patients with cancer pain controlled by oxycodone APAP, the addition of ibuprofen resulted in a significant reduction in the number of doses of the opioid when compared to placebo control. In this study the placebo group actually demonstrated statistically significant increases in opioid intake. The maximal beneficial effects of ibuprofen occurred at 48 hours, demonstrating a delay in the additive effects of the NSAIDs.

optimal use of the NSAIDs in cancer pain, it is apparent that the NSAIDs should play a significant role in cancer pain management, and should be more widely used.

SELECTION OF AN NSAID: DOSAGE REGIMENS, PEAK EFFECT, PHARMACOKINETICS

PEAK EFFECT

The NSAIDs that are currently available in the United States are shown in Appendix C, Table 1, along with recommended dosing regimens, maximum dosages, and selected pharmacokinetic parameters.[48-53] A more complete description of the pharmacokinetics of individual drugs can be found in the cited references. Although each of the NSAIDs has different pharmacokinetic parameters, overall effects on pain and inflammation appear to be similar. A peak or "ceiling" effect for analgesia has been demonstrated for aspirin, acetaminophen, and the NSAIDs. This is defined as the dosage at which a maximum analgesic response is observed, and beyond which only further anti-inflammatory effects or increased toxicity occur. Regardless of the agent chosen, the maximum dosage or peak analgesic effect dosage should always be used, except when dose-limiting toxicity supervenes. This dosage should serve as the basis for the pyramid analgesic schema suggested above. Suboptimal analgesic doses (*eg*, over-the-counter preparations of ibuprofen taken intermittently) will not produce the maximum analgesic effect required for optimal control of cancer pain, and are likely to lead to early and inappropriate discontinuation of the NSAID. It is preferred to select an NSAID for which the peak analgesic dose has been described (*eg*, ibuprofen 800 mg, ketoprofen 50 mg, fenoprofen 200 mg), and to prescribe accordingly. It has been suggested that although a ceiling dose exists for each NSAID, it may differ in individual patients,[54] thus reflecting our incomplete understanding of ceiling doses vis-à-vis each of the NSAIDs. As a result, selected patients may benefit from attempts to titrate the dosage of a given NSAID upward beyond the usual recommended dose, especially if the maximum dose or ceiling dose is unknown, while observing for improved analgesia without added toxicity.

PHARMACOKINETICS

The pharmacokinetics of the NSAIDs are one important factor in defining dosage guidelines for individual agents. The importance of the pharmacokinetics is highly apparent in patients with compromised hepatic or renal function. Dose modification is often necessary, and guidelines have been described for many of the NSAIDs. By the same token, it is important to use a reduced dosage of the NSAIDs in elderly patients because of altered pharmacokinetic parameters, especially renal clearance. Long-acting NSAIDs facilitate once- or twice-daily dosing, and are therefore favored in patients already taking multiple drugs. Newer parenteral agents should facilitate NSAID use in patients with advanced disease for whom oral administration is impractical because of gastrointestinal dysfunction.

DRUG INTERACTIONS

Drug interactions play an extremely important role in the use of NSAIDs, as shown in Figure 7–5. The route of elimination of the NSAIDs is via hepatic metabolism, and reduced hepatic function, whether due to chemotherapy, radiation toxicity, liver metastasis, or preexisting insufficiency, should result in corresponding dose reductions. The concurrent administration of drugs that effect hepatic microsomal activity also alter NSAID pharmacokinetics. The chronic use of agents that stimulate microsomal function (*eg*, phenobarbital) increases the metabolism of the NSAIDs, decreases their overall effects, and calls for increasing the dose of the NSAID. Similarly, the coadministration of agents that block microsomal metabolism (*eg*, some chemotherapeutic agents) decreases NSAID clearance from the plasma and prolongs the effect of the NSAIDs, suggesting that dosage intervals should be increased.

The kidney is partially responsible for NSAID elimination, and alterations in renal function may increase or decrease the overall effects of the NSAIDs. Although the NSAIDs can cause renal toxicity by their actions on renal prostaglandins, the primary effect of the NSAIDs on the kidney is that of competition for active renal tubular secretion at the proximal tubule. Interaction at the proximal tubal between certain NSAIDs and methotrexate has recently been described. The concomitant administration of fenoprofen, naproxen, and tolmectin could increase the risk of methotrexate toxicity. It appears that ibuprofen and other NSAIDs can be used more safely.[53,55] The NSAIDs decrease lithium clearance, probably as a result of competition at renal binding sites, and concomitant administration may result in increased plasma levels of lithium.

TOXICITY

Toxicity resulting from the use of the NSAIDs remains the most significant factor limiting their role in cancer pain management, and serves as another important guide to selecting the most appropriate agent in a given patient. NSAID-associated toxicity results primarily from the effect of this class of drugs on the arachidonic acid cascade, and specifically to the blockade of the formation of prostaglandins in all organs. The relative side effect profile of members of the NSAID class of drugs is depicted in Figure 7–6.

Gastrointestinal toxicity is mediated by reversal of the gastrointestinal prostaglandins, resulting in increased gastric acid secretion, a decrease in gastric mucin production and mucosal resistance, and a decrease in sphincter tone. Gastrointestinal upset results from a combination of these factors. The risk of hemorrhagic gastropathy is further increased by the additional thromboxane-decreasing effect of the NSAIDs, with subsequent platelet dysfunction, and is a major limiting side effect. Microscopic bleeding is usually less severe with the NSAIDs than with aspirin.[56,57] The nonacetylated salicylates (sodium salicylate, choline magnesium trisalicylate) are less

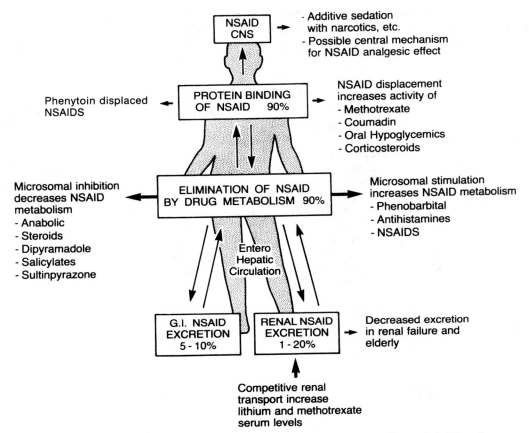

Figure 7–5. Multiple interactions have been described when NSAIDs are administered concurrently with other drugs. This figure depicts the more important and potentially serious sites of interaction. A high proportion of cancer patients receive multiple medications including phenytoin, methotrexate, corticosteroids, hypoglycemics, coumadin, and as a result drug reactions or suboptimal therapy may occur. These interactions must be clearly understood and considered when prescribing NSAIDs for cancer pain.

potent *in vitro* inhibitors of cyclo-oxygenase than aspirin, but clinically appear to have comparable efficacy,[58] and a more favorable toxicity profile. Nonacetylated preparations do not affect *in vitro* tests of platelet aggregation,[59] are associated with less gastrointestinal bleeding and side effects,[60–62] and may be better tolerated than aspirin in patients with asthma.

A variety of strategies have been used in an attempt to improve gastrointestinal tolerance and reduce the risk of bleeding. NSAIDs may be used concomitantly with histamine receptor antagonists; such combined usage limits the development of gastrointestinal upset or bleeding, thereby allowing expanded or long-term use of the NSAID. Recent reports showing a favorable interaction between NSAIDs and H_2 receptor antagonists would appear to be applicable to clinical practice.[63] Such use of H_2 antagonists should significantly reduce gastrointestinal toxicity due to the NSAIDs. Patients with a history of gastritis or prior gastrointestinal intolerance of

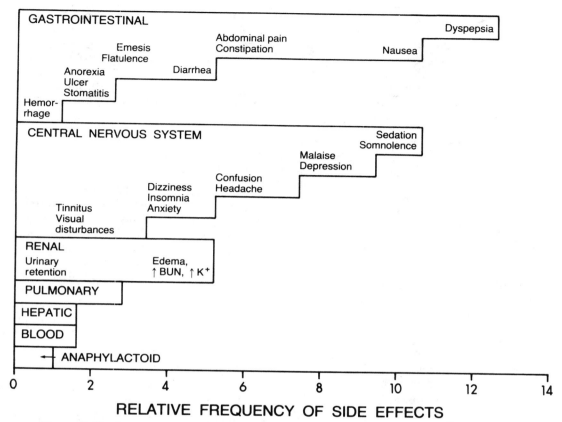

Figure 7–6. As a group, the NSAIDs have well-defined toxicity profiles. The NSAIDs vary in terms of the degree to which such effects occur (see Appendix C), providing a rationale for the exclusion of some agents from cancer pain therapy (eg, phenylbutazone, mefenamic acid). Side effects may go unrecognized in multisymptomatic patients.

NSAIDs should also benefit from the addition of antacids and newer antireflux agents on a prophylactic basis. Patients with a history of peptic ulcer disease specifically associated with the NSAIDs are usually not considered candidates for NSAID therapy. Currently, the literature does not support the use of the NSAIDs in patients with known peptic ulcer disease, and until more effective antiulcer regimens can be identified for these individuals, the NSAIDs should be avoided.

Central nervous system (CNS) mechanisms of NSAID toxicity are unclear, but are believed to be related to local prostaglandin inhibition. Some reported side effects, such as headache and depression, may also result from serotonin-like reactions, which can be pronounced with some of the NSAIDs. Subtle cognitive impairment has been reported in elderly patients taking some NSAIDs. Aseptic meningitis and reversible toxic amblyopia are rare, apparently idiosyncratic events that have been reported after the administration of ibuprofen. Central nervous system side effects have been observed with various NSAIDs and in some cases are dose limiting, or may require a trial of an alternative agent. The CNS sequelae of aspirin overdose are well known.

NSAIDs interfere with renal prostaglandin

synthesis, and as a result may produce marked vasoconstriction, decreased renal blood flow, hyperkalemia, and edema. Alternate renal effects have been previously described.[64] Renal impairment may be somewhat more common for indomethacin than other drugs. Factors predisposing to renal injury include the presence of congestive heart failure, chronic renal insufficiency, cirrhosis with ascites, lupus, intravascular volume depletion, atherosclerosis, and concurrent diuretic use.[65] A report of acute renal failure in two patients with multiple myeloma as an apparent consequence of naproxen administration has appeared recently.[66] Although renal impairment is rare overall, long-term use may lead to chronic renal damage and carcinogenesis.

NSAID administration results in reduced levels of pulmonary prostaglandins, which increases leukotrienes and can exacerbate underlying asthma and chronic lung disease, rarely leading to bronchospasm, pulmonary edema, and respiratory failure.

NSAID administration may be associated with mild, generally reversible elevations in hepatic enzymes. Significant hepatic damage as a result of treatment with currently available agents is rare. Advanced age, decreased renal function, multiple drug use, and higher drug doses may be associated with an increased risk of hepatotoxicity.[67] Hepatocellular injury, cholestasis, and granulomatous hepatitis have been reported in association with the use of phenylbutazone, usually within the first 6 weeks of therapy.[68] An association between severe hepatic toxicity and several previously available agents has resulted in their withdrawal from the market.

The administration of the NSAIDs is associated with reversible inhibition of platelet aggregation. In contrast, aspirin acetylates platelet cyclo-oxygenase, resulting in permanent effects that persist for the duration of affected platelets. Nonacetylated salicylates have little or no effect on platelet function. Blood dyscrasias have been reported as a side effect of therapy with the NSAIDs, but are rare. Significant bone marrow toxicity can ensue with the continued use of some NSAIDs, particularly phenylbutazone, and, as a result, limited or short-term use is recommended for these drugs.

Anaphylactoid reactions to the NSAIDs are rare, but allergic reactions, skin rashes, vasculitis, angioedema, and tissue necrolysis have been reported with some frequency.

DRUG CLASSIFICATION, PRIOR EXPERIENCE, COST

Beaver has characterized the NSAIDs as a heterogenous group of drugs considered together because of common indications and mechanisms, rather than a similarity of structure or even pharmacologic action.[69] The NSAIDs can be grouped by chemical structural similarities (see Appendix C, Table 1). Despite the existence of limited supportive data, it has been suggested that if inadequate analgesia or toxicity results from one NSAID, and a trial of another agent is being considered, it may be prudent to select the new agent from a distinct chemical class.[54,65]

When considering initiating NSAID therapy, a history of prior drug use should be obtained. If a patient has had a prior positive experience with a given NSAID, it is reasonable to consider its repeated use, and, by the same token, if toxicity has occurred in the past, it is reasonable to avoid the offending agent.

More recently released agents tend to be more costly, and in the absence of specific indications or contraindications for a specific agent, the cost is a factor to be taken into account when selecting an NSAID.

CONCLUSION

The overall favorable risk-to-benefit ratio of NSAID administration has resulted in their widespread clinical acceptance, and is further evidenced by over-the-counter labeling of ibuprofen based on its safety/usage records. The choice of an appropriate NSAID for cancer pain management should be based on the above parameters, namely, toxicity (including age, concurrent disease, and concomitant drug administration), ease of dosing, prior experience, cost, (possibly) drug classification, as well as clinician familiarity.

CONCLUSIONS REGARDING NSAID USE IN CANCER PAIN

The above discussion provides a rationale for the inclusion of the NSAIDs as a component of therapy for cancer pain, and outlines guidelines for their optimal use. Applying an analgesic pyramid or a ladder model is best achieved by including an NSAID as a part of the initial therapeutic regimen. The selected agent should be used at its peak or maximum analgesic dose, whether it is used as a sole agent or is combined with an opioid. Careful titration of the doses of both agents is intended to take advantage of their additive properties and to produce a balanced analgesia, ultimately limiting overall toxicity and requirements for opioids. This type of approach may inhibit the development of tolerance and opioid-induced side effects. The clinical parameters described for the use of the NSAIDs, including their provision in maximum analgesic doses, reducing doses for organ dysfunction and age, and avoiding the combined use of agents with known potential for interaction, are extremely important in clinical cancer pain regimens.

Although analgesic effects are observed after single doses, cumulative effects and peak analgesia are not observed until up to 48 hours after the initiation of treatment with an NSAID.[29] Overall efficacy should be assessed only after several days of treatment has elapsed, and then, only when a carefully documented record of side effects has been reviewed. When possible, the addition of opioids should be instituted after repeated dosing with the NSAIDs to gain a clearer understanding of the potential for additive analgesia and combined toxicity. The formulation of a carefully controlled and calculated combined dosage regimen should result in optimum control of cancer pain with currently available agents.

REFERENCES

1. Twycross RG: The management of pain in cancer: A guide to drugs and dosages. Primary Care and Cancer 1988;15–20.
2. Stambaugh JE: Studies in chronic pain models: Cancer pain model. In Max M, Laska E, Portenoy R (eds): Advances in Pain Research and Therapy. New York, Raven Press, 1991.
3. Coyle N, Foley K: Pain in patients with cancer: Profile of patients and common pain syndromes. Seminars in Oncology Nursing 1985;1(2):93.
4. Taddeini L, Rotschafer J: Pain syndromes associated with cancer. Postgrad Med 1984;75:101.
5. McGinney WT, Crooks G: The care of patients with severe chronic pain in terminal illness. JAMA 1984;251:1182.
6. Massie MJ, Holland JC: The cancer patient with pain: Psychiatric complications and their management. Med Clin North Am 1987;71:243.
7. Portenoy RK: Treatment of cancer pain. Mediguide to Pain 1987;8(1):1.
8. Ventafridda V, Caraceni A, Gamba A: Filed testing of the WHO guidelines for cancer pain relief: Summary report of demonstration projects. In Foley KM, Bonica JJ, Ventafridda V (eds): Advances in Pain Research and Therapy, vol 16. New York, Raven Press, 1990.
9. Foley KM: Pain syndromes in patients with cancer. In Bonica JJ, Ventafridda V (eds): Advances in Pain Research and Therapy, vol 2, p 59. New York, Raven Press, 1979.
10. Bonica JJ: Cancer pain. In Bonica JJ (ed): Pain, p 335–362. New York, Raven Press, 1979.
11. Ahles TA, Ruckdeschel JC, Blanchard EB: Cancer related pain: Prevalence in an outpatient setting as a function of stage of disease and type of cancer. J Psychosom Res 1984;28:115–119.
12. Walsh TD: Oral morphine in chronic cancer pain. Pain 1984;18:1–3.
13. Twycross RG: The use of narcotic analgesics in terminal illness. J Med Ethics 1975;1:10–17.
14. Kanner RM, Foley K: Patterns of narcotic drug use in a cancer pain clinic. Ann NY Acad Sci 1978;161:172.
15. Hill CS: The difficult job of managing pain in a drug dependent patient. Primary Care and Cancer 1987;29–32.
16. Stambaugh JE: The management of the patient with chronic pain due to advanced malignancy. J Med 1982;13:183–190.
17. Ferreira SH, Vane JR: New aspects of the mode of

action of nonsteroidal, anti-inflammatory drugs. Ann Rev Pharmacol 1974;4:57.

18. Goodwin JS: Mechanism of action of nonsteroidal anti-inflammatory agents. Am J Med 1984:77(1A):57.

19. Wolf RE: Nonsteroidal anti-inflammatory drugs. Arch Intern Med 1984;144:1658.

20. Boynton CS, Dick CF, Mayor GH: NSAIDS, an overview. J Clin Pharmacol 1988;28:512.

21. Newcombe DS: Leukotrienes: Regulation of biosynthesis, metabolism and bioactivity. J Clin Pharmacol 1988;28:530.

22. Ventafridda V, Martino G, Mandelli V et al: Indoprofen, a new analgesic and anti-inflammatory drug in cancer pain. Clin Pharmacol Ther 1974;17:284.

23. Stambaugh JE, Trejada F, Trudnowski RJ: Double blind comparison of zomepirac and oxycodone with APC in cancer pain. J Clin Pharmacol 1980;20:261.

24. Ventafridda V, Fochi C, DeConno D et al: Use of nonsteroidal anti-inflammatory drugs in the treatment of pain in cancer. J Clin Pharmacol 1980;10:3435.

25. Weingart WA, Sorkness CA, Earhart RN: Analgesia with oral narcotics and added ibuprofen in cancer patients. Clin Pharmacol 1985;4:53.

26. Ferrer-Brechner T, Ganz P: Combination therapy with ibuprofen and methadone for chronic cancer pain. Am J Med 1984;78–83.

27. Martino G, Ventafridda V, Parini J et al: A controlled study on the analgesic activity of indoprofen in patients with cancer pain. In Bonica JJ, Albe-Fessul D, (eds): Advances in Pain Research and Therapy, p 573. New York, Raven Press, 1976.

28. Stambaugh JE: The analgesic efficacy of zomepirac sodium in patients with pain due to cancer. J Clin Pharmacol 1981;21:501.

29. Stambaugh JE, Drew J: The combination of ibuprofen and oxycodone acetaminophen in the management of chronic cancer pain. Clin Pharmacol Ther 1988; 44:665.

30. Ventafridda V, DeConno F, Panerai AE et al: Nonsteroidal anti-inflammatory drugs as the first step in cancer pain therapy: Double-blind, within patient study comparing nine drugs. J Int Med Res 1990; 18:21.

31. Kantor TG: The control of pain by nonsteroidal anti-inflammatory drugs. Med Clin North America 1982; 66:1053–1059.

32. Moertel CG: Treatment of cancer pain with orally administered medications. JAMA 1980;244:2448.

33. Walsh TD: Control of pain and other symptoms in advanced cancer. Oncology 1987;1:5.

34. Payne R: Oral and parenteral drug therapy for cancer pain. Current Management of Pain 1989;3:11–32.

35. Cleeland CS: Pain control in cancer. In Brain MC, Cerlone PO, (eds): Current Therapy in Hematology–Oncology–3, p 255. Current Therapy Series. Toronto, BC Decker, 1988.

36. Kanner RM: Pharmacological management of pain and symptom control in cancer. Journal of Pain and Symptom Management 1987;2 (Suppl 1):9.

37. Stambaugh JE: The use of nonsteroidal anti-inflammatory drugs in cancer bone pain. Orthopaedic Review 18:54–60.

38. Ventafridda V, Fochi C, DeConno D et al: Use of nonsteroidal anti-inflammatory drugs in the treatment of pain in cancer. Br J Clin Pharmacol suppl 1980;10:343S–346S.

39. Portenoy RK: The management of cancer pain. Compr Ther 1990;16:53.

40. American Pain Society: Principles of Analgesic Use in the Treatment of Acute Pain and Chronic Cancer Pain. 1987, Natl Hd Am Pain Society, 1615 L Street, NW, Washington, DC, 20036.

41. World Health Organization: Cancer Pain Relief. Geneva, World Health Organization, 1986.

42. Chapman CR, Casey KL, Dubner R et al: Pain measurement: An overview. Pain 1985;22:1.

43. Stambaugh JE, McAdams J: Comparison of intramuscular dezocine with butorphanol and placebo in chronic cancer pain: A method to evaluate analgesia after both single and repeated doses. Clin Pharmacal Ther 1987;42:210.

44. Max MB, Schafer SC, Culnanne M et al: Association of pain relief with drug side effects in post-herpetic neuralgia: A single dose study of clonidine, codeine, ibuprofen and placebo. Clin Pharmacol Ther 1988; 43:363.

45. Beaver WT: Combination analgesics. Am J Med 1984;38.

46. Houde RW, Wallenstein SL, Beaver WT: Clinical measurement of pain. In de Stevens G (ed): Analgetics, p 75. New York, Academic Press, 1965.

47. Beaver WT: Aspirin and acetaminophen as constituents. Arch Intern Med 1981;141:293.

48. Lombardino JG: Medicinal chemistry of acidic nonsteroidal anti-inflammatory drugs. In Lombardino JG (ed): Nonsteroidal Anti-Inflammatory Drugs, p 253. New York. John Wiley and Sons, 1985.

49. Verbeech RK, Blackburn JL, Loewen GR: Clinical pharmacokinetics of nonsteroidal anti-inflammatory drugs. Clin Pharm 1983;8:297.

50. Graham GG, Day RO, Champion GD et al: Aspects of the clinical pharmacology of nonsteroidal anti-inflammatory drugs. Clinics in Rheumatic Diseases 1984;10:229.

51. Amadio P: Peripherally acting analgesics. Am J Med 1984;17.

52. Denson DD, Mather LE: Nonsteroidal anti-inflammatory agents. Practical Management of Pain. 1986; 29:521.

53. Brater DC: Clinical pharmacology of NSAIDS. J Clin Pharmacol 1988;28;518.
54. Portenoy R: Drug therapy for cancer pain. American Journal of Hospice and Palliative Care 1990;7:10.
55. Nurenberg DW: Competitive inhibition of methotrexate accumulation in rabbit kidney slices by nonsteroidal anti-inflammatory drugs. J Pharmacol Exp Ther 1983;226:1–6.
56. Schlegel SI, Paulus HE: Nonsteroidal and analgesic use in the elderly. Clin Rheum Dis 1986;12:245.
57. Lussier A, Arsenault A: Gastrointestinal blood loss induced by ketoprofen, aspirin and placebo. J Rheumatol 1976;5 (Suppl 14):73.
58. Ferrera SH: Prostaglandins and non-steroidal anti-inflammatory drugs. In Bert F, Samuelson B, Velvo GP (eds): Prostaglandins and Thromboxanes, p 353. New York, Plenum Press, 1976.
59. Morris HG: Effects of salsalate (nonacetylated salicylate) and aspirin on serum prostaglandins in humans. Ther Drug Monit 1985;7:435.
60. Rothwell KG: Efficacy and safety of a non-acetylated salicylate, choline magnesium trisalicylate in the treatment of rheumatoid arthritis. J Int Med Res 1983;11:343.
61. Leonards JR, Levy G: Gastrointestinal blood loss from aspirin and sodium salicylate tablets in man. Clin Pharmacol Ther 1973;14:62.
62. Goldenberg A, Rudnicki RD, Koonce ML: Clinical comparison of efficacy and safety of choline magnesium trisalicylate and indomethacin in treating osteoarthritis. Curr Ther Res 1978;24:245.
63. Delhotal-Landes B, Flouvat B, Liote F et al: Pharmacokinetic interactions between NSAIDS (indomethacin or sulindac) and H2-receptor antagonists (cimetidine or ranitidine) in human volunteers. Clin Pharmacol Ther 1988;44:442.
64. Carmichael J, Shankel SW: Effects of nonsteroidal anti-inflammatory drugs on prostaglandins and renal function. Am J Med 1985;78:992.
65. Sunshine A, Olson NZ: Non-narcotic analgesics. In Wall PD, Melzack R (eds): Textbook of Pain, 2nd ed, p 670. Edinburgh, Churchill Livingstone, 1989.
66. Wu MJ, Kumar KS, Kulkarni G et al: Multiple myeloma in naproxen-induced acute renal failure. N Engl J Med 1987;317:170.
67. Paulus HE: Governmental affairs: FDA Arthritis Advisory Committee meeting. Arthritis Rheum 1982; 25:1124.
68. Benjamin SB: Phenylbutazone liver injury: A clinical pathologic survey of 23 cases and review of the literature. Hepatology 1981;1:255.
69. Beaver WT: Maximizing the benefits of the weaker analgesics. In IASP Refresher Courses on Pain Management, p 1. Hamburg, Germany, International Association for the Study of Pain, 1987.

Chapter 8

Inadequate Outcome of Opioid Therapy for Cancer Pain: Influences on Practitioners and Patients

Russell K. Portenoy

INTRODUCTION

The influence of the hospice movement during the past three decades has resulted in a broad-based consensus that opioid drugs are appropriate treatment for the pain associated with advanced cancer.[1-4] Surveys have suggested that the optimal administration of opioid therapy can provide adequate pain relief to more than three-quarters of patients.[5,6] Although complete relief is seldom attained, at least among those with far-advanced disease, the degree of relief experienced by these patients is usually sufficient to substantially improve quality of life.[7]

The clinical acceptance of opioid therapy for patients with cancer pain among experts in palliative care has not been accompanied by sustained improvement in therapeutic outcome among the larger population of patients who are not treated by these specialists. Surveys that have evaluated prevalence rates for pain consistently demonstrate that the proportion of patients with unrelieved pain in routine clinical settings is far higher than would be expected if optimal therapeutic approaches were applied.[8–10] For example, a survey of 1,103 consecutive admissions to a specialty acute care hospital devoted to the care of patients with advanced cancer revealed that on presentation 73% had pain and 38% had severe pain.[8] Similarly, a survey of 100 admissions to a hospice in the United Kingdom reported that before admission, 90 patients had experienced unrelieved pain for 4 weeks, and 77 patients had inadequate relief for more than 8 weeks; most of these patients had described their pain intensity during this period as severe or excruciating.[10] Thus, the available data portray a disheartening picture in which a large group of patients with cancer pain who could obtain meaningful relief from opioid drugs do not, even during the terminal phase of the disease, when the use of opioids is fully sanctioned.

Continuing efforts to improve the outcome of opioid therapy for cancer pain must be based on a detailed analysis of the factors that may be limiting the efficacy and application of this approach. Specific hypotheses that clarify the causes of ineffective treatment can then be developed, and they may serve as guides for educational programs and clinical trials of therapeutic advances. This analysis does not deny the existence of patients who have truly refractory pain—pain that fails to respond adequately to optimal therapy—but assumes that the proportion of these patients is relatively small among those whose pain is currently unrelieved. The considerations discussed herein relate specifically to factors that can, and should, be addressed to yield a higher rate of successful treatment among patients with inadequately controlled cancer pain.

FACTORS ASSOCIATED WITH INADEQUATE OPIOID THERAPY

From the broadest perspective, it may be postulated that the determinants of inadequate opioid therapy derive from two sets of factors: 1) those primarily related to clinician behavior, and 2) those primarily related to the pa-

TABLE 8–1.
Factors Contributing to Inadequate Relief of Cancer Pain with Opioid Drugs

Clinician-Related Factors

Uncertainty about the role of opioid therapy
1. Patients with early disease
2. Patients with indolent metastatic disease
3. Patients with treatment-related pain
Undertreatment
1. Caused by deficiencies in knowledge of opioid therapy
2. Caused by failure of assessment
3. Caused by overestimation of risks
   • risk of adverse pharmacologic outcomes
   • risk of addiction
4. Caused by physician fear of sanctions

Patient-Related Factors

Ineffectual pain reporting
1. Caused by desire to focus on treatment of tumor
2. Caused by stoicism
3. Caused by desire to please the staff
4. Caused by use of pain to follow course of disease
Fear of opioid drugs
1. Fear of adverse pharmacologic outcomes
2. Fear of addiction
Inadequate understanding of dosing guidelines

Other Factors

Pharmacies that fail to maintain opioid supply
Excessive cost

tient (Table 8–1). Although these factors will be discussed in turn, it should be recognized that the outcome of opioid therapy in any individual patient most likely involves a complex interplay of multiple factors.

CLINICIAN-RELATED FACTORS

Clinician-related factors that eventuate in unrelieved pain can be divided into those that reflect appropriate uncertainty about the role of opioid therapy and those that lead to inappropriate undertreatment of pain. The available evidence suggests that the latter factor, inappropriate undertreatment, is more important by far.

Uncertainty About the Role of Opioid Therapy

The degree of relief that may be attained through optimal administration of an opioid drug will, of course, not be realized if clinicians purposely withhold therapy in the belief that it is not appropriate. As noted, this attitude has been largely eliminated in the setting of far-advanced cancer. In this population, humane considerations and the poor prognosis for long-term survival appear to alter the perceived risk-to-benefit ratio for treatment, such that the risks believed to exist, whether supported by the evidence or not, diminish in importance relative to the desire to provide comfort. Moreover, the pain of these patients is usually clearly caused by an underlying organic process that produces persistent tissue injury; this situation parallels acute traumatic or surgical pain, for which opioids are considered to be acceptable treatment, thereby increasing the clinician's comfort with the approach.

The relative acceptance of chronic opioid therapy for those with far-advanced disease does not, however, imply that clinicians have lesser concerns about the use of these drugs. Given the common clinical perception that substantial risks are inherent in opioid treatment, it is not surprising that support for the liberal administration of these agents does not fully generalize to other clinical situations. Three types of cancer patients are most affected by the perception of risk: 1) patients with limited neoplastic disease; 2) patients with indolent metastatic disease; and 3) patients with treatment-related pains and no current evidence of neoplasm. In each of these groups, clinician uncertainty about the appropriate role of opioid treatment contributes to reticence in the administration of these drugs, which in turn limits the overall efficacy of therapy.

The sources of clinician uncertainty can be clarified by noting the similarities between the concerns raised by opioid therapy in these groups and the continuing controversy surrounding the use of opioids for chronic nonmalignant pain. Clinicians have traditionally rejected opioid treatment in the latter population because of persistent concerns about adverse outcomes, particularly addiction, and doubts about long-term analgesic efficacy. The long life expectancies of patients with nonmalignant pain and the need to emphasize rehabilitation, as well as comfort, increase the salience of these concerns. Proponents of chronic opioid therapy cite evidence that strongly suggests that the risks have been overstated.[11] Even proponents, however, note the deficiencies in studies of this approach, and agree that caution must be exercised in the decision to implement chronic opioid therapy in individuals with chronic pain and disability. To the extent that cancer patients with early disease, indolent metastatic disease, or treatment-related pain mirror those with chronic nonmalignant pain, the same issues may temper enthusiasm for aggressive opioid therapy.

From this perspective, it is evident that limited opioid prescribing due to clinical uncertainty about the appropriate role of this treatment is most justifiable in patients with treatment-related pains, many of whom are presumed to be cured of cancer. There have been no studies that specifically address the safety and efficacy of chronic opioid therapy in such patients. In the absence of such data, it is indeed reasonable to apply treatment principles prudently in this population, and clinical experience suggests that guidelines for the administration of opioid drugs to patients with nonmalignant pain[11] are appropriate in this group. These guidelines include careful patient selection, recognition that partial analgesia is a reasonable goal of therapy, concurrent administration of other treatments (some dedicated to rehabilitative goals, rather than analgesia), and the need for ongoing monitoring. Given the unresolved controversy about the role of long-term opioid therapy in chronic treatment-related pain, inadequate pain relief from opioid drugs in this population cannot be considered a result of inappropriate undertreatment.

The clinical uncertainty about the role of opioid therapy that supports limited intervention in patients with treatment-related pain and an absence of demonstrated disease is more difficult to justify in cancer patients with limited or indolent metastatic disease. Hesitancy about the use of opioid drugs in these populations presumably relates to the potential for cure in the first group, and the prognosis for long survival that characterizes both. It may be speculated that this potential for long survival, combined with a relatively good performance status, leads clinicians to perceive a connection between these patients and those with nonmalignant pain. This connection is not, however, endorsed by most cancer pain specialists, who usually respond to these patients as if a more profound link exists with those whose cancer is far-advanced than with those whose pain is nonmalignant. For experienced practitioners, the greater functional status of patients with limited cancer or indolent metastatic disease may influence the approach to opioid therapy (eg, greater attention to the potential for cognitive impairment that may compromise function), but does not justify withholding treatment. Thus, although studies are needed to confirm the favorable risk-to-benefit ratio of aggressive opioid therapy in patients with limited or indolent disease, most experts have little clinical uncertainty about the value of the approach. The perspective expressed herein is that the purposeful withholding of opioid drugs from the latter groups cannot be justified on the basis of legitimate clinical uncertainty, but should rather be construed as inappropriate undertreatment.

Undertreatment

There is substantial evidence that the undertreatment of pain is a far more common cause inadequate relief than is appropriate medical uncertainty about the proper role of opioid therapy.[12-17] The data indicate that there is a very large group of patients who could obtain adequate pain relief from optimal opioid therapy, but are not provided the opportunity to achieve this outcome. Although there has been no systematic study of the causes of undertreatment, several are well accepted on the basis of clinical experience, and are discussed below.

Deficiencies in the Knowledge of Opioid Pharmacology

It is apparent that physicians and nurses are ill-prepared by their training to manage long-term opioid therapy in patients with chronic cancer pain. Although there have been clear improvements since 1982, when one review noted that 9 medical textbooks published in the United States contained only 17 pages devoted to pain,[13] there continues to be remarkably little attention devoted to pain management in medical education. Furthermore, the availability of didactic material related to pain management and opioid pharmacology does not ensure salutary changes in clinical behavior.[18] Indeed, studies have repeatedly confirmed that the exchange of information in lectures or written material does not reliably lead to behavior change.[19] Clinical behaviors are far more likely to be determined by the influence of role models during training than by other modes of education.[18] In this way, misconceptions are sustained across generations of trainees, and the techniques that result in inadequate pain management are perpetuated.

Deficiencies in the knowledge of opioid pharmacology have several distinct elements, each of which may be amenable to appropriate interventions. For example, there appears to be widespread ignorance of pharmacokinetic and pharmacodynamic factors that may have profound influences on treatment. Several surveys have documented the high prevalence of inaccurate information about opioid drugs among physicians and nurses.[15,17,20,21] The doses needed to provide relief are typically underestimated, and the risk of adverse effects is exaggerated. The duration of opioid effects following a dose is often perceived to be longer than is actually the case, and individual differences among patient response, the recognition of which is essential to effective management, are not adequately appreciated. These deficiencies represent a major obstacle to improved outcome.

Inadequate knowledge of pharmacokinetics and pharmacodynamics is often greatly compounded by confusion about guidelines for opioid administration in the cancer population. Although dosing guidelines are empirical, their importance to the efficacy of therapy is widely accepted.[3,4,22] Given the degree to which successful therapy depends on such guidelines, it is disheartening to note that the method for dosing opioid drugs described in popular compendia, such as the *Physicians' Desk Reference*, are directed toward the management of acute pain in the nontolerant patient, and are therefore irrelevant to the treatment of cancer pain. Thus, opioid pharmacotherapy for cancer pain differs from other types of drug treatment in that appropriate dosing guidelines are not immediately accessible.

Failure of Adequate Assessment

Comprehensive assessment is prerequisite to the optimal management of opioid therapy. This assessment has numerous objectives, and often provides information that substantially influences the treatment approach, including the nature of the underlying lesion, characteristics of the pain, associated psychosocial or medical problems, and the presence of symptoms other than pain. Pain assessment by physicians and nurses is generally inadequate, and this undoubtedly contributes to poor outcome. A recent survey, for example, found that 63% of patients referred to a cancer pain service had previously unrecognized lesions discovered through the assessment provided by the pain consultant; in almost 20% of these cases, this information provided an opportunity for primary therapy, either antineoplastic or antibiotic.[23]

Overestimation of the Risk of Therapy

An assessment of risk is an appropriate element in all therapeutic decision making. There are certainly risks associated with chronic opioid therapy, and these must be carefully weighed throughout treatment. This truism, however, should not obscure the adverse consequences that may result from undertreatment that occurs from an inappropriate overestimation of risk.

The perception of risk has many aspects, any of which may predominate in clinical decision making. Two of the most important are 1) concern about adverse pharmacologic reactions, and 2) concern about the potential for addiction.

Adverse Pharmacologic Reactions. The major concerns about opioid toxicity expressed by clinicians relate to the potential for respiratory depression, which is perceived to be a threat to life, and cognitive impairment, which is perceived to limit the patient's ability to function. The available evidence suggests that these concerns are overstated.

Serious respiratory compromise is exceedingly rare in cancer patients treated with chronic opioid therapy. The risk is greatest during the initiation of treatment with methadone in relatively nontolerant patients.[24] Presumably, prolonged gradual escalation of plasma drug concentration, a well recognized phenomenon associated with the regular administration of methadone or other long half-life agents, predisposes to this outcome. Clinical experience suggests that respiratory depression is a very unlikely outcome with any opioid, including methadone, if appropriate methods of dose titration are used. Respiratory depression has also been observed in patients on high doses of opioids who undergo a procedure that abruptly eliminates pain by interrupting afferent input from the painful site (*eg*, cordotomy or neurolytic block), and in patients who develop an intercurrent cardiac or pulmonary process, such as pneumonia, pulmonary embolism, or congestive heart failure. In the latter group, partial reversal of the respiratory compromise can usually be produced by the administration of naloxone, and this may cause the clinician to assume mistakenly that opioid therapy is the primary cause of the problem.

A more substantive concern of clinicians relates to the possibility of significant cognitive impairment occurring as a result of opioid therapy. Encephalopathy is extremely common among hospitalized patients with advanced cancer,[25] and opioid therapy may augment concomitant cognitive impairment and thereby further compromise physical and psychological functioning. The possibility of this outcome is particularly important among patients with more limited disease, whose desire to maintain normal function may be as compelling as the need for pain relief. Indeed, opioid-induced impairment of function, which may compromise quality of life, represents a legitimate reason to limit the administration of these drugs. The available data cannot entirely resolve this issue, but there is evidence that the cognitive capabilities of most patients on stable doses of opioids are not impaired in a clinically significant way. Although recent studies note that reaction time may be abnormal in patients on stable opioid doses,[26,27] the impact of this observation on functional capabilities and lifestyle is not clear. A recent study of patients with advanced cancer demonstrated that the cognitive impairments that could be discerned in patients soon after an incremental increase in the opioid dose could not be identified in patients whose last dose increase occurred a week earlier.[28] Equally important, extensive clinical experience with opioid therapy in the cancer population also suggests that the individual differences in the effects on cognition, affect, and perception produced by the various opioid drugs are so large that even if cognitive impairments occur with one drug, they may not be reproduced with the administration of another, similar drug.

Thus, these observations support the view that serious adverse pharmacologic reactions are rare in patients who undergo prudent dose titration. Other side effects are usually manageable, especially when a preventative approach is adopted. Given the low incidence of severe or prolonged problems, and the potential reversibility of any adverse effects that do occur, it is more reasonable to implement aggressive therapy early and monitor any adverse outcomes than to withhold treatment for fear of adverse events, and thereby risk the experience of unrelieved pain.

Concerns About Addiction. It is extremely important to address the concern that opioid administration to patients with cancer pain may eventuate in iatrogenic addiction. Obvi-

ously, if the risk of this outcome was in fact substantial, it would indeed justify caution in the use of these drugs in patients with long survival. Fortunately, extensive clinical experience and survey data provide a firm basis for the conclusion that addiction is an extraordinarily rare outcome of the therapeutic use of opioids. As a result, experienced clinicians rarely consider this outcome during management, but rather perceive the fear of addiction as perhaps the most significant cause of undertreatment in the cancer population.[29]

Overestimation of the risk of addiction presumably originates from an inadequate understanding of the characteristics that define this syndrome, and inappropriate extrapolation of information derived from the addict population. Addiction is a psychological and behavioral syndrome defined by overwhelming involvement with the drug (psychological dependence), compulsive drug use (which may be characterized by intense efforts to maintain a supply, unsanctioned dose escalation, and continued use of the drugs despite harm to the user), and any of numerous aberrant drug-taking behaviors that are well recognized by clinicians.[11,30,31] The latter include manipulation of the medical system to obtain drugs, acquisition of drugs from nonmedical sources, use of the drugs to treat symptoms not targeted by the therapy, drug hoarding or sales, or obtaining the drug by an unprescribed route.

The phenomenon of addiction is often confused with two other concepts, physical dependence and tolerance. Tolerance refers to the need to increase the dose of a drug over time in order to maintain a given pharmacologic effect. In the clinical setting, it is a complex and poorly understood phenomenon with protean manifestations. Any patient who has required dose escalation, or who has demonstrated an opioid effect (*eg*, sedation) that has disappeared with repetitive dosing, has manifested evidence of tolerance. However, it is now widely accepted that increased drug requirements are usually associated with tumor progression, which presumably produces increased tissue injury and pain. Indeed, the need for escalating doses in the absence of tumor progression, which would suggest the primary influence of pharmacologic tolerance, is so uncommon that the potential for loss of analgesic efficacy due to this process need not be considered during routine clinical practice. Tolerance is also independent of addiction, even in those unusual patients in whom tolerance appears to be the driving force for dose escalation.

Like tolerance, physical dependence refers to another physiologic phenomenon distinct from addiction. Physical dependence is characterized by the development of an abstinence syndrome (withdrawal) after reduction or cessation of dosing or the administration of an opioid antagonist. Although the intensive effort to avoid withdrawal has been considered to be important in the genesis of addiction,[32] the vast majority of patients who receive opioids chronically, and are therefore physically dependent, never manifest any of the aberrant behaviors associated with addiction.[11,30–40] Thus, when addiction is defined appropriately as a psychological and behavioral disorder, there is no evidence that a substantial liability for this outcome exists after the therapeutic administration of opioids.

These data strongly suggest that the development of addiction is not a problem inherent to opioid therapy *per se*, but rather results from an interaction between the potential reinforcing properties of these compounds and characteristics of the individual, which may be psychological, situational, or genetic. Additional evidence for this view can be adduced from studies of the affective responses to opioid drugs, which have demonstrated that the euphoric state experienced by addicts after the administration of an opioid is rarely experienced by normal volunteers or medical patients[41]; patients more often experience dysphoria from opioids. Addicts also have modal personality traits that differ from patients,[42,43] again suggesting that individuals who develop addiction after exposure to opioid drugs are fundamentally unlike the typical patient with cancer pain. Together, these data strongly support the view that the fear of addiction should not interfere with the early institution of opioid therapy,

or with aggressive dose titration once treatment has begun.

Physician Fear of Sanctions

It has been proposed that undertreatment with opioid drugs derives in part from concern on the part of physicians that the prescription of these drugs may place them at personal risk of sanctions from overzealous regulators intent on stemming drug abuse.[11,29] Although this concern is more salient in the controversial application of chronic opioid therapy for nonmalignant pain, there is reason to believe that clinicians who prescribe these drugs to patients with cancer also react to the perceived scrutiny from regulatory agencies by limiting the prescription of opioid drugs.[44,45] This concern is presumably increased during the treatment of specific types of patients, including those who are young; those who require very high doses, rapid escalation of doses, or concurrent administration of more than one opioid; and those who need injections. Again, these concerns appear to be most likely to interfere with therapy in patients with relatively limited disease.

In recognition that the fear of sanctions may negatively influence the management of cancer pain, there has recently been some attempt to provide regulatory and statutory reassurances to clinicians who administer these drugs for therapeutic purposes. In the United States, for example, Texas and California have recently passed statutes establishing the right of physicians to prescribe opioid drugs or other controlled substances to patients who may benefit from this treatment.[46] Likewise, new guidelines issued by the International Narcotics Control Board note for the first time that opioids are essential, and that the need to regulate opioid drugs and reduce drug abuse should not undermine licit medical uses.[47]

Notwithstanding, there continues to be little appreciation for the possibility that the perceived risk of sanctions on the part of the clinician may contribute to undertreatment. The degree to which this phenomenon influences prescribing practices should be investigated, and, where clearly appropriate, efforts should be made to reassure prescribers about the acceptability of opioid therapy for patients with cancer pain.

PATIENT-RELATED FACTORS LEADING TO INADEQUATE OPIOID THERAPY

It is a commonly observed irony that patients with cancer pain may not behave in a way that optimizes the likelihood of effective opioid therapy.[48] Numerous reasons can be proposed to explain this phenomenon, as discussed below.

Ineffectual Pain Reporting

Like many of the clinicians treating them, patients often view the primary goal of therapy as palliation or eradication of the tumor, rather than control of the symptoms. Patients often have a very limited period of time to spend with a physician, and in the exchange of information that ensues, may purposely focus on the status of the disease rather than an explication of symptoms. Some patients may believe that it is not in their best interest to distract the physician from the effort to treat the tumor by forcing attention away from the neoplasm.

Other reasons for inadequate reporting of symptoms may also be observed. Patients may believe that stoicism is intrinsically valued, and that persistent complaints are undignified. Some may be concerned that continued reports of pain will lead to disappointment or lack of attention from the staff. Others feel the need to be liked, and may withhold bad news from the staff. Others desire to be more amiable. Finally, some patients perceive pain as an indicator of the status of disease, and express concern that "masking" pain will limit their ability to follow the course of disease.

Fear of Opioid Drugs

Patients also experience an intense fear of opioids, and usually focus on the same issues that concern clinicians: specifically, the risk of side effects and the potential for addiction. It must be recognized that these concerns are experienced by both the patient and significant others in the patient's environment. Patients who are otherwise willing to undertake a trial of opioid therapy suggested by the physician may be dissuaded from doing so by family members concerned about the potential for cognitive impairment or addiction. Unless specific queries are made by the clinician, these concerns may not be expressed openly, and the refusal to participate in therapy may be believed to originate from the patient alone. The genesis of these fears must be clarified, and appropriate reassurances provided.

Inadequate Understanding of Dosing Guidelines

Similar to any other pharmacologic treatment, poor compliance with opioid therapy may relate to inadequate understanding of the dosing guidelines suggested by the physician. In some cases, the utility of an opioid regimen is undermined by its complexity. Noncompliance may be more likely among patients with cancer pain who require treatment with multiple drugs, each administered many times per day. For example, a study that compared immediate-release morphine with controlled-release morphine noted that pain relief improved during the period of treatment with the latter drug, because patients missed fewer doses and consequently consumed more morphine.[49] Should the complexity of treatment appear to contribute to a lack of compliance, efforts must be made to simplify treatment by reducing the number of drugs or number of drug administrations daily.

OTHER FACTORS THAT MAY CONTRIBUTE TO INADEQUATE OPIOID THERAPY

Surveys have revealed that pharmacies often fail to stock opioid drugs.[50] This may result in delays in implementing therapy or dose changes. In some patients, these difficulties further compromise the efficacy of the treatment approach.

Cost may be another important factor. The expenditures required to provide drugs to patients on high doses may be very substantial. In some cases, the clinician can have a favorable influence on the course of therapy merely by identifying the least costly approach or by expediting reimbursement by insurers, if this is available.

CONCLUSIONS

The available evidence suggests that the inadequacies currently perceived to exist in the treatment of cancer pain can be ascribed largely to patients who potentially could respond to optimal opioid therapy. Although reticence in prescribing may be appropriate for the small group with chronic treatment-related pain, the most important causes of inadequate management relate to either inappropriate undertreatment on the part of clinicians or maladaptive behaviors on the part of patients. The likelihood of successful therapy will undoubtedly improve if efforts are made to assess these processes more fully and intervene to change them. It must be recognized, however, that routine educational programs have thus far failed to have dramatic impact on the delivery of analgesic therapies. This experience is consistent with studies that demonstrate the limited efficacy of education in altering clinician behavior.[19] Such data imply that more innovative approaches will be needed to effect significant change in prescribing practices. These approaches may include the implementation of quality assurance programs in hospitals,[51] programs of patient education, and expanded opportunity for advanced clinical training in cancer pain. Combined with efforts to reassure physicians of the acceptability of opioid therapy for the management of cancer pain and to reduce the regulatory burden in prescribing controlled substances, these types of programs may be able to yield benefits to the large proportion of cancer patients with unrelieved pain.

REFERENCES

1. McGivney WT, Crooks GM: The care of patients with severe chronic pain in terminal illness. JAMA 1984;251:1182.
2. Health and Public Policy Committee, American College of Physicians: Drug therapy for severe chronic pain in terminal illness. Ann Intern Med 1983;99:870.
3. World Health Organization: Cancer Pain Relief. Geneva, World Health Organization, 1986.
4. Foley KM: The treatment of cancer pain. N Engl J Med 1985;313:84.
5. Ventafridda V, Tamburini M, DeConno F: Comprehensive treatment in cancer pain. In Fields HL, Dubner R, Cervero F (eds): Advances in Pain Research and Therapy, vol 9, p 617. New York, Raven Press, 1985.
6. Ventafridda V, Oliveri E, Caraceni A et al: A retrospective study on the use of oral morphine in cancer pain. Journal of Pain and Symptom Management 1987;2:77.
7. Ferrell BR, Wisdon C, Wenzl C: Quality of life as an outcome variable in management of cancer pain. Cancer 1989;63:2321.
8. Brescia FJ, Adler D, Gray G et al: A profile of hospitalized advanced cancer patients. Journal of Pain and Symptom Management 1990;5:221.
9. Daut RL, Cleeland CS: The prevalence and severity of pain in cancer. 1982;50:1913.
10. Twycross RG, Fairfield S: Pain in far-advanced cancer. Pain 1982;14:303.
11. Portenoy RK: Chronic opioid therapy in nonmalignant pain. Journal of Pain and Symptom Management 1990;5:S46.
12. Portenoy RK: Cancer pain: Epidemiology and syndromes. Cancer 1989;63:2298.
13. Bonica JJ: Treatment of cancer pain: Current status and future needs. In Fields HL, Dubner R, Cervero F (eds): Advances in Pain Research and Therapy, vol 9, p 589. New York, Raven Press, 1985.
14. Portenoy RK, Kanner RM: Patterns of analgesic prescription and consumption in a university-affiliated, community hospital. Arch Intern Med 1985;145:439.
15. Marks RM, Sacher EJ: Undertreatment of medical patients with narcotic analgesics. Ann Intern Med 1973;78:173.
16. Shine D, Demas P: Knowledge of medical students, residents and attending physicians about opiate abuse. J Med Educ 1984;59:501.
17. Charap AD: The knowledge, attitudes and experience of medical personnel treating pain in the terminally ill. Mt Sinai J Med 1978;45:561.
18. Morgan JP: American opiophobia: Customary underutilization of opioid analgesics. Adv Alcohol Subst Abuse 1985–86;5:163.

19. Cleeland CS: Evaluating interventions to improve analgesic practice. In Max MB, Portenoy RK, Laska EM (eds): Advances in Pain Research and Therapy, vol 18, p 631. New York, Raven Press, 1991.

20. Grossman SA, Sheidler VR: Skills of medical students and house officers in prescribing narcotic medications. J Med Educ 1985;60:552.

21. Sheidler VR, McGuire DB, Gilbert MR et al: Nurses' inability to recognize safe narcotic orders. Oncology Nursing Forum 1989;16:195.

22. Portenoy R:. Pharmacological approaches to pain control. Journal of Psychosocial Oncology 1990;8:75.

23. Gonzales GR, Elliott KJ, Portenoy RK, Foley KM: The impact of a comprehensive evaluation in the management of cancer pain. Pain, 1991;47:141.

24. Ettinger DS, Vitale PJ, Trump DL: Important clinical pharmacologic considerations in the use of methadone in cancer patients. Cancer Treat Rep 1979; 63:457.

25. Massie MJ, Holland JC: The cancer patient with pain: Psychiatric complications and their management. Med Clin North Am 1987;71:243.

26. Sjogren P, Banning A: Pain, sedation and reaction time during long-term treatment of cancer patients with oral and epidural opioids. Pain 1989;39:5.

27. Banning A, Sjogren P: Cerebral effects of long-term oral opioids in cancer patients measured by continuous reaction time. Clinical Journal of Pain 1990;6:91.

28. Bruera E, MacMillan K, Hanson JA et al: The cognitive effects of the administration of narcotic analgesics in patients with cancer pain. Pain 1989;39:13.

29. Hill CS: Relationship among cultural, educational and regulatory agency influences on optimum cancer pain treatment. Journal of Pain and Symptom Management 1990;5:536.

30. Rinaldi RC, Steindler EM, Wilford BB et al: Clarification and standardization of substance abuse terminology. JAMA 1988;259:555.

31. Jaffe JH: Drug addiction and drug abuse. In Gilman AG, Goodman LS, Rall TW et al (eds): The Pharmacological Basis of Therapeutics, 7th ed, p 532. New York, Macmillan, 1985.

32. Wikler A: Opioid Dependence: Mechanisms and Treatment. New York, Plenum Press, 1980.

33. Taub A: Opioid analgesics in the treatment of chronic intractable pain of non-neoplastic origin. In Kitahata LM, Coolins D (eds): Narcotic Analgesics in Anesthesiology, p 199. Baltimore, Williams and Wilkins, 1982.

34. France RD, Urban BJ, Keefe FJ: Long-term use of narcotic analgesics in chronic pain. Soc Sci Med 1984;19:1379.

35. Tennant FS, Robinson D, Sagherian A et al: Chronic opioid treatment of intractable non-malignant pain. Pain Management 1988;1:18–28.

36. Portenoy RK, Foley KM: Chronic use of opioid analgesics in non-malignant pain: Report of 38 cases. Pain 1986;25;171.

37. Chapman CR: Giving the patient control of opioid analgesic administration. In Hill CS, Fields WS (eds): Advances in Pain Research and Therapy, vol 11, p 339. New York, Raven Press, 1989.

38. Porter J, Jick H: Addiction rare in patients treated with narcotics. N Engl J Med 1980;302:123.

39. Perry S, Heidrich G: Management of pain during debridement: A survey of U.S. burn units. Pain 1982;13:267.

40. Medina JL, Diamond S: Drug dependency in patients with chronic headache. Headache 1977;17:12.

41. Jaffe JH: Misinformation: Euphoria and addiction. In Hill CS, Fields WS (eds): Advances in Pain Research and Therapy, vol 11, p 163. New York, Raven Press, 1989.

42. Hill HE, Haertzen CA, Davis H: An MMPI factor analytic study of alcoholics, narcotic addicts and criminals. Quarterly Journal of Studies in Alcoholism 1962;23:411.

43. Hill HE, Haertzen CA, Glaser R: Personality characteristics of narcotic addicts as indicated by the MMPI. J Gen Psychol 1960;62:127.

44. Joranson DE: Federal and state regulation of opioids. Journal of Pain and Symptom Management 1990;5:S12.

45. Angarola RT: National and international regulation of opioid drugs: Purpose, structures, benefits and risks. Journal of Pain and Symptom Management 1990;5:S24

46. Senate Bill 20, 71st Legislature, 1st Called Session, State of Texas, July 18, 1989.

47. Joranson DE: A new drug law for the states: An opportunity to affirm the role of opioids in cancer pain relief. Journal of Pain and Symptom Management 1990;5:333-336.

48. Cleeland CS: Barriers to the management of pain. Oncology 1987;1:19.

49. Portenoy RK, Maldonado M, Fitzmartin R et al: Controlled-release morphine sulfate: Analgesic efficacy and side effects of a 100 mg tablet in cancer pain patients. Cancer 1989;63:2284

50. Kanner RM, Portenoy RK: Unavailability of narcotic analgesics for ambulatory cancer patients in New York City. Journal of Pain and Symptom Management 1986;1:87.

51. Committee on Quality Assurance Standards, American Pain Society: American Pain Society quality assurance standards for relief of acute pain and cancer pain. In Bond MR, Charlton JE, Woolf CJ (eds): Proceedings of the VIth World Congress on Pain. Amsterdam: Elsevier, 1991, pp. 185–190.

Chapter 9

Oral Opioid Analgesics

C. Stratton Hill, Jr.

GENERAL CONSIDERATIONS

Opioids are effective pain relievers when administered by mouth, and patients prefer this route of administration to all others because of its ease and convenience. If the basic pharmacokinetic properties of opioids are observed, the same pain control generally can be achieved with oral medication as with any other route of administration. Transient, undesirable side effects that may occur after oral administration, as well as with any other route of administration, are too frequently attributed to the route of administration *per se*, and it is abandoned. Since the oral administration of opioids is effective and convenient, and parenteral administration is more cumbersome and often more expensive, every effort should be made to ensure that oral administration is successful.

Oral opioid administration should not be abandoned because nausea, vomiting, or sedation occur when treatment is initiated. In most instances, these side effects are transitory, and they may in fact not even be true side effects. For example, many patients with unrelieved pain are unable to sleep, and when this sleeplessness persists over weeks or months, chronic sleep deprivation ensues. When the pain is relieved, they are able to sleep, and may do so for many hours until the sleep deprivation has been compensated. Unfamiliarity with this phenomenon may cause the physician, nurse, or family to interpret this prolonged sleeping as oversedation and an undesirable side effect. Additionally, many patients with pain may be constipated for various reasons before opioid therapy is initiated, and as a result may be predisposed to nausea or vomiting. Constipation rather than opioid treatment may account for the nausea and vomiting, and oral opioids should not be abandoned until constipation has been treated. Persistent unexplained nausea and vomiting may be treated with antiemetics during the initiation of oral opioid therapy. After a week or more of antiemetic therapy, the nausea and vomiting frequently disappear, and oral opioid therapy may proceed without the need of an antiemetic.

True allergy to the opioid drugs is an extremely rare phenomenon. It is much more common that a patient reports an allergy when he or she previously experienced a transitory side effect associated with the initiation of opioid therapy. True allergic symptoms such as skin eruptions, urticaria, or bronchospasm should be present before an allergy is diagnosed. Persistent side effects may occur with any opioid, but can usually be corrected by simply substituting an alternate opioid.

Lack of effect with oral opioids may also be advanced as a rationale to change the route of administration. This reason requires careful pharmacodynamic evaluation.[1] As long as side effects from oral administration are acceptable to the patient, lack of effect due solely to oral administration does not occur. There are certain painful states in which the type of pain (eg, neuropathic pain) is thought to influence response to opioids (see Chapters 1–3, 8, and 10). In these patients, opioids seem to be less effective.[3] There is no evidence that changing the route of administration in such patients enhances the therapeutic response to opioids.[4,5] Gastrointestinal dysfunction is a relatively common event in patients with advanced disease (see Chapters 12, 13, and 30), particularly in association with the development of dysphagia, bowel obstruction, cognitive failure, or coma, and this should be regarded as the most important element influencing a decision to seek an alternate route to oral administration (see Chapter 11).

Oral opioid therapy should be abandoned only after every effort has been made to overcome whatever problems might occur with this route of administration. The potential benefits to the patient certainly justify the effort to overcome them.

PHARMACOLOGIC CONSIDERATIONS IN THE CLINICAL USE OF OPIOIDS

CLASSIFICATION OF OPIOIDS

One useful classification of opioids divides them into three categories based on their predominant pharmacologic action: 1) pure agonists, 2) mixed agonist/antagonists, and 3) partial agonists. All opioids have a dual action of producing analgesia (agonism) and reversing it (antagonism) to varying degrees.[6] The prototype agonist is morphine. The prototype antagonist is naloxone, a drug that will reverse analgesia and all the other pharmacologic actions of opioids, and, in opioid-dependent patients, will precipitate an abstinence, or withdrawal, reaction. Mixed agonist/antagonists and partial agonists have predominantly agonist actions, but also have a potentially significant antagonist action. The practical significance of this classification relates to changing a patient's medication from one category to another. Patients who have been treated with pure agonists should not be changed to either mixed agonist/antagonists or partial agonists, because of the possibility of precipitating a withdrawal reaction. However, patients who have been treated with mixed or partial agonist/antagonists may be switched to pure agonists with impunity, because there is no danger of a withdrawal reaction.

Table 9–1.*
Pharmacologic Classification of Opioids

Classification	Opioid
Pure Agonists	Propoxyphene
	Codeine
	Dihydrocodeine
	Oxycodone
	Hydrocodone
	Morphine
	Hydromorphone
	Methadone
	Levorphanol
	Meperidine
Mixed Agonist/Antagonists	Pentazocine
	Butorphanol
	Nalbuphine
Partial Agonist	Buprenorphine

* See also Appendix C, Table 1

A number of readily available and commonly used drugs are classified in Table 9–1 and Appendix C, Table 1, and will be discussed in this chapter.

Mixed agonist/antagonists are not recommended for the treatment of chronic pain because they are associated with an increased incidence of psychotomimetic side effects, and because most can be administered only by injection.[6] The partial agonist buprenorphine will also precipitate withdrawal in patients who are tolerant to morphine-like agonists, and the respiratory depression caused by this drug is not easily reversed by naloxone.[7]

Another practical classification of opioids separates them into weak and strong agents, based on their capacity to relieve mild, moderate, or severe pain. Perhaps all narcotics could relieve any pain, but the side effects accompanying the necessary dose to accomplish this make it impractical to use the weaker narcotics for the treatment of severe pain. Drugs falling into these categories are listed in Table 9–2 and Appendix C, Table 1.

MECHANISM OF ACTION

Exogenous opioids act as ligands that bind to stereospecific and saturable receptors in the central nervous system (CNS) and other tissues (eg, the large bowel) (see Chapter 18).[8] These receptors also serve an endogenous opioid system, the endorphins, enkephalins, and dynorphins. There is reasonably firm evidence for four major categories of CNS receptors: mu, kappa, delta, and sigma. It is thought that drug activity at the level of these receptors accounts for the various attributes of the opioids, such as analgesia and changes in mental status. The affinity with which an opioid binds to one or more of these receptors may account for its characteristic action. For example, dysphoria and psychotomimetic effects are associated with opioids that have a stronger affinity for sigma receptors, whereas potent analgesia is associated with opioids that have a stronger affinity for mu receptors.[9]

Because all opioids act by this mechanism, it is seldom advantageous to combine them in significant numbers to treat pain. For example, morphine, hydromorphone, and levorphanol administered simultaneously to the same patient provide no therapeutic benefit over treatment with an adequate dose of only one of these drugs. Such polypharmacy is not infrequently practiced, probably because of a reluctance simply to increase the dose of a single opioid to an effective one, which may exceed the "usual" or "recommended" dose. Unfortunately, most standard pharmacology texts limit discussion on opioids to their applications for acute pain (see Chapter 8). Fear of censure by state and federal regulatory agencies may also contribute to the practice of polypharmacy (see Chapter 8). However, when a single agent is used in an adequate dose, it is less confusing to the patient, and similar results are achieved.

Nevertheless, combining drugs with a similar mechanism of action is rational when a specific characteristic of one drug is used to advantage. For example, methadone has a long half-life, and, as a result, its dosing interval may be 6 hours. When methadone is used as the primary or basal analgesic, it is often advisable to supplement its administration with a complementary short-acting drug, such as immediate-release morphine or hydromorphone, for "breakthrough" pain that occurs before the end of 6 hours.

Table 9–2.*
Classification of Opioids Based on Analgesic Potency

Classification	Opioid
Weak Opioids	Propoxyphene
	Codeine
	Oxycodone
	Hydrocodone
Strong Opioids	Morphine
	Hydromorphone
	Methadone
	Levorphanol
	Meperidine

* See also Appendix C, Table 1

Taking advantage of the additive or synergistic action between opioids and analgesics with other mechanisms of action (see Chapters 7 and 10) is a rational therapeutic maneuver, and will be discussed subsequently.

CLINICAL USE OF OPIOIDS

WHEN TO BEGIN STRONG OPIOID THERAPY

When does one initiate treatment of pain with strong opioids? Most often, the severity of pain experienced by the patient determines when strong opioids should be used. Pain of such severity that it can be relieved only by opioids obviously is an indication for their use, independent of whether the pain occurs in the early, or localized stage of the disease, or in the advanced stage. Too often, opioids are reserved for pain accompanying advanced disease rather than used to treat severe pain regardless of the stage of disease (see Chapter 8). A common practice is to continue treatment with a weak opioid, or a combination of a weak opioid and a non-narcotic analgesic such as acetaminophen or a nonsteroidal anti-inflammatory drug (NSAID), in an ineffective polypharmacy regimen, simply to avoid the use of a strong opioid. Physicians seem to be more comfortable using strong opioids after they are convinced that death is imminent and narcotic use will be confined to a finite period of time (see Chapter 8). Imminent death is not a valid criterion for the use of strong opioids. The strong opioids should be used whenever they are required to provide adequate pain relief.

PROTRACTED USE OF OPIOIDS

Certain tumors, such as some soft-tissue sarcomas, breast cancer, gastrointestinal malignancies, and hematologic malignancies, tend to be associated with a protracted clinical course (months to years), and are often accompanied by pain that is characteristically persistent and chronic. When pain is adequately controlled, many of these patients are able to function in their usual jobs and live relatively normal lives. Even when disease limits physical activity and normal functional capacity, adequate pain control promotes an improved quality of life that would not be otherwise possible.

Opioid therapy is frequently delayed in patients with the potential for a protracted, painful illness because of concerns about the development of tolerance and physical and psychological dependency (addiction) (see Chapters 8 and 12). Prognosis and survival time should not be determining factors for initiating or maintaining opioid therapy. Similarly, tolerance should not be a deterrent to possible long-term use. Tolerance in cancer patients, if it occurs clinically at all, develops slowly, and the need to escalate the dose occurs infrequently.[10] If there is a need for a larger opioid dose, it is usually due to progression of disease causing an increase in the intensity of pain. Physical dependence is inevitable, but is associated with no adverse consequences, unless the need for the opioid no longer exists and it is discontinued abruptly or a narcotic antagonist is administered. When opioid therapy is no longer required, withdrawal symptoms can be obviated by simply administering a lower dose of drug in a graded, gradual fashion until it is discontinued. Psychological dependence (addiction) seldom occurs when opioids are used for legitimate medical purposes (see Chapters 8 and 12).[11,12] Therefore, the possibility of opioid addiction occurring in cancer patients is remote.

In summary, it is not logical to postpone therapy with the opioids because of the possibility of long-term use and fears that tolerance, physical dependency, or addiction may develop.

CHOOSING AN OPIOID

Once the decision has been made to use an opioid, the next decision is the selection of an appropriate drug. This process begins with assessing the pain (see Chapters 1–5). The importance of assessment and reassessment of pain during the course of the patient's disease cannot be overemphasized. Severe pain requires a strong opioid for control, mild pain requires a weak opioid, and moderate pain requires either a weak or a strong opioid.

WEAK OPIOIDS

Propoxyphene

Propoxyphene is one of the four stereoisomers of methadone, the only one of which has analgesic activity (ie, it binds to opioid receptors). When administered orally, its analgesic potency is approximately one-half to two-thirds that of codeine. Various conflicting studies indicate that this drug cannot be demonstrated to be more effective than appropriate doses of aspirin, acetaminophen, or the NSAIDs.[13] A trial is, nonetheless, useful in patients with mild pain. It should not necessarily be considered a "step up" the analgesic ladder for patients whose pain is no longer relieved by aspirin or acetaminophen, notwithstanding the fact that it is technically an opioid.

Codeine

Codeine, probably the most frequently prescribed opioid for treating cancer pain, is effective in controlling mild pain. It is used most often with either aspirin or acetaminophen, a combination that produces a greater analgesic effect than the mere sum of the two types of analgesics.[14] Continuing the use of codeine, either alone or in combination, after it is no longer adequate to relieve pain is a common practice. Usually, the number of tablets is increased and/or the interval of administration is decreased to provide more codeine and to avoid using a stronger narcotic. When a fixed combination preparation of codeine and a non-narcotic is used in this manner, the patient may unintentionally receive a toxic dose of the non-narcotic.

Oxycodone

Until recently, oxycodone was not available in the United States, except in combination with either aspirin or acetaminophen (Percodan [DuPont, Wilmington, DE]; Percocet [Du Pont]; and Tylox [McNeil, Spring House, PA]. (See Appendix C, Table 2) Oxycodone is now available separately as a 5-mg tablet and as a liquid (1 mg/ml and 20 mg/ml). When prescribed in a fixed-combination preparation with aspirin or acetaminophen, the same potential problem exists as mentioned for codeine—namely, possible toxic doses of the non-narcotic may be achieved as the number of tablets is increased or the interval of administration is decreased as a part of an ill-advised attempt to avoid the use of a stronger opioid. The availability of oxycodone as a sole drug preparation obviates this problem, and makes available a useful drug for the treatment of mild to moderate pain.

Oxycodone is reported to have a relative potency of 7.7 times greater than that of codeine, using a multivariate potency statistical method.[15] It therefore can be considered a step up the analgesic ladder after codeine. Because it only recently has become available as a sole, uncombined agent, this formulation has not yet enjoyed widespread clinical use in the United States. However, it is a useful addition to the clinician's pain therapy armamentarium, and the clinician should gain experience in its use.

The fixed-combination forms of oxycodone are used extensively (see Appendix C, Table 2). Major problems with their use relate to continued administration when a strong opioid is actually needed to provide adequate pain relief, and their use as a component of inappropriate polypharmacy regimens of weak analgesics to avoid the use of strong opioids.

Hydrocodone

Hydrocodone is used extensively in antitussive compounds, and its cough-suppressant effect is slightly greater than that of codeine (see Chapter 13).[16] It is also used in fixed combinations with acetaminophen for the treatment of mild to moderate pain (see Appendix C, Table 2). Hydrocodone is not currently available as a separate analgesic. No studies comparing hydrocodone's potency with that of other analgesics are available. It is generally considered comparable with combination oxycodone products. The major misuses of hydrocodone are identical to those of oxycodone. An added precaution for fixed-combination hydrocodone products, however, is that some of them contain as much as 650 to 750 mg of acetaminophen (Anexsia 7.5/650 [Beecham, Bristol, TN], Vicodin ES [Knoll, Whippany, NJ]) in a single tablet, and toxic doses of acetaminophen will be reached more quickly if the number of tablets is increased or the interval of administration is decreased to avoid the use of a stronger opioid.

In states requiring multiple-copy prescriptions (currently nine states) for schedule II controlled substances, the use of combination hydrocodone products is popular because it is a schedule III drug, and is therefore exempt from the multiple-copy requirement. In these states, one copy of the prescription is sent to the state narcotic control agency or bureau, and this has a "chilling," inhibitory effect on physicians using schedule II drugs, even though they are clinically indicated.[17] Regrettably, this can serve as an impetus for physicians to continue prescribing a drug that is not as highly regulated, even though the medication does not provide adequate pain relief (see Chapter 8). Despite these considerations, ethical concerns dictate that physicians meet their obligations to their patients, and that they provide them with proper means to achieve pain relief regardless of their perception that legal vulnerability exists.

STRONG OPIOIDS

Morphine

Morphine is the prototype for strong opioids. It is the most widely used opioid world-wide, and has been more extensively studied than any other opioid; consequently, there is more clinical experience and investigational data available for morphine than any other opioid. Despite this wealth of experience and data, myths and misconceptions about morphine abound, and play a major role in its suboptimal usage (see Chapter 8).[18,19] Most myths stem from the association of morphine with opium (morphine was the first alkaloid purified from opium), and from cultural and societal concepts about morphine that have influenced its use by physicians (eg, "Mother must be going to die, the doctor has given her morphine," or "I can't give you any more morphine because I don't want you to become addicted").[19,20]

Pharmacokinetics of Morphine. Morphine is readily absorbed from the gastrointestinal tract. It is metabolized to morphine-3-glucuronide and morphine-6-glucuronide. Morphine-6-glucuronide is a potent analgesic, but morphine-3-glucuronide may antagonize its analgesic effect.[21–23] The role of these metabolites in analgesia is a focus of current research, and remains to be determined.

Metabolism in the liver, through a first-pass effect, basically inactivates approximately two-thirds of the orally administered dose (ie, two-thirds of a given oral dose does not possess analgesic capabilities). Parenterally administered doses (see Chapter 11) are not subject to this first-pass effect because they reach binding sites before the liver reduces their effectiveness, and as a result clinicians often perceive parenterally administered opioids to be more effective than opioids administered orally. To overcome the first-pass effect with oral opioids, the dose administered must be adjusted upward to compensate for this effect. If this pharmacokinetic principle is applied clinically, successful treatment with oral administration of opioids occurs in the vast majority of patients.

Pharmacodynamics of Morphine. Morphine has major and important effects on the central nervous system (CNS) and the bowel. Central nervous system effects differ in individuals who are experiencing pain versus individuals who are not.[24] Pain antagonizes the analgesic and respiratory depressant effects of opioids, and as a result the dose of opioid necessary to control pain is often higher than might otherwise be expected. Respiratory depression does not occur so long as the increased dose does not greatly exceed that which is necessary to control pain. Confusion about this point and irrational fears of respiratory depression often result in patients with pain receiving inadequate doses of morphine or other opioids (see Chapter 8).

Morphine's effects on the CNS are diverse, and include analgesia, drowsiness, alterations in mood, decreased mental acuity, nausea, vomiting, and endocrine and autonomic nervous system dysfunction. Effects on the bowel occur primarily in the small and large intestine, where propulsive contractions and peristaltic waves are markedly decreased or abolished. Tolerance to effects on the bowel does not occur, or occurs extremely slowly, and as a result it is extremely important to institute a bowel-cleansing program when morphine is prescribed, especially when prolonged use is anticipated (see Chapters 10 and 12). Another action of morphine in the gastrointestinal tract is an increase in biliary pressure.

Morphine may also affect urinary bladder function, causing both urgency and difficulty on voiding because of increased sphincter tone. Cardiovascular effects may include reductions in blood pressure due to peripheral arteriolar and venous dilatation.

The pharmacodynamics of the other opioids are essentially the same as for morphine. Significant clinical differences are discussed subsequently.

Dose of Morphine. The dose of morphine usually recommended for the treatment of severe pain is 10 mg given intramuscularly.[25] This dose was determined by single-dose studies in postoperative patients.[26] Pain from other causes may require more or less morphine. Cancer pain and pain in many chronic nonmalignant conditions may be more severe than postoperative pain, in which case doses greater than 10 mg will be required. A maxim about the proper dose of morphine is, "The proper dose of morphine is whatever it takes to relieve the pain without inducing intolerable side effects." A 10-mg intramuscular dose

or an equianalgesic oral dose may be a reasonable starting dose, but the results of this dose should be rapidly evaluated, and it should be titrated upward until pain is relieved. Probably the most common error that occurs in dosing with opioids is underdosing.[27,28] Daily doses of morphine required to relieve cancer pain adequately may vary from 60 to 3,000 mg in divided doses.[29] There is no "ceiling" effect for morphine; an increase in the dose will always produce a concomitant increase in pain relief. Caution is appropriate when such increases do not appear to result in further relief of pain. There is evidence that opioids are less effective in treating pain that originates from nerve damage (neuropathic pain) (see Chapters 1–3, 8, and 10).[3] Increasing the opioid dose under these circumstances may simply result in increased side effects without additional analgesia.

The duration of action for morphine is 3–4 hours, and undertreatment of pain occurs when greater dosing intervals are used. Morphine is now available in a controlled-release form that extends its effectiveness to 8–12 hours. A method of pain control using combined immediate-release and controlled-release morphine will be described subsequently.

OTHER STRONG OPIOIDS

The pharmacodynamics of other opioid drugs are similar to those described for morphine, although an individual may experience more or fewer side effects when exposed to different drugs, and the same drug may cause different effects in different patients. For example, morphine may cause nausea and vomiting in one patient but not another. These so-called side effects may occur with any of the opioids, and changing from one to another may be necessary in a given patient. There are, however, pharmacologic differences among the opioids that will be discussed below.

Hydromorphone

Hydromorphone is readily absorbed from the gastrointestinal tract, and controls severe pain when it is administered orally in adequate doses. It is more potent by weight than morphine, with 1.3 mg hydromorphone being equianalgesic to 10 mg morphine when both are administered intramuscularly. Because of biotransformation in the liver (first-pass effect), the oral dose must be four to five times the parenteral dose to produce an equianalgesic effect.[30] When administered orally, hydromorphone reaches its peak effect slightly more rapidly than does morphine, and also has a slightly shorter duration of action. It may be necessary to administer hydromorphone at 2- to 3-hour intervals.

Methadone

Methadone is as potent an analgesic as morphine in comparable doses when administered intramuscularly. However, because of its favorable oral-to-parenteral ratio of 2:1 (first-pass effect is slighter), the equianalgesic oral dose is only twice the parenteral dose. The most important clinical considerations in the use of methadone relate to its long half-life (see Chapter 8). Although the duration of analgesic effectiveness of single oral doses is approximately 4 hours, its terminal elimination half-life varies from 13 to 51 hours.[31,32] When repeated doses are given every 4 hours, the drug accumulates, and the blood concentration may reach toxic levels. Initial dosing must be carefully monitored to avoid this complication. After the first 3 to 4 days, the interval of administration can be extended, which effectively reduces the total 24-hour dose while maintaining the same analgesic level. Methadone may be effective when administered every 6 to 8 hours chronically.

Methadone may be difficult to use in older patients and in cancer patients with rapidly progressive disease and frequent changes in pain intensity. Also, some patients associate methadone with treatment for drug addiction, and are afraid that taking methadone will stigmatize them as being drug addicts.

Levorphanol

Levorphanol is an effective oral agent for the control of severe pain. It is readily absorbed from the gastrointestinal tract, and has a fa-

vorable oral-to-parenteral ratio of approximately 1:1.[33] It has a half-life of approximately 11 hours, and therefore some accumulation occurs, and dosing intervals of greater than 4 hours may be possible. The same potential problems described with the initial titration of methadone apply for levorphanol as well.

Meperidine

Meperidine, although extensively used for postoperative pain, is not recommended for the treatment of chronic pain. It is readily absorbed from the gastrointestinal tract, but has a low oral-to-parenteral ratio (4:1). Meperidine is the weakest of the "strong" opioids when compared with morphine. A 75- to 100-mg dose of meperidine is equianalgesic to a 10 mg dose of morphine when both are administered intramuscularly. Orally, 300 mg is equianalgesic to 30 mg morphine. Meperidine's duration of action is approximately 3 hours, making frequent dosing necessary.

The most serious drawback to the chronic administration of meperidine is the accumulation of the metabolite normeperidine. Its half-life is longer than that of the parent compound. Normeperidine is a CNS stimulant, and may cause tremor, muscle twitches, and seizures. Toxicity is more likely to occur in patients with renal failure.[34]

Table 9–3 and Appendix C, Table 1 show the oral-to-parenteral dose ratios and the equianalgesic doses for commonly used opioids. This table can be used to convert the dose of one opioid to that of another, and is useful to convert between routes of administration. The reference standard is 10 mg morphine administered intramuscularly for treatment of severe pain.

OPIOIDS WITH MIXED AGONIST/ ANTAGONIST ACTIVITY AND PARTIAL AGONISTS

Opioids with mixed agonist/antagonist activity and partial agonists are not recommended for the treatment of chronic cancer pain. These opioids tend to produce a higher incidence

Table 9–3.*

Oral-to-Parenteral Dose Ratios and Equianalgesic Doses for Various Opioids (Reference Dose 10 mg Morphine Intramuscularly to Treat Severe Pain)

Drug	Oral Dose	Oral-to-Parenteral Dose Ratio	Parenteral Dose
Morphine			
Single dose	60 mg	6 : 1	10 mg
Repeated dose	30 mg	3 : 1	10 mg
Hydromorphone	8 mg	5 : 1	1.6 mg
Methadone hydrochloride	20 mg	2 : 1	10 mg
Levorphanol	2 mg	1 : 1 (approx)	2 mg
Meperidine hydrochloride	300 mg	4 : 1	75 mg
Codeine	200 mg	1.5 : 1	130 mg

* See also Appendix C, Table 1

of psychotomimetic reactions than the pure agonists, and only pentazocine is available for oral administration in the United States. Differential binding to opioid receptor sites is thought to account for the higher incidence of psychotomimetic reactions.[9] Patients being treated with pure agonist drugs should not be switched to treatment with an agonist/antagonist or a partial agonist because of the latter group's potential to precipitate a withdrawal reaction by their antagonist action.

SIDE EFFECTS OF OPIOIDS

Many clinicians assume that all drug side effects are *prima facie* undesirable. If a broader view is adopted, it can be seen that this does not hold true for the opioids. Patients being treated for pain who also have diarrhea will appreciate the "constipating" effects of the opioids. The same is true for the antitussive effects of the opioids in patients with cough (see Chapters 12, 13, and 30).

Side effects may be transitory or persistent. Side effects that are usually transitory and associated with the initiation of opioid therapy are sedation, mental clouding (including transient hallucinations), dizziness, urinary retention, nausea, vomiting, and itch-

ing. A careful pharmacodynamic evaluation should be made of these side effects before it is concluded that opioids or a particular opioid or route of administration must be abandoned. There can be multiple causes for these symptoms, and the opioid should not be implicated unless a definite relationship can be established.

Sometimes these side effects persist after the initiation of opioid therapy, and are sufficiently severe to impede overall function. Sedation can be managed with the concurrent administration of CNS stimulants such as dextroamphetamine sulfate or methylphenidate. Synergistic analgesic effects have been observed for dextroamphetamine sulfate and morphine, and concurrent administration may not only correct sedation but enhance pain relief.[35] Mood may be affected in a positive way as well. Nausea and vomiting can be controlled with antiemetics, which often can be discontinued after 1 to 2 weeks without a recurrence of nausea and vomiting. Patients with problems urinating can be taught to catheterize themselves, and after several days normal function generally resumes. Many of the transient side effects are dose dependent, and once the dose is adjusted properly the side effects are minimized or resolve entirely.

The most consistent and persistent side

effect of opioids is constipation (see Chapters 10, 12, and 13). It occurs with all opioids, including the weak ones, especially codeine, and with all routes of administration. A bowel-cleansing program should be instituted at the same time that a narcotic is prescribed, especially when treatment is likely to be chronic. This program should most often initially include a stool softener and mild laxative. Just as pain must be frequently reassessed, so must the presence and severity of side effects, and treatment should be altered accordingly.

Some clinicians confuse the intrinsic attributes of opioids with their side effects. Tolerance and physical dependence are two attributes of opioids that occur inevitably with long-term opioid administration (see Chapters 8 and 12). As was stated previously, in cancer patients clinical tolerance occurs very slowly, if at all. Physical dependence occurs, but is of no consequence because it does not cause symptoms or undesirable effects until opioid therapy is no longer needed. Abrupt discontinuation will produce symptoms of an abstinence or withdrawal reaction that is not only distressing, but in some circumstances can be life-threatening. This outcome can be avoided by reducing the opioid dose in a graded manner. There is ample evidence that patients taking opioids for pain relief do not develop psychological dependence (addiction).[11,36,37] Cancer patients taking opioids for pain relief welcome the discontinuation of these drugs when pain abates. Additionally, addiction to a drug has been shown to involve more complex factors than mere exposure to the drug.[11,12,37,38] The likelihood of a cancer patient who takes opioids for pain becoming a drug abuser or typical street drug "addict" is remote.[11,37,39] Many clinicians have an irrational fear of this outcome, and, consequently, many patients suffer needlessly because the use of strong opioids is postponed or treatment is provided with doses that are inadequate to achieve adequate relief of pain.

Most patients can be treated successfully with oral opioids, even for extremely severe pain, if dosing guidelines are observed and adequate attention is paid to the recognition and treatment of side effects. Patience and persistence on the part of both the physician and patient in overcoming side effects are essential elements to achieving optimal, cost-efficient pain relief.

TREATMENT PLANS

The observation of two principles is an essential component of any pharmacologically based treatment plan: 1) the use of an analgesic that will control the pain; and 2) frequent reassessment of the outcome of the plan to determine its success. A corollary to these principles is that side effects resulting from treatment must be documented and treated.

The first step in establishing a plan is to assess the severity and other characteristics of the pain. The analgesic selected should be no stronger than is needed to bring about pain relief (ie, mild pain requires a mild analgesic and severe pain requires a strong analgesic). The stage of disease is irrelevant in making this determination (see Chapter 8). For example, severe pain can occur at the onset of cancer, in which case treatment with a strong narcotic will be required early in the disease course.

"ANALGESIC LADDER" APPROACH

The World Health Organization (WHO) recommends an "analgesic ladder" approach to pain treatment (see Chapters 7 and 27)[40]: patients with pain that is initially mild and progresses in a crescendo fashion to more severe pain are treated with a ladder approach using increasingly stronger analgesics. Mild pain is treated with a nonopioid analgesic, such as acetaminophen, aspirin, or another NSAID, with or without an adjuvant drug such as an antidepressant or anticonvulsant. For moderate pain, a weak opioid alone or in combination with acetaminophen, aspirin, or another NSAID is recommended, again with the option of adding an adjuvant drug. For severe pain, the strong opioids should be used alone or in combination with a nonopioid analgesic and an adjuvant drug. The minimum dose of opioid employed for any degree of pain intensity should be that which is adequate to relieve the pain. The so-called usual or recommended doses found in pharmacology texts, or other standard sources or references, will frequently need to be exceeded in order to provide adequate relief of pain.

MORPHINE TEST

Unfortunately, pain intensity does not always progress in a predictable crescendo fashion. Frequently, pain is severe at the outset, as in the case of a pathologic fracture of a long bone or a collapsed vertebra, and in other cases it may begin as mild and progress quickly to a severe pain, skipping the moderate step. For this reason, the WHO-recommended ladder approach requires a complementary approach to accommodate these clinical situations. The proper dose of morphine may be determined by a simple "morphine test," performed as described below.

After the initial pain assessment, a small-gauge butterfly needle attached to a plastic catheter is inserted into an upper extremity vein, or, when available, a permanent venous access device may be used. The initial test dose of morphine (5 to 15 mg) is administered essentially as a "push" over an interval of 30 to 90 seconds, and is selected based on the clinician's subjective assessment of pain intensity. After the morphine is delivered, the catheter is flushed with 5 ml normal saline to ensure that the bolus immediately enters the venous circulation. When definite and significant pain relief follows the initial injection, the procedure is repeated until the patient is relatively pain-free (usually after two injections separated by a 15-minute interval). When pain relief is equivocal and indefinite, injections are repeated until no further pain relief is experienced or troublesome side effects arise (usually after three to five injections separated by 15-minute intervals).

For patients in whom oral opioid therapy is appropriate, an oral dose of morphine is then calculated based on the intravenous dose required to relieve the subject's pain using a 3:1 oral-to-parenteral ratio. For example, if 10 mg intravenous morphine produced complete pain relief, the correct oral dose would be 30 mg every 4 hours. Other opioids the patient might be taking are not considered in this calculation, since these failed to relieve the pain. The advantage of applying this type of test is that unnecessarily long titration intervals are avoided, and patients are more likely to benefit from immediate relief of pain.[41]

COMBINATION THERAPY WITH CONTROLLED-RELEASE AND IMMEDIATE-RELEASE MORPHINE

Morphine is available in a resin matrix that slowly dissolves in the gastrointestinal tract, releasing the morphine over a 12-hour interval. This allows patients to be dosed with controlled-release morphine at 8- to 12-hour intervals.[42,43] Adequate pain control frequently can be achieved using this 8- to 12-hour regimen alone. Should "breakthrough" pain occur between doses, it can be treated with immediate-release (regular) morphine. By using a combination of controlled-release and immediate-release morphine, a treatment regimen can be devised that is analogous with that used in treating an insulin-dependent diabetic with long-acting insulin supplemented by short-acting insulin.

The first consideration in formulating this treatment regimen is to determine the amount of morphine necessary to control the patient's pain over a 24-hour period. The 24-hour dose is determined by the size of the individual dose times the number of doses of immediate-release morphine a patient requires to maintain the pain-free state over a 24-hour period. For example, if 30 mg of oral morphine is required every 4 hours, there would be six such intervals in a 24-hour period, and the 24-hour dose would be 180 mg. The patient's pain could be controlled by giving 90 mg of controlled-release morphine every 12 hours instead of 30 mg every 4 hours, thus affording the patient greater convenience. Psychologically, the patient also benefits, because when fewer doses are taken, he or she is reminded less often of the pain.

Immediate-release morphine is always prescribed along with controlled-release morphine in case breakthrough pain should occur. This "escape" dose is usually one-sixth of the total 24-hour dose, but should be titrated to meet the goal of adequate pain relief. This method is analogous to prescribing regular, short-acting insulin along with long-acting insulin to cover the contingency of insulin-need during the interval that the long-acting insulin is predicted to provide adequate blood sugar control. Combination therapy produces optimum diabetic control because all contingencies affecting blood sugar control are covered. Similarly, the immediate-release morphine is available should additional pain occur during the 12-hour interval that the controlled-release morphine dose is expected to provide adequate pain control.

After the patient starts taking controlled-release morphine, the number of doses of immediate-release morphine required to maintain pain control serves as a monitor to determine when the dose of controlled-release morphine should be increased. As pain intensity increases, pain will be controlled less readily with the same dose of controlled-release morphine administered over a 24-hour period. Consequently, the patient will require more doses of breakthrough pain medication. When the number of doses of breakthrough medication exceeds two during the daytime interval and one during the nighttime interval, the dose of controlled-release morphine should be increased. The amount of increase can be calculated simply by adding the total amount of immediate-release morphine taken for breakthrough pain during a 24-hour period, dividing by two, and adding the result to the current controlled-release dose. Again, this is analogous to methods used to adjust the dose of long-acting insulin for patients with diabetes.

Any immediate-release, short-acting opioid (eg, hydromorphone, oxycodone) can be used in conjunction with controlled-release morphine for treating breakthrough pain, but the use of immediate-release morphine obviates the necessity to convert a nonmorphine breakthrough opioid dose to a morphine dose when the controlled-release morphine dose needs to be increased. Also, keeping the number of different medications a patient takes to a minimum simplifies the process. The mechanism of action for all opioids is the same (ie, binding to opioid receptor sites in the CNS). Except when taking advantage of other pharmacologic differences discussed earlier, there is little need to administer more than one opioid at a time.

This combination regimen has many important advantages. It is convenient, and ambulatory patients can carry their medication with them in out-of-sight containers. Frequent dosing is unnecessary, and as a result patients are not conspicuous when taking medication. In addition, pain is controlled throughout the night, and neither pain nor the need to awaken to take medicine interferes with sleep. For these reasons, this type of pain management should be considered for all patients with oncologic pain that is relatively constant.

REFERENCES

1. Portenoy RK, Foley KM, Inturrisi CE: The nature of opioid responsiveness and its implication for neuropathic pain: New hypotheses derived from studies of opioid infusions. Pain 1990;43:273.
2. Twycross RG: Opioid analgesics in cancer pain: Current practice and controversies. Cancer Surv 1988;7:29.
3. McQuay HJ. Pharmacological treatment of neuralgic and neuropathic pain. Cancer Surv 1988;7:141.
4. Arner S, Arner B: Differential effects of epidural morphine in the treatment of cancer related pain. Acta Anaesthesiol Scand 1983;29:32.
5. Arner S, Meyerson BA: Lack of analgesic effect of opioids on neuropathic and idiopathic forms of pain. Pain 1988;33:11.
6. Houde RW: Analgesic effectiveness of the narcotic agonist/antagonists. Br J Clin Pharmacol 1979;1 (Suppl 3):297S.
7. Inturrisi CE: Management of cancer pain: Pharmacology and principles of management. Cancer 1989; 63:2308.

8. Snyder SH: Drug and neurotransmitter receptors in the brain. Science 1984;224:22.

9. Martin WR: Pharmacology of opioids. Pharmacol Rev 1984;35:283.

10. Foley KM: Controversies in cancer pain: Medical perspectives. Cancer 1989;63:2257.

11. Porter J, Jick H: Addiction rare in patients treated with narcotics. N Engl J Med 1980;302:123.

12. Morgan JP: American opiophobia: Customary under-utilization of opioid analgesics. In Hill CS Jr, Fields WS (eds): Advances in Pain Research and Therapy, vol 11: Drug Treatment of Cancer Pain in a Drug-Oriented Society, p 181. New York, Raven Press, 1989.

13. Cooper SA, Beaver WT: A model to evaluate mild analgesics in oral surgery patients. Clin Pharmacol Ther 1976:20;241.

14. Beaver WT: Combination analgesics. Am J Med 1984;77:38.

15. Sunshine A, Laska EM, Olson NZ: Analgesic effects of oral oxycodone and codeine in the treatment of patients with postoperative, postfracture, or somatic pain. In Foley KM, Inturrisi CE (eds): Advances in Pain Research and Therapy, vol 8: Opioid Analgesics in the Management of Clinical Pain, p 225. New York: Raven Press, 1986.

16. Jaffe JH, Martin WR: Opioid analgesics and antagonists. In Goodman LS, Gilman A (eds): The Pharmacological Basis of Therapeutics, 7th ed, p 505. New York, Macmillan, 1985.

17. Jorenson DE: Federal and state regulation of opioids. Journal of Pain and Symptom Management. 1990;5 (Suppl 1):S12

18. Twycross RW, Lack SA: Symptom control in far advanced cancer: Pain Relief, p 112. London, Pittman, 1983.

19. Musto DF: The American Disease: Origins of Narcotic Control, p 30. New York, Oxford University Press, 1987.

20. Hill CS: Relationship among cultural, educational, and regulatory agency influences on optimum pain treatment. Journal of Pain and Symptom Management 1990;5 (Suppl 1):S37.

21. Yoshimura H, Ida S, Oguri K et al: Biochemical basis for analgesic activity of morphine-6-glucuronide: I. Penetration of morphine-6-glucuronide in the brain of rats. Biochem Pharmacol 1983;22:1423.

22. Sawe J: Morphine and its 3- and 6-glucuronides in plasma and urine during chronic administration in cancer patients. In Foley KM, Inturrisi CE (eds): Advances in Pain Research and Therapy, vol 8: Opioid Analgesics in the Management of Clinical Pain, p 45. New York, Raven Press, 1986.

23. Smith MT, Watt JA, Cramond T: Morphine-3-glucu-ronide: A potent antagonist of morphine analgesia. Life Sci 1990;47:579.

24. Hanks GW, Twycross RG, Lloyd JW: Unexpected complication of successful nerve block. Anaesthesia 1981;36:37

25. Houde RW: Misinformation: Side effects and drug interactions. In Hill CS, Fields WS (eds): Advances in Pain Research and Therapy, vol 11: Drug Treatment of Cancer Pain in a Drug-Oriented Society, p 145. New York, Raven Press, 1989.

26. Twycross RG: The management of pain in cancer: A guide to drugs and dosages. Oncology 1988;2:35.

27. Marks RM, Sachar EJ: Undertreatment of medical inpatients with narcotic analgesics. Ann Intern Med 1973;78:173.

28. Sriwatanakul K, Weis OF, Alloza JL et al: Analysis of narcotic usage in the treatment of postoperative pain. JAMA 1983;250:926.

29. Kaiko RF, Grandy RP, Oshlack B et al: The United States experience with oral controlled-release morphine. Cancer 1989;63:2348.

30. Houde RW: Clinical analgesic studies of hydromorphone. In Foley KM, Inturrisi CE (eds): Advances in Pain Research and Therapy, vol 8: Opioid Analgesics in the Management of Clinical Pain, p 129. New York, Raven Press, 1986.

31. Inturrisi CE, Colburn WA: Pharmacokinetics of methadone. In Foley KM, Inturrisi CE (eds): Advances in Pain Research and Therapy, vol 8: Opioid Analgesics in the Management of Clinical Pain, p 191. New York, Raven Press, 1986.

32. Nilsson MI, Anggard E, Holmstrand J et al: Pharmacokinetics of methadone during maintenance treatment: Adaptive changes during the induction phase. Eur J Clin Pharmacol 1982;22:343.

33. Dixon R: Pharmacokinetics of levorphanol. In Foley KM, Inturrisi CE (eds): Advances in Pain Research and Therapy, vol 8: Opioid Analgesics in the Management of Clinical Pain, p 217. New York, Raven Press, 1986.

34. Inturrisi CE, Umans JG: Meperidine biotransformation and central nervous system toxicity in animals and humans. In Foley KM, Inturrisi CE (eds): Advances in Pain Research and Therapy, vol 8: Opioid Analgesics in the Management of Clinical Pain, p 143. New York, Raven Press, 1986.

35. Forrest WH, Brown BW Jr, Brown CR et al: Dextroamphetamine with morphine for the treatment of postoperative pain. N Engl J Med 1977;296:712.

36. Foley KM: The ''decriminalization'' of cancer pain. In Hill CS, Fields WS (eds): Advances in Pain Research and Therapy, vol 11: Drug Treatment of Cancer Pain in a Drug-Oriented Society, p 7. New York, Raven Press, 1989.

37. Perry S, Heidrich G: Management of pain during debridement: A survey of U.S. burn units. Pain 1982;13:267.

38. Robins LN, David DH, Nurco DN: How permanent was Vietnam drug addiction? Am J Public Health 1974;64:38.

39. Peele S: Ain't misbehavin': Addiction has become an all-purpose excuse. The Sciences, NY Acad Sci, July/August 1989 p 14.

40. World Health Organization: Cancer Pain Relief, 2nd ed. Geneva, World Health Organization, 1989.

41. Hill CS, Thorpe DM, McCrory L: A method for attaining rapid and sustained pain relief and discriminating nociceptive from neuropathic pain in cancer patients. Pain 1990;5 (Suppl 1):S498.

42. Hanks GW, Twycross RG, Bliss JM: Controlled release morphine tablets: A double-blind trial in patients with advanced cancer. Anaesthesia 1987;42:840.

43. Hanks GW: Controlled-release morphine (MST Contin) in advanced cancer: The European experience. Cancer 1989;63:2378.

Chapter 10

Adjuvants to Opioid Analgesics

Eduardo Bruera

Carla Ripamonti

INTRODUCTION

Opioid analgesics are widely acknowledged as the most important drugs for the treatment of chronic pain (see Chapters 8, 9, 11, and 12).[1,2] Although these drugs can, in most cases, control severe pain, even when they are used appropriately they may produce new symptoms or exacerbate preexisting symptoms, most notably nausea and somnolence (see Chapters 9 and 12).[1-3] This aspect of treatment with opioid compounds is particularly problematic in patients with advanced cancer. The combination of severe pain, anorexia, chronic nausea, asthenia, and somnolence is a frequent finding in patients with advanced cancer (see Chapters 12, 13, and 30).[3]

The term "adjuvant drug" has been used in a variety of ways even in the context of cancer pain management. For the purposes of this chapter, an adjuvant drug meets one or more of the following criteria: 1) increases the analgesic effect of narcotics (adjuvant analgesia); 2) decreases the toxicity of narcotics; or 3) improves other symptoms associated with terminal cancer. When epidemiologic data suggest patients are at a high risk for developing toxicity as a consequence of commencing chronic treatment with narcotics (*eg*, constipation), consideration should be given to initiating adjuvant treatment in advance of clinical evidence of toxicity.

Claims have been made for the adjuvant analgesic effects of many drugs (Table 10–1), but, unfortunately, most of the evidence for these effects is anecdotal. Controlled clinical trials are needed to define better

Table 10–1.
Drugs Suggested to Have Adjuvant Effects

Nonsteroidal anti-inflammatories	Antibiotics
	Baclofen
Antiemetics	Amphetamines
Phenothiazines	Corticosteroids
Benzodiazepines	Diphosphonates
Tricyclic antidepressants	Calcitonin
Clonidine	Nifedipine
Anticonvulsants	

the indications and risk:benefit ratios of these agents, some of which have the potential to produce significant toxicity, and can aggravate the toxicity of narcotics. Research is complicated by the need to measure multiple end points during such a trial (see below). Some of these end points are likely to remain constant (eg, constipation or pain), but others are likely to change as a function of time (sedation, nausea), and results tend to be confounded by the effects of tumor progression, which often are not well quantified. The duration of the clinical trial and its design will also be affected by the characteristics of the adjuvant drugs being tested (see below).

This chapter summarizes the current use of adjuvant drugs and contemporary approaches to clinical trial design. Emphasis will be placed on those drugs that should be the focus of future research.

PART I: CURRENT USE OF ADJUVANT DRUGS

Treatment for most patients with cancer pain includes adjuvant drug therapy.[1,4–6] Our group studied the prescribing patterns for narcotics and adjuvant drugs in 100 consecutive patients admitted to a cancer center during 1980, 1984, and 1987. All patients were consecutive admissions under the Department of Medicine, and none had prior consultation with a pain specialist or palliative care physician.[4,5] Table 10–2 summarizes the pattern of use of adjuvant drugs during 1980, as compared to 1984 and 1987. The results show that more than two-thirds of patients received laxatives and non-narcotic analgesics, almost half received hypnotics and antiemetics, and approximately one-third received psychoactive drugs. In a separate survey, we observed that prescribing patterns for adjuvant drugs also differ between countries. Patients admitted to a South American cancer center received significantly fewer prescriptions for laxatives, hypnotics, and nonpharmacologic treatment, and were more often treated with tricyclic antidepressants and non-narcotic analgesics as compared to patients admitted to a North American cancer center (see Chapter 27).[7]

Thus, in addition to narcotics, most symptomatic cancer patients receive more than one or two adjuvant drugs. Unfortunately, very few of these drugs have been subjected to controlled clinical trials.

NONSTEROIDAL ANTI-INFLAMMATORY DRUGS (NSAIDs)

Tumor growth produces inflammatory and mechanical effects in adjacent tissue that can trigger the release of prostaglandins (PG), bradykinin, and serotonin, which in turn may precipitate or exacerbate pain in the surrounding tissues.[8–10] Prostaglandin-mediated actions on peripheral nociceptors probably include both direct activation and sensitization to other algesic substances (see Chapter 7).

Prostaglandins are frequently associated with painful bone metastasis because of their involvement in bone reabsorption.[11] Prostaglandin synthesis has been observed in bone metastasis of rats and rabbits,[12] and in malignant breast tumors. An increased production of PG-analogue material has been found in malignant breast tumors as compared to benign tumors and healthy breast tissue. Increased in vitro synthesis of PG has been observed in bone metastases, as well.[13]

The nonsteroidal anti-inflammatory

Table 10–2.
Use of Adjuvant Drugs in 100 Consecutive Patients Admitted to a North American Cancer Center[4,5]

No. of Patients Receiving	1980	P	1984	P	1987
Laxatives	65	NS	69	NS	66
Corticosteroids	8	NS	11	NS	14
Antiemetics	49	NS	54	NS	53
Psychoactive drugs	22	<0.05	36	NS	39
Hypnotics	47	NS	49	NS	48
Non-narcotic analgesics	50	<0.01	77	NS	71

P, Probability; NS, Not significant

agents seem to exert their analgesic, anti-pyretic, and anti-inflammatory actions by blocking the synthesis of PG. This occurs via the inhibition of cyclo-oxygenase, an enzyme that catalyzes the conversion of arachidonic acid into endoperoxide, the substrate for PG, thromboxanes, and prostacyclins.[14]

By virtue of their different mechanisms of action and toxicity profiles, the NSAIDs and narcotics are often administered together. Commercial preparations containing codeine or oxycodone and acetaminophen or aspirin are among the most widely prescribed scheduled analgesics, and are frequently administered to cancer patients. This is appropriate, because a synergistic effect has been observed when the NSAIDs and mild opioids are combined to treat pain.[15] Unfortunately, when in response to increased pain, patients are advanced to more potent analgesics (morphine, hydromorphone, levorphanol, etc.), non-narcotics are usually not prescribed concurrently, and the potential advantageous effect of these medications is lost.[4,5]

Peripheral PG inhibitors may be more difficult to use than acetaminophen, because cancer patients are predisposed to NSAID-induced toxicity based on advanced age and concurrent hematologic and renal disorders. The most common NSAID-related side effects involve the gastroenteric tract, the liver, the kidneys, the skin, and the blood.[16,17]

Gastrointestinal complications include gastric pain, nausea, vomiting, hemorrhage, and, in extreme cases, perforation. Gastrointestinal damage is mediated by PG inhibition. The most common form of nephrotoxicity associated with the use of NSAIDs is renal failure, related to PG inhibition and consequent vasodilation. Clinical conditions such as congestive heart failure, cirrhosis, diuretic-induced hypovolemia, and the nephrotic syndrome have been observed to activate NSAID-mediated toxicity.[18] Hepatic injury has been reported with the use of aspirin, benoxaprofen, and phenylbutazone, and less commonly with diclofenac, ibuprofen, indomethacin, naproxen, pirbrofen, and sulindac. Sulindac, however, seems to be associated with a higher incidence of cholestasis.[19,20]

NSAID use is also associated with a variety of hypersensitive reactions involving the skin (rash, eruption, itching), blood vessels (angioneurotic edema, vasomotor disorders), and the respiratory system (rhinitis, asthma). In particular, aspirin may cause anaphylactic crisis, a syndrome characterized by dyspnea, sudden weakness, sweating, and collapse.[19] Undesirable hematologic effects of NSAIDs include platelet dysfunction, aplastic anemia, and agranulocytosis. The latter effects have been reported mostly with the use of phenylbutazone.[20] Stevens–Johnson syndrome has been reported with the use of benoxaprofen, diflusinal, sulindac, fenclofenac, and other less commonly used NSAIDs. Although untoward central nervous effects effects are rare, headache has been reported after treatment with dimethylxanthine.[20] Factors often considered in the empirical selection of an NSAID for a given patient include their relative toxicity, cost, dosage schedule, and prior experience. The use of certain aspirin analogues (sodium salicylate, choline magnesium trisalicylate) has been suggested to be associated with a low incidence of gastropathy and platelet dysfunction.[21–24]

Controlled trials conducted in cancer pain patients receiving opioids have demonstrated that the addition of non-narcotics can provide additive analgesia.[25] Other reports suggest a particularly important role for these agents in the treatment of patients with metastatic bone pain,[26] and in individuals whose pain has a prominent inflammatory component. Used as single agents in the management of cancer pain, the effects of the NSAIDs are characterized by a ceiling effect, beyond which further increases in dose do not enhance analgesia.[27] Portenoy has suggested, however, that the dosage at which this ceiling effect occurs may differ among individuals, and that it may be desirable to titrate the dose of the NSAID, often to twice its recommended dose, until the ceiling dose is arrived at empirically.[28]

A large retrospective study of 292 cancer patients treated according to the sequential analgesic ladder proposed by the World Health Organization (see Chapters 9 and 27) reported that the average length of treatment with NSAIDs alone was only 19 ± 24 days. Treatment with the NSAIDs was either discontinued due to their side effects (48%), or supplemented with narcotic analgesics because of incomplete relief of pain (52%).[29] There are no conclusive studies that demonstrate which non-narcotic agents are most effective for managing cancer pain, nor have the proper doses or routes of administration been established in prospective trials.

TRICYCLIC ANTIDEPRESSANTS

Despite the frequent use of these agents in hospice care,[30] South American cancer centers,[7] and some European centers,[31] their use in North American cancer centers has been infrequent, at least historically.[4–7,32] A recent study suggests, however, that the use of tricyclics has increased significantly in recent years in North American centers, and that pain is the main indication for 40% of prescriptions.[33]

The tricyclic antidepressants have been found to be useful in a variety of neuropathic pain syndromes, especially when pain has a prominent dysesthetic or burning character. Both amitriptyline and desipramine have been found to be effective in the management of postherpetic neuralgia in separate prospective, double-blind, placebo-controlled trials.[34,35] Cross-over, placebo-controlled trials of chlorimipramine and nortriptyline have demonstrated their efficacy in the management of central pain syndromes.[36] Imipramine, clomipramine, and desipramine have all been found to be useful in the management of diabetic neuropathy in controlled, double-blind studies.[37,38] There is, however, only very limited evidence for a significant analgesic effect in other types of cancer pain. In one placebo-controlled study of terminal patients, the administration of imipramine was accompanied by decreased requirements for morphine.[39] The mechanism by which the tricyclic antidepressants relieve pain has been suggested to involve potentiation of descending inhibitory pathways.[40] The results of other studies have suggested that the concurrent administration of the tricyclics may increase plasma levels of morphine[41,42] and methadone[43] by enhancing their bioavailability.

In support of a distinction between modulation of pain and affect, most clinicians using the tricyclics for pain relief do so in doses inadequate to combat depression.[1,6] At least in patients with postherpetic neuralgia, their effect appears to be unrelated to altered mood.[34] Clinical experience suggests that the tricyclics constitute a useful treatment for pain of central, deafferentation, or neuropathic origin, particularly when pain has a prominent dysesthetic or burning character, although the optimal drug and dosing regimen are unknown. Specific syndromes in which their use may be potentially beneficial include postherpetic neuralgia, postablative anesthesia dolorosa, post-treatment neuritis and neuropathy, and invasion of neural structures by tumor. A trial of tricyclic antidepressants may be useful in any patient whose pain has responded inadequately to standard pharmacologic management with opioids. It should be recalled that relief of pain is often not well established until 1 to 3 weeks of treatment have elapsed. Potentially beneficial side effects include the restoration of a normal pattern of nighttime sleep and improved mood.

The toxic effects of these drugs are mainly autonomic (dry mouth, postural hypotension) and centrally mediated (somnolence, confusion). Because their use may contribute to symptoms already present in debilitated patients, they should be administered cautiously in susceptible patients.

ANTICONVULSANTS

Carbamezepine, phenytoin, valproic acid, and clonazepam, alone or in combination with the tricyclic antidepressants, have been used successfully to treat pain of neuropathic origin.[44] On the basis of well documented efficacy for the treatment of trigeminal neuralgia (tic douloureux),[45] considerable anecdotal experience has accumulated for the use of these agents for neuropathic cancer pain syndromes, including neural invasion by tumor, radiation fibrosis or surgical scarring, herpes zoster, and deafferentation.[7,46] Based on clinical observations, improvement can be expected in a proportion of patients whose predominant complaint is pain of a lancinating, burning, or hyperesthetic nature.[7,47] There is a need for controlled clinical trials to determine the optimal drug, dose, and indications for use.

Side effects of therapy are potentially serious, particularly in patients with advanced cancer, and can include bone marrow depression, hepatic dysfunction, ataxia, diplopia, and lymphadenopathy. Periodic monitoring of complete blood count and liver function tests are recommended.

CORTICOSTEROIDS

Uncontrolled studies suggest that the administration of corticosteroids to selected patients with advanced cancer results in decreased pain and improved appetite and activity.[48] In 1974, Moertel randomized 116 patients with advanced gastrointestinal cancer to receive dexamethasone, 0.75 and 1.5 mg, four times daily or placebo in a double-blind trial. Significant tumor regression was not observed in the treated group, but symptomatic improvement (mainly appetite and strength) was significant after 2 weeks of treatment. These benefits were, however, no longer apparent after 4 weeks of treatment. Serious toxicity was low, and consisted only of one case of gastrointestinal hemorrhage.[49] We randomized 31 patients to methylprednisolone, 16 mg twice daily, versus placebo for 1 week.[50] After that period a cross-over took place, and patients received the alternative treatment for a second week. At the end of this double-blind trial, a significant improvement in pain, appetite, and activity was observed. Seventy-five percent of subjects blindly chose methylprednisolone as a more effective drug than placebo. Subsequently, treatment with methylprednisolone was continued in an open-label trial. After 3 weeks of treatment, all parameters with the exception of pain intensity had returned to near-baseline values. These results suggest that the effects of corticosteroids are significant but short-lasting.[50] Neither the Moertel nor the Edmonton study established whether the observed lack of long-term benefits was due to a decremental effect of corticosteroids over time, or to the natural progression of the underlying disease. Della Cuna et al randomized 403 patients with terminal cancer to receive daily intravenous injections of methylprednisolone sodium succinate (MPSS) 125 mg for a total of 8 weeks, versus placebo.[51] Most patients were hospitalized. Various symptoms were measured with instruments that included a nurse's observational scale and self-assessment by linear analogue. In addition, a physician's global evaluation scale was used to define overall symptom control as excellent, good, fair, poor, or none. At each weekly follow-up evaluation, MPSS produced significantly more improvement than placebo in the total symptom score and in pain, appetite, vomiting, and well-being scores. All these parameters were measured blindly. In the physician's blinded judgment, MPSS was significantly more effective than placebo in affecting an improved quality of life. Mortality rate was significantly higher for patients receiving MPSS, which was accounted for by a significantly lower mortality for female placebo-treated patients. Eleven patients dropped out of the study due to side effects (10 patients on MPSS and 1 patient on placebo). The principal untoward effects were abdominal pain, hypotension, hyperglycemia, hypoalbuminemia, and, in two instances, gastrointestinal bleeding. The total incidence of side effects was 38.2% in MPSS-treated patients versus 28.1% in placebo-treated patients. The authors concluded that MPSS appears to significantly improve the quality of life in this patient population, but expressed concern over the significant decreases in survival time observed in steroid-treated female patients. Subsequently, Popiela et al performed a similar study that randomized 173 female terminal cancer patients to daily infusions of 125 mg MPSS versus placebo for 8 consecutive weeks.[52] The findings of significant benefit in relief of nausea, vomiting, and improvements in sensation of well-being, and total symptom score were replicated; however, no significant differences emerged when comparing overall mortality during the 8 week follow-up period. Although a trend for steroid-treated patients to die earlier than their placebo-treated counterparts was observed, differences between treatments with regard to time to death were not significant. Patients receiving MPSS had a significantly higher incidence of gastrointestinal and cardiovascular side effects compared to the placebo group.

The mechanism by which corticosteroids appear to produce beneficial effects in patients with terminal cancer is unclear, but may involve their euphoriant effects or the inhibition of prostaglandin metabolism. Presumably, at least in some cases, reductions in peritumoral edema and inflammation, with consequent relief of pressure and traction on nerves and other pain-sensitive structures, contributes to relief of pain, although it is difficult to quantify the degree to which the beneficial effects of steroids on mood, appetite, and weight contribute to improved subjective pain reports. The optimal drug and dosing regimens have not been established (see Appendix C). For the treatment of painful conditions, prednisone and dexamethasone are often administered in doses totaling 30–60 mg/day and 8–16 mg/day, respectively, sometimes chronically and sometimes followed by a gradual "taper," although it should be reemphasized that neither the selection of drug nor its dosage have been the subject of controlled trials. Although long-term side effects are not an important consideration, treatment may produce limiting side effects in cancer patients, particularly immunosuppression (candidiasis will occur in most patients), proximal myopathy, and psychiatric symptoms. The incidence of psychological disturbances ranges from 3% to 50%, with severe symptoms occurring in about 5% of patients. The spectrum of disturbances ranges from mild to severe affective disorders (depression, mania), psychotic reactions (steroid psychosis), and global cognitive impairment (delirium).[53]

Finally, local and perilesional injections of water-soluble steroids have a time-tested role in the treatment of nonmalignant back pain,[54] and have been anecdotally reported as providing good temporary relief in various neuropathic cancer pain syndromes (see Chapters 1 and 3).[55] The comparative analgesic effects of oral versus intralesional steroid administration have not yet been investigated.

PHENOTHIAZINES AND BENZODIAZEPINES

Although these drugs have been frequently used in association with narcotics, there is very little evidence that drugs in either class have major adjuvant analgesic effects. Benzodiazepines do not appear to produce clinically useful analgesia, aside from their benefits as muscle relaxants in patients with muscle spasms.[56] The benzodiazepines, however, are useful for short-term administration in situations characterized by anxiety and sleep disturbances, such as surgery,[57] labor, or myocardial infarction.[56] Although inappropriate as substitutes for opioid analgesics or appropriate psychosocial intervention, the judicious use of anxiolytics in cancer patients with anticipatory pain or a prominent underlying component of anxiety is useful. With the exception of methotrimeprazine, the phenothiazines have not shown consistent analgesic effect, or potentiation of narcotics.[58,59] Methotrimeprazine, a parenteral phenothiazine derivative with potent antiemetic effects, has been shown to produce analgesia comparable to that of morphine.[60,61] A mechanism of action distinct from that of the opioids (alpha adrenergic blockade) has been suggested, implying a potential role for its use in opioid-tolerant and opioid-intolerant patients.[62] Sedation and orthostatic hypotension are common when treatment is first started, even in low doses (5 mg every 6 hours), but tend to resolve over time, permitting upward titration.[63] Hydroxyzine, an anxiolytic with antihistaminic and antiemetic properties, has been demonstrated to potentiate opioid analgesia,[64] but because of the need for parenteral administration its use is primarily restricted to the management of patients with acute pain. The phenothiazines can produce Parkinson-like symptoms, and both groups of drugs can exacerbate narcotic-induced sedation, thereby limiting the dose of narcotics that a patient is able to tolerate. Unless indications other than pain are present, these drugs should not be considered useful adjuvant analgesics at the present time.

AMPHETAMINES

Somnolence is a frequent symptom in cancer patients, and is most often multifactorial. Treatable metabolic disorders, such as hypercalcemia, sometimes play a role, but in the majority of cases, medications, most commonly the narcotic analgesics, are contribu-

tory. The main aim in titrating a patient's dose of narcotic is to reach a "therapeutic window," a dose range at which pain relief is achieved without unwanted sedation. Unfortunately, in many patients such a window does not exist, and the dose needed for adequate analgesia exceeds the dose that is associated with undesirable somnolence.

Early research reported that amphetamine derivatives increase analgesia and decrease sedation in animals[65] and human volunteers,[66] and increase arousal and decrease fatigue in normal adults.[67] In 1977, Forrest et al conducted a double-blind study of dextroamphetamine administered to patients recovering from anesthesia and cholecystectomy. They found that a single dose of 5 and 10 mg of dextroamphetamine significantly potentiated the analgesic effects of morphine, while decreasing sleepiness and increasing intellectual performance.[68] In 1982, an open study in 18 cancer patients suggested that dextroamphetamine could improve pain control, activity, and appetite in cancer patients, and thereby "enhance the comfort of terminally ill patients with cancer."[69]

Our group compared mazindol (a mild amphetamine derivative); 1 mg with breakfast, lunch, and at 4 PM versus placebo in a double-blind, cross-over trial in a group of 26 patients with advanced cancer.[70] Although pain intensity and analgesic consumption were significantly reduced, a significant decrease in appetite and food intake, and increase in anxiety was observed, and serious toxicity (delirium) occurred in two cases. Encouraged by the findings of improved analgesia, we studied patients receiving higher doses of narcotics and methylphenidate, a different amphetamine derivative. The design was again double-blind, cross-over, with a 3-day treatment period.[71] Methylphenidate was selected as the study drug because of its shorter half-life, and evidence that it might be well tolerated in geriatric patients.[72] Significantly decreased pain and sedation, and increased activity were observed in methylphenidate-treated patients. Toxicity was not significantly different from placebo, and patients chose methylphenidate blindly as being more effective in 20 cases (70%).

These data suggest that whereas amphetamines should not be used indiscriminately in efforts to enhance the comfort of terminal cancer patients, a subset of patients will benefit from their administration; these drugs may decrease sedation and increase activity by antagonizing the sedating side effects of narcotics. We have since used methylphenidate in an open trial (10 mg at 8:00 AM, 5 mg at noon) in 50 patients with narcotic-induced sedation with good results.[73] Toxic effects were very uncommon, but the induction of delirium and paranoid reactions in three patients confirmed the necessity for selective use. We routinely check cognitive function, and review the past history for paranoid behavior before use. The presence of neoplastic or other causes of organic brain dysfunction represents another relative contraindication to the use of amphetamines.

ORAL LOCAL ANESTHETICS

In 1986, Kastrup observed that intravenous infusions of lidocaine administered over 30 minutes resulted in significant relief of pain in patients with diabetic neuropathy.[74] Bach reported similar findings in another controlled clinical trial in patients with painful diabetic neuropathy.[75] Petersen treated two patients with Dercum's disease with intravenous lidocaine, and observed immediate relief of pain lasting for 8 and 25 days, respectively.[76] Positive findings were not, however, reproduced in one study of patients with neuropathic cancer pain syndromes treated in a similar fashion.[77]

The development of sodium channel blocking agents (oral analogues of the amide local anesthetics) for the treatment of cardiac arrhythmias prompted trials of these drugs in patients with various neuropathic pain syndromes. Mexiletine and tocainide have been found to be useful in the management of painful diabetic neuropathy[78] and the lancinating pain of trigeminal neuralgia,[79] respectively. Although no controlled trials of their use in

cancer pain have been completed, these drugs may also be useful for the treatment of neuropathic cancer pain syndromes. Flecainide is absorbed well when administered rectally, and may have a potential indication in terminal cancer patients when oral drugs cannot be administered.[80]

ANTIEMETICS

Chemotherapy-induced emesis has been well studied in cancer patients, and effective treatments have been developed for acute emesis, delayed emesis, and anticipatory nausea. However, patients with advanced cancer frequently suffer severe chronic nausea, and only limited research has taken place in this field (see Chapters 12, 13, and 30). Chronic nausea correlates with cardiovascular[81] and gastrointestinal[82] autonomic disturbances. Narcotic analgesics can aggravate nausea by central and peripheral effects.[83] Antidopaminergic agents, such as metoclopramide or haloperidol, have been used to treat chronic nausea, both orally and as continuous subcutaneous infusions.[84,85] Unfortunately, because of the absence of studies that specifically address the problem of chronic nausea, most treatment is adapted from trials for chemotherapy-induced emesis, and this may compromise optimal therapy. For example, phenothiazines and antihistamines, common interventions for acute nausea, can potentiate the sedating effects of narcotics, and thus may be undesirable for chronic use. Newer, powerful antiemetics such as the modified benzamides[86] and antiserotonergics[87] have not yet been investigated for the treatment of chronic nausea or narcotic-induced emesis. Currently, the best type and dose of antiemetic for the treatment of these symptoms are unknown.

LAXATIVES

Although there is a general consensus that laxatives are needed in patients receiving narcotic therapy, the best type or combination and dose are unknown.[88,89] Over time, tolerance usually develops to opioid-induced sedation and nausea, but may not develop to their constipating effects, and most authors recommend the continued use of laxatives as long as patients continue to receive narcotics. The sequelae of undertreated constipation are potentially serious, and include increased anxiety and pain, decreased appetite, intestinal pseudo-obstruction, and even colonic perforation. A preventative approach is recommended. Consideration should be given to prescribing a laxative at the time an opioid is initially prescribed, rather than waiting for constipation to occur (see Chapters 12, 13, and 30).

OTHER DRUGS

Other drugs have been suggested to have analgesic effects in patients with specific pain syndromes. For example, clonidine has been used in neuropathic pain,[90] and antibiotics for the sudden aggravation of pain in ulcerated tumors.[91] Studies are currently being conducted on drugs such as clonidine, calcium channel blockers, calcitonin, and baclofen. Most of the evidence available for the effects of these drugs results from anecdotal reports or open trials.

PART II: FUTURE RESEARCH

Numerous studies of various adjuvant drugs are needed. Some of the most important areas of interest are discussed below.

NON-OPIOID ANALGESICS

A clearer definition of the effects and roles of these agents in different types of pain is needed (eg, visceral, neuropathic, incidental). A comparison between acetaminophen and NSAIDs in cancer pain would be useful because of their different side effect profiles and mechanisms of action. Among the NSAIDs,

the best drug or class of drug and dose have not yet been defined.

TRICYCLICS

Research on these drugs is complicated by the long latency of some of their effects and the high incidence of associated side effects. Although several controlled trials were started on these drugs as adjuvants for cancer pain, only one was published in abstract form.[39] A potential study of these agents will be further complicated by recent suggestions that their administration may affect the bioavailability of morphine.[41] Because the tricyclics are frequently used as adjuvants by some groups and rarely by others, they deserve more intensive study in a controlled trial. Such a study could very likely require a multicenter effort.

CORTICOSTEROIDS

The nature and duration of the effects of these drugs need to be better characterized. The optimum choice of drug and its dosage should also be established. Since the potential for additive toxicity suggests that steroids should not be administered concomitantly with the NSAIDs, a comparison of both classes of drugs as adjuvants to the narcotic analgesics would be desirable.

AMPHETAMINES

Indications for use, as well as the best type and dose of amphetamine should be more clearly defined.

ANTIEMETICS

Comparative trials to assess effectiveness and toxicity should be performed among metoclopramide, haloperidol, prochlorperazine, and the corticosteroids. The newer antiemetics, such as modified benzamides[86] and antiserotonergic drugs,[87] should be considered as narcotic adjuvants. This is an area in which prospective studies are almost nonexistent.

LAXATIVES

Prospective comparative trials should be designed in narcotic-induced constipation to assess effectiveness, toxicity, patient satisfaction, and compliance. The last two end points are important, given the need for long-term use of laxatives in patients receiving narcotics.

OTHER DRUGS

The rest of the drugs included in Table 1 have been suggested to have adjuvant analgesic effects. Osteoclast-inhibiting agents, such as the diphosphonates[92] and calcitonin,[93] are potentially useful but under-studied drugs for the treatment of bone pain. Antibiotic trials should be performed in patients with sudden aggravation of pain to ulcerated tumors.[91] Because information on the potential adjuvant effects of these drugs is extremely limited, uncontrolled trials of their administration in different dosages should be instituted before long-term, more expensive, controlled trials are initiated. Uncontrolled trials would help to define the type, duration, and end points of a controlled trial.

GUIDELINES FOR CLINICAL TRIALS OF ADJUVANT DRUGS

Clinical research on adjuvant drugs presents the investigator with a series of unique obstacles related to the characteristics of the drug under investigation, the patient population, and the nature of the effects to be measured.

THE DRUG

As discussed previously, an adjuvant drug may be useful because it potentiates the analgesic effects of the opioid (eg, NSAIDs), be-

cause it decreases opioid-induced toxicity (eg, laxatives), or both (eg, amphetamines). Thus, one constant characteristic of these trials is that patients are already receiving narcotic drugs. The interaction between the adjuvant drug and the opioid is therefore a critical aspect of these studies. For example, the adjuvant drug may have effects on the bioavailability of the opioid, as suggested in recent reports demonstrating that chlorimipramine and amitriptyline interact with morphine pharmacokinetics and pharmacodynamics.[41,42] By the same token, a recent study of metoclopramide, a properistaltic antiemetic, also showed a change in the rate of absorption of orally administered opioids.[94]

In these two cases, the interaction between the opioid and the adjuvant drug may significantly affect a study's final results. In the second case (antiemetics that enhance gastric emptying), the potential bias can easily be eliminated by studying the antiemetic effects in patients receiving parenteral opioids. In the first case (drugs that could increase the bioavailability of opioids), one way of evaluating the potential for bias is to measure plasma opioid levels in patients until steady state is approached before and after the addition of the adjuvant. Another method is to use a patient-controlled analgesia system to allow patients to adjust their dose to a stable degree of analgesia before and after addition of the adjuvant. In the latter case, if a lower dose of the opioid yields a similar level of pain control in the absence of any change in blood level of the drugs, it can be assumed that the adjuvant opioid only works by increasing the bioavailability of the opioid. Alternatively, if less drug is needed to provide similar symptom control in the presence of a lower steady-state blood level of the opioid, it can be assumed that there is a genuine analgesic potentiating effect.

One of the most sensitive areas of interaction between an opioid and an adjuvant drug is that of potentiating sedation or confusion by the addition of the adjuvant. Comparisons between oral morphine solutions and the Brompton's cocktail[95] showed that the addition of other drugs in the cocktail did not result in analgesic potentiation, but did result in an increased incidence of central side effects. An increased level of obtundation or confusion in patients may result in decreased demand for analgesic drug, regardless of residual pain. Therefore, the simple measurement of "narcotic-sparing effect" (ie, the degree of narcotic dose reduction after treatment with the adjuvant) is not necessarily an adequate measure of analgesic efficacy, particularly when symptom assessment and the administration of the drugs are done by a third person. If possible side effects of the adjuvant drug include sedation or confusion (eg, benzodiazepines, phenothiazines, antihistaminics), it is important to assess prospectively the cognitive status and the level of sedation of the patient during administration of the study drug and control. If the "narcotic-sparing effect" or the "blinded" choice by the patient and investigator are accompanied by significant cognitive deterioration or increased sedation, it is possible that the effects are just a consequence of increased central toxicity produced by the adjuvant drug.

If the adjuvant drug is likely to potentiate narcotic-induced sedation, patients should be asked at the end of the trial if they believe that they had received the adjuvant drug or placebo, and why, in order to assess the effectiveness of the blinding. For example, our group found it necessary to cancel a double-blind, placebo-controlled, cross-over study of cyproheptadine after 13 consecutive patients easily recognized the drug treatment phase because of somnolence. This failure might have been avoided by instituting a pilot study in a small number of patients. Some studies have attempted to mask the sedative effects of a study drug by controlling the results not only with a placebo, but also with other drugs with sedative effects.[96,97] This is likely to improve blinding, but tends to make the trial longer and more complicated.

Long-Acting Drugs

For drugs with a long latency to maximal effect, such as the tricyclic antidepressants, several days of drug or placebo administration is necessary before a valid assessment can take place. If a cross-over design is used under these conditions, the status of the patients' symptoms may change significantly before the completion of the trial. Changes may be related to the development of tolerance to opiate-induced effects, including analgesia, sedation, or nausea, or to the development of new complications of the disease, such as confusion or bowel obstruction. In trials performed in advanced cancer patients, the number of nonevaluable patients at the end of a study may be large enough to invalidate the results. For these reasons, some investigators (eg, Walsh[39]) use a parallel group design. There are problems associated with this choice as well, including: 1) the power of the trial decays very significantly; 2) a deterioration in the cognitive status or the presence of sedation in the patient population receiving the study drug may not be easily perceived; and 3) the role of the patient and investigator in overall assessment of satisfaction is lost. Finally, it is important to consider that all the effects of the drug may not be characterized by a long latency. For example, although the antidepressant effects of the tricyclics are usually not apparent for 2 to 3 weeks after starting treatment, analgesic effects in patients with postherpetic neuralgia have been observed between 48 and 72 hours after the start of treatment.[34] Similarly, although the maximal effect of an NSAID in the treatment of rheumatic conditions usually takes several weeks, their effect on cancer pain usually may be measurable after just a few days.[25]

Before embarking on a long and expensive controlled trial of a new adjuvant, it is recommended to perform an uncontrolled pilot trial in a small number of patients. This preliminary study can determine the onset of action and duration of the different effects of the new adjuvant. During the pilot trial, it is also possible to test different doses of the drug under study. Although the influence of a placebo effect is not systematically evaluated in these trials, information is provided about the characteristics of the drug and both the power and appropriateness of the trial that is being designed. Comparing the results of this trial with historical controls provides information that can be extremely useful in planning the controlled trial.

Short-Acting Drugs

Design tends to be much more simple when short-acting drugs are being evaluated. A double-blind, cross-over trial is almost mandatory for proper assessment of these drugs. The power of this design is much higher than that of a parallel design, and it allows for a blinded choice by patients and investigators. This blinded choice provides overall estimations of satisfaction with the new agent.

Some drugs should not be tested in a double-blind, cross-over trial, despite a short effect. Drugs with sedating effects are probably not best evaluated in this fashion, since the patient and investigator are much more likely to discriminate the effects and side effects of drugs in a cross-over trial. Therefore, drugs with clinically significant side effects may need to be administered in very low doses, or be tested in a parallel group design in which the patient is not given the opportunity to compare the study drug with placebo. Other drugs for which the choice of a short-term cross-over trial design would be inappropriate are those that have a rapid onset of action, but a long-lasting effect. For example, a study of antibiotics on the pain of ulcerated tumors could not be designed as a cross-over trial because of the significant effect that 3 or 4 days of antibiotic therapy would have on the natural history of local infection.

THE PATIENT POPULATION

Clinical trials ideally should be performed in a population that resembles the population that will be likely to benefit clinically from the use of the drug. Unfortunately, in efforts to better characterize the biologic effects of certain agents, and to simplify the clinical trial, investigators frequently study patients who are more stable than those who would ultimately benefit from the new treatment. One example of this problem is research that con-tributed to the development of sustained-release morphine preparations. Most of the studies on these agents were performed in a population of very stable patients requiring an overall low dose of narcotics.[98–100] The results from these trials cannot readily be applied to populations of patients with severe pain, who require much higher doses of narcotics and have significant impairment of gastrointestinal motility. The bioavailability of long-acting preparations may be significantly different in patients with advanced disease than in those in an earlier stage of the disease.

At times, the characteristics of the drug being studied preclude evaluation in the population in which it would most likely be used. If this is the case, the investigators should report this fact in the "methods" section, and should discuss both the possible impact of the selection of the patient population on the final results of the study, and possible implications on the application of the drug for other populations.

The patient population should be well characterized, using all known prognostic parameters. In the case of a cross-over trial, this will help other investigators and clinicians to understand the population in which the trial was performed. In the case of a parallel group trial, this information is of even greater importance. These patients should be stratified according to the most important prognostic factors before randomization takes place. Factors that should be considered include pain mechanism (neuropathic versus non-neuropathic pain), temporal features of the pain (incident versus continuous pain), the need for high or rapidly increasing doses of narcotics, and severe psychological distress. A staging system has been proposed that considers all these prognostic factors.[101] Patients with a history of severe alcoholism or drug addiction, or who are cognitively impaired should be screened before admission to the trial, and considered ineligible. The statement "pain due to cancer," which is, regrettably, considered an acceptable characterization of the pain syndrome by most medical journals,[102] must be carefully qualified in the reported results of these trials.

It is important to consider how many potentially eligible patients can be entered in a trial within a reasonable period of time. The assistance of a biostatistician is invaluable at this stage of the planning. By postulating what would be considered to be a clinically relevant difference between study drug and control, the number of cases needed reliably to reject a Type 2 error (the possibility that a real adjuvant effect exists even if the study does not find it) can be estimated. The probability that the study will be able to reject this Type 2 error is defined as the "power" of the study. As noted, study power is relatively less with a parallel group design than a cross-over design.

In some studies, the inclusion of large numbers of patients is required to answer fundamental questions concerning the effects of different drugs. Even the largest individual centers may not be able to perform such trials. In oncology, this problem has been overcome successfully by the creation of cooperative groups. These groups have been able to design a multitude of clinical trials, and all the member institutions cooperate by entering patients. Unfortunately, no such formalized group exists for clinical research in pain.

If the problem under study occurs very rarely, and patients remain stable for long periods of time, the "n of 1" design can be used.[103]

THE END POINTS OF THE STUDY

An adjuvant drug given to a patient who is already receiving a narcotic analgesic can have multiple effects. It may change the effects of the opioid on the patient (*eg*, analgesia, nausea, sedation, constipation, etc.), or have therapeutic effects and side effects of its own. In the case of a tricyclic antidepressant, for example, antidepressant effects occur, together with autonomic effects, sedation, dry mouth, hypotension, and the potential for cardiac arrhythmias. For these reasons, the interpretation of the effects of an adjuvant drug on a patient who is already receiving a narcotic can be extremely complex. Moreover, the effects may vary in their latency, duration, and intensity. In the case of a tricyclic, dry mouth and sedation usually occur immediately, analgesia may require 3 to 4 days or more before it is apparent, and effects on mood can accrue over weeks.

From this, it is evident that no single study is able fully to characterize the adjuvant effects of a given drug. Short-term, intensive, cross-over trials will provide ample information on the acute effects of an adjuvant drug, but inevitably miss some of potentially important long-term effects. Less intensive, long-term studies will determine more accurately long-term effectiveness and side effects, but potentially will miss early effects. Research on amphetamines provides a useful example of these problems. In an elegant double-blind study, Forrest et al demonstrated that a single dose of dextroamphetamine was able to potentiate morphine-induced analgesia and decrease sedation.[68] However, it is not possible to conclude from their study that repeated doses of amphetamines are useful adjuvants for chronic cancer pain, nor can conclusions be drawn about long-term toxicity. Conversely, in two short-term, cross-over trials, our group determined that amphetamines could decrease narcotic-induced sedation and potentiate analgesia in cancer patients,[70,71] but significant toxicity and a rapid development of tolerance were detected. Although the results of our studies suggest that amphetamines can be useful adjuvants, at least for the short term, in some patients with pain due to advanced cancer, it cannot be inferred from the results of these studies alone that amphetamines will be efficacious or safe during long-term administration.

The finding of a significant improvement in one or more isolated variables does not necessarily mean that an adjuvant drug will be clinically useful. For example, at the end of our double-blind, cross-over trial of mazindol, patients had significantly better pain control and lower analgesic consumption on mazindol compared to placebo,[70] but their overall preferences were equally distributed between "drug," "placebo," and "no choice." In the case of mazindol, the low level of patient satisfaction with the drug was probably due to the significant anxiety and anorexia associated with its use.[70] This fact could be determined only because several variables in addition to pain were measured as a part of the study. However, even the simultaneous measurement of several variables will not always provide an explanation for the observed global satisfaction. It is always possible for deterioration to occur in an unmeasured variable, or that the patient's judgment reflects improvement or deterioration of several variables combined, none of which when measured independently reach statistical significance. A recent trial of clonidine in the treatment of anticipatory nausea in patients receiving chemotherapy is illustrative: although clonidine was able to decrease anticipatory nausea, patients preferred not to receive it in subsequent courses of chemotherapy for reasons that remain unclear.[104]

Although it is useful to combine assessment of objective variables (daily dose of narcotic, number of rescue doses, number of vomiting episodes, etc.) and subjective variables (pain intensity, nausea, somnolence, confusion, etc.) in trials, the clinical utility of an adjuvant drug will depend on its ability to modify the subjective parameter. A "narcotic-sparing effect" is only important for the patient's comfort if it is associated with decreased toxicity (ie, decreased narcotic-induced toxicity without significant toxicity by the adjuvant), or improved pain control.

SUMMARY AND CONCLUSIONS

Patients with chronic cancer pain experience many distressing symptoms in addition to pain. Opioid analgesics are very likely to improve pain, but will not improve and may actually worsen some of the other symptoms, and as a result, multidrug treatment is the rule in this population. Unfortunately, despite their frequent use, evidence for the efficacy of most of the adjuvant drugs is anecdotal. During recent years, efforts have been made to characterize better the effects of some of the adjuvant drugs. Although some improvement in our knowledge base has occurred, prospective, well designed clinical trials are badly needed in this area.

REFERENCES

1. Foley K: The treatment of cancer pain. N Engl J Med 1985;313:84.
2. Cancer Pain: A Monograph on the Management of Cancer Pain. Ottawa, Canada, Health and Welfare Canada: Minister of Supply and Service, H42-2/5-1984E.
3. Foley K, Portenoy R, MacDonald RN et al: Cancer Pain. American Society of Clinical Oncology Educational Booklet, p 79. American Society of Clinical Oncology, 1988.
4. Bruera E, Fox R, Chadwick S et al: Changing patterns in the treatment of pain and other symptoms in cancer patients. Journal of Pain and Symptom Management 1987;2:139.
5. Bruera E, Brenneis C, Michaud M et al: Influence of the Pain and Symptom Control Team (PSCT) on the patterns of treatment of pain and other symptoms in a cancer center. Journal of Pain and Symptom Management 1989;4:112.
6. Twycross R, Lack S: Symptom Control for Advanced Cancer: Pain Relief. London, Pitman, 1984.
7. Bruera E, Navigante A, Barugel M et al: Treatment of pain and other symptoms in cancer patients: Patterns in a North American and South American hospital. Journal of Pain and Symptom Management 1990;5:78.
8. Beck PW, Handwerker HO, Zimmerman M: Nervous block from the cat's foot during noxious radiant heat stimulation. Brain Res 1974;67:373.
9. Mense S: Nervous outflow from skeletal muscle following chemical noxious stimulation. J Physiol Lond 1977;267:75.
10. Hick VE, Koley J, Morrison JFB: The effect of bradykinin on afferent units in intraabdominal nerve trunks. Q J Exp Physiol 1977;62:19.
11. Editorial: Osteolytic metastases. Lancet 1976;ii:1063.
12. Powles TJ, Alexander P, Millar JL: Enhancement of anticancer activity of cytotoxic chemotherapy with protection of normal tissue by inhibition of prostaglandin synthesis. Biochem Pharmacol 1978;27:1389.
13. Bennet A, Charlier EM, McDonald AM et al: Prostaglandins and breast cancer. Lancet 1977;ii:624.
14. Flower RJ, Moncada S, Vane JR: Analgesic–antipyretic and antiinflammatory agents. In Goodman A, Goodman LS, Rall TW, Murad F (eds): The Pharma-

cological Basis of Therapeutics, p 674. New York, Macmillan, 1985.

15. Beaver WT: Combination analgesics. Am J Med 1984;77 (Suppl 3A):38.

16. CSM Update: Nonsteroidal anti-inflammatory drugs and serious gastrointestinal adverse reactions: I. Br Med J 1986;292:614.

17. CSM Update: Nonsteroidal anti-inflammatory drugs and serious gastrointestinal adverse reactions: II. Br Med J 1986;292:1190.

18. L'E Orme M: Non-steroidal anti-inflammatory drugs and the kidney. Br Med J 1986;292:1621.

19. Rainsford K: Side-effects of anti-inflammatory analgesic drugs: Renal, hepatic and other systems. TIPS May 1984;205.

20. Rainsford KD, Velo GP: Side Effects of Anti-Inflammatory Analgesic Drugs. New York, Raven Press, 1983.

21. Morris HG, Sherman NA, McQuain C, et al: Effects of salsalate (nonacetylated salicylate) and aspirin on serum prostaglandins in humans. Ther Drug Monit 1985;7:435.

22. Rothwell KG: Efficacy and safety of a non-acetylated salicylate, choline magnesium trisalicylate in the treatment of rheumatoid arthritis. J Int Med Res 1983;11:343.

23. Leonards JR, Levy G: Gastrointestinal blood loss from aspirin and sodium salicylate tablets in man. Clin Pharmacol Ther 1973;14:62.

24. Goldenberg A, Rudnicki RD, Koonce ML: Clinical comparison of efficacy and safety of choline magnesium trisalicylate and indomethacin in treating osteoarthritis. Curr Ther Res 1978;24:245.

25. Ferrer-Brechner T, Ganz P: Combination therapy with ibuprofen and methadone for chronic cancer pain. Am J Med 1984;77:78.

26. Brodie G: Indomethacin and bone pain. Lancet 1988;ii:1180.

27. Portenoy RK: Pharmacologic management of chronic pain. In Fields HL (ed): Pain Syndromes in Neurology, vol 10, p 260. London: Butterworths, 1989.

28. Portenoy R: Drug therapy for cancer pain. American Journal of Hospice and Palliative Care 1990;7:10.

29. Ventafridda V, Tamburini M, Caraceni A et al: A validation study of the WHO method for cancer pain relief. Cancer 1987;59:850.

30. Walsh T, Saunders C: Hospice care: The treatment of pain in advanced cancer. Recent Results Cancer Res 1984;89:201.

31. Magni G, Arsie D, De Leo D: Antidepressants in the treatment of cancer pain: A survey in Italy. Pain 1987;29:347.

32. Derogatis L, Feidstein M, Morrow G et al: A survey of psychotropic drug prescriptions in an oncology population. Cancer 1979;44:1919.

33. Stiefel FC, Kornblityh AB, Holland JC: Changes in the prescription patterns of psychotropic drugs for cancer patients during a 10 year period. Cancer 1990;65:1048.

34. Watson C, Evans R, Reed K et al: Amitryptiline versus placebo in post-herpetic neuralgia. Neurology 1982;32:671.

35. Kishore-Kumar R, Max MB, Schafer SC et al: Desipramine relieves post-herpetic neuralgia. Clin Pharmacol Ther 1990;47:305.

36. Panerai AE, Monza G, Mouilia P et al: A randomized, within-patient, crossover, placebo-controlled trial on the efficacy and tolerability of the tricyclic antidepressants chlorimipramine and nortriptyline in central pain. Acta Neurol Scand 1990;82:34.

37. Sindrup SH, Ejlertsen B, Froland A et al: Imipramine treatment in diabetic neuropathy: Relief of subjective symptoms without changes in peripheral and autonomic nerve function. Eur J Clin Pharmacol 1989;37:151.

38. Sindrup SH, Gram LF, Skjold T et al: Clomipramine vs desipramine vs placebo in the treatment of diabetic neuropathy symptoms: A double-blind crossover study. Br J Clin Pharmacol 1990;30:683.

39. Walsh TD: Controlled study of imipramine and morphine in chronic pain due to cancer (abstract). Proc Am Soc Clin Oncol 1986;5:237.

40. Feinman C: Pain relief by antidepressants: Possible modes of action. Pain 1985;23:1.

41. Ventafridda V, Ripamonti C, De Conno F et al: Antidepressants increase bioavailability of morphine in cancer patients. Lancet 1987;i:1204.

42. Ventafridda V, Bianchi M, Ripamonti C et al: Studies on the effects of antidepressant drugs on the antinociceptive action of morphine and on plasma morphine in rat and man. Pain 1990;43:155.

43. Liu SJ, Wang RIH: Increased analgesia and alterations in distribution and metabolism of methadone by desipramine in the rat. J Pharmacol Exp Ther 1975;195:94.

44. Swerdlow M: The use of anticonvulsants in the management of cancer pain. In Erdmann W, Oyamma T, Pernak MJ (eds): The Pain Clinic, vol 1, p 9. Utrecht, The Netherlands, VNU Science Press, 1985.

45. Sweet WH: Treatment of trigeminal neuralgia (tic douloureux). N Engl J Med 1986;315:174.

46. Hatangdi VS, Boas RA, Richard EG: Postherpetic neuralgia: Management with antiepileptic and tricyclic drugs. In Bonica JJ, Albe-Fessard D (eds): Advances in Pain Research and Therapy, vol 1, p 583. New York, Raven Press, 1976.

47. Payne R, Max M, Inturrisi C et al (eds): Principles of

Analgesic Use in the Treatment of Acute Pain and Chronic Cancer Pain. Washington, DC, American Pain Society, 1986.

48. Shell H: Adrenal corticosteroid therapy in far-advanced cancer. Geriatrics 1972;27:131.
49. Moertel C, Shutte A, Reitemeir R et al: Corticosteroid therapy in pre-terminal gastro-intestinal cancer. Cancer 1974;33:1607.
50. Bruera E, Roca E, Cedaro L et al: Action of oral methylprednisolone in terminal cancer patients: A prospective randomized double-blind study. Cancer Treat Rep 1985;69:751.
51. Della Cuna GR, Pellegrini A, Piazzi M: Effect of methylprednisolone sodium succinate on quality of life in preterminal cancer patients: A placebo-controlled, multicenter study. Eur J Cancer Clin Oncol 1989;25:1817.
52. Popiela T, Lucchi R, Giongo F: Methylprednisolone as palliative therapy for female terminal cancer patients. Eur J Cancer Clin Oncol 1989;25:1823.
53. Stiefel FC, Breitbart WS, Holland JC: Corticosteroids in cancer: Neuropsychiatric complications. Cancer Invest 1989;7:479.
54. White AH, Derby R, Wynne G: Epidural injections for diagnosis and treatment of low-back pain. Spine 1980;5:78.
55. Abram SE: The role of nonneurolytic blocks in the management of cancer pain. In Abram SE (ed): Cancer Pain, p 67. Boston, Kluwer Academic, 1988.
56. Stimmel B: Barbiturates, nonbarbiturate hypnotics and minor tranquilizers. In Stimmel B (ed): Pain, Analgesia and Addiction, p 170. New York, Raven Press, 1983.
57. Artru A: Midazolam potentiates the analgesic effect of morphine in patients with postoperative pain. Clinical Journal of Pain 1986;2:92.
58. McGee JL, Alexander MR: Phenothiazine analgesia: Fact or fantasy. Am J Hosp Pharm 1979;36:633.
59. Stimmel B: Tranquilizers. In Stimmel B (ed): Pain, Analgesia and Addiction, p 190. New York, Raven Press, 1983.
60. Lasagna RG, DeKornfeldt TJ: Methotrimeprazine: A new phenothiazine derivative with analgesic properties. JAMA 1961:178:887.
61. Beaver WT, Wallenstein SL, Houde RW et al: A comparison of the analgesic effect of methotrimeprazine and morphine in patients with cancer. Clin Pharmacol Ther 1966;7:436.
62. Breitbart W, Holland J: Psychiatric aspects of cancer pain. In Foley KM, Bonica JJ, Ventafridda V (eds): Advances in Pain Research and Therapy, vol 16, p 73. New York, Raven Press, 1990.
63. Rodgers A: personal communication.
64. Beaver WT, Feise G: Comparison of analgesic effects

of morphine, hydroxyzine, and their combination in patients with postoperative pain. In Bonica JJ, Albe-Fessard D (eds): Advances in Pain Research and Therapy, vol 1, p 553. New York, Raven Press, 1976.
65. Evans W, Beryner D: A comparison of the analgesic effect of morphine, pentazocine, and a mixture of metamphetamine and pentazocine in the rat. Journal of New Drugs 1964;4:82.
66. Ivy A, Goetzl F, Burril D: Morphine-dextro-amphetamine analgesia. War Medicine 1984;6:67.
67. Weiner N: Amphetamines. In Goodman A, Goodman L, Gilman A (eds): The Pharmacological Basis of Therapeutics, p 159. New York, Macmillan, 1980.
68. Forrest W, Brown B, Brown C et al: Dextro-amphetamine with morphine for the treatment of postoperative pain. N Engl J Med 1977;296:712.
69. Joshi J, de Jongh C, Schnapper N et al: Amphetamine therapy for enhancing the comfort of terminally ill patients with cancer (abstract). Proc Am Soc Clin Oncol 1982;1:C213.
70. Bruera E, Carraro S, Roca E et al: Double-blind evaluation of mazindol in enhancing the comfort of terminally ill cancer patients. Cancer Treat Rep 1986; 70:295.
71. Bruera E, Chadwick S, Brenneis C et al: Methylphenidate associated with narcotics for the treatment of cancer pain. Cancer Treat Rep 1987;71:67.
72. Katon W, Raskind M: Treatment of depression in the medically ill elderly with methylphenidate. Am J Psychiatry 1980;137:963.
73. Bruera E, Brenneis C, Michaud M et al: Association between asthenia and nutritional status, lean body mass, anemia, psychological status and tumor mass in patients with advanced breast cancer. Journal of Pain and Symptom Management 1989;4:59.
74. Kastrup J, Petersen P, Dejgard A et al: Intravenous lidocaine infusion: A new treatment of chronic painful diabetic neuropathy. Pain 1987;28:69.
75. Bach FW, Jensen TS, Kastrup J et al: The effect of intravenous lidocaine on nociceptive processing in diabetic neuropathy. Pain 1990;40:29.
76. Petersen P, Kastrup J: Dercum's disease (adiposis dolorosa): Treatment of the severe pain with intravenous lidocaine. Pain 1987;28:77.
77. Ellemann K, Sjogren P, Banning AM et al: Trial of intravenous lidocaine on painful neuropathy in cancer patients. Clinical Journal of Pain 1989;5:291.
78. Dejgard A, Petersen P, Kastrup J: Mexiletine for treatment of chronic painful diabetic neuropathy. Lancet 1988;i:9.
79. Lindstrom P, Lindblom U: The analgesic effect of tocainide in trigeminal neuralgia. Pain 1987;28:45.
80. Lie-A-Huen L, Proost JH, Kingma JH et al: Absorp-

tion kinetics of oral and rectal flecainide in healthy subjects. Eur J Clin Pharmacol 1990;38:595.

81. Bruera E, Chadwick S, Fox R et al: Study of autonomic insufficiency in advanced cancer patients. Cancer Treat Rep 1986;70:1383.

82. Bruera E, Catz Z, Hooper R et al: Chronic nausea and anorexia in advanced cancer patients: A possible role for autonomic dysfunction. Journal of Pain and Symptom Management 1987;2:19.

83. Manara L, Bianchetti A: The central and peripheral influence of opioids on gastrointestinal propulsion. Ann Rev Pharmacol Toxicol 1985;75:249.

84. Bruera E, Brenneis C, Michaud M et al: Continuous subcutaneous infusion of metoclopramide for the treatment of the narcotic bowel syndrome. Cancer Treat Rep 1987;71:1121.

85. Billings A: Nausea and vomiting. In Billings A (ed): Outpatient Management of Advanced Cancer, p 45. Philadelphia, JB Lippincott, 1985.

86. Smaldone L, Fairchild C, Rozencweig M et al: Dose-range evaluation of BMY-25801, a non-dopaminergic antiemetic (abstract). Proc Am Soc Clin Oncol 1988;7:280.

87. Kris M, Gralla R, Tyson L et al: Phase I study of the serotonin antagonist GR-C507 when used as an antiemetic (abstract). Proc Am Soc Clin Oncol 1988;7:283.

88. Manara L, Bianchetti A: The control and peripheral influences of opioids on gastrointestinal propulsion. Ann Rev Pharmacol Toxicol 1985;25:249.

89. Billings A: Constipation, diarrhea and other gastro-intestinal problems. In Billings A (ed): Outpatient Management of Advanced Cancer, p 69. Philadelphia, JB Lippincott, 1985.

90. Maciewicz R, Boukons A, Martin J: Drug therapy of neuropathic pain. Clinical Journal of Pain 1985;1:39.

91. Bruera E, MacDonald RN: Intractable pain in patients with advanced head and neck tumors: A possible role for local infection. Cancer Treat Rep 1986;70:691.

92. June A, Chantraine A, Donath A, et al: Use of diphosphonate in metastatic bone disease. N Engl J Med 1983;308:1499.

93. Vaughn C, Vaitkevicius K: The effects of calcitonin in hypendiemia in patients with malignancy. Cancer 1974;34:1268.

94. Manara A, Shelly M, Quinn K et al: The effect of metoclopramide on the absorption of oral controlled release morphine. Br J Clin Pharmacol 1988;25:518.

95. Twycross R: Effect of codeine in the Brompton Cocktail. In Bonica J, Ventafridda V (eds): Advances in Pain Research and Therapy, vol 3, p 627. New York, Raven Press, 1979.

96. Woodcock A, Gross E, Gellery A: A comparison of diazepam and promethazine in the treatment of breathlessness in patients with chronic obstructive lung disease. Br Med J 1982;1:96.

97. Woodcock A, Gross E, Gellery A et al: Effects of dihydrocodeine, alcohol and caffeine on breathlessness and exercise tolerance in patients with chronic obstructive lung disease. N Engl J Med 1981;305:1611.

98. Hanks G, Twycross R, Bliss J: Controlled release morphine tablets: A double-blind trial in patients with advanced cancer. Anaesthesia 1987;42:840.

99. Walsh TD: Clinical evaluation of slow release morphine tablets (abstract). Proc Am Soc Clin Oncol 1985;4:266.

100. MacDonald RN, Bruera E, Brenneis C et al: Long acting morphine in the treatment of cancer pain: A double-blind, crossover trial (abstract). Proc Am Soc Clin Oncol 1987;6:1054.

101. Bruera E, Macmillan K, MacDonald RN et al: The Edmonton staging system for cancer pain: Preliminary report. Pain 1989;37:203.

102. MacDonald RN, Bruera E: Clinical trials in cancer pain research. In Foley K, Ventafridda V (eds): Advances in Pain Research and Therapy, vol 16, p 443. New York, Raven Press, 1990.

103. Gordon H, Guyatt MD, Keller JL et al: The n-of-1 randomized controlled trial: Clinical usefulness: Our three-year experience. Ann Intern Med 1990;112:293.

104. Fetting J, Stefanek M, Sheidlen J et al: Noradrenergic activity in anticipatory nausea (abstract). Proc Am Soc Clin Oncol 1988;7:284.

Chapter 11

Alternate Routes of Administration of Opioids for the Management of Cancer Pain

Eduardo Bruera

Carla Ripamonti

INTRODUCTION

Approximately 60%–80% of patients with advanced cancer develop significant pain before death. In these patients, maintenance of the oral route for drug treatment is preferable because of its overall safety, efficacy, and convenience (see Chapters 6 and 9). However, approximately 70% of patients will benefit from the use of an alternate route for opioid administration sometime before death.[1-3] The duration for which patients need alternate routes of administration varies between hours and months. When alternative routes of administration are required, regular intermittent intramuscular or intravenous injections can control cancer pain in most cases.[3,4] However, because of the short duration of action of most opioids, injections need to be repeated regularly, usually at intervals of at least every 4 hours. This method is ultimately undesirable because it becomes painful for the patient, time-consuming for nursing staff, and difficult to maintain in the home setting.

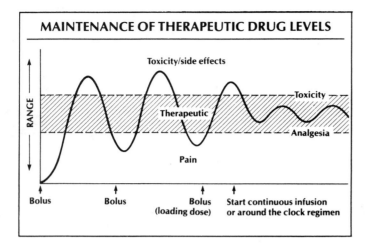

MAINTENANCE OF THERAPEUTIC DRUG LEVELS

Figure 11–1. Schematic graph of time versus blood levels of analgesic demonstrating the potential for alternating intervals of toxicity ("bolus effect") and pain often associated with traditional prn dosing (so-called "sine wave" or "roller coaster" kinetics). Note transition to more consistently maintained therapeutic levels and reduction in peaks and troughs when property titrated continuous infusion is initiated, a scenario often closely mimicked by patient-controlled analgesia.

Studies have shown that intravenous infusions of narcotics produce stable blood levels of drug, thereby reducing the frequency and intensity of "peak" levels associated with acute toxicity and "trough" levels associated with recurrent pain (Fig. 11–1). These studies also suggest that continuous intravenous infusions are safe and effective for treating both postoperative and cancer pain.[5–8] The main problem associated with chronic narcotic administration by continuous infusion in cancer patients is the prolonged maintenance of an intravenous line. Targeted patients have been subject to numerous venipunctures, often have received multiple treatments with sclerosing agents, and have few accessible peripheral veins. If an intravenous cannula becomes displaced or blocked, the patient may need to be transported to a hospital to have the infusion restarted. Totally implantable central venous catheters such as the Port-A-Cath[9,10] (Fig. 11–2) represent a major improvement, permitting long-term intravenous access; however, these catheters are expensive, need to be surgically implanted, and their maintenance requires considerable nursing expertise and patient teaching.

The purpose of this chapter is to summarize the results of research and clinical experience with the alternative routes for narcotic administration that have been developed during recent years. Some of these routes appear to be approximately as effective as the intramuscular or intravenous routes, but may be associated with increased patient comfort and/or decreased toxicity.

SUBCUTANEOUS ROUTE

In 1979, Russell[11] described a method for subcutaneous administration of morphine to patients with advanced symptomatic cancer. Since then, other authors have reported on

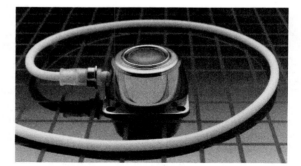

Figure 11–2. Totally implantable central venous access device with silicone and stainless steel port and Silastic tubing. Courtesy of Pharmacia Deltec, Inc.

the use of continuous subcutaneous infusions (CSCI) for the treatment of postoperative and cancer pain.[12-27] Although most reports are based on experience in a small number of patients, their results strongly suggest that CSCI is both safe and efficacious. In a consecutive series of 108 patients, we found that after 48 hours, 94% of patients preferred CSCI to an equal dose of the same analgesic administered by continuous intravenous infusion (CIVI) or intermittent injections.[23] Of the 70 patients treated with a portable pump, 33 (47%) were discharged home for a mean of 29 ± 20 days.

In a series reported by Coyle et al,[15] 13 of 15 patients (87%) reported adequate control of pain, and were maintained on CSCI from 3 to 76 days. Other reports have all suggested that excellent pain control can be achieved with this method.[12-14,20-22]

Ventafridda et al[24] reported their experience in Milan. They treated 40 patients with CSCI using an Italian-made syringe-driver. Adequacy of pain control in their review was similar to that obtained with intermittent injections, and, in addition, chronic nausea improved significantly in concert with CSCI treatment.

Kerr et al[25] treated 18 consecutive patients with CSCI using the Pharmacia 5800 pump, a device that allows for extra bolus doses for breakthrough pain (patient-controlled analgesia—see below). Improved pain control was achieved in all cases. Significant improvements in lifestyle were reported in several patients, and five patients were able to die at home with the support of their families.

A major theoretical concern with CSCI of narcotics relates to irregular absorption because of uneven skin perfusion, with the potential for excessive absorption during periods of increased perfusion. Waldmann et al[26] measured blood levels of morphine in nine patients receiving CSCI for postoperative pain and in four patients receiving CIVI at the same dose (0.05 mg/kg/hour). They found no difference between CSCI and CIVI after 5, 12, 18, and 24 hours of infusion (mean blood level, 20 ± 7 ng/ml). Nahata et al[27] measured morphine blood levels in three children receiving CSCI at a rate of 0.03 to 0.06 mg/kg/hour for the treatment of terminal cancer pain, and arrived at a median blood level of 20 ng/ml. These two studies suggest that blood levels of morphine during CSCI remain stable, and are not subject to sudden changes.

In most cases, CSCI is administered in the subclavicular region, anterior chest, or abdominal wall. Some authors have recommended a change in the infusion site every 2 to 3 days,[15,21] whereas others have suggested that the needle could stay in place for weeks.[11,12] Because of the lack of prospective studies on the optimal duration of site maintenance, we recently conducted a prospective study in 45 patients receiving CSCI of narcotics.[28] Once CSCI was started, the site of infusion was not changed until signs or symptoms of local intolerance developed (pain, redness, swelling, or leakage). Triceps skin fold was determined as an estimation of the thickness of the subcutaneous tissue. All sites were checked daily by one of the authors. After starting 119 sites in 45 patients, the mean duration of sites was 7.3 ± 5.2 days (range, 1–29 days). The duration of the site was not affected by age, sex, dose, type of narcotic, or triceps skin fold. The most frequent signs of local toxicity were redness and swelling, and no episodes of serious local toxicity were encountered. These results suggest that most patients will require a weekly change in the site of infusion. This represents an important guideline for the management of patients receiving CSCI at home.

In addition to local toxicity at the site of infusion, treatment with CSCI has the potential to induce systemic side effects similar to those associated with CIVI. However, three studies have found that the incidence of side effects (mainly sedation, nausea, and confusion) may be lower with CSCI than with intermittent administration.[12,17,20,25] Intermittent administration is associated with a high incidence of so-called "bolus effects," a phenomenon of acute, short-duration toxicity related to transient elevations in serum blood levels of narcotics (see Fig. 11–1). Patients who experience bolus effects with intermittent administration[29] are most likely to benefit from CSCI. Respiratory depression is possible whenever opioids are administered, particularly in patients with compromised renal function and other metabolic abnormalities,[30] but has not been reported as a complication of CSCI by other authors. In 78 consecutive patients we have observed only one case of respiratory depression. This occurred in an 85-year-old patient with normal renal and liver function, whose respiratory status subsequently improved after opioids were discontinued for 2 hours and were restarted at a lower dose. Respiratory depression is unlikely in cancer patients who, as a rule, have been chronically exposed to opioids before starting CSCI, and have therefore developed a certain degree of tolerance.

Some authors have suggested that tolerance might develop at an accelerated pace in patients receiving parenteral opioids, particularly when they are administered by continuous infusion.[4,6,8,31,32] We measured the daily increase of opioid dose in 54 consecutive patients who received CSCI for less than 4 days and underwent no other procedures aimed at relieving pain. The mean daily increase was 2.4% ± 1.6% of the initial dose. Only eight patients (15%) had a daily increase of greater than 5%. In these eight patients, adequate pain control was maintained by frequent dose increases.[23] These results suggest that tolerance is not a clinically relevant problem in cancer patients receiving CSCI. Moreover, in cancer patients, it may be impossible to differentiate genuine tolerance from an increase in nociceptive stimulation caused by tumor growth (see Chapters 7–9).

PATIENT-CONTROLLED ANALGESIA

Most available evidence suggests that CSCI is safe and effective for cancer pain. However, some patients' clinical course is characterized by varying levels of pain, and as a result a fixed rate of infusion may produce effects that are excessive in a particular period and insufficient in another period. Patient-controlled intravenous analgesia has been used successfully in patients with postoperative pain.[33,34] In postoperative studies, opioids typically are administered intravenously, the amount of drug per self-injection is very small, and patients are expected to self-inject every 15 to 60 minutes. These methods are of limited value in the long-term management of cancer pain because of their reliance on the intravenous route and need for frequent administration. We decided to test patient-controlled analgesia using the subcutaneous route (PCSCA) with a dose per injection equivalent to 4 hours of infusion.[35]

Twenty-five consecutive patients with cancer pain who required parenteral hydromorphone were randomized to 3 days of treatment with hydromorphone administered by CSCI or PCSCA using a Pharmacia 5800 pump. Each dose of PCSCA was the equivalent of that delivered during 4 hours of CSCI. After 3 days, all patients were crossed over to the alternate treatment for 3 days. During both phases of the study, patients could request additional doses of hydromorphone from their nurses. In 22 evaluable patients, pain intensity (visual analogue scale 0–100) at 9 AM and 4 PM was 28 ± 17 and 27 ± 17 on PCSCA, versus 31 ± 23 and 28 ± 18 on CSCI, respectively (**P** = not significant). The total doses of hydromorphone (milligrams) were 168 ± 197 and 181 ± 239 on PCSCA and CSCI, respectively (**P** = not significant). There were no significant differences in nausea, drowsiness, or number of hours of sleep. The total number of extra doses of hydromorphone was 6 ± 7 on CSCI versus 2.2 ± 3 on PCSCA (**P** = 0.007). At the end of the study, patients preferred PCSCA and CSCI in 7 and 10 cases, respectively (**P** = not significant; 5 patients expressed no preference).

These results suggest that PCSCA can be a useful alternative to CSCI in some patients. Although this could be seen as a type of prn (as needed) administration of narcotics, it has major differences compared with the usual manner in which the prn modality is used: patients assess their own level of pain, and there is no need to contact a second person (nurse) to request analgesics, and hence independence is maintained and delays are decreased. Moreover, in contrast to oral administration, drugs are administered as injections, thereby shortening the latency period between pain and relief quite significantly. After this initial study, we treated several patients with PCSCA using the Edmonton Injector (see below).[36] Our results suggest that this method is safe and effective in some patients.

A major limitation of this method relates to the cognitive failure that frequently is manifest in preterminal patients.[37] When this occurs, self-administration is likely to be unreliable, necessitating greater involvement of family members. Patients with a history of drug addiction or alcoholism may be poor candidates for PCSCA. More studies are necessary to address issues such as long-term effectiveness, toxicity, and the development of tolerance to opioids. Simpler and less expensive infusion devices for PCSCA are also badly needed. Preliminary results, however, suggest that PCSCA is effective and safe for the treatment of cancer pain.

GUIDELINES FOR CSCI OF OPIOIDS

Patient Selection

Patients in whom the administration of oral opioids (see Chapter 9) is unreliable because of nausea, vomiting, or malabsorption are candidates for CSCI, as are individuals who require extremely large doses of oral opioids, which are awkward and uncomfortable to administer. Although these patients could be managed with regular injections, it seems clear that CSCI is more effective, simpler, possibly associated with fewer side effects than intermittent injections, and certainly more convenient for the patients and their families.

Patients in whom bolus effects are prominent are also likely to benefit from CSCI (see Fig. 11–1). Administration by CSCI is preferable to CIVI in patients being prepared for discharge home. Patients who are already receiving an intravenous infusion with drugs that are compatible with opioids can, however, be managed easily with CIVI. Before discharging a patient on CSCI, it is important to ensure that the patient and family have been instructed properly on all aspects of care, that a responsible care provider is at home, and that the patient and family have access to professional consultation on an around-the-clock basis. In part, because of the high prevalence of cognitive disorders in terminal cancer patients,[37] we have found it useful to admit our patients for 48 hours at the beginning of the infusion to provide training and to permit practice time for the patient and family.

Patients with pain that is unlikely to respond to the administration of opioids, independent of the route or method selected, are poor candidates for treatment with CSCI. These include individuals with neuropathic or episodic pain, and those in whom psychological suffering is prominent.

Severe sedation and respiratory depression may occur when morphine is administered chronically to patients with renal failure, because of the potential for the accumulation of morphine metabolites.[31] These patients may develop toxicity with any regular form of administration of opioids, including CSCI. We recently treated severe bone pain in a 41-year-old patient with multiple myeloma and renal failure (creatinine clearance, 20 ml/minute). Severe pain persisted despite prn bolus injections of morphine, and CSCI of hydromorphone (50 mg/day) was initiated. Within 72 hours of the introduction of CSCI infusion, the patient developed severe sedation and confusion that improved completely after a 96-hour drug-free period. Hydromorphone was restarted at 8 mg administered intravenously every 4 hours by regular injection, and severe sedation and confusion were again noted after the passage of 24 hours. Similar symptoms were noted after a trial of regular intravenous injections of morphine. Finally, adequate pain control without excessive sedation was achieved with hydromorphone administered 4 mg intravenously as needed (intervals between doses averaging 18–24 hours). This case suggests that hydromorphone, as well as morphine, can cause severe toxicity in patients with renal failure. The presence of renal failure represents one of the few relative indications for the as-needed (prn) administration of opioids.

During recent years, numerous series have reported excellent results with subcutaneous opioids administered for chronic pain.[17,24,25,38] As experience has accrued and many groups have come to rely on CSCI or PCSCA as the principal means for administering parenteral opioids, guidelines for patient selection have become less rigid than when the first experimental reports on the use of this technique were published.

Choice of Drug and Dosage

Most published reports of clinical experience with subcutaneous opioid administration have used morphine, hydromorphone, or diamorphine. These drugs are all characterized by a short half-life, and as a result steady-state plasma levels (four to five half-lives) are achieved rapidly. Drugs with longer half-lives, such as methadone[25] and levorphanol,[15] have also been used, but are associated with the potential for poor pain control at the beginning of treatment, and the risk of delayed toxicity days after the infusion has started as a result of slowly escalating blood levels (see Chapters 8 and 9). These hazards are increased in elderly patients. For these reasons, morphine and its congeners should be the first-choice drugs for CSCI. If treatment is to be administered by a portable infusion pump, convenience dictates the use of a highly concentrated solution infused at a very slow rate, and hydromorphone is usually preferred because of its higher solubility. In countries where it is readily available, diamorphine (heroin) is occasionally used when even more concentrated solutions are required.

Dose selection commences with a determination of the total daily dose of narcotic that the patient is receiving. The daily dose is translated into an equivalent dose in milligrams of parenteral morphine (morphine equivalents) using an appropriate conversion table (see Chapter 9 and Appendix C, Table 1). If pain control was adequate before conversion, then the new dose is simply divided by 24, and the result is administered hourly by the subcutaneous route. In patients with a history of inadequate pain control, an increase of 20% to 30% in the daily dose is considered at the start of treatment with CSCI. An initial bolus dose equivalent to 2 hours of infusion is a useful option to increase blood levels of the narcotic rapidly, thereby reducing the time interval before steady state is achieved. Orders should also be provided for the administration of escape (prn) doses of opioids for breakthrough pain. The usual escape dose used at our center is equivalent to the dose of drug that would be administered in 2 hours of regular infusion. The regular infusion site can be used for the subcutaneous administration of both the initial bolus and escape doses by means of a three-way stopcock. This practice does not decrease the duration of the site.[23] Once an infusion has been started with morphine or hydromorphone, steady-state blood levels will be reached within 24 hours, and, therefore, if neither adequate pain control nor toxicity occur in 1 day, neither event is likely to occur subsequently at the same dose. Initially, in most patients daily dose changes are needed until the goal of adequate pain control and minimal toxicity is achieved. Once patients are discharged, our experience in 183 patients suggests that changes are needed only every 8 ± 7 days. Less than 20% of the patients will need rapid dosage increases, a pattern that is demanding when patients are managed at home.

Method of Infusion

Once the proper drug and dosage have been determined, the infusion is started using a 25- or 27-gauge butterfly needle that is usually inserted under the skin of the anterior chest or abdominal wall, as illustrated in Figure 11–3. A three-way stopcock can be placed in the system to facilitate the administration of the initial bolus and extra doses of narcotics, as well as for the administration of steroids or metoclopramide if these are needed.[39]

Other groups prefer to use a perpendicular needle such as the Travenol needle,[26] a device specifically designed for subcutaneous use. These needles are considerably more expensive than standard butterflies, and their use does not result in significantly longer duration of the infusion site.

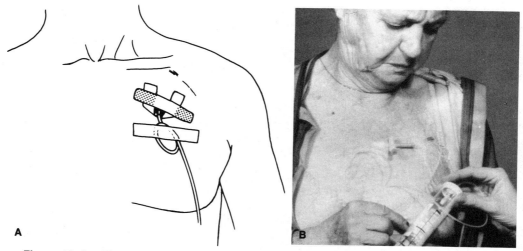

Figure 11–3. Placement of 25–27-g butterfly needle for continuous subcutaneous administration of opioids is depicted schematically in **A** and demonstrated in actual patient in **B**.

A number of different methods of infusion may be used, and are discussed below.

Use of Nonportable Pumps. The opioid solution is prepared in a 48-cc bag and is infused at a rate of 2 cc/hour using a standard hospital bedside pump, such as the IVAC or IMED pump. Our data suggest that the rate of infusion can be increased up to 10 cc/hour without producing pain at the site of infusion. This is the most cost-effective method for the administration of subcutaneous opioids in hospitalized patients. However, because of the slow rates of infusion, it is necessary to use a flow-calibrated infusion pump, and in small hospitals and in most developing countries, these pumps are not available.

Hypodermoclysis. Hypodermoclysis refers to the subcutaneous administration of large volumes of fluid, a practice that was used regularly for hydration from the 1930s to the 1950s, before intravenous administration was well accepted. Hypodermoclysis is facilitated by the addition of hyaluronidase, an enzyme that hydrolyzes hyaluronic acid, causing rapid diffusion and absorption of injected fluids by temporarily lysing the normal interstitial barrier, which mainly consists of hyaluronic acid. As a result of research conducted in geriatric patients, hypodermoclysis has been repopularized in recent years.[40,41]

Hays[42] has recently demonstrated that it is possible to administer morphine and hydromorphone safely with CSCI at rates of 20 to 80 cc/hour supplemented by the addition of hyaluronidase (Wydase) to the infusion (600 unit/liter of 2/3:1/2 solution). This method allows the nurse to control the rate of infusion without mechanical aids (flow-calibrated pump), simply by manually adjusting flow through the drip chamber. Because of the high rates of infusion, it can also be used to promote hydration. When a solution containing dextrose, with or without hyaluronidase, is administered by hypodermoclysis, fluid is drawn from the surrounding tissues into the site of injection. This effect may persist for several hours, causing unnecessary pain and decreased plasma volume. This scenario can be avoided by using a dextrose solution that contains electrolytes. The cost of hyaluronidase and occasional sensitivity reactions are the only drawbacks of this technique.

Intermittent Injections. When neither a nonportable pump nor hyaluronidase are avail-

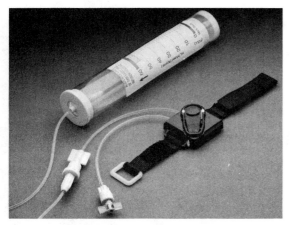

Figure 11–4. PCA Infusor System: cost-effective, lightweight disposable device. Delivers medication via a balloon reservoir system and sustained internal pressure after activation from wrist band demand module. Courtesy of Baxter Healthcare Corporation.

able, it is still possible to administer subcutaneous opioids by means of a butterfly needle placed under the skin. The butterfly needle can be left in place for as long as 7 days without special care, and injections of opioids can be administered by the nursing staff, relatives, or the patient intermittently with only minimal discomfort. The technique of repeated injection through an *in situ* butterfly needle is less painful and simpler to teach than intermittent percutaneous, subcutaneous, or intramuscular injection. The former method is more cost-effective, and can also be used for the administration of metoclopramide and corticosteroids.

Portable Infusors. Portable infusion devices are often considered for the management of patients who are ambulatory or house-bound. Many different devices are currently available, and new entrants to the market are commonplace. It is important to consider which of the different portable pumps is most suitable for a given patient. Several of the more commonly used portable pumps are discussed below.

Travenol Infusor: This is a disposable plastic cylinder that measures 16 cm in length and 3 cm in diameter (Fig. 11–4). Its weight is 90 g when full. It infuses a total volume of 48 ml in 1 day at a fixed rate of 2 ml/hour, and has a reserve of 12 ml for emergencies. Its main advantage is its extreme simplicity and convenient size. Patients generally fasten the device to their clothes with a pin. Nursing staff and patients are readily instructed in its use. The patient or a relative connects a new, disposable infusor to the butterfly needle daily. We usually provide a 1-week supply at a time. Disadvantages include its cost (Canadian, $22), and the fact that after a single day's use it must be disposed of and cannot be reused. Also, flexibility of administration is limited. Patient-controlled analgesia (PCA) is not possible, and, since the rate of infusion cannot be altered, changes in dosage require substitution of a differently concentrated drug. Plans are underway for our group to begin testing a 5-day infusor that is the same size, but which functions at a fixed rate of 0.5 ml/hour.

Pharmacia 5800: This is a battery-operated, computer-driven pump, designed specifically for the purpose of pain control (Fig. 11–5). It not only administers a continuous infusion, but also allows the patient to self-administer extra injections at preset intervals and volumes (PCA). We tried this pump in a number of patients and found it safe and reliable. Currently, we are conducting a comparative trial between this pump and the Travenol Infusor. It can be used with 50- and 100-ml bags. It is both heavier and bulkier that the Travenol Infusor, but is readily transported in an over-the-shoulder holster. Its main drawbacks are its cost (Canadian, $3,600 plus $14–$22 for cassettes) and its complexity, which requires more intensive training for patients and nursing staff. We think that it is necessary to have a specially trained nurse to operate a program with this pump, and therefore it might be unsuitable for small programs with limited staffing.

Syringe Driver: Syringe-drivers (Fig. 11–6) are used primarily in Britain.[11–18] Important advantages are cost (Canadian, $1,900) and simple operation, compared with more complex mechanized devices like the Pharmacia models. The syringe driver, however, is bulky, and as a result uncomfortable to trans-

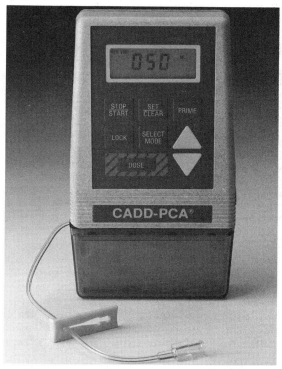

Figure 11–5. CADD-PCA Model 5800: example of a reliable, portable, computer-driven infusion device intended specifically for pain control. Courtesy of Pharmacia Deltec, Inc.

virtually limited to North America and Britain. Most European countries and almost all of the developing countries have no access to these devices because of their cost and complexity. At the University of Alberta, we decided to design a system that would allow safe and simple administration of subcutaneous narcotics at a very low cost.

The Edmonton Injector (Fig. 11–7) is a plastic device that allows the patient, a relative, or a nurse to administer intermittent 1-cc boluses of a narcotic analgesic by the subcutaneous route. It provides intermittent PCSCA but not CSCI. It has been tested in 223 patients admitted to the Cross Cancer Institute for periods of 1 to 60 days. Seventeen patients were discharged home for periods of 1 to 60 days. The system can be assembled by an untrained nurse in less than 5 minutes, and patients can be trained in its use in less than 5 minutes. Its use in more than 450 patient-days resulted in no serious accidents. Daily operational costs are less than 10% of those for other portable injection devices. This device may be extremely useful for the management of patients with cancer pain in community hospitals, small cities, or developing countries.

port, even with a fitted holster. They are relatively unsafe. An ambulatory patient could accidentally self-administer an overdose of narcotics, and even for bedridden patients they may not be very safe during night hours. Changing the syringe is a relatively complicated procedure that may pose difficulties for the patient or relative.

Edmonton Injector: All of the previously described infusors, as well as at least five more that are available, can be used for the subcutaneous administration of opioids. They all, however, have in common high initial and operational costs (bags, tubings), as well as the need for specially trained personnel to provide supervision and teaching. Regrettably, these characteristics have made the availability of ambulatory subcutaneous analgesia

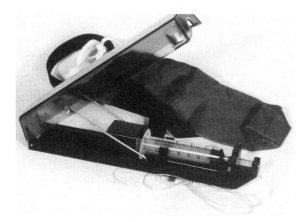

Figure 11–6. Contemporary version of syringe driver for subcutaneous or intravenous administration of opioids. See text for advantages and disadvantages relative to other means of administration.

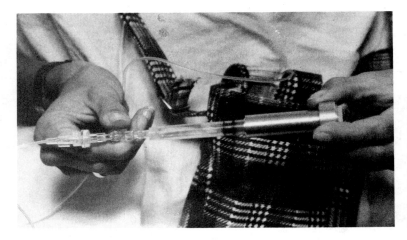

Figure 11–7. The Edmonton Injector, a simple, reliable, cost-effective and portable device that allows the patient, a relative, or a nurse to administer intermittent 1-cc boluses of an opioid analgesic by the subcutaneous route. Device permits delivery of patient-controlled boluses, but not continuous administration.

Choice of Pumps

With the current trend toward high-technology machinery, miniaturization, and patient-controlled analgesia, new, small portable pumps are being developed continuously. Each institute should make their decision regarding which pump is appropriate for them according to multiple factors, listed in Table 11–1.

Most complicated, mechanized devices have more options (CSCI plus PCSCA, etc.), but are generally significantly more expensive and require specially trained personnel to maintain them. The elements to consider in the cost-effectiveness equation are listed in Table 11–2.

When CSCI is indicated for outpatient management, it is desirable to start the infusion during a 48-hour admission period. The admission permits dose titration, teaching, and assessment of the patient's and family's ability to manage the technique to take place in a supervised environment. However, admission for these purposes may not always be feasible or desirable. We initiated treatment with CSCI in 12 outpatients with good results using the Travenol Infusor, and in two patients with PCSCA using the Edmonton Injector.

When an intervention has been undertaken that is anticipated to relieve long-standing pain (ie, radiation therapy, chemotherapy,

nerve block, neurosurgery), and the patient is presumed to be able to make a transition to treatment with oral opioids, we usually first decrease CSCI to the minimum dose that provides adequate analgesia over 3 to 4 days, and then convert the patient to treatment with oral opioids over 5 days (eg, day 1: CSCI 80%, oral 20%; day 2: CSCI 60%, oral 40%; day 3: CSCI 40%, oral 60%; day 4: CSCI 20%, oral 80%; and day 5: CSCI 0%, oral 100%). Finally, when an admitted patient has good pain control with CSCI, we increase the daily dose by 10% to 20% before discharge, because of the likelihood of increased activity at home.

In summary, the use of the subcutaneous route for opioid administration provides analgesia that is equivalent to that achieved by the intravenous route, and is associated with increased patient comfort and less potential toxicity. Subcutaneous administration also permits patients who otherwise would need prolonged hospitalization to be safely discharged. The optimum method and means of administration must be decided according to patient needs and characteristics of the institution where treatment takes place. More research is needed on CSCI to define better the pharmacokinetics and the clinical effects of drugs administered with this technique, and to compare CSCI to new methods such as patient-controlled analgesia.[35] The administration of other drugs such as steroids or anti-

Table 11–1.
Factors Influencing an Institution's Selection of Infusion Device

1. **Cost:** Is the initial expense of a computerized high-technology pump affordable? Will the volume of patient use justify its cost? If it is estimated that the pump will be used only occasionally, consideration should be given instead to employing a disposable infusor that requires no initial investment, only daily maintenance costs.
2. **Flexibility:** Will the pump allow "escape" doses to be administered for "breakthrough" or "incident" pain?
3. **Education of health professionals:** Is the pump simple or complex to program, operate, and troubleshoot? A trial period is recommended before purchasing a high-technology pump. This will allow time for involved health professionals to make an informed evaluation.
4. **Patient/family education and safety:** Can a teaching program for this pump realistically be implemented for your population? Does the pump have the safety features you desire (accuracy, dependability, occlusion, and low battery alarms)?

emetics[39] via CSCI should also be explored further.

RECTAL ROUTE

RECTAL ABSORPTION OF DRUGS

The surface area of the human rectum is relatively limited (200–400 cm^2) because of the absence of intestinal villi. The pH of its fluid contents ranges between 7–8.[43] The main mechanism of absorption from the rectum is passive diffusion, which is probably no different from that which occurs in the proximal gastrointestinal tract, despite differing pH, fluid content, and surface characteristics in these regions.[44]

The rectum is drained by the superior rectal vein into the portal system, and by the middle and inferior rectal veins into the systemic circulation. Extensive anastomoses exists among these three veins,[45] and as a result it is impossible to predict what proportion of

Table 11–2.
Factors Influencing the Cost-Effectiveness of Infusion Therapy

1. **Capital costs:** Purchase and lease costs differ dramatically among devices and regions.
2. **Maintenance costs:** Includes the cost of bags, tubings, connections, and other supplies.
3. **Cost of the medications to be administered to outpatients:** In some localities these costs are covered by the local government or insurance agencies, whereas in others they must be paid for by the patients or absorbed by the treatment facility. Infusion therapy may even result in dramatic savings to the patient, because in some cases pharmacy-prepared injectable drugs are covered by insurance, but oral medications are not.
4. **Pharmacy and biomedical engineering time:** Some pumps can be evaluated for accuracy and set up in a very short time, whereas others require a considerable amount of time.
5. **Nursing time:** Some pumps require a considerable amount of teaching time with the patient, family, and other nurses, as well as a specially trained person to be on call 24 hours a day for possible complications.
6. **Intensity of usage:** The hospital loses money each day a costly pump that requires a costly support structure goes unused. In the case of simple, disposable devices, the hospital incurs expense only when the pump is in use.

drug will avoid or be subject to the hepatic first-passage elimination.

Rectal drug vehicles may be liquid or solid.[46] The absorption of aqueous and alcoholic solutions occurs very rapidly, but the absorption of suppositories is generally slower, and highly dependent on the nature of the suppository base, the use of surfactants, and other factors such as the presence or absence of feces and the total volume content within the rectum.[44]

The pharmacokinetics of rectally administered drugs is incompletely understood. For example, despite evidence of an almost complete absence of metabolism before systemic absorption for intrarectal lidocaine administered to humans,[47] several other drugs have been found to be metabolized equally or more with rectal than oral administration.[48–50] Also, in animal studies, morphine, buprenorphine, and etorphine have been demonstrated to undergo conjugation within the gut wall, although it is not known if a similar effect exists in humans.[51]

PHARMACOKINETICS

Studies demonstrate considerable interindividual variation in the bioavailability of rectally administered morphine.[52–54] After administering 10-mg aliquots of rectal and intravenous morphine chloride to eight patients for 24 hours, Johnson et al[53] found that the bioavailability of morphine after rectal administration was 53 ± 18% of the values obtained after intravenous administration. These data, combined with results of a previous study suggesting that the bioavailability of oral morphine is 37%,[55] caused the authors to conclude that first-passage elimination of morphine may be reduced by rectal administration. Investigating six cancer patients, Breda et al[56] found comparable bioavailability for free morphine and morphine-6-glucuronide after acute administration of 10 mg of morphine via the oral and rectal routes. Pannuti et al have reported similar results also in cancer patients.[57]

Ellison et al[58] compared the administration of 10 mg of morphine sulfate in oral solution versus rectal suppository in 10 patients with cancer pain. Significantly higher mean concentrations of free morphine were obtained with the rectal suppository compared to the oral solution at all time points during the study, whereas there were no differences in mean morphine-3-glucuronide concentrations between routes. These data reinforce the concept that first-passage metabolism may be partially averted when morphine is administered rectally.

Moolenaa et al[59] studied the rectal absorption of aqueous solutions of morphine hydrochloride with different pH in seven volunteers. The rectal absorption of morphine appeared to be dependent on the pH of the solution: a significant improvement in absorption was observed when the pH of the rectal solution was adjusted to 7–8.

Westerling[52] found a wide variation in bioavailability of rectal morphine (12%–61%) administered as an aqueous solution to healthy female patients undergoing gynecologic operations. In another study by the same author, morphine premedication was administered rectally or intramuscularly. The mean availability of rectally administered morphine hydrogel was 48% (range, 31%–72%). Compared to rectal administration, the mean plasma concentration of morphine after intramuscular injection was significantly lower 90 minutes after administration.[60] Rectal premedication with diazepam, morphine, and hyoscine has been reported for children undergoing minor surgery. Peak plasma levels of diazepam and morphine were reached within 30 minutes, and plasma levels decreased after 2 hours.[61]

Kaiko et al[62] carried out a randomized, multidose, cross-over study in 14 healthy male subjects to investigate the comparative bioavailability of 30-mg tablets of sustained-release morphine (MS Contin, Purdue Frederick, Norwalk, CT) administered orally and rectally. There was no significant difference in morphine absorption between the two methods of administration. The 24-hour area under the curve was 90% of oral for the rectal treatment group. However, the rectally administered sustained-release morphine was associated with a lower peak plasma level. Furthermore, the time of occurrence of the largest observed plasma morphine concentrations was significantly delayed from 2.46 hours after oral ingestion to 5.38 hours after rectal administration. The results suggest a slower rate of absorption for sustained-release morphine administered rectally than when given orally.

Hojsted et al[63] compared the absorption of morphine hydrochloride suppositories rectally and after administration into a colostomy. The bioavailability after colostomy administration showed a very wide variation, but the mean value as compared to rectal administration was 43% (range 0%–127%). After transcolostomy administration, low plasma concentrations occurred in three patients, and a higher plasma concentration occurred in one patient. The authors concluded that transcolostomy administration is unreliable and cannot be recommended. They suggested that the reasons for the low and variable bioavailability observed may be poor vascularization of the colostomy, absorption of morphine in feces, and the influence of first-pass elimination.

CLINICAL EXPERIENCE

The majority of the experience reported in the literature is with the short-term use of rectal opioids for the management of acute pain syndromes. For example, Lindahl et al[61] used rectal suppositories with diazepam, morphine, and hyoscine for premedication in 20 children undergoing minor surgery, and satisfactory sedation was achieved in the majority of children. In the Westerling experience,[60] all patients became sleepy within 30 minutes after premedication with morphine hydrogel.

Brook-Williams et al[64] prepared morphine suppositories by putting morphine sulfate tablets (15 and 30 mg) into #1 gelatin capsules. Good pain control was achieved in 10 patients with a variety of malignant diseases. In five patients the suppositories were used for 1 to 4 weeks. Four patients received them for periods of up to 3 days immediately before death, and one patient received them immediately after surgery for 4 days. In a prospective, nonrandomized trial, Pannuti et al[57] treated cancer patients with oral morphine chlorhydrate (37 patients), rectal morphine as a 5 mg/cc aqueous solution every 4 hours (37 patients), or sublingual morphine as a 20 mg/cc aqueous solution administered every 4 hours (28 patients). Pain was assessed using a visual analogue scale. The authors concluded that pain control was achieved more rapidly and was significantly better with the sublingual route followed by the rectal and oral routes. The incidence and severity of side effects were not different between the three different routes of administration. Six percent of patients needed to discontinue the intrarectal route because of local intolerance. Brumley[65] treated 30 patients with cancer pain who had good pain control on oral morphine tablets with an equianalgesic dose of the same tablets inserted rectally in #2 gelatin capsules. Up to six tablets were inserted into each gelatin capsule, and several patients required the use of several gelatin capsules at a given time. The capsules were administered regularly every 4 hours. Twenty-six of 30 patients achieved effective pain control without the need for further titration of dose. The highest dose was 330 mg every 4 hours in one patient. The home-made morphine sulfate suppositories were found to be much more economical and better tolerated by patients than were commercially prepared suppositories.

Maloney[66] reviewed his experience with 39 terminally ill patients who received slow-release morphine as a rectal suppository. All patients had terminal cancer, and 38 patients were receiving oral slow-release morphine before starting the rectal administration. Good pain control was reported in all cases. In two cases, the slow-release morphine tablets were administered into a colostomy stoma, and in one case a female patient with diarrhea received the tablets intravaginally. A standard commercial preparation of 30 mg slow-release morphine tablets was used, and there were no local side effects reported. Patients were treated for an average of 11.5 days (range, 1–30 days).

In summary, preliminary evidence suggests that morphine sulfate and morphine chlorhydrate can be administered rectally in a variety of forms, including aqueous solution, suppositories, and commercially available tablets intended for oral use (sustained-release and short-acting preparations). Although considerable interindividual variability exists, acceptable absorption has been observed for all these different preparations. Unfortunately, the data on clinical use are extremely limited. There are no controlled trials on the long-term use of rectal morphine for cancer pain. Some of the obvious advantages of the rectal route compared to the subcutaneous or intravenous routes are the absence of the need for the insertion of needles and the use of portable pumps. Among the disadvantages are that frequent rectal administration can be uncomfortable, absorption may be decreased by the presence of stool in the rectum, diarrhea, or simply by normal bowel movements, and progressive titration can be difficult because of the limited availability of different commercial preparations. Future research should focus on the relative role of the rectal route as compared to the subcutaneous and other alternative routes, on patient satisfaction and compliance, on the possibility of use of this route for "rescue doses" of opioids and on the possibility of administering other opioids by this route.

SUBLINGUAL AND BUCCAL ROUTE

ABSORPTION

The surface of the buccal and sublingual area is small (200 cm^2), and the ambient pH is 6.2–7.4.[67] However, due to the rich vascularity and lymphatic drainage of this region, there is the potential for rapid drug absorption and direct passage into the systemic circulation with avoidance of hepatic first-pass metabolism.[45,68] The best preparations are probably tablets because liquids and pastes spread through the whole mouth, increasing the pos-

sibility that the drug will be swallowed. Dilution by saliva adversely affects the absorption of the drug, and increases the likelihood that the drug will be swallowed before it is maximally absorbed. In the case of buccal administration, it is important to locate the tablet on the mucosa of the gum above the gingival margin on the upper buccal sulcus.[45] Polar (hydrophilic) drugs are poorly absorbed, whereas drugs that are moderately lipophilic are well absorbed.[69–71] Drugs with a very high partition coefficient are too water-soluble to achieve high concentrations in saliva.[72] The oral mucosa appears to behave in a manner similar to other biologic lipoidal membranes.[73] Therefore, the amount of drug absorbed will depend on multiple factors, including the pKa, rate of partition of the un-ionized form of the drug, the lipid–water partition coefficient and molecular weight of the drug, passive diffusion, and the pH of the solution in the mouth.[74]

PHARMACOKINETICS

Bell[75] studied 40 patients with postoperative pain in a prospective, double-blind, double-dummy study comparing intramuscular and buccal morphine. All patients received a dose of 13.3 mg of intramuscular or buccal morphine. Peak plasma levels were slightly higher after intramuscular morphine, but declined more slowly after buccal morphine. The area under the curve was significantly greater for buccal morphine, and the overall bioavailability was 40%–50% greater for buccal than intramuscular morphine. Fisher et al[76] were not able to reproduce the results of Bell's study. They treated 11 volunteers with 25 mg of buccal morphine, and 5 preoperative surgical patients with 10 mg of intramuscular morphine. The morphine serum concentrations observed by high-pressure liquid chromatography after intramuscular morphine administration were similar to those found by Bell. However, the mean maximum morphine concentration was eight times lower after buccal administration than after intramuscular injection, and occurred at a mean of 4 hours later. The area under the curve was significantly greater after intramuscular administration. These authors concluded that serum morphine concentrations are significantly lower after buccal than intramuscular morphine, and that buccal administration is an unpredictable mode of delivery because of extreme interindividual variability.

Pannuti et al[57] found that higher plasma concentrations were achieved more rapidly for sublingual morphine than with oral or rectal morphine. They observed a second peak in the plasma levels near the third hour after the administration of the drug. The authors concluded that the drug absorption takes place initially at the oral mucosa, and is then later absorbed in the gastrointestinal tract. Al-Sayed-Omar[77] studied the absorption of morphine sulfate and morphine-3-glucuronide at various buffer pH values (4–10) over 5 minutes in four normal healthy volunteers. Their results suggest that increasing pH caused an increase in buccal absorption for both drugs. The maximum mean absorption for morphine was 37% at a pH of 10, and for morphine-3-glucuronide, 19% at a pH of 8. The lower uptake at lower pH values is consistent with morphine's basic nature. A water-soluble metabolite such as morphine-3-glucuronide is less well absorbed by the buccal membrane, and shows a markedly lower buccal absorption over the pH range studied.

Breda et al[56] found that the bioavailability of free morphine and morphine-6-glucuronide was similar after administration by the oral, buccal, rectal, and subcutaneous routes. There was no significant change in the area under the curve of free morphine or its metabolite after acute administration by the four routes in six cancer patients.

Weinberg et al[78] studied the absorption of nine different narcotic drugs in healthy volunteers after sublingual administration. In all cases, the drug was administered as a 1-cc solution placed via pipette under the tongue, and maintained there for 10 minutes without swallowing. They studied the bioavailability of each drug, but also the concentration of drug in the solution expectorated from the oral cavity after 10 minutes without swallowing. The study confirmed that lipophilic drugs are better absorbed than hydrophilic drugs. Morphine concentration/time profiles suggested that the apparent sublingual bioavailability for morphine was only 9% ± 11% of that after an intramuscular administration. When the oral cavity was buffered to pH 8.5, methadone absorption was increased to 75%. Therefore, an alkaline pH microenvironment that favors the un-ionized fraction of opioids increased sublingual drug absorption. Their results indicate that although the sublingual absorption and apparent sublingual bioavailability of morphine (a hydrophilic drug) appear to be poor, the sublingual absorption of methadone, fentanyl, and buprenorphine (lipophilic drugs) is relatively high under controlled conditions.

Osborne et al[79] studied the pharmacokinetic parameters of morphine, morphine-6-glucuronide, and morphine-3-glucuronide after the administration of a single dose of morphine by five different routes. Their findings suggest that sublingual, buccal, and sustained-released buccal morphine result in delayed absorption, with attenuation and delay of peak morphine and metabolite levels compared to intravenous morphine. However, the bioavailability of morphine and morphine glucuronide production was not altered by the use of these alternate routes. After an administration of oral morphine, very low morphine levels were observed, and the morphine-6-glucuronide plasma area under the curve exceeded that of morphine by a factor of 9:1.

CLINICAL EXPERIENCE

There are very few reports on the clinical effects of sublingual and buccal morphine, as is the case for other alternative routes. Most of the reports are related to one-time dosage or anecdotal experience. Whitman et al[80] reported that 70%–80% of 150 patients with cancer pain treated with sublingual morphine obtained "adequate to good pain control." Patients were treated with morphine sulfate tablets in a dose of 10–30 mg every 3–4 hours around the clock. The main side effects reported were intolerance to the taste of the drug and occasional confusion or unpleasant dreams. Pannuti et al[57] treated 28 patients with cancer pain with sublingual drops of morphine hydrochloride administered every 4 hours for an average of 5 weeks. Although the authors reported more rapid and significant remission of pain with treatment by the sublingual route compared to the rectal and oral routes, no significant differences in the incidence or severity of side effects were reported. No patient required discontinuation of sublingual treatment because of toxicity. In summary, there is still considerable controversy regarding the absorption and bioavailability of morphine and other narcotic preparations when they are administered by the buccal or sublingual route. Future research should focus on further characterizing the absorption and bioavailability of different narcotic preparations, and on determining the clinical effects and toxicity of these drugs.

TRANSDERMAL ROUTE

ABSORPTION

The skin allows for transdermal permeation of topically applied creams and ointments in quantities sufficient to have systemic action.[81] Many substances with adequate solubility in oil and water, and with molecular weights below 800–1,000 daltons can permeate across the skin.[82] Absorption varies in accordance with multiple factors, such as the vehicle selected, the integrity of the skin, the presence or extent of skin inflammation, age, ethnic differences, and regional differences in skin permeability in different areas of the body.[83] Most transdermal delivery systems consist of films of an explicit surface area that deliver medicine to the intact skin at a preprogrammed rate. In this way, the system and not the skin determines the rate for drug absorption. The use of these transdermal therapeutic systems provides a predictable rate of administering topical drugs, eliminating many of the variables associated with the con-

ventional use of ointments and creams.[83] A number of drugs, including hyoscine, nitrates, clonidine, and estradiol have been found to be effective when administered in this fashion.[84]

Usually, transdermal delivery systems should not cover an area much larger than 50 cm^2 because of the potential for toxicity. Drugs such as nitroglycerin, which penetrate the skin rapidly, do so at rates of 10–15 $\mu g/cm^2/$ hour.[85] In general, drugs with the potential for successful transdermal administration are those in which the daily dose does not exceed a few milligrams.[86]

Fentanyl citrate (a synthetic narcotic analgesic about 75 times more potent than morphine) is suitable for rate-controlled transdermal delivery, based on its high potency, skin compatibility, relatively low molecular weight, and high solubility.

PHARMACOKINETICS

Transdermal fentanyl has been evaluated in multiple studies of patients with postoperative pain, administered as a membrane-modulated drug delivery system programmed to release 1.8 mg of drug per day (Fig. 11–8).

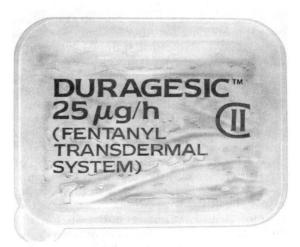

Figure 11–8. Transdermal Fentanyl Delivery System ("Patch"). Designed to deliver constant levels of analgesic continuously over a 72-hour period. Available in 25, 50, 75, and 100 $\mu g/hr$ sizes.

Steady-state plasma concentrations oscillate between 0.93 and 2.16 μg/liter; however, the steady-state concentration is not reached until at least 8 hours after initial application.[87–90] In addition to its long latency of onset, transdermal fentanyl's pharmacokinetic profile is characterized by a slow decline in plasma concentration after the removal of the system, resulting in prolonged clinical effects, probably reflecting the formation of a skin depot. In each study, once equilibrium was reached, the patch maintained analgesic concentrations of fentanyl similar to those found with constant intravenous infusion.

Fentanyl was administered intravenously and transdermally to eight surgical patients. Serum fentanyl concentrations reached a plateau about 14 hours after the application of the transdermal delivery system, and this plateau was maintained until its removal at 24 hours. After removal of the patch, the decrease in serum fentanyl concentrations took considerably longer than with intravenous administration in the same patients (terminal half-life of 17.0 ± 2.3 hours vs. 6.1 ± 2.0 hours).

The rate of absorption measured from 4–8 hours after placement of transdermal fentanyl until removal of the system after 24 hours was relatively constant, and continued at a declining rate after removal of the system. The authors concluded that the long terminal half-life of serum fentanyl concentrations after transdermal system removal is due to continued slow absorption of fentanyl, probably from a cutaneous depot of drug at the site of prior transdermal system placement.[91]

Duthie et al[92] measured plasma fentanyl concentration during and after transdermal fentanyl administration in 34 patients undergoing general surgical procedures. Concentrations measured at 8 and 12 hours did not differ from those observed in a matched group of patients receiving fentanyl by intravenous infusion. At 24 hours, the concentration of fentanyl was significantly lower in the transdermal group. The plasma fentanyl clearance did not differ significantly between the groups. However, as in other studies, the plasma fentanyl concentration decreased slowly after the removal of the transdermal patch.

Holley et al[93] found morphine requirements in eight patients with postoperative pain receiving transdermal fentanyl to be similar to those of 39 patients receiving a continuous intravenous infusion of fentanyl. After patch application, the serum concentration of fentanyl increased slowly and reached a plateau at 15 hours, then decreased slowly (apparent half-life of 21 hours).

Gourlay et al[94] found a mean delay time of 12.7 hours before minimum effective blood fentanyl concentration was obtained with fentanyl patches in 13 surgical patients. A pseudo-steady state was reached at between 36 and 48 hours, and a decay time of 16 hours was observed after the systems were removed (time for fentanyl concentration to decrease to a level below the mean effective concentration for the control of postoperative pain). There was a marked variability between patients in the actual hourly fentanyl dose rate. The authors concluded that the transdermal fentanyl system provides a significant contribution to postoperative pain relief, but at the dose rates used (50–125 μg/hour), supplementary doses of meperidine were required by all patients, probably to control "incident" pain. In a double-blind comparison of fentanyl and placebo for postoperative pain, the same authors found that there was no significant difference in visual analogue measurements of pain intensity between fentanyl and placebo-treated patients assessed at 0–12, 12–24, 24–36, and 36–48-hour intervals after surgery, suggesting a similar quality of pain relief for fentanyl and placebo.[95] However, significantly less supplementary meperidine was administered to the fentanyl group in the 12–24, 24–36, and 36–48-hour periods. These clinical findings are consistent with the pharmacokinetic data obtained by these investigators in their first trial.

CLINICAL EXPERIENCE

Rowbotham compared transdermal fentanyl with placebo in a double-blind study of postoperative pain.[96] All patients received intravenous morphine on demand for supplementary analgesia. The transdermal systems were applied 2 hours before induction of anesthesia, and were left in place for 24 hours. Pain scores were significantly lower, peak expiratory flow rates significantly higher, and demand for supplementary morphine significantly less in the treatment versus the control group.

Miser et al[97] treated five patients with cancer pain with transdermal fentanyl for periods of 3–156 days. Doses were adjusted to individual patient needs, and varied from 75 μg/hour to 350 μg/hour (median, 225 μg/hour). Two patients experienced intermittent vomiting that continued during treatment, one patient experienced transient somnolence and respiratory depression at the peak dose that resolved with dose reduction, and one patient presented with both intermittent vomiting that persisted during fentanyl therapy and transient lethargy and respiratory depression after dose escalation. Somnolence responded to treatment with amphetamines in this patient.

Simmonds et al[98] treated a total of 39 patients with cancer pain with a fentanyl transdermal therapeutic system. Patients were converted from oral morphine to fentanyl plus immediate-release morphine for breakthrough pain. The median starting dose of fentanyl was 50 μg/hour, and the median final dose was 100 μg/hour (range 25–525 μg/hour). Patients wore the patch for a median of 84 days (range, 5–365 days). The median supplementary dose of morphine was 105 mg/day (range 0–720 mg/day). Transdermal treatment was readily maintained through a series of common events such as surgery, herpes zoster infections, and chemotherapy infusions. Patient compliance was considered excellent. No significant toxicity was described by the authors.

SUMMARY

In summary, pharmacokinetic data suggest that transdermal fentanyl is well absorbed, although there is a considerable delay in reaching steady-state plasma levels, and a slowly declining plasma concentration after removal of the patch. These characteristics are potential obstacles for its regular clinical use, particularly in unstable patients. Although clinical experience is still very limited, treatment appears to be well tolerated. Future research will need to focus on comparisons between the transdermal route and long-acting morphine preparations and continuous subcutaneous infusions of opioids.

INHALATION ROUTE

Studies have suggested that in using standard nebulizers or pressurized aerosols, only 7%–30% of inhaled drugs actually reaches the lung.[99,100] In the case of opioids, a large but variable percentage of drug remaining at the buccal level could later be absorbed, either directly or after being swallowed.

Chrubasik et al[101] randomized 20 patients with postsurgical pain to a continuous-plus-on-demand "infusion" of inhaled morphine from the oxygen supply's nebulization reservoir, versus morphine administered by intravenous infusion. No significant difference in pain control was found for intravenous versus inhaled morphine. Pharmacokinetic data indicated that only a proportion of the inhaled morphine reached the systemic circulation via the mucous membranes and the lung. The authors suggested that a potent analgesic derivative might be derived during the passage of morphine via the respiratory tract. The authors concluded that because of relative ease of administration and a lower incidence of side effects, morphine administered by the inhaled route might be preferable to intravenous morphine.

Oliver[102] described three cases of bronchospasm after street use of inhaled heroin by drug addicts. All patients responded readily to standard treatment for bronchospasm. Because heroin is often mixed with a variety of powdered carrier substances, impurities are inevitably inhaled, and might have contributed to the bronchospasm in this population.

Tandberg et al[103] described successful endotracheal absorption of naloxone in a patient with respiratory failure and severe bradycardia after a heroin overdose. Serial serum naloxone levels obtained over the 3 hours after administration showed a similar pharmacokinetic pattern to that previously reported for intravenous naloxone.

Chrubasik[104] compared the pharmacokinetic behavior of 10 mg of morphine injected into the nebulization reservoir placed between the endotracheal tube and the anesthetic circle in seven postoperative patients, versus 10 mg of morphine administered intramuscularly in the same patients 5 days later. There was marked individual variation in the serum morphine concentrations produced between routes of administration. The maximum serum morphine concentration after inhaled morphine was approximately six times lower than that after intramuscular morphine, and the time of occurrence differed significantly. The individual relative bioavailabilities of inhaled morphine varied from 9% to 35% of the intramuscular administration, with a mean of 17%.

Young et al[105] treated 11 adult patients with advanced chronic lung disease whose exercise endurance was limited by dyspnea, in a double-blind, randomized, cross-over study comparing inhaled low dose morphine versus placebo. The mean endurance time was significantly greater after subjects had inhaled morphine than after placebo. The mean dose of morphine nebulized was 1.7 mg, achieving a mean inhaled dose of about 0.6 mg (on the assumption of 30% retention of the nebulized dose by each patient). No side effects were reported. The authors suggest that small amounts of morphine delivered to the lungs might act directly on lung afferent nerve endings to reduce dyspnea.

Fuller[106] studied the systemic effects of inhaled morphine and codeine on cough and increased respiratory resistance provoked by inhaled capsaicin in 13 healthy subjects. Both morphine (10 mg) and codeine (50 mg) significantly reduced increases in respiratory resistance after inhaled capsaicin. However, neither drug altered the cough response. In contrast, oral codeine (60 mg) significantly reduced the number of coughs at 1 and 2 hours, and intravenous morphine (0.15 mg/kg) significantly reduced the sensitivity of the cough response, an effect that was observed to be reversed by naloxone administration. However, there was no significant drug effect on either the baseline respiratory resistance or its increase after capsaicin. The authors concluded that whereas "systemic" doses of opiates seem to be required to reduce the cough reflex, inhaled opiates may reduce the increased respiratory resistance after inhaled capsaicin.

Masters et al[107] treated five male volunteers with 8 mg of morphine and 5 mg of diamorphine, administered by inhalation. Both drugs appeared to be absorbed rapidly. The plasma morphine concentration was similar in magnitude to values reported after oral, intravenous, and intramuscular administration of morphine. Although the dose of diamorphine was lower, higher blood levels were achieved, probably due to the fact that diamorphine is considerably more lipophilic than morphine.

In summary, the current level of knowledge about the absorption and pharmacokinetics of morphine administered by the inhaled route is still quite limited. Future research should focus on further characterizing the absorption and pharmacokinetics of different nebulized narcotics before reliable clinical trials can be designed.

POTENTIAL CLINICAL APPLICATION OF ALTERNATIVE ROUTES

Table 11–3 summarizes some of the potential clinical applications of these drugs in patients with cancer pain. Although a significant volume of clinical information exists on the use of the subcutaneous route, very limited information is available on the clinical use of the rectal, sublingual, buccal, transdermal, and inhalatory routes of administration in patients with cancer pain.

However, available pharmacokinetic data and limited clinical experience suggest specific applications for these routes in some clinical situations. All of these routes are likely to be useful for patients in whom the oral route must be bypassed because of bowel obstruc-

Table 11–3.
Potential Applications for Alternative Routes of Narcotic Administration

Feature	R	SL*	B*	TD	SC	I*
Emesis	++	++	++	++	++	++
Bowel obstruction	++	++	++	++	++	++
Dysphagia	++	++	++	++	++	++
Cognitive failure	++	0	0	++	+	0
Comatose patients	++	0	0	++	++	0
Diarrhea	0	++	++	++	++	++
Colostomy	0	++	++	++	++	++
Hemorrhoids, anal fissures	0	++	++	++	++	++
Coagulation disorders	++	++	++	++	0	++
Severe immunosuppression	++	++	++	++	0	++
Generalized edema	++	++	++	0	++	++
Frequent dose changes	++	++	++	0	++	++
Initial titration	+	++	++	0	++	++
Breakthrough pain	++	++	++	0	++	++

Key: R = rectal, SL = sublingual, B = buccal, TD = transdermal, SC = subcutaneous, I = inhalatory
* Not enough information available to recommend clinical use.

tion, severe emesis, or severe dysphagia. The buccal, sublingual, and inhalatory routes will not be useful in patients with severe cognitive failure or comatose states, whereas the rectal route will not be useful in patients with diarrhea, colostomy, hemorrhoids, or anal fissures. The transdermal route is likely to be less useful in patients with generalized edema, and in patients who are medically unstable or who require initial titration of the analgesic dose, frequent dose changes, or when there is a high incidence of breakthrough pain. The subcutaneous route is less desirable in patients with coagulation disorders or severe immunosuppression. Because of their simplicity of administration, most of these routes are likely to become useful for long-term management. The rectal route may be more difficult to use on a long-term basis if short-acting medications requiring frequent administration are used, and, conversely, more useful for long-term use if long-acting morphine preparations are used. Because of their ease of administration, all these routes except the transdermal are likely to become useful in the management of breakthrough pain. Further definitive research is needed before any recommendation for clinical use can be made on treatment by the sublingual, buccal, and inhalatory routes. Research on these three routes should attempt to establish the absorption and bioavailability of different narcotic preparations, and the ideal solutions and concentrations. In the case of rectal and transdermal administration, enough information is available to suggest that some narcotics are well absorbed, and therefore controlled clinical trials in cancer patients should be designed.

Finally, the subcutaneous route has been shown to be associated with reliable absorption, and has been demonstrated to be safe and effective in cancer pain management. On this basis, it should be considered the standard alternative route against which all newer alternative routes of administration should be tested.

REFERENCES

1. Foley K: The treatment of cancer pain. N Engl J Med 1984;313:84.
2. Cancer Pain: A Monograph on the Management of Cancer Pain. Ottawa, Canada, Health & Welfare Canada: Minister of Supply and Services, H42-2/5-1984E.
3. Bruera E: Subcutaneous administration of opioids in the management of cancer pain. In Foley K, Ventafridda V (eds): Advances in Pain Research and Therapy, vol 16, p 203. New York, Raven Press, 1990.
4. Beaver W: Management of cancer pain with parenteral medication. JAMA 1980;244:2653.
5. Fraser D: Intravenous morphine infusion for chronic pain. Ann Intern Med 1980;93:781.
6. Portenoy RK, Mouline DE, Rogers A et al: IV infusion of opioids for cancer pain: Clinical review and guidelines for use. Cancer Treat Rep 1986;70:575.
7. Citron M, Johnston-Early A, Fossieck B et al: Safety and efficacy of continuous intravenous morphine for severe cancer pain. Am J Med 1984;77:199.
8. Rutter P, Murphy F, Dudley H: Morphine: Controlled trial of different methods of administration of post-operative pain relief. Br Med J 1980;1:12.
9. Hagle M: Implantable devices for chemotherapy: Access and delivery. Seminars in Oncology Nursing 1987;3:96.
10. Niederhuber J, Ensminger W, Gyves J et al: Totally implanted venous and arterial access system to replace external catheters in cancer treatment. Surgery 1982;92:706.
11. Russell P: Letter: Analgesia in terminal malignant disease. Br Med J 1979;1:1561.
12. Dickson R, Russell P: Letter: Continuous subcutaneous analgesia for terminal care at home. Lancet 1982;i:165.
13. Campbell C, Mason J, Weiler J et al: Continuous subcutaneous infusion of morphine for the pain of terminal malignancy. Ann Intern Med 1983;98:51.
14. Wright B, Callan K: Slow drug infusions using a portable syringe driver. Br Med J 1979;2:582.
15. Coyle N, Mauskop A, Maggard J et al: Continuous subcutaneous infusion of morphine for post-operative pain relief. Anaesth Analg 1985;40:1086.
16. Bruera E, Chadwick S, Bacovsky R et al: Continuous subcutaneous infusion of narcotics using a portable disposable pump. Journal of Palliative Care 1985;1:45.
17. Goudie T, Allan M, Lonsdale M et al: Continuous subcutaneous infusion of morphine for post-operative pain relief. Anaesth Analg 1985;40:1086.
18. Miser A, Davis D, Hughes C et al: Continuous subcutaneous infusion of morphine in children with cancer. Am J Dis Child 1983;137:383.
19. Bruera E, Brenneis C, Michaud M et al: Continuous sc infusion of narcotics using a portable disposable device in patients with advanced cancer. Cancer Treat Rep 1987;71:635.
20. Hutchinson H, Leedham G, Knight A: Continuous subcutaneous analgesia and antiemetics in domicillary terminal care. Lancet 1981;ii:1279.
21. Sheehan A, Sauerbier G: Continuous subcutaneous infusion of morphine. Oncology Nursing Forum 1986;13:92.
22. Jones V, Hanks G: New portable infusion pump for prolonged subcutaneous administration of opioid analgesics in patients with advanced cancer. Br Med J 1986;1:1496.
23. Bruera E, Brenneis C, Macmillan K et al: The use of the subcutaneous route for the administration of narcotics. Cancer 1988;62:407.
24. Ventafridda V, Spoldi E, Caraceni A et al: The importance of continuous sc morphine administration for cancer pain control. The Pain Clinics 1986;1:47.
25. Kerr I, Sone M, DeAngelis C et al: Continuous narcotic infusion with patient-controlled analgesia for chronic cancer pain in outpatients. Ann Intern Med 1988;108:554.
26. Waldmann C, Eason J, Rambohul E et al: Serum morphine levels: A comparison between continuous subcutaneous and intravenous infusion in postoperative patients. Anaesth Analg 1984;39:768.
27. Nahata M, Miser A, Reuning R: Analgesic plasma concentrations of morphine in children with terminal malignancy receiving a continuous subcutaneous infusion of morphine to control severe pain. Pain 1984;18:109.
28. Brenneis C, Michaud M, Bruera E et al: Local toxicity during subcutaneous infusion of narcotics: A prospective study. Presented at the VIth World Congress on Care of the Terminally Ill, Montreal, Canada, September 1986. Cancer Nursing 1987; Vol 10(4):172–176.
29. Portenoy R: Continuous infusion of opioid drugs in the treatment of cancer pain: Guidelines for use. Journal of Pain and Symptom Management 1986; 1:223.
30. Inturrisi C, Foley K: Narcotic analgesics in the management of pain. In Kuhar M, Pasternak G (eds): Analgesics: Neurochemical, Behavioral, and Clinical Perspectives, p 257. New York, Raven Press, 1984.
31. Osborne R, Joel S, Selvin M: Morphine intoxication in renal failure: The role of morphine-6-glucuronide. Br Med J 1986;2:296.
32. Inturrisi C: Role of opioid analgesics. Am J Med 1984;77:27.
33. Tamsen A, Sjoestroems S, Hartvig P: The Uppsala experience of patient-controlled analgesia. In Foley

KM, Inturrisi C (eds): Advances in Pain Research and Therapy, vol 8, p 435. New York, Raven Press, 435.

34. Bullingham R, Jacobs O, McQuay H et al: The Oxford system of patient-controlled analgesia. In Foley KM, Inturrisi C (eds): Advances in Pain Research and Therapy, vol 8, p 319. New York, Raven Press, 1986.

35. Bruera E, Brenneis C, Michaud M et al: Patient-controlled subcutaneous hydromorphone versus continuous subcutaneous infusion for the treatment of cancer pain. JNCI 1988;80:1152.

36. Bruera E, Macmillan K, Perry B: The Edmonton injector: A safe and simple device for subcutaneous patient-controlled analgesia. Journal of Palliative Care 1988;4:70.

37. Bruera E, Chadwick S, Weinlick A et al: Delirium and severe sedation in patients with terminal cancer. Cancer Treat Rep 1987;71:787.

38. Bruera E, Brenneis C, MacDonald RN: Continuous SC infusion of narcotics for the treatment of cancer pain: An update. Cancer Treat Rep 1987;71:953.

39. Bruera E, MacDonald M, Brenneis C et al: Letter: Metoclopramide infusion with a disposable portable pump. Ann Intern Med 1986;104:896.

40. Shen R, Arieli S: Administration of potassium by subcutaneous infusion in elderly patients. Br Med J 1982;285:1167.

41. Shen R, Singer M: Subcutaneous infusions in the elderly. J Am Geriatr Soc 1981;29:583.

42. Hays H: Hypodermoclysis for symptom control in terminal care. Canadian Family Physician 1985; 31:1253.

43. Wilson TH: Intestinal Absorption. Philadelphia, WB Saunders, 1962.

44. De Boer AG, Moolenaar F, De Leede LGJ et al: Rectal drug administration: Clinical pharmacokinetic considerations. Clin Pharmacokinet 1982;7:285.

45. De Boer AG, De Leede LGJ, Breimer DD: Drug absorption by sublingual and rectal routes. Br J Anaesth 1984;56:69.

46. Cole L, Hanning CD: Review of the rectal use of opioids. Journal of Pain and Symptom Management 1990;118.

47. De Boer AG, Breimer DD, Mattie H et al: Rectal bioavailability of lidocaine in man: Partial avoidance of first-pass metabolism. Clin Pharmacol Ther 1979;26:701.

48. Moolenaar F, Olthof L, Huizinga T: Absorption rate and bioavailability of paracetamol from rectal aqueous suspensions. Pharmaceutisch Weekbload Scientific Edition 1979;1:25.

49. Moolenaar F, Oldenhof NJJ, Goenewoud W et al: Absorption rate and bioavailability of acetyl salicylic acid and its calcium salt after oral and rectal administration. Pharm Weekbl (Sci) 1979;1:243.

50. Moolenaar F, Stuurman-Bieze AGG, Visser J et al: Biopharmaceutics of rectal administration of drugs in man: 1. Introduction of benzoic acid as a test drug. Int J Pharmacol 1978;1:323.

51. Rance MJ, Shillingford JS: The metabolism of opiates by the gut. In Alder ML, Manara L, Samanin R (eds): Factors Affecting the Action of Narcotics, p 359. New York, Raven Press, 1978.

52. Westerling D, Lindahl S, Anderson KE et al: Absorption and bioavailability of rectally administered morphine in women. Eur J Clin Pharmacol 1982;23:59.

53. Johsson T, Christensen CB, Jordening H et al: The bioavailability of rectally administered morphine. Pharmacol Toxicol 1988;62:203.

54. Moolenaar F, Visser J, Leuvermann A et al: Bioavailability of morphine from suppositories. Int J Pharmacol 1988;45:161.

55. Sawe J, Dahlstrom B, Paalzow L et al: Morphine kinetics in cancer patients. Clin Pharmacol Ther 1981;30:629.

56. Breda M, Bianchi M, Ripamonti C et al: Plasma morphine and morphine 6-glucuronide patterns in cancer patients after oral, subcutaneous, sublabial and rectal acute administration. International Journal of Clinical Pharmacology Research (in press).

57. Pannuti F, Rossi AP, Iafelice G et al: Control of chronic pain in very advanced cancer patients with morphine hydrochloride administered by oral, rectal, and sublingual route. Pharmacol Res Commun 1982;14:369.

58. Ellison NM, Lewis GO: Plasma concentrations following single doses of morphine sulfate in oral solution and rectal suppository. Clin Pharm 1984;3:614.

59. Moolenaar F, Yska JP, Visser J et al: Drastic improvement in the rectal absorption profile of morphine in man. Eur J Clin Pharmacol 1985;29:119.

60. Westerling D, Anderson KE: Rectal administration of morphine hydrogel: Absorption and bioavailability in women. Acta Anaesthesiol Scand 1984;28:540.

61. Lindahl S, Olsson AK, Thomson D: Rectal premedication in children. Anaesthesia 1981;36:376.

62. Kaiko RF, Healy N, Pav J et al: The comparative bioavailability of MS Contin tablets (controlled-release oral morphine) following rectal and oral administration. In Doyle D (ed): The Edinburgh Symposium on Pain Control and Medical Education, 1989: Royal Society of Medical Services International Congress and Symposium Series Number 149. London, Royal Society of Medical Services, 1989.

63. Hojsted J, Rubeck K, Peterson H et al: Comparative bioavailability of a morphine suppository given rectally and in a colostomy. Eur J Clin Pharmacol 1990;39:49.

64. Brook-Williams P, Hoover LH: Morphine suppositories for intractable pain. Can Med Assoc J 1982; 126:14.

65. Brumley RD: Home made rectal morphine sulphate suppositories. Hospice Journal 1988;4:95.

66. Maloney CM, Kesner RK, Klein G et al: The rectal administration of MS Contin: Clinical implications of use in end stage cancer. American Journal of Hospice Care 1989;6(4):34.

67. Danhof M, Breimer DD: Therapeutic drug monitoring in saliva. Clin Pharmacokinet 1978;3:39.

68. Hollinshead WH: The head and neck. In Anatomy for Surgeons, vol 1, p 426. New York, Harper and Row, 1968.

69. Taraszka MJ: Absorption of clindamycin from the buccal cavity. J Pharm Sci 1970;59:873.

70. Beckett AH, Moffat AC: Correlation of partition co-efficients in n-heptane-aqueous systems with buccal absorption data for a series of amines and acids. J Pharm Pharmacol 1969;21 (Suppl):1445.

71. Beckett AH, Moffat AC: Kinetics of buccal absorption of some carboxylic acids and the correlation of the rate constants and n-heptane: Aqueous phase partition coefficients. J Pharm Pharmacol 1970;22:15.

72. Gibaldi M, Kaning L: Absorption of drugs through the oral mucosa. Journal of Oral Therapeutics and Pharmacology 1965;1:440.

73. Beckett AH, Hossie R: In Brodie BB, Gilette JR (eds): Handbook of Experimental Pharmacology Vol XX VII/1. Concepts in Biochem Pharmacol Part 1, vol 3, p 25. New York, Springer, 1979.

74. Beckett AH, Triggs EJ: Buccal absorption of basic drugs and its application as an in vivo model of passive drug transfer through lipid membranes. J Pharm Pharmacol 1967;19 (Suppl):31S.

75. Bell MDD, Mishra P, Weldon BD et al: Buccal morphine: A new route for analgesia? Lancet 1985; i:71.

76. Fisher AP, Fung C, Hanna M: Serum morphine concentrations after buccal and intramuscular morphine administration. Br J Clin Pharmacol 1987;24:685.

77. Al-Sayed-Omar O, Johnston A, Turner P: Influence of pH on the buccal absorption of morphine sulphate and its major metabolite, morphine-3-glucuronide. J Pharm Pharmacol 1987;39:934.

78. Weinberg DS, Inturrisi CE, Reidewberg B et al: Sublingual absorption of selected opioid analgesics. Clin Pharmacol Ther 1988;44:335.

79. Osborne R, Joel S, Trew D et al: Morphine and metabolite behavior after different routes of morphine administration: Demonstration of the importance of the active metabolite morphine-6-glucuronide. Clin Pharmacol Ther 1990;47:12.

80. Whitman HH: Sublingual morphine: A novel route of narcotic administration. Am J Nurs 1984;84:939.

81. Schenplein RJ, Blank IH: Permeability of the skin. Physiol Rev 1971;51:702.

82. Michaels AS, Chandrasekaran SK, Shaw JE: Drug permeation through human skin: Theory and in vitro experimental measurement. American Institute of Chemical Engineers 1975;21:985.

83. Shaw JE, Urquhart J: Transdermal drug administration: A nuisance becomes an opportunity. Br Med J 1981;283:875.

84. Price NM, Schmitt LG, McGuire J et al: Transdermal scopolamine in the prevention of motion sickness at sea. Clin Pharmacol Ther 1981;29:414.

85. Good WR: Transderm-nitro controlled delivery of nitroglycerin via the transdermal route. Drug Development and Industrial Pharmacy 1983;9:647.

86. Guy RH, Hadgraft J: Transdermal drug delivery: The ground rules are emerging. Pharmacupoea Internationalis 1985;6:112.

87. Caplan RA, Ready LB, Olsson GL et al: Transdermal delivery of fentanyl for post-operative pain control (abstract). Anesthesiology 1986;65:196.

88. Holley FO, Van Steeins C: Transdermal administration of fentanyl for post-operative analgesia (abstract). Anesthesiology 1986;65:548.

89. Nimmo WS, Duthie DJR: Plasma fentanyl concentrations after transdermal or IV infusion of fentanyl (abstract). Anesthesiology 1986;65:559.

90. Plezia PM, Linford J, Kramer H et al: Transdermal therapeutic system (fentanyl) for post-operative pain: An efficacy, toxicity and pharmacokinetic trial (abstract). Anesthesiology 1986;65:210.

91. Varvel JR, Shafer SL, Hwang SS: Absorption characteristic of transdermally administered fentanyl. Anesthesiology 1989;90:928.

92. Duthie DJR, Rowbotham DJ, Wyld R et al: Plasma fentanyl concentrations during transdermal delivery of fentanyl to surgical patients. Br J Anaesth 1988; 60:614.

93. Halley FO, van Steennis C: Post-operative analgesia with fentanyl: Pharmacokinetics and pharmacodynamics of constant-rate IV and transdermal delivery. Br J Anaesth 1988;60:608.

94. Gourlay GK, Kowalski SR, Plummer JL et al: The transdermal administration of fentanyl in the treatment of post-operative pain: Pharmacokinetics and pharmacodynamic effects. Pain 1989;37:193.

95. Gourlay GK, Kowalski SR, Plummer JL et al: The efficacy of transdermal fentanyl in the treatment of post-operative pain: A double-blind comparison of fentanyl and placebo systems. Pain 1990; 40:21.

96. Rowbotham DJ, Wyld R, Peacock JE: Transdermal fentanyl for the relief of pain after upper abdominal surgery. Br J Anaesth 1989;63:56.

97. Miser AW, Narang PK, Dothage JA et al: Transdermal fentanyl for pain control in patients with cancer. Pain 1989;37:15.

98. Simmonds MA, Payne R, Richenbaucher J et al: TTS (fentanyl) in the management of pain in patients with cancer (abstract). Proc Am Soc Clin Oncol 1989;8:324.

99. Gaensler EA, Beakey JF, Segal MS: Pharmacodynamics of pulmonary absorption in man: I. Aerosol and intratracheal penicillin. Ann Intern Med 1949;31:582.

100. Newman SP, Pavia D, Moren F et al: Deposition of pressurised aerosols in the human respiratory tract. Thorax 1981;36:52.

101. Chrubasik J, Geller E, Niv D et al: Morphine inhalation versus intravenous infusion of pain treatment after abdominal surgery (abstract). Anesth Analg 1987;66 (Suppl):S29.

102. Oliver RM: Broncho-spasm and heroin inhalation. Lancet 1986;i:915.

103. Tandberg D, Abercrombie D: Treatment of heroin overdose with endotracheal naloxone. Ann Emerg Med 1982;11:443.

104. Chrubasik J, Wust H, Griedrich G et al: Absorption and bioavailability of nebulized morphine. Br J Anaesth 1988;61:228.

105. Young IH, Daviskas E, Keena VA: Effect of low dose nebulised morphine on exercise endurance in patients with chronic lung disease. Thorax 1989;44:387.

106. Fuller RW, Karlsson JA, Choudry NB et al: Effect of inhaled and systemic opiates on responses to inhaled capsaicin in humans. J Appl Physiol 1988;65:1125.

107. Masters N, Heap G, Wedley J et al: Inhaled nebulised morphine and diamorphine: Useful in general practice? Practitioner 1988;232 (Pt I):910.

Chapter 12

Opioid Analgesics for Cancer Pain: Toxicities and Their Treatments

Neil M. Ellison

Misinformation regarding the side effects and potential toxicities of the opioid analgesics is common. It is a primary reason for the underuse and misprescription of these agents for the management of cancer pain. Such misinformation commonly is possessed by physicians, other health care workers, caregiver families and friends, and patients themselves.[1-3]

Fortunately, most adverse effects of opioid analgesics can easily be controlled with readily available means. The perceived incidence of opioid-mediated toxicities, in general, far exceeds their actual occurrence.

This chapter reviews the side effects of opioid analgesics prescribed appropriately for the relief of cancer-related pain, and presents a preventative approach for treating potential side effects of treatment. It is imperative to realize that the management of opioid side effects is a fundamental component of competent opioid analgesic therapy.

SIDE EFFECT VERSUS ALLERGY

Dorland's Medical Dictionary defines a side effect as "a consequence other than the one(s) for which an agent or measure is used . . . especially on a tissue or organ system other than the one sought to be benefited by its administration." Side effects may be desirable, but are usually undesirable. For example, the antitussive effects of an opioid may be viewed as beneficial in a patient with pain and cough due to bronchogenic carcinoma, but to the contrary, the obstipation produced by these same drugs is usually quite troublesome.

Allergy refers to a hypersensitivity of the body cells to a specific antigen that results in various types of reactions, such as bronchospasm, hives, or anaphylaxis. Opioid-induced allergic reactions are infrequent. They are usually manifested by urticaria or other skin reactions such as rashes. Anaphylaxis is rare.[4] It is, however, quite common for patients who have experienced an opioid-associated adverse effect, such as nausea or vomiting, to state that they have an "allergy" to that drug, and consequently this "allergic history" is perpetuated in the medical record. This error often precludes the administration of an appropriate analgesic that could be co-administered with a regimen to counteract the toxicity that was mislabeled as an allergy. Caregivers should carefully question a history of opioid allergy, and correct any miscommunication in the medical record. Such clarification of a patient's allergic status permits the opioid drugs to be prescribed appropriately.

THE MYTHS OF OPIOID USE FOR THE CONTROL OF CANCER-RELATED PAIN

Misconceptions regarding opioid use for the control of cancer-related pain are common among lay citizens as well as health care providers (see Chapters 8 and 9). Public misunderstanding is evidenced by the results of a telephone survey of 496 randomly selected individuals in Wisconsin.[5] The respondents' major concerns related to mental confusion associated with the use of opioids (58%), the development of tolerance resulting in the need for increasing amounts of opioids (56%), and the development of addiction (45%). Health care providers predominantly fear opioid-induced addiction and respiratory depression.[6,7]

Efforts to promote patient and family education and to enhance physician and nurse familiarity with the appropriate use of these drugs are essential to dispel the pervasive myths that interfere with effective cancer pain management.

OPIOID-INDUCED RESPIRATORY DEPRESSION

The inordinate fear by nurses and physicians of the infrequent occurrence of opioid-induced respiratory depression is an important impediment to adequate control of cancer pain. All opioid agonists have similar depressant effects on the brain-stem respiratory center.[4] This effect is less with agonist–antagonist drugs. At first exposure there is an initial decrease in responsiveness of the medullary respiratory center to carbon dioxide tension, but over time tolerance to this effect develops.[8–10] Natural sleep has a similar effect on the respiratory center, and may be additive to that produced by the opioids. A resultant decrease in respiratory rate, tidal volume, and minute ventilatory volume occurs. The maximum effect is observed 5–10 minutes after the administration of intravenous morphine, and 30–90 minutes after intramuscular or subcutaneous administration.

Rarely, high doses of opioid analgesics can have a bronchoconstricting effect, probably through bronchial histamine release. Their administration is therefore relatively contraindicated during an episode of acute bronchial asthma. Inhibition of the medullary cough center also occurs, which may be a beneficial side effect in some circumstances.

Clinically significant respiratory depression is an uncommon problem when opioids are used appropriately. Pain acts as an antagonist to respiratory depression. An individual in pain or an easily arousable patient taking opioid analgesics rarely has significant respiratory depression. In contrast, the somnolent patient with complete control of pain who continuously receives opioids with inattention to their increasing sedative effects is at greatest danger for respiratory depression. This adverse effect is rapidly reversible with either noxious stimuli, such as sternal pressure, or intravenous naloxone hydrochloride.[2,10] In general, pharmacologic reversal of opioid-induced respiratory depression is not necessary if peak plasma levels of the opioid have already been reached, and the patient is just somnolent and is not cyanotic or unarousable. In such cases, the patient can be observed and the opioid withheld until somnolence improves. The interval of administration can then be lengthened or the dose decreased to prevent further problems. If rapid reversal of the respiratory depression is necessary, a dilute solution of naloxone should be administered carefully in small increments.[11,12] The administration of a large bolus dose of naloxone can precipitate profound withdrawal, seizures, or painful crises in an opioid-dependent patient, and is contraindicated. For example, naloxone 0.4 mg in 10 cc saline can be administered in 0.5-cc aliquots at 2-minute intervals safely. The pharmacologic half-life of naloxone is only about 30 minutes, which is much shorter than that of most opioids. As a result, either repetitive dosing or a slow infusion of naloxone may be necessary to manage effectively opioid-induced respiratory depression.

No contraindication exists to the use of opioid analgesics in patients with underlying or preexisting pulmonary disease. These drugs may be prescribed cautiously for such individuals. Particular care is indicated in the continued management of patients receiving high doses of opioids who undergo a neurosurgical or anesthetic procedure that abruptly reduces nociceptive input. The absence of the respiratory center-stimulating effect of preexisting pain leads to an unopposed opioid-mediated respiratory depressant effect that may result in somnolence or abrupt respiratory depression or arrest. In the case of a successful procedure, the dose of opioids should be tapered gradually, and patients should be observed carefully for increased sedation and possible respiratory depression.

ADDICTION, PHYSICAL DEPENDENCE, AND TOLERANCE

Addiction (psychological dependence) (see Chapters 7–9) may be defined as an aberrant behavior manifesting as an overwhelming involvement in the use or acquisition of the drug for nonmedical purposes. This occurs with a frequency of less than 1:10,000 in patients with cancer-related pain for whom opioids are prescribed appropriately to relieve pain.[7,13,14] Regrettably, health care professionals often do not realize that patients who "demand" opioids for cancer pain relief, due to the inappropriate administration of the drug on a prn (as needed) schedule or at nontherapeutic doses, are not addicted.[15] Such behavior, so-called "pseudoaddiction," is iatrogenically induced, and although manipulative behavior may be present, these patients are merely seeking appropriate pain control. Correct adjustment of opioid dosage and around-the-clock administration in such situations should eliminate this situation.

Physical dependence (see Chapters 7–9) is defined as an altered physiologic state resulting in withdrawal symptoms when opioids are abruptly discontinued or an opioid antagonist is administered. Physical dependence occurs within 3–4 weeks in most patients receiving daily opioid analgesics. Infrequently, it may occur more rapidly. Cessation of opioid therapy is still achieved easily in the physically dependent patient when indicated. Halving or quartering the dose of opioid every 1 to 2 days until the daily equivalent of about 15 mg of oral morphine is reached should allow complete discontinuation without symptoms of withdrawal.[10]

Tolerance (see Chapters 7–9), the need for an increasing amount of drug to achieve a given effect, normally occurs in most individuals using opioids chronically. It has been suggested that tolerance is induced more rapidly with parenteral administration than with oral use, but this point is controversial. When tolerance does occur, increasing the dose of opioid usually restores adequate analgesia. Current opinion suggests that clinically significant tolerance is a less frequent event than was previously believed. Increased pain in patients with cancer whose symptoms have been well controlled on stable doses of opioids is usually due not to tolerance, but to increased tumor invasion and tissue injury. A common decision-making error in such a setting is a failure to recognize the need simply to increase the dose of the prescribed drug. Instead, it is often assumed that the prescribed opioid is no longer effective, and that the analgesic formulation should be altered. There is no advantage to changing opioid preparations for the development of tolerance or new pain alone; increasing the dose of the administered opioid is preferred, and is usually effective.

CONSTIPATION

Opioid analgesics bind directly to peripheral receptors in the gastrointestinal tract, with resultant decreased peristalsis, diminished biliary, pancreatic, and intestinal secretions, and increased anal sphincter tone. Stool transit time increases, and desiccation of feces results.[16,17]

This problem is often compounded by decreased fluid intake, decreased ambulation, and poor dietary fiber ingestion in many patients with symptomatic cancer. Tolerance to the constipating effects of narcotics is slow to develop, and often does not occur. The goal of bowel management for patients taking opioids should be prevention of constipation rather than treatment of constipation. The average number of bowel movements for a general population ranges from three stools per day to one stool every 3 days.[18] Therefore, the expectations and goals for evacuation vary greatly between patients, and should be individualized. Patients may have bowel movements but still feel constipated because of changes in the caliber, consistency, or quantity of the passed stool.

Any bowel program should begin with encouraging the intake of fluids and bulk-forming foods. A stool softener hydrates and softens the stool, but has little cathartic effect, and should not be used alone.[4] Stool softeners may be of modest benefit when given in conjunction with a peristaltic stimulant such as senna.

Few controlled studies exist that evaluate the effects of various cathartics for opioid-induced constipation in cancer patients.[19] As a result, recommendations are based primarily on anecdotal experience. A typical regimen would consist of a senna compound–stool softener combination administered initially in increasing dosages in conjunction with increments in the dose of opioid prescribed.[19–21] Senna compounds are purported to cause less abdominal cramping than other peristaltic stimulants because they selectively stimulate Auerbach's plexus in the colon. The result is passage of a formed soft stool 6 to 12 hours after their ingestion.

Other peristaltic stimulants, bulk-forming and osmotic laxatives, with suggested dosing, are reviewed in Table 12–1. Often, substantial doses of individual agents or combinations of these medications are necessary to promote regular evacuation in opioid-treated patients. Enemas or disimpaction may be necessary, but are less desirable than oral or rectal administration of laxatives, both from the patient's and health care provider's point of view.

Since constipation can be considered to be practically a universal occurrence with the administration of opioid analgesics for the control of cancer pain, a prophylactic approach to this problem is strongly recommended. A prophylactic bowel regimen should be instituted along with the initiation of opioid therapy. Plans to continue this regimen indefinitely and to increase the laxative dose with increasing opioid doses can prevent patient frustration, discomfort, and morbidity. If tolerance does develop to the obstipatory effects of opioids, administration of the cathartics can be decreased or discontinued.

NAUSEA AND VOMITING

Opioid-induced nausea and vomiting is a common cause of patient-perceived "narcotic allergy." This side effect is more common in ambulatory patients. Nausea has been estimated to occur in up to 40% and vomiting in 15% of ambulatory patients treated with opioids.[4,22] These symptoms can occur with all opioid agonists, and are not predictably more common with any single drug. The mechanisms of opioid-induced nausea and vomiting are complex. Centrally, direct stim-

Table 12–1.
Recommendations for Pharmacological Management of Opioid-Induced Constipation

Doses

Stimulant laxatives	
Senokot S	1 tab hs—4 tab tid given orally
Dulcolax	1 tab hs—3 tab tid given orally
	(rectal suppositories may also be used)
Bulk-forming laxatives	
Metamucil	1 teaspoonful in 8 oz water qd-tid
Bran	
Saline or osmotic cathartics	
Milk of magnesia	15–40 ml qd-bid
Magnesium citrate solution	240 ml qd

Recommendations

1. Adequate activity, fluid intake, and bulk-forming foodstuffs should be recommended whenever possible.
2. Begin with a stimulant laxative administered around-the-clock with the opioid analgesic. Increase laxative dose as necessary, titrating to effect. Increased laxative doses often are required in conjunction with increased dosage of opioids. Add other agents, if necessary, when maximum tolerated dose is reached.
3. This list is not meant to be all-inclusive. Various combinations of these or other drugs may be used.

ulation of the medullary vomiting center and chemoreceptor trigger zone occurs. A peripheral effect results in increased gastric antral tone, decreased gastrointestinal motility, and delayed gastric emptying. These occurrences can be additive to the constipatory effect of the opioids, and symptoms of gastric outlet obstruction symptoms may result. Finally, opioid-induced increased vestibular sensitivity, especially in the ambulatory patient, can also be emetogenic.[4]

Since the majority of patients will not develop nausea or vomiting while taking opioids, prophylactic treatment is not indicated. However, patients should have ready access to antiemetics in case nausea or vomiting occur. The narcotic and antiemetic regimen should then be administered concurrently in an around-the-clock fashion for 3 to 7 days. After this period of time, tolerance to the nausea and vomiting effect of narcotics usually develops, and the antiemetics can be gradu-

ally tapered. Patients commonly err by taking opioids and antiemetics sporadically rather than regularly and concurrently. Intermittent use of opioid drugs impairs the development of tolerance to their side effects.

If nausea and vomiting remain intractable despite aggressive therapy with antiemetics, changing to treatment with a different opioid may overcome this problem. The amelioration of side effects that is sometimes observed when a different opioid analgesic is used is explained by "incomplete cross-tolerance," a term that refers to the unpredictable variations in side effects observed from drug to drug in the same individual. When applied systematically and aggressively, these strategies are usually successful.

Inpatient care nevertheless is occasionally necessary for the administration of parenteral narcotics, antiemetics, and hydration in an attempt to manage this side effect until tolerance occurs. Rectal or transdermal administra-

Table 12–2.
Presumed Site of Action of Antiemetics

Medullary vomiting center
  Phenothiazines
  Antihistamines
  Anticholinergics
Medullary chemoreceptor trigger zone
  Butyrophenones
  Phenothiazines
  Trimethobenzamide
  Metoclopramide
Higher CNS
  Cannabinoids
  Benzodiazepines
  Corticosteroids
Periphery
  Metoclopramide
  Corticosteroids
Vestibular
  Scopolamine
  Meclizine

tion of an opioid with concurrent antiemetics may also be considered until tolerance to emetogenesis develops, or effective therapy is established.

Few, if any, controlled therapeutic studies of narcotic-induced nausea or emesis have been carried out. Available references recommending antiemetic therapies are primarily extrapolated from the vast literature pertaining to chemotherapy-induced nausea and vomiting.[23,24] Table 12–2 lists antiemetics with their presumed or known sites of action. Table 12–3 lists recommendations for specific drug therapy to control nausea. When symptoms do not resolve with single-agent therapy, a polypharmaceutical approach similar to that used to treat chemotherapy-related nausea is applied. A therapeutic addition unusual to the treatment of chemotherapy-induced nausea and vomiting is the use of drugs acting on the vestibular apparatus. This approach may be of particular benefit in the ambulatory patient complaining of dizziness or vertigo and associated nausea while taking opioid analgesics.

SEDATION

Sedation is a common adverse effect of treatment with the opioid analgesics (see Chapters 10 and 30). It is most commonly an acute event associated with the onset of therapy or with escalations in dosage. Few studies support any prolonged cerebral effects related to chronic opioid administration.[25,26] Further elucidation of this issue by well controlled studies is necessary before any definitive statements can be made regarding the effect of chronic opioid use on mentation or motor function. In general, ambulatory and functioning patients should be advised not to drive or perform potentially dangerous activities for several days after the initiation of treatment or escalation of opioid doses. Tolerance to the sedative effect of opioids usually occurs fairly rapidly, and enables many patients to resume normal activities.

Somnolence is reversible with cessation of treatment or decreasing the dose. Patients with recent inadequate control of pain are often sleep-deprived, and experience catch-up sleep for several days when adequate analgesia is obtained. This phenomenon should not be confused with excessive somnolence, because sleep-deprived patients are easily arousable.

If sedation persists and pain control is adequate, a 10%–25% reduction of the dose of opioid or continuation of the same total daily

Table 12–3.
Outpatient Treatment of Opioid-Induced Nausea and Emesis

1. Relieve constipation.
2. Prescription for oral prn use—polypharmacy is often necessary.
  Prochlorperazine or thiethylperazine 5–10 mg q 4–6 h. Available as suppository also.
  Metoclopramide 10–40 mg q 6–8 h.
  Halperidol 0.5–2 mg q 4–12 h.
  Lorazepam 1 mg q 6–12 h.
  Diphenhydramine 25–50 mg q 6–8 h.
  Meclizine 12.5–25 mg q 6–8 h, or scopolamine transdermal 1 disk q 3 d.

dose administered in smaller but more frequent intervals (*eg*, 40 mg morphine solution every 4 hours may be changed to 20 mg morphine solution every 2 hours) may result in improvement. Alternatively, substituting different opioid formulations at equianalgesic doses may alter the central nervous system (CNS) side effect profile in a given patient.

Despite limited human data regarding the use of dextroamphetamine sulfate or methylphenidate hydrochloride to ameliorate the CNS effects of narcotics, this approach has proved quite useful in clinical practice (see Chapter 10). Oral doses of 10 mg on awakening and 5 mg at noon of either drug are effective and safe in most patients, although the development of tolerance may increase dose requirements over time. Reports describing beneficial effects of these drugs on opioid-induced somnolence and/or motor skill testing pertain either to the immediate postoperative situation or relatively short-term use in cancer patients. These stimulant drugs also appear to potentiate the analgesic effect of the opioids, thus allowing lower doses to be administered with an equianalgesic effect and perhaps fewer side effects such as somnolence.[27-29] Mazindol, an amphetamine derivative of mild potency possessing a low addictive potential, did not effect activity or depressive symptoms when given to cancer patients in conjunction with propoxyphene.[30]

CONFUSION

Confusion caused by treatment with opioid analgesics, like sedation, is predominantly an acute problem, to which tolerance usually develops rapidly. Euphoria and dysphoria are also acute and usually evanescent problems that are infrequent when opioids are used in the treatment of chronic cancer-related pain. In the case of persistent confusion, there are usually multifactorial etiologies compounding the opioid's possible effect. The majority of cancer patients will experience some degree of delirium during the last week of life, a phenomenon that is an almost universal occurrence during the final 48 hours. In this context, disorientation can usually be attributed more to organic encephalopathy from multisystem failure rather than opioid use.[31-33] It is imperative that analgesia be continued in these situations to assure a pain-free death.

If confusion occurs acutely in concert with the administration of opioids, it is most appropriately treated with calm reassurance and reorientation. Haloperidol (0.5–2 mg every 6–8 hours) can be used when necessary. Changing opioid preparations may be of benefit, since this side effect is also idiosyncratic. Although it cannot be assumed to be universally less common with one formulation than another, this may be the case in a given patient.

Bruera et al described the cognitive effect of narcotic analgesic dose escalation of the opioids ($\geq$30% baseline dose in past 3 days) in 20 patients with cancer-related pain.[34] A control group consisted of 20 similar patients receiving a stable dose of opioids. The patients with recent increases in dosing demonstrated more cognitive dysfunction after the administration of the drug than the similarly tested group on the steady dose. This difference was no longer present after several days on the increased but then stable dose of narcotics. It was also determined that the impaired group of patients did not recognize their loss of cognitive or motor skills. The investigator's conclusion was that cognitive dysfunction occurs acutely with elevation of opioid dosing, but tolerance develops rapidly.

Patients who achieve adequate analgesia from opioid therapy, but who experience significant sedation or confusion that persists may be considered for other interventions. Anesthetic blocks, neurosurgical procedures, or other means of management such as intraspinal opioid therapy, are only a few examples of many approaches available. A report by Sjogren and Banning failed to demonstrate any difference in cognitive effect in patients receiving systemic or epidural opioids for cancer pain control.[26] This finding needs further clarification by more prospective studies.

CARDIAC AND VASCULAR EFFECTS

Opioid analgesics have no significant effect on normal myocardium, although patients with coronary artery disease may experience a decrease in myocardial oxygen consumption, cardiac work, left ventricular pressure, and diastolic blood pressure with opioid administration.[35] A vasodilating effect on peripheral vasculature with resultant orthostatic hypotension has also been demonstrated.[18] Blood pressure changes are minimal in the supine patient. When hypotension does occur in the supine individual, the cause should not be attributed to opioids, and other etiologies should considered. Opioid-induced orthostasis can be additive to that caused by other drugs such as phenothiazines. Rarely, sudden death has been reported in patients with cor pulmonale who have received opioid analgesics. Opioids therefore should be used cautiously in this setting.

There is no direct effect of opioid analgesics on the cerebrovascular circulation. However, if significant respiratory depression occurs, carbon dioxide retention may result in cerebrovascular vasodilation, which may in turn lead to intracranial hypertension in individuals with preexisting CNS pathology. Caution in the use of opioids in patients with brain injury or head trauma is therefore advised.

URINARY EFFECT

Although opioid analgesics may cause increased tone and amplitude of ureteral contraction, increased urinary bladder detrusor muscle tone, and increased vesicle sphincter tone,[4] clinically significant urinary retention occurs infrequently, and then usually in men. Tolerance to this effect usually develops rapidly. Intermittent bladder catheterization may be necessary for a short time after the initiation of these drugs in affected patients.

MYOCLONUS AND SEIZURES

Central nervous system hyperexcitability and myoclonus are infrequent side effects of treatment with the opioid analgesics. These symptoms occur most often with the chronic administration of high doses, and may be more common when the opioids are administered in conjunction with other drugs.[9,36] Myoclonic jerks are usually more troubling to the family and staff observers than to patients. Concern that myoclonic spasms represent a prelude to a seizure usually is not warranted. Reassurance regarding the etiology and self-limited nature of this symptom is indicated. Both oral steroids and the benzodiazepines (especially clonazepam) have been reported anecdotally to be beneficial in the management of opioid-induced myoclonus.[37]

Morphine, methadone, and d-propoxyphene have been shown to be capable of producing convulsions in animal models when administered in very high doses. Seizures are reversible with the administration of naloxone and anticonvulsant drugs. The threshold for induced seizures from these agents is much higher than the threshold for analgesia, and therefore the actual potential for this problem is of little clinical relevance.[4] In contrast to these findings, the chronic administration of meperidine more commonly results in myoclonus and seizures due to accumulation of a metabolite, normeperidine, particularly in patients with renal insufficiency. These convulsions are not readily reversible with naloxone.[38] Although meperidine is eliminated from plasma rapidly (half-life of 3–4 hours), the half-life of normeperidine is 15–30 hours. Because of this prolonged excretion time and the relatively high incidence of CNS stimulation, the repetitive administration of meperidine is contraindicated in the treatment of chronic cancer-related pain.

CUTANEOUS EFFECTS

Opioids may induce dilation of cutaneous blood vessels with resultant flushing.[9] Pruritus, primarily limited to the face, palate, and torso, occurs most frequently with the administration of intraspinal opioids.[4] These effects are thought to be centrally mediated, and can be controlled with very small, carefully titrated doses of naloxone.

CONCLUSION

The purpose of this review of the side effects associated with the administration of the opioid analgesics is to facilitate the appropriate, effective, and safe use of these drugs in the treatment of cancer-related pain. Although some toxicities are common and bothersome, almost all can be managed medically without sacrificing adequate analgesia. The primary obstacle to optimal use of the opioids continues to relate to patient and health care provider educational issues. Patients and their families must be reassured of the relative safety and effectiveness of treatment for cancer pain. They must be given the opportunity and taught how to communicate possible drug toxicities or lack of efficacy to their physician. The prophylactic use of cathartics and availability of antiemetics should coincide with the initial prescription of the opioid analgesics. It is important to remember that the side effect profile of different opioids is relatively unpredictable. If, with one drug regimen, analgesic efficacy cannot be achieved without intolerable side effects, then alternate opioid preparations should be tried. If treatment is still ineffective, then rapid consultation regarding other means of pain control is indicated.

To provide adequate analgesia for patients with cancer-related pain, physicians and other health care workers must often overcome their own prescribing hesitancies, based on exaggerated misconceptions of toxicity. This is especially true for the ''industrial-strength'' doses of opioids that are necessary in some cancer patients. The right dose of opioid analgesics for cancer pain control is the dose that is effective with manageable or no toxicity.

The health care team should then be reassured that tolerance develops to their own anxiety associated with the appropriate use of the opioids in even very difficult clinical situations. The next prescription is easier, and patients will continue to benefit greatly from effective palliation of their cancer-related pain.

REFERENCES

1. Hill CS, Fields WS (eds): Advances in Pain Research and Therapy, vol 11: Drug Treatment of Cancer Pain in a Drug-Oriented Society. New York, Raven Press, 1989.
2. Hill CS, Chairman: Guidelines for Treatment of Cancer Pain. Texas Cancer Council's Work Group on Pain Control in Cancer Patients, Texas Cancer Council, State of Texas, 1990.
3. Twycross RG, Lack SA: Symptom Control in Far Advanced Cancer: Pain Relief. London, Pitman, 1983.
4. Gilman AG, Rall TW, Niles AS et al (eds): The Pharmacologic Basis of Therapeutics, 8th ed. New York: Pergamon Press, 1990.
5. Levin DN, Cleeland CS, Dar R: Public attitudes toward cancer pain. Cancer 1985;56:2337.
6. Marks RM, Sachar J: Undertreatment of medical inpatients with narcotic analgesics. Ann Intern Med 1973;78:173.
7. Angell M: The quality of mercy. N Engl J Med 1982;306:98.
8. Walsh TD: Recent Results in Cancer Research, vol 89. New York, Springer-Verlag, 1984.
9. Bonica JJ: The Management of Pain. Philadelphia, Lea and Febiger, 1990.
10. Foley KM, Inturrisi CE: Analgesic drug therapy in cancer pain: Principles and practice. Med Clin North Am 1987;71:207.
11. Bradberry JC, Raebel MA: Continuous infusion of naloxone in the treatment of narcotic overdose. Drug Intell Clin Pharm 1981;15:945.
12. Citron ML: How would you treat narcotic overdoses in cancer patients? Drug Therapy 1984;9:85.
13. Porter J, Jick H: Addiction rare in patients treated with narcotics. N Engl J Med 1980;302:123.
14. Kanner RM, Foley KM: Patterns of narcotic drug use in a cancer pain clinic. Ann NY Acad Sci 1981;362:161.
15. Weissman DE, Burchman SL, Dinndorf PA et al: Handbook of Cancer Pain Management. University of Wisconsin Medical School, Wisconsin Cancer Pain Initiative, 1988.
16. Twycross RG: Managing constipation: A not-so-easy problem in cancer patients. Primary Care and Cancer August 1989:23.
17. Portenoy RK: Constipation in the cancer patient. Med Clin North Am 1987;71:303.
18. Connell AM, Hilton C, Irvine G et al: Variation of bowel habit in two population samples. Br Med J 1965;2:1095.
19. Izard MW, Ellison FS: Treatment of drug-induced constipation with a purified senna derivative. Conn Med 1962;26:589.

20. Maguire LC, Yon JL, Miller E: Prevention of narcotic-induced constipation. N Engl J Med 1981;305:1651.

21. Cimprich B: Symptom management: Constipation. Cancer Nurs 1985;8 (Suppl 1):39.

22. Levy MH: Pain management in advanced cancer. Semin Oncol 1985;12:394.

23. Craig JB, Powell BL: Review: The management of nausea and vomiting in clinical oncology. Am J Med Sci 1987;293:34.

24. Gralla RJ, Tyson LB, Kris MG: The management of chemotherapy-induced nausea and vomiting. Med Clin North Am 1987;71:289.

25. Banning A, Sjogren P: Cerebral effects of long-term oral opioids in cancer patients measured by continuous reaction time. Clinical Journal of Pain 1990;6:91.

26. Sjogren P, Banning A: Pain, sedation, and reaction time during long-term treatment of cancer patients with oral and epidural opioids. Pain 1989;39:5.

27. Forrest WH, Brown BW, Brown CR et al: Dextroamphetamine with morphine for the treatment of postoperative pain. N Engl J Med 1977;296:712.

28. Joshi JH, Jongh CA, Schnaper N et al: Amphetamine therapy for enhancing the comfort of terminally ill patients with cancer. American Society of Clinical Oncology Abstracts 1982;vol 23:C213.

29. Bruera E, Chadwick S, Brennels C et al: Methylpheni-date associated with narcotics for the treatment of cancer pain. Cancer Treat Rep 1987;71:67.

30. Bruera E, Carraro S, Roca E et al: Double-blind evaluation of the effects of mazindol on pain, depression, anxiety, appetite, and activity in terminal cancer patients. Cancer Treat Rep 1986;70:295.

31. Bruera E, Chadwick S, Weinlick A et al: Delirium and severe sedation in patient with terminal cancer. Cancer Treat Rep 1987;71:787.

32. Zimberg M, Berenson S: Delirium in patients with cancer: Nursing assessment and intervention. Oncology Nursing Forum 1990;17:529.

33. Kellar M: Oral morphine solution: Effect on pain, confusion, drowsiness, and nausea for the terminally ill patient. Hospice Journal 1988;4:55.

34. Bruera E, MacMillan K, Hanson J: The cognitive effects of the administration of narcotic analgesics in patients with cancer pain. Pain 1989;39:13.

35. Lowenstein E, Hollowell P, Levine FH et al: Cardiovascular response to large doses of intravenous morphine in man. N Engl J Med 1969;281:1389.

36. Potter JM, Reid DB, Shaw RJ et al: Myoclonus associated with treatment with high doses of morphine: The role of supplemental drug. British Medical Journal 1989;299:150.

37. Portenoy R: Personal communication.

38. Kaiko RF, Foley KM, Grabinski PY et al: Central nervous system excitatory effects of meperidine in cancer patients. Ann Neurol 1983;13:180.

Non-Pharmacologic Treatment and Novel Approaches to Management

13

Treatment of Related Symptoms

Ina Cummings Ajemian

INTRODUCTION

Quality of life is a concern for all cancer patients, and as a result should influence every therapeutic decision. In newly diagnosed disease, some symptoms result inevitably from anticancer therapy, and aggressive management will ensure better compliance with treatment recommendations. In advanced disease, quality of life is inarguably the sole consideration guiding management. As a malignancy progresses, multiple organ systems may become involved. Previous therapy may have produced troublesome sequelae. As has been stressed, pain is common, and ongoing analgesic therapy is often associated with side effects that, if poorly controlled, will further compromise well-being. Most patients with advanced disease will suffer simultaneously from four or five different symptoms. Most of these symptoms can be controlled, and call for the same detailed, aggressive approach to management as does pain.

APPROACH TO SYMPTOM MANAGEMENT

Although pragmatic and useful guidelines have been developed, treatment must necessarily be highly individualized, and as a result there are no rigid protocols for appropriate symptom management in patients with advanced cancer. Interventions such as surgery, that might be considered if cure or remission were realistic goals, rarely are indicated when quality of life is regarded as the sole therapeutic aim, but might be considered, for example, in a patient with intestinal obstruction resulting from a single bypassable lesion. A blood transfusion that may help to maintain the independent functioning of an ambulatory patient will have little effect on the quality of life of a bed-bound patient, and is therefore generally inappropriate in the latter. Antibiotic therapy may reduce painful inflammation associated with head and neck tumors,[1] but is not indicated for asymptomatic urinary tract infections, or for pulmonary congestion in a moribund patient. Each proposed treatment should be subjected to a "cost–benefit analysis": will the intervention improve the current quality of life, and what is the anticipated associated morbidity of the proposed intervention? Useful principles when problems related to symptom management are encountered include the following[2,3]:

1. As is true in other disciplines, careful assessment forms the basis for therapeutics: a problem-solving approach to symptom diagnosis is essential so that the most effective therapy can be instituted. For example, vomiting associated with increased intracranial pressure requires a very different approach to management than does vomiting associated with the initiation of opioid therapy (see Chapter 9). It should be recalled that not all symptoms are related to the underlying malignancy. Also, regular review is necessary since cancer is a dynamic process, and as the disease state evolves, symptoms can change rapidly.

2. Symptoms that can be eliminated or reduced should be aggressively treated. The perception of enhanced well-being that comes from even incremental improvement often makes residual symptoms seem less troublesome.

3. Treatment of multiple concurrent symptoms usually requires combination pharmacotherapy. At the same time, polypharmacy should be avoided whenever possible to minimize the likelihood of adverse drug interactions and additive side effects. A regular review of each patient's medication regimen aimed at eliminating those agents no longer required for the management of current symptoms is essential.

4. Consider all possible treatment options. In most cases, the primary approach will be pharmacologic in nature, but more invasive procedures may be helpful in selected cases.

5. The review of medical symptoms should take place in the context of an interdisciplinary case review. The perspective that symptoms are often multifactorial and are not always wholly physical in origin is an extremely important one. For example, insomnia may reflect the anxiety of family stress, or nausea may be exacerbated by underlying spiritual torment. Successful management requires a coordinated approach to all symptoms—physical, psychosocial, and spiritual.

6. Anticipate events. Symptoms that are persistent and amenable to pharmacologic management should be managed proactively with medications administered regularly by the clock. Side effects that are sufficiently common to be anticipated in a high proportion of cases, such as constipation secondary to opioid therapy, should be managed prophylactically, or patients and their families should be instructed to recognize the onset of a problem so that therapy can be instituted at the first sign of a problem.

7. Involve the patient and family in discussions. Whenever possible, the patient should be provided with the opportunity to identify which symptoms are most distressing at a given moment, and to evaluate whether the continued presence of the symptom or the morbidity of the proposed treatment would be preferable. The family needs to understand the goals of therapy if they are to assist the patient and help monitor the results of treatment.

FREQUENCY OF SYMPTOMS

The incidence of symptoms in reported series varies due to a number of factors, probably including the influences of 1) proximity of death; 2) whether the patient population under study is ambulatory or institutional; 3) whether the program is an independent hospice program or is one associated with an acute care referral center; and 4) whether the data are based on patient self-report or actions observed by staff. Twycross has summarized information obtained from the medical accounts of patients admitted to St. Christopher's Hospice, and lists the 19 most commonly documented symptoms.[2] Using self-report measures, Coyle et al reported on the incidence of various symptoms at 4 weeks before death in a series of 90 consecutive patients followed by the Supportive Care program at a major cancer hospital.[4] Also based on self-report measures, Dunlop has presented data on a series of 50 hospice and hospital inpatients,[5] and in another report Bedard et al summarized the symptoms observed in 952 hospice patients.[6] These results are summarized in Table 13–1. Although the incidence of symptoms varies in these surveys, all reflect a cluster of symptoms that predominates among patients with advanced cancer. The discussion in this chapter is limited to those symptoms most commonly encountered in patients with malignant disease. The reader is referred to one of the many excellent published reviews on symptom management for more comprehensive and detailed information.[7–12]

ASTHENIA, WEAKNESS, AND FATIGUE

Asthenia is regarded as including the syndromes of fatigue and generalized weakness. Fatigue is defined as easy tiring and a decreased capacity to perform normal activity, whereas generalized weakness refers to the perception of difficulty in initiating certain activities.[13] This symptom complex is most distressing to patients and their families, and occurs in as many as 50%–75% of individuals with advanced cancer. Although many potential causes exist for generalized weakness, in the majority of cancer patients weakness is related to the cancer and cancer-induced metabolic abnormalities.[14] Malnutrition and ane-

mia often contribute to asthenia, although the syndrome can exist in their absence.[15]

Lacking more specific therapy, management focuses on helping patients reorganize their activity to retain maximum independence in the face of diminishing strength. Simple measures can be useful, such as the provision of a hospital bed, bedside commode, and consultation with a physical or occupational therapist regarding the applicability of assistive devices that might help conserve energy. Simple explanation and reassurance is valuable. Advise patients to alternate periods of rest and activity, and, if they are inclined, to supplement their diet with liquid supplements. Small, frequent meals as well as assistance in their preparation may be helpful. Drug therapy with the potential to improve patients' sense of well-being includes corticosteroids (methylprednisolone 15–30 mg/day),[16] and central nervous system stimulants (methylphenidate 15 mg/day).[17]

ANOREXIA AND CACHEXIA

Anorexia or diminished appetite is very common in cancer patients, and leads to weight loss with reduced tissue mass, and thus to cachexia. This cycle becomes self-perpetuating, and often results in the common picture of an emaciated, malnourished cancer patient, a scenario that is particularly common as death approaches.[18] The etiology of this process is complex and incompletely understood. Contributing factors include: 1) the mechanical or obstructive local effects of tumor mass; 2) the effects of previous therapy (eg, radiation-induced mucositis, or surgical bowel resection); 3) associated symptoms such as cough, pain, ascites, and hiccups; and 4) metabolic changes induced by circulating tumor-related humoral agents. Alterations in desire for specific types of foods has been observed in cancer patients, such that patients may favor foods that they have ignored for a lifetime, and may abhor traditional choices. This is often manifested as an increased threshold for sweets and a decreased threshold for bitter tastes. Meat aversion is common, perhaps sec-

Table 13–1.
Common Symptoms (Percentages) in Patients with Advanced Disease

	Twycross[2]	Coyle et al[4]	Dunlop[5]	Bedard[6]
Weight loss	77	—	—	—
Pain	71	54	46	Almost all
Anorexia	67	8	58	14
Dyspnea	51	17	30	9
Cough	50	6	28	9
Constipation	47	4	36	12
Weakness	47	43	82	—
Nausea/vomiting	40	12	42	15
Edema/ascites/pleural effusion	31	—	—	6
Insomnia	29	7	46	—
Urinary symptoms	23	3	—	5
Dysphagia	23	3	—	—
Decubitus ulcer	19	—	—	—
Hemorrhage	14	—	—	—
Drowsiness	10	24	4	5
Paralysis	8	—	—	—
Jaundice	6	—	—	6
Colostomy	4	—	—	—
Diarrhea	4	—	4	—
Confusion	—	24	30	4
Pruritus	—	—	8	—
Mouth lesions	—	—	—	14

ondary to the (masked) bitterness of urea. Specifically, exposure to *cis*-platinum may result in diminished taste acuity.[12]

The management of anorexia begins with the treatment of exacerbating symptoms, in particular stomatitis, nausea/vomiting, and constipation. A dietician can advise on how to modify the diet to maximize nutrition.[19] Family members often equate food with health, and require explanation if they are to avoid making mealtime a struggle. If the patient is troubled by these symptoms, drug therapy may be a useful adjunct:

1. Corticosteroids (prednisone 5–10 mg three times daily) may improve appetite and well-being, but do not lead to consistent weight gain or improved nutritional status.[16,20]

2. Megestrol acetate (160 mg each day) has recently been evaluated,[21] and was shown to stimulate appetite and food intake, resulting in weight gain in a proportion of treated patients. This approach appears promising, but treatment is costly.[22]

CONSTIPATION

Constipation (see Chapter 12) is one of the most prevalent symptoms in terminally ill patients, especially in individuals receiving opioid analgesics for the management of pain. Despite its potentially serious sequelae, constipation tends to be considered in an inappropriately light-hearted manner, and unfortunately often is treated as an afterthought.

Constipation may result in increased anxiety and pain, decreased appetite, intestinal pseudo-obstruction, and even colonic perforation. An episode of fecal impaction is long remembered. The effects of constipation may be so extended that many patients will endure some degree of pain rather than risk becoming constipated from opioid therapy. Persistent constipation often results in suboptimal use of analgesics, and may provoke a cycle of persistent pain and increased inactivity, exacerbating the patient's suffering. As in chronic pain, the causes of chronic constipation can seldom be removed, and the goal of therapy is symptomatic management.

Constipation refers to the infrequent or difficult passage of stool. A stool that is difficult to pass is usually hard and dry. In the presence of marked weakness or neurogenic bowel dysfunction, the rectum may be full of soft stool, but the patient will still be constipated. As is the case with the symptom of pain, the definition is personal and subjective, and the diagnosis requires a careful history of the patient's individual habits. As a rule, patients will not discuss constipation spontaneously, and need to be prompted. The common causes of constipation in the cancer patient are summarized in Table 13–2.

Although constipation may stem from a variety of causes, and, like most symptoms in cancer patients, is often multifactorial, the use of opioid drugs is the most frequent factor contributing to constipation in the cancer patient with chronic pain. Although opioid-induced constipation appears to be dose-related, there is large individual variation.[23] Tolerance develops very slowly, and most patients will have to take laxatives as long as they take opioids.[24] The exact mechanisms by which narcotics induce constipation are unclear, but appear to be mediated through opioid receptors in the central nervous system and the gastrointestinal tract. The administration of opioids results in decreased secretory activity in the stomach and marked motor inhibition, with emptying delayed as long as 12 hours.[25] The tone and the nonpropulsive motility of the ileum and colon are increased, thus slowing transit time. As stool remains

Table 13–2.
Common Causes of Constipation in the Cancer Patient

1. Factors directly related to the tumor
   Structural
     Intraluminal or extraluminal partial bowel obstruction from tumor, postoperative adhesions, or strictures
   Neurologic
     Spinal cord or cauda equina compression from epidural metastases
2. Factors related to symptom therapy
   Drugs
     Opioids
     Anticholinergics (tricyclic antidepressants, phenothiazines, antispasmodics)
     Diuretics
     NSAIDs
     Antacids containing aluminum, calcium
     Some anticonvulsants
     Chemotherapy (vincristine-induced neuropathy)
     Iron
3. Factors indirectly related
   Physiologic
     Age, weakness, dyspnea
     Decreased dietary bulk
     Decreased fluid intake
     Dehydration (vomiting, fever)
     Decreased activity
     Depression
     Absence of privacy, routine, comfortable position
   Metabolic
     Hypercalcemia
     Hypokalemia
     Uremia
     Diabetes (Autonomic neuropathy)
     Hypothyroidism
   Painful inhibition
     Hemorrhoids
     Anal fissure

in the bowel for a longer period, a greater percentage of the water is absorbed.

Common symptoms of constipation include abdominal discomfort, anorexia, nausea, and vomiting. Restlessness and confusion may be induced or exacerbated, especially in the elderly patient. Occasionally, pressure on the floor of the bladder may cause urinary retention. A careful history of recent

Table 13–3.
Sample Bowel Management Protocol

1. Mild constipation
   Increase fluid, fiber, activity if possible
   Docusate 100 mg/bid
2. Mild/moderate constipation
   Docusate 100–200 mg/bid
   Bisacodyl 5 mg or Senekot 1–4 tablets qd
3. No BM × 3 days, no stool in rectum
   Add milk of magnesia 30 ml po hs
4. No BM ×3 or more days, stool in rectum
   Above medications
   Glycerin with or without Bisacodyl suppository
   Phosphate (Fleet) enema if unsuccessful with
      suppository
5. Impacted stool in rectum[28]
   Above medications
   Oil retention enema
   Manual disimpaction—using local anesthetic on
      finger, sedation, or nitrous oxide inhalation to re-
      duce discomfort
   Follow-up cleansing saline or phosphate enema
   Repeat daily until no further hard stool
6. Chronic constipation with absent rectal sensation
   Drugs as above to maintain soft stool
   Bisacodyl suppository qd
   Phosphate enema (Fleet) q3 days to empty rectum
      and avoid incontinence

bowel habits and a rectal examination usually confirm a diagnosis.

In the very ill patient it is difficult to modify the contributing factors of decreased dietary and fluid intake, and decreased activity. A commode by the bedside may conserve strength, permitting avoidance of the very difficult task of defecating in the horizontal position on a bedpan. Scheduling time after breakfast or dinner will take advantage of the gastrocolic reflex. When risk factors exist, bowel function should be monitored daily, and constipation should be treated in a progressive manner (Table 13–3). Laxative therapy will need to be prescribed for most patients (Table 13–4).

Additional dietary fiber is desirable, but may be difficult to achieve. Bulk laxatives such as psyllium should be avoided, for to be effective they require a larger fluid intake than is usually possible in patients who are unwell. If these agents are administered with insufficient quantities of water, fecal impaction, small bowel obstruction, or a gastric bezoar may result.[25] Those patients able to eat small amounts may use a natural laxative spread on bread or toast (equal amounts of softened dates, figs, raisins, and pitted prunes, chopped and blended with prune nectar to make a spread that can be refrigerated).[26]

Table 13–4.
Laxative drugs.

1. Bulk-forming laxatives.
   Bran
   Methylcellulose
   Psyllium (Metamucil)
   Action: increase the stool bulk, soften the stool
      consistency by increased water content; reduce
      transit time
2. Lubricants
   Mineral oil (Agarol, Magnolax)
   Glycerine suppositories
3. Osmotic (saline) cathartics
   Magnesium salts
      Magnesium citrate (Citormag)
      Magnesium sulphate (Epsom salts)
      Magnesium hydroxide (Milk of Magnesia)
   Sodium Salts
      Sodium phosphate (Fleet enema)
   Lactulose (Chronulac)
      Action: osmotic particles draw fluid into bowel,
         and semiliquid stool has decreasd transit time
4. Contact cathartics
   a) Docusate (Dioctyl sulfosuccinate: Regulex,
         Colace)
      Action: anionic surface-active agents that facili-
         tate the penetration of the fecal mass by water
         and fats; promote the secretion of fluid in large
         and small bowels; weak effect on gut motility
   b) Anthraquinones: Cascara, Senna
      Action: stimulation of myenteric plexus to in-
         crease propulsive peristalsis
   c) Diphenylmethanes
      Phenolthalein (several proprietary prepara-
         tions)
      Bisacodyl (Ducolax)
5. Special Action
   Metoclopramide
   Polyethylene glycol electrolyte lavage solution

Lubricant laxatives containing mineral oil are best avoided, except for transient use in the "well" patient. Mineral oil decreases the absorption of fat-soluble vitamins, and should aspiration occur, can lead to lipoid pneumonia.

If the stool is hard and dry, docusate or one of the osmotic cathartics will help. Docusate is well tolerated, and patients can be taught to adjust the dose in response to the consistency of their stool. One of the magnesium or sodium salts may be substituted or added to the treatment regimen when constipation persists and there is no renal failure. All agents may cause cramping or bloating. Lactulose, a nonabsorbed disaccharide, is effective and safe, but may cause nausea, and it is relatively more costly than other drugs in its class.

The contact cathartics, such as senna preparations and bisacodyl, act on the colon, affecting mucosal electrolyte transport and stimulating propulsive peristalsis. These agents are helpful where there is a decreased response to the stimulus of increased luminal bulk, as in the elderly or the very ill, and in countering the diminished peristalsis induced by opioids. Metoclopramide may be helpful in the presence of neurogenic or opioid-induced bowel paresis.

Bowel obstruction may result from impaction of stool at any level in the colon. Stool in the rectum can be removed manually. Stool higher in the colon needs to be softened and brought down to the rectum to be removed. Usually, increased doses of an osmotic cathartic such as lactulose are effective. A modified use of the balanced electrolyte colonic lavage solution, Golytely (Braintree Laboratories, Braintree, MA), has been observed to be successful 90% of the time in the elderly,[27] but the required fluid intake (2 liters/day for 2 days) is often impossible in very ill patients.

Diarrhea is unusual in advanced cancer. The most frequent cause is overzealous use of laxatives. A rectal examination should always be performed to rule out fecal impaction, with spurious diarrhea resulting from bacterial liquefaction of the more proximal feces and fecal leakage.[28]

NAUSEA AND VOMITING

Nausea (see Chapter 12) occurs frequently and is one of the most demoralizing symptoms of advanced cancer. There are numerous causes, and symptomatic management must be undertaken at the same time as an evaluation to identify potentially treatable etiologies.

Nausea is a well established side effect of opioid drugs. Contributing mechanisms include: 1) activation of the chemoreceptor trigger zone in the brain-stem, 2) changes in vestibular function, and 3) direct effects on the stomach and bowel.[29] Nausea may occur in up to a quarter of patients initially treated with morphine, and many patient reports of "allergy" to morphine in fact reflect nausea that was not promptly treated. It appears that tolerance develops quickly, and only a small proportion of patients will experience chronic opioid-induced nausea.

A reasonable approach to managing opioid-induced nausea is as follows:

1. All patients being initiated on an opioid should be given a prescription for an antiemetic that they can begin at the first evidence of nausea. Given the potential for additive side effects (primarily sedation) and the incomplete prevalence of nausea, prophylactic treatment is not recommended.[30]
2. If nausea occurs, vigorous treatment is indicated to avoid compromising management with analgesics.
3. Antiemetics of choice include those acting at the chemoreceptor trigger zone (phenothiazines—haloperidol, droperidol; metoclopramide).
4. The presence of bloating and early satiety suggests delayed gastric emptying secondary to opioid-induced gastroparesis. In this setting, metoclopramide will be most effective due to its local action on the stomach and upper small bowel.
5. Patients may be comfortable at rest and still complain of nausea that is exacerbated

by movement. This finding suggests a vestibular component, and lends itself to management with an antihistamine or anticholinergic antiemetic (cyclizine, dimenhydrinate, scopolamine).

6. As with pain, if symptoms are refractory to the above measures, then combination pharmacotherapy is indicated.
7. If vomiting precludes the use of oral medications, antiemetics in suppository form or, in even more resistant cases, by continuous subcutaneous infusion will be temporarily required.
8. When nausea has been controlled for 1 to 2 weeks, antiemetics should be tapered and discontinued, and reinstituted only if nausea recurs.

Occasionally, nausea occurs in a patient whose symptoms previously have been well controlled on a stable dose of an opioid. Renal function should be evaluated in this setting, since it has recently been recognized that mild renal insufficiency can predispose to the accumulation of morphine-6-glucuronide, a relatively toxic metabolite of morphine.[31] When such a phenomenon is suspected, patients may benefit from transition to an alternative opioid analgesic.

Other common factors that contribute to nausea include: 1) oral infection or irritation; 2) constipation and partial or complete bowel obstruction; 3) metabolic factors, including uremia, hypercalcemia, and hepatic failure; 4) increased intracranial pressure; 5) other concurrently administered drugs such as chemotherapeutic agents, antidepressants, and nonsteroidal anti-inflammatory drugs; and 6) unpleasant sights, smells, and emotional associations. In all instances, a correct diagnosis of the etiology will facilitate treatment and supportive therapy that are specific to the symptom's underlying causes, as outlined above.

An extremely important clinical observation is that constant and persistent nausea is usually perceived as a much more distressing phenomenon than is intense but occasional vomiting. If nausea is relieved, which is usually an achievable goal, then occasional vomiting will usually be accepted without undue distress. Thus, as Baines et al have demonstrated, malignant bowel obstruction (see Chapter 29), even when complete, can be managed effectively without the discomfort of prolonged nasogastric suction and intravenous fluid administration.[32] Many patients will require a continuous subcutaneous infusion of antiemetics and analgesics to control nausea and crampy abdominal pain, but patients may continue to eat and drink, with only the occasional brief distress of periodic vomiting.

DYSPNEA

Dyspnea is the subjective experience of difficult breathing, and is a common sensation in patients in whom the demand for oxygen is greater than the body's ability to supply it. Dyspnea tends to be multifactorial, and its severity does not always correlate with the degree of demonstrable underlying organic pathology. The intensity of dyspnea should always be assessed in terms of the patient's expression of distress. Much of the focus in treating dyspnea is in altering the patient's perception.

Dyspnea is always associated with panic and fear. The subjective element can be modified in a variety of ways: 1) reassurance and explanation; 2) slow rhythmic movements in all aspects of bedside care; 3) massage; 4) music; 5) increased air movement with an open window or fan; and 6) a comfortable chair placed in the semireclining position.

Treatment of dyspnea should be directed at altering the underlying pathologic process insofar as this is possible. Some of the more common causes of dyspnea in advanced cancer are listed below, along with suggested approaches to management.[33,34]

Airway Obstruction by Tumor and Its Sequelae. Local tumor masses may be shrunk by radiotherapy. Corticosteroids (dexamethasone 8–12 mg/day, followed by decreasing doses) may be of benefit, presumably due to reductions in peritumoral edema. Antibiotics will reduce swelling secondary to infection.

Superior vena caval syndrome (see Chapter 29), marked by head, neck, and upper limb edema, plethora, and hoarseness, may result from mediastinal obstruction. Corticosteroids and radiotherapy are the treatments of choice.

Pleural Effusion (see Chapter 29). Small effusions rarely cause dyspnea. Symptomatic effusions should be drained completely, and, if recurrent, a sclerosant such as tetracycline should be instilled into the pleural space.

Lymphangitic Carcinomatosis. Radiographic changes occur late, and the degree of dyspnea is often in excess of what would be expected from radiographic findings. Over half of such patients will respond to corticosteroids (dexamethasone 4–8 mg/day or an equivalent dose of prednisone).

Pneumonia. Treatment depends on the patient's status before infection. In advanced disease, oral antibiotics usually will control the production of troublesome sputum, whereas in moribund patients, therapy aimed at eradicating the infection achieves little.[35] In this scenario, low doses of opioids administered regularly usually will control dyspnea.[36]

Pulmonary Embolism. In advanced disease, the risk of bleeding from anticoagulation therapy often outweighs the risk of repeated embolism. When the prognosis of life expectancy is sufficient to justify anticoagulation, the initiation of heparin therapy often relieves dyspnea and pleuritic pain.

Anemia. Dyspnea is usually associated with congestive heart failure, and is rare in bedbound patients except when anemia is profound. Transfusion may be indicated if dyspnea appears to be related to low counts or if hypoxia-induced confusion is a problem.

Palliation. Symptomatic management of dyspnea is indicated whenever the underlying disease process cannot be modified. Bronchodilator drugs are useful in the presence of reversible airway obstruction. Despite a mechanism of action that is unclear, regularly administered low doses of opioids will reduce dyspnea in terminal cancer patients without altering respiratory rate or oxygen saturation.[36] The provision of oxygen is controversial, and rarely is associated with objective benefit, although its positive placebo effect in many patients must be weighed against the high probability of dependency. Anxiolytic drugs may produce beneficial sedation, but have no intrinsic action on dyspnea.

COUGH

Persistent cough is troublesome, contributes to fatigue, insomnia, and anorexia, and may cause chest wall pain. Reversible causes should be sought and treated. Discontinuation of smoking should be encouraged. Humidification and hydration may prove beneficial by reducing sputum viscosity, and patients may benefit from maintenance of a semi-upright position. Standard expectorants and mucolytics are of little value. Antibiotic therapy may control sputum production, even if the underlying causes are not relieved. Dry, nonproductive cough can be exhausting, and may be suppressed with the administration of low-dose opioids or nebulized local anesthetics.[33]

ORAL SYMPTOMS

The condition of the mouth is too often overlooked while symptoms with more serious implications and of a more obvious nature are addressed. Symptoms of a dry, coated, or painful mouth are very common in cancer patients, and are almost universally present in patients with advanced disease. The condition of the mouth will influence ability to communicate, ability to eat, and total well-being, and merits attentive management.[37] Numerous risk factors predispose to mouth care problems: cachexia, relative dehydration, reduced saliva secondary to previous radiotherapy or medications (morphine,[38] diuretics, antidepressants, anticholinergics), mucositis secondary to chemotherapy or radiotherapy, depressed immune response, and mouth breathing. Treatment is symptomatic:

1. Dry mouth—frequent sips of water or juice, artificial saliva, sugar-free chewing gum, citrus fruit.
2. Painful mouth—2% viscous lidocaine before meals, or gargle with a solution of one part diphenhydraine, two parts sucralfate suspension.
3. Crusted mouth or adherent plaques—soften with lubricating jelly, clean with a toothette moistened in a solution of one part 3% hydrogen peroxide and three parts saline. Treat candidiasis with topical mycostatin or ketoconazole,[39] ensuring that dentures are also cleaned.
4. Loose dentures—refer for soft reline.

PRESSURE SORES

Pressure sores are painful and demoralizing, and may lead to life-threatening infections, more complex nursing management, and prolonged hospital stays. The focus is solidly on prevention, for rehabilitation after ulcers have developed is slow or impossible. Many excellent reviews are available,[40-45] and the variety of proposed treatments suggests that success rests with compulsive attention to care, and not with a particular treatment regimen. Patients with advanced cancer are predisposed to developing pressure sores due to decreased mobility, compromised peripheral circulation, poor nutritional status, and the possibility of incontinence or draining wounds. Decreased sensation due to neurolytic block or neurologic disease removes pain as a stimulus to alter position, and further increases risk. Successful prevention and management require the collaboration of the interdisciplinary team—patient and family, nurse, physiotherapist, and physician.

HICCUPS

Although an uncommon symptom, when severe, intractable hiccups (singultus) can be extremely distressing because of their propensity to interfere with nutrition and sleep, and to produce pain and extreme fatigue. Hiccup consists of a sudden, involuntary, reflex spasm of the muscles of inspiration (diaphragm, intercostals, and scalenes) against a closed glottis. The mechanism of hiccup remains incompletely understood.

Neoplastic causes of hiccup include tumors of the brain, neck (especially distal esophagus), chest (especially base of the lung and diaphragm), and abdomen (especially gastric carcinoma and hepatomegaly). Other causes to bear in mind include uremia, pneumonia, pericarditis, myocardial infarction, gastric distention, gastritis or ulcer, peritonitis, pancreatitis, and nervous system disorders (trauma, cerebrovascular insufficiency, infection, nerve impingement).

A variety of home remedies and pharmacologic regimens has been suggested to be effective.[2,12] Therapeutic options include metoclopramide 10 mg four times daily to correct gastric distension, chlorpromazine 10–25 mg four times daily[2] or prn during an attack, amitriptyline 10 mg three times daily,[46] nifedipine 20 mg three times daily,[47] or methylphenidate 10–20 mg intravenously. Phrenic nerve block may be considered in the rare instance of truly intractable hiccups.

URINARY SYMPTOMS

Urinary infections are frequent, and generally respond to the administration of an appropriate antibiotic. In advanced illness, catheterization is frequently required for a variety of reasons, including incontinence secondary to infection, tumor invasion of the base of the bladder, and neurologic dysfunction. Secondary infection requires treatment only when symptomatic. Urinary retention may be precipitated by anticholinergic drugs, but if associated with back pain, should call attention to the possibility of metastatic spinal cord compression, one of the true emergencies of symptom management (see Chapter 25).

CONCLUSION

Symptom control in patients with cancer should not be confined to the terminal stages of disease. An aggressive approach applied to symptom management throughout the disease process will allow many patients to undergo better specific anticancer therapy.[3] Successful management will enable patients to live as fully as possible, regardless of prognosis. If symptoms are controlled, the way is opened for patients to focus on those things that give meaning to life and lead to personal growth.

REFERENCES

1. Bruera E, MacDonald N: Intractable pain in patients with advanced head and neck tumors: A possible role of local infection. Cancer Treat Rep 1986;70:691.
2. Twycross RG: Symptom Control in Terminal Cancer: Lecture Notes. Oxford, Sir Michael Sobell House, 1988.
3. Walsh TD: Symptom control in patients with advanced cancer. American Journal of Hospice and Palliative Care 1990;7, no. 6:20.
4. Coyle N, Adelhardt J, Foley KM et al: Character of terminal illness in the advanced cancer patient: Pain and other symptoms during the last four weeks of life. Journal of Pain and Symptom Management 1990;5:83.
5. Dunlop GM: A study of the relative frequency and importance of gastrointestinal symptoms, and weakness in patients with far advanced cancer: Student paper. Palliative Medicine 1990;4:37.
6. Bedard J, Dionne A, Dionne L: The experience of La Maison Michael Sarrazin (1985-1990): Profile analysis of 952 terminal-phase cancer patients. Journal of Palliative Care 1991;7:42.
7. Billings JA (ed): Outpatient Management of Advanced Cancer. Philadelphia, JB Lippincott, 1985.
8. Doyle D, Benton TE: Pain and Symptom Control in Terminal Care, 2nd ed. Edinburgh, St. Columba's Hospice, 1988.
9. Kaye P: Notes on Symptom Control in Hospice and Palliative Care. Essex, CT, Hospice Education Institute Inc., 1989.
10. Saunders Dame C (ed): The Management of Terminal Malignant Disease, 2nd ed. London, Edward Arnold, 1984.
11. Twycross RG, Lack SA: Therapeutics in Terminal Cancer, 2nd ed. Edinburgh, Churchill Livingstone, 1990.
12. Walsh TD (ed): Symptom Control. Oxford, Blackwell Scientific, 1989.
13. Bruera E, MacDonald RN: Asthenia in patients with advanced cancer. Journal of Pain and Symptom Management 1988;3:9.
14. Lichter I: Weakness in terminal illness. Palliative Medicine 1990;4:73.
15. Bruera E, Brenneis C, Michaud M et al: Association between asthenia and nutritional status, lean body mass, anemia, psychological status and tumor mass in patients with advanced breast carcinoma. Journal of Pain and Symptom Management 1989;4:59.
16. Bruera E, Roca E, Cedaro L et al: Action of oral methylprednisolone in terminal cancer patients: A prospective randomized double-blind study. Cancer Treat Rep 1985;69:751.
17. Bruera E, Chadwick S, Brenneis C: Methylphenidate associated with narcotics for the treatment of cancer pain. Cancer Treat Rep 1987;71:120.
18. Enck RE: Anorexia and cachexia. American Journal of Hospice Care 1987;4, no. 5:13.
19. D'Agostina NS: Managing nutrition problems in advanced cancer. Am J Nur 1989;89:51.
20. Wilcox JC, Corr J, Shaw J et al: Prednisolone as an appetite stimulant in patients with cancer. Br Med J 1984;288:27.
21. Loprinzi CL, Ellison NM, Schaid DJ et al: Controlled trial of megestrol acetate for the treatment of cancer anorexia and cachexia. JNCI 1990;82:1127.
22. Enck RE: Anorexia and cachexia: An update. American Journal of Hospice and Palliative Care 1990;4:13.
23. Twycross RG, Harcourt JMV: The use of laxatives at a palliative care center. Palliative Medicine 1991;5:27.
24. Portenoy RK: Constipation in the cancer patient. Med Clin North Am 1987;71, no. 2:303.
25. MacCara ME: The uses and abuses of laxatives. Can Med Assoc J 1982;126:780.
26. Skelton D: Designing a management program to regulate bowel function. Canadian Journal of Geriatrics 1988;4, no. 2:27.
27. Fox RA: Taking the logical approach to managing constipation. Geriatric Medicine 1986;2:85.
28. Wrenn K: Fecal impaction. N Engl J Med 1989;321:658.
29. Baines M: Nausea and vomiting in the patient with advanced cancer. Journal of Pain and Symptom Management 1988;3:81.
30. Portenoy RK, Coyle N: Controversies in the long-term management of analgesic therapy in patients with advanced cancer. Journal of Pain and Symptom Management 1990;5:307.
31. Hagen NA, Foley KM, Cerbone DJ et al: Nausea and morphine-6-glucuronide. Journal of Pain and Symptom Management 1991;6:125.
32. Baines M, Oliver DJ, Carter RL: Medical management of intestinal obstruction in patients with advanced

malignant disease: A clinical and pathological study. Lancet 1985;ii:990.

33. Cowcher K, Hanks GW: Long-term management of respiratory symptoms in advanced cancer. Journal of Pain and Symptom Management 1990;5:320.

34. Regnard C: Dyspnea in advanced cancer: A flow diagram. Palliative Medicine 1990;4:311.

35. Hoy A: Dyspnoea. In Bates TD (ed): Contemporary Palliation of Difficult Symptoms, p 277. London, Bailliere Tindale, 1987.

36. Bruera E, Macmillan K, Pither J et al: Effects of morphine on the dyspnea of terminal cancer patients. Journal of Pain and Symptom Management 1990; 5:341.

37. Regnard C: Mouth care: A flow diagram. Palliative Medicine 1989;3:67.

38. White ID, Hoskin PJ, Hanks GW et al: Morphine and dryness of the mouth. Br Med J 1989;298:1222.

39. Epstein JB: Oral and pharyngeal candidiasis: Topical agents for management and prevention. Postgrad Med 1989;85:257.

40. Reuler JB, Cooney TG: The pressure sore: Pathophysiology and principles of management. Ann Intern Med 1981;94:661.

41. Seiler WO, Stahelin HB: Decubitus ulcers: Preventive techniques for the elderly patient. Geriatrics 1985;40:53.

42. Seiler WO, Stahelin HB: Decubitus ulcers: Treatment through five therapeutic principles. Geriatrics 1985; 40:30.

43. Seiler WO, Stahelin HB: Recent findings on decubitus ulcer pathology: Implication for care. Geriatrics 1986;41:47.

44. Low AW: Prevention of pressure sores in patients with cancer. Oncology Nursing Forum 1990;17:179.

45. Dolinger RD: Pressure sores and optimum skin care. Journal of Palliative Care 1990;6:50.

46. Stalnikowicz R, Fich A, Troudard T: Amitriptyline for intractable hiccups. N Engl J Med 1986;315:64.

47. Muchopadhyay P, Osman MR, Wajima T et al: Nifedipine for intractable hiccups. N Engl J Med 1986; 314:1256.

Chapter 14

Diagnosis and Treatment of Psychiatric Complications in the Cancer Patient with Pain

William Breitbart

INTRODUCTION

The cancer patient encounters many stressors during the course of cancer illness, including fears of painful death, disability, disfigurement, and dependency. Although such fears are universal, corresponding levels of psychological distress are quite variable, depending on personality, coping ability, social support, and medical factors.[1] Pain is one of the most feared consequences for the patient with cancer. The presence of pain has a profound impact on levels of emotional distress, and, clearly, psychological factors such as mood, anxiety, and the patient's internalized meaning of pain may intensify the cancer pain experience.[2] The pain specialist who undertakes the management of patients with cancer pain encounters complex diagnostic and therapeutic challenges, including the challenge of clarifying the physical and psychological issues involved in cancer pain. Appropriate management of cancer pain requires the application of a multidimensional concept of pain, and often a multidisciplinary approach that recognizes the importance of diagnosis and treatment of concurrent psychological symptoms and psychiatric syndromes.[3] This chapter reviews the common psychological issues and psychiatric complications (anxiety, depression, and delirium) seen in cancer pain patients, and provides guidelines for their assessment and management. In addition, psychiatric intervention strategies that can improve pain control in cancer patients are presented.

PSYCHOLOGICAL IMPACT OF CANCER

A diagnosis of cancer often leads to a rather characteristic set of responses that have been well described by Holland, Massie, and others.[1,3–5] This characteristic emotional response often consists of an initial period of shock, denial, and disbelief, followed by a period of anxiety, depression, disturbed sleep, altered appetite, and irritability. Concentration is poor, and intrusive thoughts about cancer and fears about the future intrude and interfere with daily activities. These "stress responses" tend to occur at predictable points in the course of cancer and its treatment—at the time of diagnosis, with relapse, before diagnostic tests or surgery, before chemotherapy or radiation, and, surprisingly, even as treatments end. Symptoms of emotional distress usually begin to resolve over a period of weeks, and patients return to their prior levels of stability once a treatment plan has been proposed and accepted, and support from family and friends ensues. Generally, psychiatric intervention is not necessary in such patients, although anxiolytic or sedative medications and relaxation techniques may be helpful in restoring sleep and minimizing distress (see Chapter 5). Usually, the support of clergy, social workers, nurses, physicians, family, and friends is sufficient to help patients through these crisis periods.

The degree of psychological distress encountered in cancer patients can be quite variable, however, and some patients continue to have high levels of depression and anxiety that persist for weeks to months, and interfere with their ability to function or even comply with cancer treatment. Often, this variability

is due to some unique medical factor (often the presence of pain or advanced disease), social factor (lack of available social or emotional support), or psychological factor (preexisting psychiatric disorder, coping ability, developmental stage). Such high levels of distress are often a result of psychiatric disorders that have developed as a complication of cancer, and usually require psychiatric intervention. For the most part, the physician treating cancer patients is interacting with psychologically healthy individuals who are reacting to the stresses imposed by cancer and its treatment. Nearly 90% of the psychiatric disorders seen in cancer patients are reactions to or manifestations of disease or treatments.[1,5,6] The spectrum of psychiatric disorders seen in cancer patients is reviewed and discussed below.

PSYCHOLOGICAL FACTORS AND PAIN IN CANCER

Cancer is perceived by the public as an extremely painful disease, and pain is perhaps the most feared of cancer's complications.[7] The magnitude of the problem of pain in cancer is great. Some 15% of patients with non-metastatic cancer have significant pain.[8,9] In advanced cancer, 60%–90% of patients report debilitating pain, and up to 25% of all patients with cancer die in pain.[10–12] Appropriate management of cancer pain is essential, and requires a multidisciplinary approach that includes a psychiatrist playing a major role.[3,13] The current multidimensional concept of pain that emphasizes the contribution of cognitive, motivational, behavioral, and affective as well as sensory (nociceptive) phenomena, has facilitated the acceptance of psychiatric and psychological participation in the fields of pain research, assessment, and treatment (see Chapter 5).[14] The definition of pain proposed by the International Association for the Study of Pain[15] states that "Pain is an unpleasant sensory and emotional experience associated with actual or potential tissue damage, or described in terms of such damage." In the contemporary view, pain is not viewed simply as tissue injury or a nociceptive event, but is recognized and accepted as a psycho-physiologic process involving nociception, pain perception, and pain expression. Psychological variables such as perception of control, personal meanings of pain, fear of death, depressed mood, and hopelessness contribute to the cancer pain experience and attendant suffering.[16,17] It is in these areas that psychological interventions can have their greatest impact.[3]

The psychological factors that influence the experience of pain (see Chapter 5) include anxiety, depression, and the meaning or significance that the pain has for the patient. In a study of women with metastatic breast cancer, Spiegel and Bloom[16] found that the site of metastasis did not predict level of pain, but the level of mood disturbance and beliefs about the meaning of pain in relation to illness were significant predictors. Daut and Cleeland[9] showed that cancer patients who believed their pain represented a worsening of their condition reported the greatest lifestyle interference to apparently unrelated causes. Alterations in measures of emotional disturbance have also been reported to predict pain intensity in patients with advanced cancer.[18] Bond demonstrated that cancer patients with lower levels of neuroticism, anxiety, and depression were less likely to report pain.[19]

Psychiatric Disorders in Cancer Patients With Pain

The Psychosocial Collaborative Oncology Group determined the prevalence of psychiatric disorders in 215 cancer patients treated in 3 cancer centers using criteria from the *Diagnostic and Statistical Manual III* (DSM III) classification of disorders.[6] About half (53%) of the patients evaluated were adjusting normally to the stresses of cancer, with no evidence of diagnosable psychiatric disorder; however, 47% of patients had clinically apparent psychiatric disorders. Of the 47% with psychiatric disorders, 68% had reactive anxiety and depression (adjustment disorders with depressed or anxious mood), 13% had major

depression, and 8% had an organic mental disorder (delirium). Cancer patients with pain are twice as likely to develop a psychiatric complication of cancer than are their counterparts without pain. Of the patients who received a psychiatric diagnosis, 39% reported significant pain, in contrast to only 19% of patients without a psychiatric diagnosis (Table 14–1). The psychiatric diagnoses of these patients with pain were predominantly adjustment disorder with depressed or mixed mood (69%) or major depression (15%). This finding of an increased frequency of psychiatric disturbance in cancer patients with pain has been reported by others, including Ahles et al and Woodforde.[2,20]

Cancer patients with advanced disease are a particularly vulnerable group.[3,5,11] The incidences of pain, depression, and delirium all increase in association with higher levels of physical debilitation and advanced illness.[13,21,22] Approximately 25% of all cancer patients experience severe depressive symptoms, the prevalence of which increases to 77% in individuals with advanced illness.[21] The prevalence of organic mental disorders (delirium) among cancer patients requiring psychiatric consultation independent of stage of disease has been found to range from 25% to 40%, and to as high as 85% during the terminal stages of illness.[22] The administration of narcotic analgesics is known to contribute to confusional states, particularly in elderly and terminally ill patients.[4,23]

Epidural spinal cord compression (ESCC) (see Chapter 29) is a common neurologic complication of systemic cancer that occurs in 5%–10% of patients, and results in severe pain. These patients are routinely treated with a combination of high-dose dexamethasone and radiotherapy. Patients who receive tapering high-dose regimens of steroids are exposed to as much as 96 mg a day of dexamethasone for up to a week, and generally continue on a tapering course for up to 3 or 4 weeks. Stiefel et al[24] recently described the spectrum of psychiatric complications seen in cancer patients undergoing such treatment for epidural spinal cord compression. Twenty-two percent of patients with ESCC were diagnosed with a

Table 14–1.
Incidence of DSM-III Psychiatric Disorders and Prevalence of Pain Observed in 215 Cancer Patients from Three Cancer Centers*

Diagnostic Category	Number in Diagnostic Class	Percent of Psychiatric Diagnosis	Number with Significant Pain†
Adjustment disorders	69 (32%)	68%	
Major affective disorders	13 (6%)	13%	
Organic mental disorders	8 (4%)	8%	
Personality disorders	7 (3%)	7%	
Anxiety disorders	4 (2%)	4%	
Total w/psychiatric Dx	101 (47%)		39 (39%)
Total w/no psychiatric Dx	114 (53%)		21 (19%)
Total patient population	215 (100%)		60 (28%)

* Adapted from Deragotis LR, et al: The prevalence of psychiatric disorders among cancer patients. JAMA 1983;249:754.
† Score greater than 50 mm on a 100 mm VAS for pain severity

major depressive syndrome, as compared to 4% in the comparison group. Also, delirium was much more common in the dexamethasone-treated patients than the comparison group (24% vs. 10%).

ASSESSMENT ISSUES

INADEQUATE PAIN CONTROL

Psychiatric symptoms in cancer pain patients initially are best viewed as a consequence of uncontrolled pain. Personality factors may be quite distorted by the presence of pain, and relief of pain often results in the resolution of a perceived psychiatric disorder.[2,3,19] Often, the psychiatrist is the very last physician to consult on a cancer patient with pain, and in that role may represent the patient's final opportunity for a comprehensive pain diagnosis and optimal medical analgesic management. Inadequate management of cancer pain is often due to the failure of clinicians to properly assess pain in all its dimensions.[3,13,25,26] All too frequently, psychological variables are

proposed to explain continued pain or lack of response to therapy, when in fact medical factors have not been addressed adequately. The causes of inadequate cancer pain management (see Chapters 6–9, 12) include: 1) failure to assess pain thoroughly; 2) lack of knowledge of current therapeutic approaches; 3) focus on prolonging life and providing cure versus alleviating suffering; 4) inadequacy of the physician–patient relationship; 5) limited expectations of patients and physicians; 6) unavailability of narcotics; 7) fear of respiratory depression; and, most important, 8) fear of addiction.

ADDICTION

Fear of addiction (see Chapters 8, 9, and 12) adversely affects both patient compliance and prescribing of narcotic analgesics, leading to the undermedication of patients with cancer pain.[25,26] Studies of patterns of the use of chronic narcotic analgesic in patients with cancer have demonstrated that whereas tolerance and physical dependence occur with relative frequency, addiction (psychological dependence) is exceedingly rare, and almost never occurs in the absence of a history of drug abuse before the cancer illness. Escalation of narcotic analgesic use by cancer patients is usually due to progression of cancer or the development of tolerance.[8] For further information on the distinctions among tolerance, physical dependence, and addiction, the reader is referred to Chapters 8, 9, and 12.

TREATING PSYCHIATRIC COMPLICATIONS

It is imperative that the patient be reassessed after pain has been controlled sufficiently to allow determination of whether a psychiatric disorder is indeed present. Psychiatric complications of cancer cause increased morbidity and mortality, and their treatment is essential for maintenance of an optimal quality of life. Interventions that help diminish mood disturbance in patients with cancer pain also help reduce pain. Our preferred method of treating psychiatric complications of cancer involves a multimodal approach using psychotherapeutic, behavioral, and psychopharmacologic interventions in combination. Treatment decisions are predicated on the assumption that a thorough medical and psychiatric assessment has led to an accurate diagnosis, thus facilitating specific and effective intervention. The management of specific psychiatric disorders such as depression, delirium, and anxiety in cancer patients (including those with pain) has been reviewed in detail by Holland, Massie, and Breitbart.[1,4,5,27,28] A brief guide to the diagnosis and management of these disorders is presented below.

DEPRESSION IN CANCER PAIN PATIENTS

The incidence of depression in cancer patients ranges from 20%–25%, and increases in correlation with levels of disability, advanced illness, and pain.[21,28,29] Certain types of cancer

are associated with an increased incidence of depression; for example, patients with pancreatic cancer are more likely to develop depression than are patients with other types of intra-abdominal malignancy.[30] The somatic symptoms of depression (*eg*, anorexia, insomnia, fatigue, and weight loss), especially when considered in isolation, are unreliable markers of depression in patients with cancer, because these symptoms are common sequelae of systemic cancer.[31] Thus, the psychological symptoms of depression (dysphoric mood, feelings of hopelessness, worthlessness, guilt, and suicidal ideation) take on greater diagnostic value in these patients.[21,28–31] A family history of depression or of previous depressive episodes further suggests the reliability of a diagnosis of depression. Coexisting organic factors related to the cancer or its therapy, such as treatment with corticosteroids,[24] chemotherapeutic agents[32–35] (vincristine, vinblastine, asparaginase, intrathecal methotrexate, interferon, interleukin), amphotericin,[36] whole-brain radiation,[37] or the presence of central nervous system metabolic–endocrine complications,[38] and paraneoplastic syndromes,[39,40] may be responsible for depression, and a thorough assessment of these factors must precede initiation of treatment.

TREATMENT OF DEPRESSION

Depressed cancer patients usually are treated with a combination of supportive psychotherapy, cognitive–behavioral techniques (see Chapter 5), and antidepressant medications.[28] Psychotherapy and cognitive–behavioral techniques specifically aimed at helping to control pain are discussed later in this chapter, in the section on psychologic interventions for cancer pain. Many of these same techniques are useful in the management of psychological distress in cancer patients, and have been applied to the treatment of depressive and anxiety symptoms related to cancer and cancer pain. Psychotherapeutic interventions, either in the form of individual or group counseling, have been shown effectively to reduce psychological distress and depressive symptoms in cancer patients.[41–43] Cognitive–behavioral interventions, such as relaxation and distraction with pleasant imagery, have also been shown to decrease depressive symptoms in patients with mild to moderate levels of depression.[44] Psychopharmacologic interventions (ie, antidepressant medications), however, are the mainstay of management for cancer patients who meet criteria for major depression.[28] The efficacy of antidepressants in the treatment of depression in cancer patients has been well established.[45–48] Our clinical experience at Memorial Sloan-Kettering Cancer Center supports the use of antidepressants in depressed cancer patients with or without pain.[4,5,28] Antidepressant medications used in cancer patients are listed in Table 14–2.

Tricyclic Antidepressants

The tricyclic antidepressants (TCAs) are the antidepressants most frequently prescribed in the setting of cancer. Treatment is initiated in low doses (10 to 25 mg at bedtime), especially in debilitated or elderly patients, and the dose is increased slowly by 10 to 25 mg every 1 to 2 days until a beneficial effect is achieved. Depressed cancer patients often have a therapeutic response at much lower doses (25 to 125 mg orally) than are usually required in patients who are in good physical condition (150 to 300 mg daily).[28] The choice of a TCA depends on side effect profiles, coexisting medical problems, the nature of the depressive symptoms, and the patient's prior experience with specific antidepressants. Tricyclic antidepressants with prominent sedative side effects like amitriptyline or doxepin are preferentially prescribed for the agitated, depressed patient with insomnia. Desipramine or nortriptyline are relatively nonanticholinergic, and as such are particularly useful to avoid exacerbating urinary retention, decreased intestinal motility, or stomatitis. Patients receiving multiple drugs with anticholinergic properties (eg, meperidine, atropine, diphenhydramine, phenothiazines) are at risk for developing an anticholinergic delirium, and as a result TCAs with potent anticholiner-

gic properties should be avoided in these patients. Amitriptyline, imipramine, and doxepin can be administered intramuscularly in patients whose condition precludes the reliable use of the oral route. Alternatively, rectal suppositories containing amitriptyline or other TCAs can also be formulated and used. Although not approved for use in the United States, TCAs such as amitriptyline have been safely administered intravenously as a slow infusion.[4,28]

Second-Generation Antidepressants

If a patient does not respond to a TCA, or is unable to tolerate their associated side effects, a second-generation (bupropion, trazodone, fluoxetine) or a heterocyclic (maprotiline, amoxapine) antidepressant can be prescribed. The second-generation antidepressants are generally considered to be less cardiotoxic than the TCAs.[49] Trazodone is relatively sedating, and in low doses (50–100 mg nightly) is a good choice in the treatment of the depressed cancer patient with insomnia. Trazodone is highly serotonergic, and its use should be considered when an adjuvant analgesic effect is required in addition to antidepressant effects. Trazodone has been associated with priapism, and should therefore be used with caution in male patients.[50] Fluoxetine, an even more highly serotonergic drug, is a selective inhibitor of neuronal serotonin uptake, and has fewer sedative and autonomic effects than the TCAs.[51] Its most common side effects are mild nausea and a brief period of increased anxiety. Fluoxetine can cause appetite suppression that usually endures for a period of several weeks, making it a good choice for overweight patients. Some of our patients have experienced transient weight loss, but weight usually returns to baseline levels, and its anorectic properties have not been a limiting factor in our use of this drug in cancer patients. In general, the side effect profile of fluoxetine may make it a more favorable treatment for depressed, medically ill patients in whom further sedation is undesirable. Bupropion has only recently been released in the United States, and as such, experience with

Table 14–2.
Antidepressant Medications Used in Cancer Pain Patients*

Drug	Therapeutic Daily Dosage PO (mg)
Tricyclic Antidepressants	
Amitriptyline	25–125
Doxepin	25–125
Imipramine	25–125
Desipramine	25–125
Nortriptyline	25–125
Clomipramine	25–125
Second-Generation Antidepressants	
Bupropion	200–450
Fluoxetine	20
Trazodone	150–300
Heterocyclic Antidepressants	
Maprotiline	50–75
Amoxapine	100–150
Monoamine Oxidase Inhibitors	
Isocarboxazid	20–40
Phenelzine	30–60
Tranylcypromine	20–40
Psychostimulants	
Dextroamphetamine	5–30
Methylphenidate	5–30
Pemoline	37.5–150
Benzodiazepines	
Alprazolam	0.75–6.00
Lithium carbonate	600–1200

* Adapted from Massie MJ, Holland JC: Depression and the cancer patient. J Clin Psychiatry 1990;51:12.

its use in patients with coexisting medical illness is limited. At present, while it is not the first drug of choice for depressed patients with cancer, we consider prescribing bupropion if patients have had a poor response to reasonably thorough trials of other antidepressants. Bupropion may be somewhat activating in medically ill patients. Its use should be avoided in patients with seizure disorders, brain tumors, and malnutrition.[52]

Heterocyclic Antidepressants

The side effect profiles of the heterocyclic antidepressants are similar to those of the TCAs. Maprotiline should be avoided in patients with brain tumors and in individuals who are at risk for seizures because of an association with an increased incidence of seizures.[53] Amoxapine has mild dopamine-blocking activity, and as a result patients taking other dopamine antagonists (*eg*, antiemetics) are at increased risk for developing extrapyramidal symptoms and dyskinesias.[54] Mianserin (not yet available in the United States) is a serotonergic antidepressant with adjuvant analgesic properties that is widely used in Europe and Latin America. Costa and colleagues[48] have demonstrated that mianserin is a safe and effective drug for the treatment of depression in patients with cancer.

Psychostimulants

The psychostimulants, (dextroamphetamine, methylphenidate, and pemoline) have been shown to be effective antidepressants in cancer patients and other medically ill populations.[55–59] These agents are most helpful in the treatment of depression in cancer patients with advanced disease, and in those individuals in whom dysphoric mood is associated with severe psychomotor slowing and even mild cognitive impairment. Psychostimulants have been shown to improve attention, concentration, and overall performance on neuropsychological testing in the medically ill.[60] In relatively low doses, psychostimulants stimulate appetite, promote an improved sense of well-being, and reduce feelings of weakness and fatigue in cancer patients. Treatment usually begins with doses of dextroamphetamine (2.5–5.0 mg) or methylphenidate (10 mg) administered at 8:00 AM and at noon. The dosage is slowly increased over several days until either the desired effect is achieved or side effects (overstimulation, anxiety, insomnia, paranoia, confusion) intervene. Typically, doses greater than 30 mg per day are not necessary, although occasionally patients require up to 60 mg per day. Patients usually are maintained on methylphenidate for 1 to 2 months, after which the drug can be withdrawn in approximately two-thirds of patients without a recurrence of depressive symptoms. When symptoms recur, patients can be maintained on a psychostimulant for up to 1 year without significant abuse problems. Tolerance will develop, and dose adjustments may be necessary. An additional benefit of such stimulants as methylphenidate and dextroamphetamine is that they have been shown to reduce sedation secondary to opioid analgesics, and to provide adjuvant analgesia.[61]

Pemoline is a unique psychostimulant that is chemically unrelated to amphetamine, and is a less potent stimulant with little abuse potential.[59] The advantages of pemoline as a psychostimulant in cancer patients include its lack of potential for abuse, and an absence of strict regulatory restrictions, its mild sympathomimetic effects. Also, it is available in a chewable tablet form that can be absorbed through the buccal mucosa, which is beneficial in patients with gastrointestinal dysfunction. In our clinical experience, pemoline is as effective as methylphenidate or dextroamphetamine in the treatment of depressive symptoms in cancer patients. Treatment with pemoline can be initiated at a dose of 18.75 mg in the morning and at noon, and increased gradually over days. Typically, patients require daily doses of 75 mg or less. Pemoline should be used with caution in patients with liver impairment, and periodic monitoring of liver function tests is recommended with longer-term treatment.[62]

Monoamine Oxidase Inhibitors

The monoamine oxidase inhibitors (MAOI) should be used only cautiously in patients with cancer. Traditional restrictions on tyramine-containing foods may be poorly accepted by cancer patients who are already subject to dietary and nutritional restrictions based on their disease. Extreme caution is indicated when considering their co-administration with the opioids, a combination that has resulted in severe myoclonus and delirium.[4] The concomitant administration of meperidine and an MAOI can lead to hyperpyrexia and cardiovascular collapse, and is absolutely contraindicated. Sympathomimetic drugs and other less obvious MAOIs, such as the chemotherapeutic agent procarbazine, can precipitate hypertensive crisis in patients taking an MAOI. If a patient has responded well to an MAOI for depression in the past, its continued use is warranted, but again with caution.

Lithium Carbonate

Patients who have been receiving lithium carbonate before a cancer illness should receive maintenance therapy throughout cancer treatment, although close monitoring is necessary in surgical patients during the perioperative period, when fluids and salt may be restricted or administered intravenously. Maintenance doses of lithium may need to be reduced in seriously ill patients. Lithium should be prescribed only cautiously in patients receiving cis-platinum because both drugs are potentially nephrotoxic. Several authors have reported possible beneficial effects on white cell counts, apparently associated with the administration of lithium to neutropenic cancer patients; however, the functional capabilities of these leukocytes have not been determined. This presumed bone marrow-stimulating effect appears to be transient; no mood changes have been noted in these patients.[63]

Benzodiazepines

The triazolobenzodiazepine alprazolam has been shown to be a mildly effective antidepressant as well as an anxiolytic. Alprazolam is particularly useful in cancer patients who have mixed symptoms of anxiety and depression. The starting dose is 0.25 mg three times a day, and effective doses are usually in the range of 4 to 6 mg daily.[44]

Electroconvulsive Therapy

Occasionally, it is necessary to consider electroconvulsive therapy (ECT) for depressed cancer patients who have depression with psychotic features, or in whom treatment with antidepressants poses unacceptable risks or side effects. The safe, effective use of ECT in the medically ill has been reviewed by others.[28]

ANXIETY IN CANCER PAIN PATIENTS

The types of anxiety observed in the setting of cancer are: 1) reactive anxiety related to the stresses of cancer and its treatment; 2) anxiety that is a manifestation of a medical or physiologic problem related to cancer (organic anxiety disorder); and 3) phobias, panic, and chronic anxiety disorders that predate the cancer diagnosis but are exacerbated during illness.[5,27]

REACTIVE ANXIETY

Most patients normally become anxious at critical moments during the work-up and treatment of cancer—while waiting to hear of diagnosis or possible recurrence, before procedures, diagnostic tests, surgery, or while awaiting test results. If, however, the anxiety is so great that it disturbs a patient's functioning or ability to understand or cooperate, the judicious prescription of anxiolytics such as alprazolam, oxazepam, or lorazepam may be beneficial. If levels of anxiety are relatively mild, and if there is sufficient time for the patient to learn a behavioral technique, relaxation and imagery exercises can be useful in reducing levels of distress (see Chapter 5).[44] The combined use of benzodiazepines and relaxation exercises has been a successful approach in our hands.

ORGANIC ANXIETY

Patients in acute pain and those with acute or chronic respiratory distress usually appear anxious. Anxiety that accompanies acute pain is best treated with analgesics; anxiety that accompanies severe respiratory distress is usually relieved by oxygen and the judicious use of mild sedation or morphine. Many patients on corticosteroids have insomnia and symptoms of anxiety, which vary from mild to severe in intensity. Since it is undesirable to discontinue steroids when they are prescribed as part of cancer therapy, a benzodiazepine or low-dose antipsychotic agent may be prescribed to relieve symptoms of anxiety that occur in this setting.[24] Patients who are developing an encephalopathy (delirium) or who are in early stages of dementia can also appear restless or anxious. Symptoms of anxiety are also features of withdrawal from narcotics, alcohol, benzodiazepines, and barbiturates. Since patients who abuse alcohol usually inaccurately report alcohol intake before admission, the diagnosis of alcohol withdrawal should be considered in all patients who develop otherwise unexplained anxiety symptoms during the early days of hospitalization. Other medical conditions that may have anxiety as a prominent or presenting symptom include hyperthyroidism, pheochromocytoma, carcinoid, primary and metastatic brain tumor, and mitral valve prolapse.[27,38]

PHOBIAS AND PANIC

Occasionally, patients have their first episode of panic or phobia while in medical settings. At Memorial Sloan-Kettering Hospital, approximately 20% of patients developed anxiety or claustrophobia so severe that they could not complete a magnetic resonance imaging scan.[64] The presence of this particular type of anxiety disorder (*eg*, panic attack, needle phobia, or claustrophobia) can complicate treatment, and thus an early psychiatric consultation is recommended. The techniques available to treat these disorders include both long-term behavioral treatment (for phobias) and short-term pharmacologic approaches for both phobias and panic. If there is the luxury of time (days to weeks), and the patient is likely to encounter repeated stressful events (venipunctures, bone marrow aspirations), relaxation therapy and distraction techniques can help many patients gain additional control over their fears. Often, however, the urgency of procedures is too acute, and an approach that combines the use of a benzodiazepine (*eg*, alprazolam 0.25–1.0 mg orally) and the provision of emotional support help the phobic patient undergo necessary procedures.

Such combination drug and behavioral treatment often provides a successful result.

PHARMACOLOGIC TREATMENT OF ANXIETY SYMPTOMS AND DISORDERS

The most commonly used drugs for the treatment of anxiety are the benzodiazepines[5,27] (Table 14–3). Other medications that are helpful include buspirone, antipsychotics, antihistamines, beta-blockers, and antidepressants. There is no place in the treatment of anxiety for barbiturates because of their high addictive potential and lethality in overdose.

Benzodiazepines

When the benzodiazepines are indicated in medically unwell patients, those with shorter half-lives (*ie*, alprazolam, lorazepam, and oxazepam) are preferred, particularly when patients are receiving other medications with sedative properties. These are better tolerated by medically ill patients, and because drug accumulation is less, patients are less likely to become oversedated. The starting dose is determined by the severity of the anxiety, the patient's physical status (respiratory and hepatic impairment), and the concurrent use of other medications (antidepressants, analgesics, antiemetics). The dose schedule depends on the half-life of the drug; the shorter-acting benzodiazepines need to be given three to four times a day, whereas longer-acting diazepam can be used on a twice-daily schedule. Anxiolytics may be given on as needed and/ or prophylactic basis to patients who have anxiety just before procedures or on a chemotherapy treatment day. However, patients with chronic anxiety should be treated with anxiolytics on an around-the-clock schedule, just as a time-contingent dosing schedule is preferred for the management of chronic pain. The most common side effects of the benzodiazepines are drowsiness, confusion, and motor incoordination. Physicians must be aware of potentially synergistic effects when these agents are used with other

Table 14–3.
Commonly Prescribed Benzodiazepines in Cancer Pain Patients*

Drug	Approximate Dose Equivalent	Initial Dosage PO (mg)	Elimination Half-Life Drug Metabolites (hours)
Short-acting			
Alprazolam	0.5	0.25–0.5 tid	10–15
Oxazepam	10.0	10–15 tid	5–15
Lorazepam†	1.0	0.5–2.0 tid	10–20
Temazepam‡	15.0	15–30 qhs	10–15
Triazolam‡	0.25	0.125–0.25 qhs	
Intermediate-acting			
Chlordiazepoxide	10.0	10–25 tid	10–40
Long-acting			
Diazepam	5.0	5–10 bid	20–100
Chlorazepate	7.5	7.5–15	30–200 bid
Clonazepam	1.0	0.5 bid	

* Adapted from Massie MJ, Holland JC: The cancer patient with pain: Psychiatric complications and their management. Med Clin North Am 1987;71:243.
† Metabolized by oxidation
‡ Metabolized by conjugation

central nervous system (CNS) depressants. If these effects occur, the dose of the benzodiazepine should be reduced. If side effects persist, the anxiolytic should be discontinued, and a medication from another class should be started. Abrupt discontinuation of benzodiazepines can precipitate a serious withdrawal syndrome similar in character to alcohol withdrawal.

Midazolam (Versed; Roche Laboratories, Nutley, NJ) is an ultra-short-acting benzodiazepine that was developed as a premedicant and component of anesthesia for surgical patients. Its use has been extended to include the provision of sedation for adult and pediatric patients undergoing other stressful procedures such as endoscopy, bone marrow aspiration, and lumbar puncture. For these purposes, it is usually administered in small, successive intravenous increments under careful observation and respiratory monitoring. It has also gained rapid acceptance ad-

ministered as an intravenous infusion in critical care settings to provide sedation in the agitated or anxious patient on a respirator. It is available in an oral formulation in some locales outside the United States.

Clonazepam, a new, longer-acting benzodiazepine, has been found to be extremely useful in our setting for the treatment of symptoms of anxiety and depersonalization or derealization in patients with seizure disorders, brain tumors, and mild organic mental disorders. Patients who experience end-of-dose failure with recurrence of anxiety on shorter-acting drugs also find clonazepam helpful. It is not uncommon for us to substitute clonazepam for alprazolam when attempting to taper off alprazolam. Clonazepam is also useful in patients with organic mood disorders who have symptoms of mania, and as an adjuvant analgesic in patients with neuropathic pain.[65,66]

Nonbenzodiazepine Anxiolytics

Buspirone is a nonbenzodiazepine anxiolytic that is useful along with psychotherapy in patients with chronic anxiety or anxiety related to adjustment disorders. The onset of its anxiolytic action is delayed in comparison to that seen with the benzodiazepines. Five to 10 days of administration is often required before its beneficial effects on anxiety are manifested. Since buspirone is not a benzodiazepine, it will not interfere with benzodiazepine withdrawal reactions, and so one must be cautious when switching from a benzodiazepine to buspirone. The recommended dose of buspirone is 10 mg orally, three times daily.[67]

Antipsychotics such as thioridazine are useful in treating severe anxiety that is unresponsive to high doses of benzodiazepines, and in treating anxiety in patients with cognitive impairment (eg, encephalopathy or dementia) in whom benzodiazepines may worsen an organic mental syndrome. Thioridazine can be started at a low dose (10–20 mg orally two to three times per day), and increased, if necessary, up to 100 mg three times per day. Antihistamines are infrequently prescribed for anxiety because of their low efficacy; hydroxyzine can be useful for anxious patients with respiratory impairment in whom benzodiazepines are contraindicated. Acute panic is best treated with alprazolam or clonazepam. For maintenance treatment of panic disorders, the tricyclic antidepressant imipramine (used in doses comparable to those for the treatment of depression), alprazolam, clonazepam, and the monoamine oxidase inhibitors (eg, phenalzine) all have demonstrated antipanic effects. Propranolol can be a useful adjunct in blocking the physiologic manifestations of anxiety in patients with panic disorders.[5,27]

DELIRIUM
(ORGANIC MENTAL DISORDERS)

Delirium, the second most common psychiatric diagnosis among cancer patients, can be due either to the direct effects of cancer on the

Table 14–4.
Causes of Delirium in Cancer Pain Patients*

Direct
Primary brain tumor
Metastatic spread

Indirect
Metabolic encephalopathy due to organ failure
Electrolyte imbalance
Treatment side effects from
   Chemotherapeutic agents, steroids,
   Radiation
   Narcotics
   Anticholinergics
   Antiemetics
Infection
Hematologic abnormalities
Nutrition
Paraneoplastic syndromes

* Adapted from: Fleishman SB, Lesko LM: Delirium and dementia. In Holland J, Rowland J (eds): The Handbook of Psychooncology: Psychological Care of the Cancer Patient p 342. New York, Oxford Press, 1989.

CNS, or to indirect CNS effects of the disease or treatments (medications, electrolyte imbalance, failure of a vital organ or system, infection, vascular complications, and preexisting cognitive impairment or dementia) (Table 14–4). About 15%–20% of hospitalized cancer patients have organic mental disorders.[68,69]

Early symptoms of delirium can be misdiagnosed as anxiety, anger, depression, or psychosis. A diagnosis of delirium should be considered in any patient with an acute onset of agitation, impaired cognitive function, altered attention span, or a fluctuating level of consciousness.[70] A common error among medical and nursing staff is to conclude that a new psychological symptom is functional without excluding all possible organic etiologies. Given the large numbers of drugs taken by cancer patients and the fragile state of their physiologic functioning, even the routine administration of mild hypnotics is often sufficient to precipitate an episode of delirium. Narcotic analgesics such as levorphanol, morphine sulfate, and meperidine are common

Table 14–5.
Neuropsychiatric Side Effects of Chemotherapeutic
Drugs

Drug	Neuropsychiatric Symptoms
Methotrexate (intrathecal)	Delirium, dementia, lethargy, personality change
Vincristine, vinblastine	Delirium, hallucinations, lethargy, depression
Asparaginase	Delirium, hallucinations, lethargy, cognitive dysfunction
BCNU	Delirium, dementia
Bleomycin	Delirium
Fluorouracil	Delirium
Cis-platinum	Delirium
Hydroxyurea	Hallucinations
Procarbazine	Depression, mania, delirium, dementia
Cytosine arabinoside	Delerium, lethargy, cognitive dysfunction
Hexylmethylamine	Hallucinations
Isophosphamide	Delirium, lethargy, hallucinations
Prednisone	Depression, mania, delirium, psychoses
Interferon	Flu-like syndrome, delirium, hallucinations, depression
Interleukin	Cognitive dysfunction, hallucinations

causes of confusional states, particularly in elderly and terminally ill patients.[23] Chemotherapeutic agents known to cause delirium include methotrexate, fluorouracil, vincristine, vinblastine, bleomycin, BCNU, cis-platinum, asparaginase, procarbazine, and the glucocorticosteroids[24,32–36] (Table 14–5). Except for steroids, most patients receiving these agents will not develop prominent CNS effects.

The spectrum of mental disturbances related to steroid use includes minor mood lability, affective disorders (mania or depression), cognitive impairment (reversible dementia), and delirium (steroid psychosis). The incidence of these disorders ranges from 3%–57% in noncancer populations, and they occur most commonly on higher doses. Symptoms usually develop within the first 2 weeks of steroid administration, but in fact can occur at any time, on any dose, even during the tapering phase.[24] Prior psychiatric illness or prior mental disturbance on steroids is not a good predictor of susceptibility to, or the nature of, mental disturbance with steroids. These disorders are often rapidly reversible on dose reduction or discontinuation.[24]

MANAGEMENT OF DELIRIUM

It is often necessary to provide treatment for a patient's agitated or disturbed behavior while simultaneously trying to determine its cause. When agitation is severe or the patient is delusional or hallucinating, one-to-one nursing observation is indicated. Pharmacologic intervention is often indicated for the delirious patient. Patients with delirium with psychotic symptoms and agitation need a medication that is rapidly effective and easily administered. If the presenting symptoms include suspiciousness, with refusal to take medications by mouth, or poor compliance secondary to agitation, an antipsychotic agent should be administered parenterally.[70–72]

Antipsychotic drugs vary in their sedating properties and likelihood of producing orthostatic hypotension, neurologic side effects (acute dystonia, extrapyramidal symptoms), and anticholinergic effects. The acutely agitated cancer patient requires a medication with sedative properties; the patient with hypotension requires a drug with lesser effects on blood pressure; the delirious postoperative patient who has mechanical ileus or urine retention should receive an antipsychotic with the least anticholinergic effects. Haloperidol is the most commonly prescribed antipsychotic agent in our setting for patients with delirium, because of its useful sedating effects and low incidence of cardiovascular and anticholinergic effects. Haloperidol can be given orally in tablet or concentrate, or by intramuscular or intravenous injection. Peak plasma concentrations are achieved 2–4 hours after an oral dose, and measurable plasma concentrations occur 15–30 minutes after intramuscular ad-

ministration. Although not yet approved by
the Food and Drug Administration for intravenous use, haloperidol is commonly and
safely administered by this route for agitation.[71,72] In cancer patients, the initial dose of
haloperidol should be low (0.5 mg to 1.0 mg
orally, intramuscularly, or intravenously),
and the dose should be repeated frequently
(every 30 to 45 minutes) until symptom
control is achieved. A drawback to the use
of haloperidol is its tendency to produce
movement disorders. Acute dystonias and
extrapyramidal side effects generally can be
controlled by the co-administration of antipar-
kinsonian medications (*eg*, diphenhydramine, trihexyphenidyl); akathisia responds either to low doses of propranolol (*eg*, 5 mg two
to three times per day), lorazepam (0.5–1.0
mg two to three times per day), or antiparkin-
sonian medications (*eg*, benzotropine 1 to 2
mg once to twice per day). A rare but sometimes fatal complication of treatment with the
antipsychotics is the neuroleptic malignant
syndrome. Neuroleptic malignant syndrome
usually occurs after prolonged, high-dose administration of neuroleptics, and is characterized by hyperthermia, increased mental
confusion, leukocytosis, muscular rigidity,
myoglobinuria, and high serum creatine
phosphokinase. Treatment consists of discontinuing the neuroleptic and the use of dantrolene sodium (0.8–10 mg/kg/day) or bromo-
criptine mesylate (2.5–10 mg three times per
day).[72]

SUICIDE AND CANCER PAIN

Uncontrolled pain is a major factor in cancer
suicide.[73,74] Cancer is perceived by the public
as an extremely painful disease relative to
other medical conditions. In Wisconsin, a
study revealed that 69% of the public agreed
that cancer pain can become so intolerable
that a person might consider suicide.[7] The
vast majority of cancer suicides had severe
pain that often was inadequately controlled
and had been poorly tolerated.[75] Although relatively few cancer patients commit suicide,
studies suggest that this population is at in-

Table 14–6.
Cancer Pain Suicide Vulnerability Factors

Pain; suffering aspects
Advanced illness; poor prognosis
Depression; hopelessness
Delirium; disinhibition
Control; helplessness
Preexisting psychopathology
Suicide history; family history

creased risk.[76] Suicidal thinking seems to occur quite frequently, however, especially in
individuals with advanced cancer.[73] Suicide is
often held as an option by the patient in order
to retain a sense of control. Patients with advanced illness are at highest risk, and are most
likely to have the complications of pain, depression, delirium, and symptoms of other
deficits.[74] Psychiatric disorders are frequently
present in hospitalized cancer patients who
are suicidal. A recent review of our consultation data at Memorial showed that one-third
of suicidal cancer patients had a major depression, about 20% had delirium, and over 50%
had an adjustment disorder.[74]

MANAGEMENT

The cancer suicide vulnerability factors (Table
14–6) should be used as a guide to the evaluation and management of suicidal patients.
Early psychiatric involvement with high-risk
individuals can often avert suicide in the cancer setting. Once the setting has been made
secure, assessment of relevant mental status
and the adequacy of pain control can be initiated. Analgesics, neuroleptics, or antidepressant drugs should be used when appropriate
to help manage agitation, psychosis, depression, or pain. A crisis intervention-oriented
psychotherapeutic approach, that mobilizes
the patient's support system, is an important
element of therapy. Although it is appropriate
to intervene when medical or psychiatric factors are clearly the driving force in a suicidal

cancer patient, there are circumstances in which overly aggressive intervention may be less helpful. This is most evident in those patients with advanced illness, for whom comfort and symptom control are the primary concerns. The goal of intervention should be to establish rapport, to develop an alliance, and to provide effective management of poorly controlled symptoms as an alternative to suicide.

ANTICIPATORY NAUSEA AND VOMITING RELATED TO CHEMOTHERAPY

During the course of chemotherapy, many patients become sensitized to treatment, develop phobic-like reactions, and even develop conditioned responses to stimuli in the hospital setting. As a result of being conditioned by the experience of profound nausea and vomiting secondary to highly emetic chemotherapy agents, patients report being nauseated in anticipation of treatment. A conservative estimate of the prevalence and anticipatory nausea and vomiting (ANV) is at least 33%.[77] The factors that increase the likelihood of developing ANV are as follows: 1) severity of post-treatment nausea and vomiting (high intensity, duration, and frequency); 2) a pattern of increasing nausea and vomiting; and 3) the administration of highly emetic drugs (*cis*-platinum) or combination chemotherapy.[78]

TREATMENT OF ANTICIPATORY NAUSEA AND VOMITING

Pharmacologic

Given the relationship between the intensity of postchemotherapy nausea and vomiting and the development of ANV, the efficacy of antiemetic regimens in the management of these symptoms is exceedingly important. The most effective preventative regimens currently combine several agents such as metoclopramide, steroids, and lorazepam. These

drugs are given a few hours before chemotherapy, and their administration is continued by intravenous infusion up to 36 hours after the completion of chemotherapy. Parenteral lorazepam reduces vomiting and produces mild amnesia for the vomiting episodes. Metoclopramide is a dopamine antagonist, and can induce extrapyramidal side effects that are reversible with treatment. There is only one reported case of tardive dyskinesia secondary to intravenous metoclopramide used as part of an antiemetic regimen.[79]

Rapid-onset, short-acting benzodiazepines are helpful in controlling ANV once it has developed. Alprazolam has been demonstrated to be clinically effective in reducing ANV in doses of 0.25 to 0.5 mg three or four times daily, given orally for 1 to 2 days before chemotherapy.[80]

Behavioral Treatment

Behavioral control of ANC, although time-intensive, has proven to be highly effective.[81,82] The techniques that have been studied include 1) relaxation training with guided imagery, 2) video game distraction (in children), and 3) systemic desensitization. It is unclear whether muscular relaxation or cognitive–attentional distraction is the key element in the efficacy of these techniques. These techniques can be administered effectively by specially trained chemotherapy nurses, often with remarkable improvement in the quality of life for chemotherapy patients.

PSYCHOLOGICAL INTERVENTIONS FOR CANCER PAIN

Optimal management of cancer pain is multimodal and may require pharmacologic, psychotherapeutic, cognitive–behavioral, anesthetic, stimulatory, and rehabilitative approaches, often in combination. Psychiatric and psychological participation in cancer pain management (see Chapter 5) involves the use of psychotherapeutic, cognitive–behavioral, and psychopharmacologic interventions.

Table 14–7.
Psychotherapy and Cancer Pain

Goals	Form
Support—provide continuity	**Individuals**—supportive/crisis intervention
Knowledge—provide information	**Family**—patient and family are the unit of concern
Skills—relaxation, cognitive coping, use of analgesics, communication	**Group**—share experiences, identify successful coping strategies

PSYCHOTHERAPY AND CANCER PAIN

The goals of psychotherapy with cancer pain patients (Table 14–7) are to provide support, knowledge, and skills. Using short-term supportive psychotherapy based on a crisis intervention model, the therapist provides emotional support, continuity, and information, and assists in adaptation to crisis. The therapist has a role in emphasizing past strengths, supporting previously successful coping strategies, and teaching new coping skills such as relaxation, cognitive coping, proper use of analgesics, self-observation, documentation, assertiveness, and communication skills. Communication skills are of paramount importance for both patient and family, particularly around issues related to pain and analgesic use. The patient and family are the unit of concern, and need a more general, long-term, supportive relationship within the health care system, in addition to specific psychological approaches to dealing with pain, that can be provided by a psychiatrist, psychologist, social worker, or nurse. Although psychotherapy in the cancer pain setting is primarily non-analytical and focuses on current issues, exploration of reactions to cancer often involve insights into earlier, more pervasive life issues. Occasionally, patients choose to continue a more exploratory mode of psychotherapy during survivorship. Group interventions with individual patients, spouses, couples, and families are a powerful means of sharing experiences and identifying successful coping strategies. Using psychotherapy to diminish symptoms of anxiety and depression, and to identify factors that can intensify pain empirically, has beneficial effects on the experience of cancer pain. In a controlled, randomized, prospective study, Spiegel and Bloom[83,84] demonstrated the beneficial effect in general of supportive group therapy for patients with metastatic breast cancer, and, in particular, the beneficial effect of hypnotic pain control exercises. Their support group focused not on interpersonal processes or self-exploration, but rather on a series of themes related to the practical and existential problems of living with cancer. Patients were divided into two groups, a treatment group and a control group. The treatment patients experienced significantly less pain than the control patients. Those in the treatment group who were taught a self-hypnosis exercise for pain experienced a slight increase, while the control group experienced a large increase in pain.

COGNITIVE–BEHAVIORAL TECHNIQUES

Cognitive–behavioral techniques that are potentially useful in cancer pain (Table 14–8) include passive relaxation with mental imagery, cognitive distraction or focusing techniques, progressive muscle relaxation, biofeedback, hypnosis (see Chapter 5), and music therapy.[85–87] The goal of such interventions is to guide the patient toward a sense of enhanced control over pain. Whereas some techniques are primarily cognitive in nature, focusing on perceptual and thought pro-

Table 14—8.
Cognitive–Behavioral Techniques Used by Cancer Pain Patients

Psychoeducation
  Preparatory information
  Self-monitoring

Relaxation
  Passive breathing
  Progressive muscle relaxation

Distraction
  Focusing
  Controlled mental imagery
  Cognitive distraction
  Behavioral distraction

Combined Techniques (relaxation and distraction)
  Passive/progressive relaxation with mental imagery
  Systematic desensitization
  Meditation
  Hypnosis
  Biofeedback
  Music therapy

Cognitive therapies
  Cognitive distortion
  Cognitive restructuring

Behavioral therapies
  Modeling
  Graded task management
  Contingency management
  Behavioral rehearsal

cesses, others are directed at modulating patterns of behavior to help cancer patients cope with pain. Cancer patients are highly motivated to learn and practice these methods, since they are often effective not only in symptom control, but in restoring a sense of self-control, personal efficacy, and active participation in their care. Importantly, these techniques must not be used as a substitute for the appropriate management of cancer pain with analgesics, but rather as part of a comprehensive multimodal approach. The lack of side effects of these techniques makes them attractive in the oncology setting as a supplement to already complicated medication regimens. The successful use of these techniques should never lead to the erroneous conclusion that the pain was of psychogenic origin, and as such was not "real." The mechanisms by which these cognitive and behavioral techniques relieve pain are unclear; however, they all seem to share elements of relaxation and distraction. Distraction or redirection of attention helps reduce awareness of pain, whereas relaxation reduces muscle tension and sympathetic arousal.[86] Most cancer patients with pain are appropriate candidates for the application of these techniques; however, the clinician should take into account the intensity of pain and the mental clarity of the patient. Ideal candidates have mild to moderate pain, whereas patients with severe pain can expect only limited benefit from psychologic interventions, unless somatic therapies can lower the level of pain to a more manageable level. Confusional states interfere dramatically with a patient's ability to focus attention, and so limit the usefulness of these techniques.[88]

BEHAVIORAL TECHNIQUES

These include methods of modifying physiologic pain reactions, respondent pain behaviors, and apparent pain behaviors. The most fundamental technique is self-monitoring. The development of the ability to monitor his or her behaviors allows a person to notice dysfunctional reactions and to learn to control them. Systematic desensitization is useful in extinguishing anticipatory anxiety that leads to avoidant behaviors, and is helpful in remobilizing inactive patients. Graded task assignment is essentially systematic desensitization applied to patients by encouraging them to take small steps gradually so as to perform activities more readily. Contingency management is a method of reinforcing well behaviors only, thus modifying dysfunctional operant pain behaviors associated with secondary gain.[85–87]

COGNITIVE TECHNIQUES

A variety of cognitive techniques for coping with pain are aimed at increasing relaxation and reducing intensity and distress qualities of the pain experience. Cognitive modification is an approach derived from cognitive therapy for depression or anxiety, and is based on how one interprets events and bodily sensation. It is assumed that patients have dysfunctional automatic thoughts about pain that are consistent with underlying assumptions and beliefs. Identifying dysfunctional automatic thoughts and pervasive underlying beliefs can allow for a more rational salutary response, thus allowing for restructuring or modification of thought processes or cognition.[85]

RELAXATION–IMAGERY

These encompass a variety of techniques that are designed to achieve a mental and physical state of relaxation. Muscular tension, autonomic arousal, and mental distress exacerbate pain.[85–87] Some specific relaxation techniques include: 1) passive relaxation, which focuses attention on sensations of warmth and decreased tension in various parts of the body; 2) progressive muscle relaxation, involving active tensing and relaxing of muscles; and 3) meditation. Other techniques that use both relaxation and cognitive methods include hypnosis, biofeedback, and music therapy (see below).

Clinically, relaxation techniques are most helpful in managing pain when they are combined with some distracting or pleasant imagery. The use of distraction or focusing involves control over the focus of attention. One can use imaginative inattention by picturing oneself on a beach, for example. Mental distraction can be used in a manner that is similar to the practice of counting sheep in order to aid sleep. Keeping oneself busy is a form of behavioral distraction. Imagery (*ie*, using one's imagination while in a relaxed state) can be used in an effort to transform pain into a warm or cold sensation. One can also imaginatively transform the context of pain (*eg*, imagine oneself in battle on the football field instead of the hospital bed). Dissociated somatization can be used by some patients, wherein they imagine that a painful body part is no longer part of their body.[85] It is important to note that not every patient finds these techniques acceptable, and that often the therapist must try out a number of approaches to select measures that are most consistent with the patient's style.

HYPNOSIS

Hypnosis has been shown to be efficacious in the treatment of cancer pain.[84,88–90] The hypnotic trance is essentially a state of heightened and focused concentration that can be used to manipulate the perception of pain. The depth of hypnotizability may determine the effectiveness as well as the strategies used during hypnosis. One-third of cancer patients are not hypnotizable, and for these patients it is recommended that other techniques be used. Of the two-thirds of patients who are identified as being low, moderately, and highly hypnotizable, three principles underlie the use of hypnosis in controlling pain: 1) the use of self-hypnosis; 2) relaxation, encouraging the patient not to fight the pain; and 3) the use of a mental filter to ease the hurt in pain. Patients who are highly or moderately hypnotizable can often alter sensations in a painful area by changing temperature sensation or substituting a sensation of tingling. Moderately hypnotizable individuals can alter sensation in a painful area by changing temperature sensation or experiencing tingling. Less hypnotizable patients can often use an alternative focus by concentrating on a sensation in a nonaffected body part or a mental image of a pleasant scene.

BIOFEEDBACK

Fotopoulous et al[91] noted significant pain relief in a group of cancer patients who were taught electromyographic (EMG) and electroencephalographic biofeedback-assisted relaxation. Only 2 of 17 patients were able to maintain analgesia after the treatment ended. A lack of generalization of effect can be a problem with biofeedback techniques. Although physical condition, especially for the terminally ill, may make a prolonged training period impossible, most cancer patients can use EMG and temperature biofeedback techniques for learning relaxation-assisted pain control.[86]

MUSIC THERAPY

Munro and Mount have written extensively on the use of music therapy with cancer patients, documenting clinical examples and suggesting mechanisms of action.[92] Music can often capture the focus of attention in a manner unlike other stimuli, and helps patients distract their perception of pain while permitting meaningful self-expression.

PSYCHOTROPIC ADJUVANT ANALGESIC DRUGS

The cancer patient with pain may gain a great deal from the appropriate use of psychotropic drugs, not only because they are more likely to develop depressive or anxious disorders than their counterparts without pain, but because some of these drugs have unique adjuvant analgesic properties (see Chapter 10). Psychiatrists often are the most experienced in the clinical use of these drugs (Table 14–9), and so can play an important role in assisting pain control.

Antidepressants

The current literature supports the use of tricyclic antidepressants in the treatment of a wide variety of chronic pain syndromes, including cancer pain (see Chapter 10).[93–97] The antidepressants are effective as adjuvants in cancer pain through a number of putative mechanisms that include antidepressant effects, potent direct analgesic effects, and the

potentiation or enhancement of opioid analgesia. The tricyclic antidepressants imipramine, amitriptyline, doxepin, and clomipramine have effects on a number of neurotransmitters and their receptors; however, it is believed that their activity as potent serotonergic agents (blockers of serotonin reuptake) is the mechanism that mediates their analgesic properties.[98] Other possible mechanisms of the analgesic actions of the antidepressants include catecholamine effects, adrenergic and serotonin receptor effects, adenosinergic effects, an antihistamine effect, anticholinergic effects, and direct neuronal effects such as inhibition of paroxysmal neuronal discharge and decreased sensitivity of adrenergic receptors of injured nerve sprouts.[66] In a placebo-controlled, double-blind study of imipramine in chronic cancer pain, Walsh demonstrated that imipramine had analgesic effects independent of its effects on mood, and was a potent co-analgesic when used along with morphine.[99]

The heterocyclic and noncyclic drugs such as trazodone, mianserin, and fluoxetine are also useful adjuvant analgesic agents.[48,66,93,100] Mianserin is not available in the United States, but is widely available elsewhere, and is a potent serotonin reuptake blocker that is associated with few adverse side effects, thus making it an attractive choice as an antidepressant or adjuvant analgesic in the medically ill.[48] Fluoxetine has rather specific activity as a serotonin reuptake inhibitor, with few other neurotransmitter or receptor effects. A potent antidepressant, it has been shown to have analgesic properties, and may be useful in the treatment of neuropathic pain, although further research is indicated.[100] Trazodone has similar antidepressant, serotonergic, and analgesic properties. The antidepressants most commonly used in clinical studies on the management of cancer pain include amitriptyline, imipramine, clomipramine, trazodone, and doxepin.[96,97,99] There is no clear indication that any particular antidepressant is more effective than the others, although perhaps the most experience has been accrued with amitriptyline.

Treatment should be initiated with a small

Table 14–9.
Psychotropic Adjuvant Analgesic Drugs for Cancer Pain

Generic Name	Trade Name	Approximate Daily Dosage Range (mg)	Route
Tricyclic antidepressants			
Amitriptyline	Elavil	10–150	PO,IM,PR
Imipramine	Tofranil	12.5–150	PO,IM
Clomipramine	Anafranil	10–150	PO
Doxepin	Sinequan	12.5–150	PO,IM
Noncyclic antidepressants			
Trazodone	Desyrel	25–300	PO
Fluoxetine	Prozac	20–60	PO
Amine precursors			
L-Tryptophan		500–3,000	PO
Psychostimulants			
Methylphenidate	Ritalin	2.5–20 bid	PO
Dextroamphetamine	Dexedrine	2.5–20 bid	PO
Phenothiazines			
Fluphenazine	Prolixin	1–3	PO,IM
Methotrimeprazine	Levoprome	10–20 q6h	IM,IV
Butyrophenones			
Haloperidol	Haldol	1–3	PO,IM,IV
Pimozide	Orap	2–6 bid	PO
Antihistamines			
Hydroxyzine	Vistaril	50 q4–6h	PO,IM,IV
Steroids			
Dexamethasone	Decadron	4–16	PO,IV
Benzodiazepines			
Alprazolam	Xanax	0.25–2.0 mg tid	PO
Clonazepam	Klonopin	0.5–4 bid	PO

Key: PO, per oral; IM, intramuscular; PR, parenteral; IV, intravenous; q6h, every 6 hours; q4–6h, every 4 to 6 hours; tid, three times a day; bid, two times a day.

dose of, for example, amitriptyline, such as 10 to 25 mg at bedtime, especially in debilitated patients, with dosages increased slowly by 10 to 25 mg every 2 to 4 days toward 150 mg, with frequent assessment of pain and side effects until a beneficial effect is achieved. Maximal effect as an adjuvant analgesic may require continuation of treatment for 2 to 6 weeks. Serum levels of antidepressant drug, when available, may also help in management to assure that significant amounts of drug are being absorbed. Both pain and depression in cancer patients often respond to lower doses (25–100 mg) of antidepressant than are usually required in the physically healthy (100–500 mg). The choice of drug depends on side effect profiles, coexisting medical problems, the nature of depressive symptoms if present, and past response to specific antidepressants. Sedating drugs like amitriptyline are helpful when insomnia complicates the presence of pain and depression. Anticholinergic properties of some of these drugs may be responsible for dose-limiting side effects, in which case a drug with less potent anticholinergic properties should be selected.

Tryptophan, a serotonin precursor, has been used for chronic pain in doses of 2 to 4 g. Nausea, however, is a common side effect with higher doses, thus limiting its usefulness in debilitated cancer patients. Monoamine oxidase inhibitors are also less useful in the setting of cancer because of dietary restrictions and potentially dangerous interactions with narcotics such as meperidine.

Psychostimulants

The psychostimulants (see Chapter 10) dextroamphetamine and methylphenidate are useful antidepressant agents prescribed selectively for medically ill cancer patients with depression.[55,57] Psychostimulants are also useful in diminishing excessive sedation secondary to opioid analgesics. Bruera et al demonstrated that a regimen of 10 mg methylphenidate with breakfast and 5 mg with lunch significantly decreased sedation and potentiated the analgesic effect of narcotics in patients with cancer pain.[61,101] Dextroamphetamine has been reported to have additive analgesic effects when used with morphine in postoperative pain.[102] A strategy we have found useful in treating cancer pain associated with depression is to start a psychostimulant (starting dose of 2.5 mg of methylphenidate at 8:00 AM and noon) and then add a tricyclic antidepressant after several days to help prolong and potentiate the short-term effects of the stimulant.

Neuroleptics

Methotrimeprazine (see Chapter 10 and Appendix C, Table 6) is a phenothiazine that is equianalgesic with morphine, but lacks the usually undesirable effects of the opioids on gut motility, and probably produces analgesia through alpha-adrenergic blockade.[103] In patients who are opioid-tolerant, it provides an alternative approach, providing analgesia by a nonopioid mechanism. It is a dopamine antagonist, and so has antiemetic as well anxiolytic effects. This drug can produce sedation and hypotension, and should be prescribed and administered cautiously. Other phenothiazines such as chlorpromazine and prochlorperazine are useful as antiemetics in cancer patients, but probably have limited efficacy as analgesics. Fluphenazine in combination with with tricyclic antidepressants has been shown to be helpful in patients with neuropathic pain. Haloperidol is the drug of choice in the management of delirium or psychoses in cancer patients, and has clinical usefulness as a co-analgesic for cancer pain. Pimozide (Orap; McNeil Pharmaceutical, Spring House, PA), a butyrophenone, has been shown to be effective as an analgesic in the management of trigeminal neuralgia, at doses of 4 to 12 mg per day.[104]

Anxiolytics

Hydroxyzine is a mild anxiolytic with sedating and analgesic properties that are useful in the anxious cancer patient with pain.[105] This antihistamine has antiemetic activity as well. One hundred milligrams of parenteral hydroxyzine has analgesic activity approaching 8 mg of morphine, and has additive analgesic effects when combined with morphine. Benzodiazepines, although potent anxiolytics, are not thought to possess specific analgesic properties, and in fact may have antianalgesic properties. Recently, Fernandez[106] showed that alprazolam, a unique benzodiazepine with mild antidepressant properties, was helpful as an adjuvant analgesic in cancer patients with phantom limb or deafferentation pain.

SUMMARY

Unfortunately, cancer patients with pain are most vulnerable to such psychiatric complications of cancer as depression, anxiety, and delirium. For the clinician who wants to provide comprehensive management of cancer pain, familiarity with psychiatric assessment and intervention, and knowledge of the indications and usefulness of psychotropic drugs will be most rewarding. Opioid analgesics are the mainstay of the pharmacologic interventions for cancer pain. There is, however, growing awareness that psychotropic drugs, in particular the antidepressants, are useful adjuvant analgesic agents in the management of cancer pain. In addition, many of these drugs are important in the treatment of psychiatric complications of cancer.

REFERENCES

1. Holland JC, Rowland J (eds): Handbook of Psychooncology: Psychological Care of the Patient With Cancer. New York, Oxford University Press, 1989.
2. Ahles TA, Blanchard EB, Ruckdeschel JC: The multidimensional nature of cancer related pain. Pain 1983;17:277.
3. Breitbart W: Psychiatric management of cancer pain. Cancer 1989;63:2336.
4. Breitbart W: Psychiatric complications of cancer. In Brain MC, Carbone PP (eds): Current Therapy in Hematology Oncology 3, p 268. Toronto, BC Decker, 1988.
5. Massie MJ, Holland JC: The cancer patient with pain: Psychiatric complications and their management. Med Clin North Am 1987;71:243.
6. Derogatis LR, Marrow GR, Fetting J et al: The prevalence of psychiatric disorders among cancer patients. JAMA 1983;249:751.
7. Levin DN, Cleeland CS, Dan R: Public attitudes toward cancer pain. Cancer 1985;56:2337.
8. Kanner RM, Foley KM: Patterns of narcotic use in a cancer pain clinic. Ann NY Acad Sci 1981;362:161.
9. Daut RL, Cleeland CS: The prevalence and severity of pain in cancer. Cancer 1982;50:1913.
10. Foley KM: Pain syndromes in patients with cancer. In Bonica JJ, Ventafridda V, Fink RB et al (eds): Advances in Pain Research and Therapy, vol 2, p 59. New York, Raven Press, 1979.
11. Twycross RG, Lack SA: Symptom Control in Far

Advanced Cancer: Pain Relief. London, Pitman Brooks, 1983.
12. Cleeland CS: The impact of pain on the patient with cancer. Cancer 1984;54:2635.
13. Foley KM: The treatment of cancer pain. N Engl J Med 1985;313:84.
14. Melzack R, Wall PD: The Challenge of Pain: New York, Basic Books, 1983.
15. IASP Subcommittee on Taxonomy Pain Terms: A list with definitions and notes on usage. Pain 1979;6:249.
16. Spiegel D, Bloom JR: Pain in metastatic breast cancer. Cancer 1983;52:341.
17. Bond MR: Psychological and emotional aspects of cancer pain. In Bonica JJ, Ventafridda V (eds): Advances in Pain Research and Therapy, vol 2, p 81. New York, Raven Press, 1979.
18. McKegney FP, Bailey CR, Yates JW: Prediction and management of pain in patients with advanced cancer. Gen Hosp Psychiatry 1981;3:95.
19. Bond MR, Pearson IB: Psychological aspects of pain in women with advanced cancer of the cervix. J Psychosom Res 1969;13:13.
20. Woodforde JM, Fielding JR: Pain and cancer. J Psychosom Res 1970;14:365.
21. Bukberg J, Penman D, Holland J: Depression in hospitalized cancer patients. Psychosom Med 1984;43:199.
22. Massie MJ, Holland JC, Glass E: Delirium in terminally ill cancer patients. Am J Psychiatry 1983;140:1048.
23. Bruera E, MacMillan K, Kuchn N et al: The cognitive effects of the administration of narcotics. Pain 1989;39:13.
24. Stiefel FC, Breitbart W, Holland JC: Corticosteroids in cancer: Neuropsychiatric complications. Cancer Invest 1989;7:479.
25. Marks RM, Sachar EJ: Undertreatment of medical inpatients with narcotic analgesics. Ann Intern Med 1973;78:173.
26. Charap AD. The knowledge, attitudes, and experience of medical personnel treating pain. Mt Sinai J Med 1978; 45:561–568.
27. Holland JC: Anxiety and cancer: The patient and family. J Clin Psychiatry 1989;50:20.
28. Massie MJ, Holland JC: Depression and the cancer patient. J Clin Psychiatry 1990;51:12.
29. Plumb MM, Holland JC: Comparative studies of psychological function in patients with advanced cancer. Psychosom Med 1977;39:264.
30. Holland JC, Hughes Korzun A, Tross S et al: Comparative psychological disturbance in pancreatic and gastric cancer. Am J Psychiatry 1986;143:982.
31. Endicott J: Measurement of depression patients with cancer. Cancer 1983;53:2243.

32. Young DF: Neurological complications of cancer chemotherapy. In Silverstein A (ed): Neurological Complications of Therapy: Selected Topics, p 57. New York, Futura, 1982.

33. Holland JC, Fassanellos, Ohnuma T: Psychiatric symptoms associated with L-asparaginase administration. J Psychiatr Res 1974;10:165.

34. Adams F, Quesada JR, Gutterman JU: Neuropsychiatric manifestations of human leukocyte interferon therapy in patients with cancer. JAMA 1984;252:938.

35. Denicoff KD, Rubinow DR, Papa MZ et al: The neuropsychiatric effects of treatment with interleukin-w and lymphokine-activated killer cells. Ann Intern Med 1987;107:293.

36. Weddington WW: Delirium and depression associated with amphotericin B. Psychosomatics 1982;23:1076.

37. DeAngelis LM, Delattre J, Posner JB: Radiation-induced dementia in patients cured of brain metastases. Neurology 1989;39:789.

38. Breitbart WB: Endocrine-related psychiatric disorders. In Holland J, Rowland J (eds): The Handbook of Psychooncology: The Psychological Care of the Patient With Cancer, p 356. New York, Oxford Press, 1989.

39. Posner JB: Nonmetastatic effects of cancer on the nervous system. In Wyngaarden JB, Smith LH (eds): Cecil's Textbook of Medicine, p 1104. Philadelphia, WB Saunders, 1988.

40. Patchell RA, Posner JB: Cancer and the nervous system. In Holland J, Rowland J (eds): The Handbook of Psychooncology: The Psychological Care of the Patient With Cancer, p 327. New York, Oxford Press, 1989.

41. Spiegel D, Bloom JR, Yalom ID: Group support for patients with metastatic cancer: A randomized prospective outcome study. Arch Gen Psychiatry 1981;38:527.

42. Spiegel D, Bloom JR: Group therapy and hypnosis reduce metastatic breast carcinoma pain. Psychosom Med 1983;4:333.

43. Massie MJ, Holland JC, Straker N: Psychotherapeutic interventions. In Holland JC, Rowland JH (eds): Handbook of Psychooncology: Psychological Care of the Patient With Cancer, p 455. New York, Oxford Press, 1989.

44. Holland JC, Morrow G, Schmale A et al: Reduction of anxiety and depression in cancer patients by alprazolam or by a behavioral technique (abstract). Proc Am Soc Clin Oncol 1988;6:258.

45. Rifkin A, Reardon G, Siris S et al: Trimipramine in physical illness with depression. J Clin Psychiatry 1985;46:4.

46. Purohit DR, Navlakha PL, Modi RS et al: The role of antidepressants in hospitalized cancer patients. J Assoc Physicians India 1978;26:245.

47. Popkin MK, Callies AL, Mackenzie TB: The outcome of antidepressant use in the medically ill. Arch Gen Psychiatry 1985;42:1160.

48. Costa D, Mogos I, Toma T: Efficacy and safety of mianserin in the treatment of depression of women with cancer. Acta Psychiatr Scand 1985;72:85.

49. Glassman AH: The newer antidepressant drugs and their cardiovascular effects. Psychopharmacol Bull 1984;20:272.

50. Sher M, Krieger JN, Juergen S: Trazodone and priapism. Am J Psychiatry 1983;140:1362.

51. Cooper GL: The safety of fluoxetine: An update. Br J Psychiatry 1988;153:77.

52. Peck AW, Stern WC, Watkinson C: Incidence of seizures during treatment with tricyclic antidepressant drugs and bupropion. J Clin Psychiatry 1983;44:197.

53. Lloyd AH: Practical consideration in the use of maprotiline (ludiomil) in general practice. J Int Med Res 1977;5:122.

54. Ayd F: Amoxapine: A new tricyclic antidepressant. International Drug Therapy Newsletter 1979;14:33.

55. Fernandez F, Adams F, Holmes VF et al: Methylphenidate for depressive disorders in cancer patients. Psychosomatics 1987;28:455.

56. Katon W, Raskind M: Treatment of depression in the medically ill elderly with methylphenidate. Am J Psychiatry 1980;137:963.

57. Kaufmann MW, Muarray GB, Cassem NH: Use of psychostimulants in medically ill depressed patients. Psychosomatics 1982;23:817.

58. Fisch R: Methylphenidate for medical inpatients. Int J Psychiatry Med 1985–86;15:75.

59. Chiarillo RJ, Cole JO: The use of psychostimulants in general psychiatry: A reconsideration. Arch Gen Psychiatry 1987;44:286.

60. Fernandez F, Adams F, Levy J et al: Cognitive impairment due to AIDS related complex and its response to psychostimulants. Psychosomatics 1988;29:38.

61. Bruera E, Chadwick S, Brennels C et al: Methylphenidate associated with narcotics for the treatment of cancer pain. Cancer Treat Rep 1987;71:67.

62. Nehra A et al: Pemoline associated hepatic injury. Gastroenterology 1990;99:1517.

63. Stein RS, Flexner JH, Graber SE: Lithium and granulocytopenia during induction therapy of acute myelogenous leukemia: Update of an ongoing trial. Adv Exp Med Biol 1980;127:187.

64. Brennan SC, Redd WH, Jacobsen PB et al: Anxiety and panic during magnetic resonance scans. Lancet 1988;ii:512.

65. Chouinard G, Young SN, Annable L: Antimanic effect of clonazepam. Biol Psychiatry 1983;18:451.

66. Walsh TD: Adjuvant analgesic therapy in cancer pain. In Foley KM, Bonica JJ, Ventafridda V (eds): Advances in Pain Research and Therapy, vol 16: Second International Congress on Cancer Pain, p 155. New York, Raven Press, 1990.

67. Robinson D, Napoliello MJ, Schenk J: The safety and usefulness of buspirone as an anxiolytic drug in elderly versus young patients. Clin Ther 1988; 10:740.

68. Posner JB: Delirium and exogenous metabolic brain disease. In Beeson PB, McDermott W, Wyngaarden JB (eds): Cecil's Textbook of Medicine, p 644. Philadelphia, WB Saunders, 1979.

69. Levine PM, Silverfarb PM, Lipowski ZJ: Mental disorders in cancer patients: A study of 100 psychiatric referrals. Cancer 1978;42:1385.

70. Lipowski ZJ: Delirium (acute confusional states). JAMA 1987;285:1789.

71. Adams F: Neuropsychiatric evaluation and treatment of delirium in cancer patients. Adv Psychosom Med 1988;18:26.

72. Fleishmann SB, Lesko LM: Delirium and dementia. In Holland J, Rowland J (eds): The Handbook of Psychooncology: Psychological Care of the Patient With Cancer, p 342. New York, Oxford Press, 1989.

73. Breitbart W: Cancer pain and suicide. In Foley KM, Bonica JJ, Ventafridda V (eds): Advances in Pain Research and Therapy, vol 16: Second International Congress on Cancer Pain, p 399. New York, Raven Press, 1990.

74. Breitbart W: Suicide in cancer patients. Oncology 1987;1:49.

75. Bolund C: Suicide and cancer: II. Medical and care factors in suicide by cancer patients in Sweden: 1973-1976. Journal of Psychosocial Oncology 1985;3:17.

76. Farberow NL, Schneidman ES, Leonard CV: Suicide among general medical and surgical hospital patients with malignant neoplasms. Medical Bulletin 9. Washington DC, U.S. Veterans Administration, 1963.

77. Morrow GR: Prevalence and correlates of anticipatory nausea and vomiting in chemotherapy patients. JNCI 1982;68:585.

78. Jacobsen PB, Andry Kowski MA, Redd WH et al: Non-pharmacologic factors in the development of post treatment nausea with adjuvant chemotherapy for breast cancer. Cancer 1988;61:379.

79. Breitbart W: Tardive dyskinesia associated with high dose intravenous metoclopramide. N Engl J Med 1986;315:518.

80. Greenberg DB, Surman OS, Clarke J et al: Alprazolam for phobic nausea and vomiting related to cancer chemotherapy. Cancer Treat Rep 1987;71:549.

81. Jacobsen PB, Redd WH: The development and management of anticipatory nausea and vomiting. Cancer Invest 1988;6:329.

82. Redd WH, Jacobsen PB, Die-Trill M et al: Cognitive attentional distraction in control of conditioned nausea in pediatric cancer patients receiving chemotherapy. J Consult Clin Psychol 1987;55:391.

83. Spiegel D, Bloom JR, Yalom ID: Group support for patients with metastatic cancer: A randomized prospective outcome study. Arch Gen Psychiatry 1981;38:527.

84. Spiegel D, Bloom JR: Group therapy and hypnosis reduce metastatic breast carcinoma pain. Psychosom Med 1983;4:333.

85. Fishman B, Loscalzo M: Cognitive-behavioral interventions in the management of cancer pain: Principles and applications. Med Clin North Am 1987; 71:271.

86. Cleeland CS: Nonpharmacologic management of cancer pain. Journal of Pain and Symptom Management 1987;2:523.

87. Cleeland CS, Tearnan BH: Behavioral control of cancer pain. In Holzman AD, Turk DC (eds): Pain Management, p 193. New York, Pergamon Press, 1986.

88. Spiegel D: The use of hypnosis in controlling cancer pain. CA 1985;4:221.

89. Redd WB, Reeves JL, Storm FK et al: Hypnosis in the control of pain during hyperthermia treatment of cancer. In Bonica JJ, Lindblom U, Iggo A (eds): Advances in Pain Research and Therapy, vol 5, p 857. New York, Raven Press, 1982.

90. Barber J, Gitelson J: Cancer pain: Psychological management using hypnosis. CA 1980;3:130.

91. Fotopoulos SS, Graham C, Cook MR: Psychophysiologic control of cancer pain. In Bonica JJ, Ventafridda V (eds): Advances in Pain Research and Therapy, vol 2, p 231. New York, Raven Press, 1979.

92. Munro S, Mount B: Music therapy in palliative care. Can Med Assoc J 1978;119:1029.

93. Getto CJ, Sorkness CA, Howell T: Antidepressants and chronic nonmalignant pain: A review. Journal of Pain and Symptom Management 1987;2:9.

94. Walsh TD: Antidepressants and chronic pain: Clin Neuropharmacol 1983;6:271.

95. Butler S: Present status of tricyclic antidepressants in chronic pain therapy. In Benedetti C, Chapman CR, Moricca G (eds): Advances in Pain Research and Therapy, vol 7, p 173. New York, Raven Press, 1986.

96. Ventafridda V, Bonezzi C, Caraceni A et al: Antidepressants for cancer pain and other painful syndromes with deafferentation component: Comparison of amitriptyline and trazodone. Ital J Neurol Sci 1987;8:579.

97. Magni G, Arsie D, DeLeo D: Antidepressants in the treatment of cancer pain: A survey in Italy. Pain 1987;23:347.

98. Spiegel K, Kalb R, Pasternak GW: Analgesic activity of tricyclic antidepressants. Ann Neurol 1983;13:462.

99. Walsh TD: Controlled study of imipramine and morphine in chronic pain due to advanced cancer (abstract). American Society of Clinical Oncology Abstract May 4–6, 1986, Los Angeles.

100. Theesen K, Marsh W: Relief of diabetic neuropathy with fluoxetine. DICP, the Annals of Pharmacotherapy 1989;3:572.

101. Bruera E, Barenneis C, Paterson AH et al: Use of methylphenidate as an adjuvant to narcotic analgesics for patients with advanced cancer. Journal of Pain and Symptom Management 1987;4:3.

102. Forrest WH et al: Dextroamphetamine with morphine for the treatment of post-operative pain. N Engl J Med 1977;296:712.

103. Beaver WT, Wallenstein SL, Houde RW et al: A comparison of the analgesic effect of methotrimeprazine and morphine in patients with cancer. Clin Pharmacol Ther 1966;7:436.

104. Lechin F et al: Pimozide therapy for trigeminal neuralgia. Arch Neurol 1989;9:960.

105. Beaver WT, Feise G: Comparison of the analgesic effects of morphine, hydroxyzine and their combination in patients with post-operative pain. In Bonica JJ, Albe-Fessard (eds): Advances in Pain Research and Therapy, vol. 2, p 553. New York, Raven Press, 1976.

106. Fernandez F, Adams F, Holmes VF: Analgesic effect of alprazolam in patients with chronic, organic pain of malignant origin. J Clin Psychopharmacol 1987;3:167.

Chapter **15**

Radiotherapy in the Palliation of Cancer

Michael Ashby

INTRODUCTION

Radiotherapy as clinical art and science has existed now for almost a century. It began with the formidable discoveries of Wilhelm Roentgen (x-rays, 1895) and Marie Curie (radium, 1898). The history and influence of radiation oncology and biology on our modern understanding of cancer is a fascinating and remarkable story.[1] For much of the twentieth century it has been the most effective, and often the only available nonsurgical tool for cancer treatment. Radiation oncologists play a key role in the palliation of incurable malignant disease, a role that has been historically undervalued. The focus of radiotherapy has been predominantly curative until quite recently. The roles and relative indications for radiotherapy have changed over recent years, in concert with a shift toward multidisciplinary and multimodal management of cancer. Improvements in technical equipment and biologic understanding have also been important influences.

A department of radiation oncology is a highly technical and scientific environment, one that has often developed historically in relative isolation from the rest of the hospital world. As such, it may seem intimidating to both patients and other health care professionals (Fig. 15–1). Medical students, junior medical staff, and nurses are taught little about what occurs there, and as a result much more education and outreach by the radiation oncology community is required. Patients

235

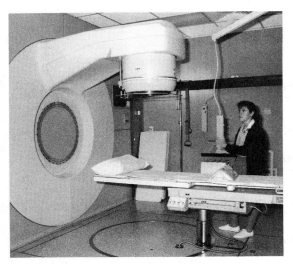

Figure 15–1. A modern megavoltage radiotherapy machine and treatment room.

PRINCIPLES AND DEFINITIONS OF TERMS USED IN RADIATION ONCOLOGY

GENERAL PRINCIPLES

Radiotherapy is the delivery of ionizing radiation into a defined volume of the body in order to eradicate (sterilize) or substantially depopulate the tumor cells in that volume, within the tolerance of normal tissues. The different physical ways of administering radiotherapy are summarized in Table 15–1. Ionizing radiation is broadly delivered either as a beam directed into the target volume within the body, or as an injected or ingested isotope, which may be delivered either as a sealed source that is unsealed once the treatment dose is delivered, or unsealed as an injection or orally, with rapid decay after the target organ(s) have been treated. Throughout the history of the technical development of radiotherapy, efforts have been directed at generating a sharply focused beam of radiation of adequate penetration into the target volume, which is often situated deep within the body. Ways of increasing the voltage at which electrons are accelerated into the target to generate the treatment beam have been devised, and this generating voltage often ex-

may maintain negative impressions from prior experience within their communities, where a friend or relative may have undergone radiotherapy and subsequently appeared very ill and died. The radiotherapy may be perceived as the cause, although in reality the disease process may have been advanced, and the aims of the radiotherapy and its side effects misunderstood. In the past some practices were suboptimal (often because of technologic limitations), and have left lasting negative impressions on communities, impressions that require correction in the light of modern techniques and attitudes. Most departments now make considerable efforts to ensure that patients and their families served by them are educated, counseled, and supported throughout the treatment process (Fig. 15–2). The majority of patients acclimatize well after their initial encounters. These perceptual and attitudinal aspects are important: it is most unfortunate if fear of high technology or negative experiences of others prevents patients from having access to the benefit of appropriate palliative radiotherapy.

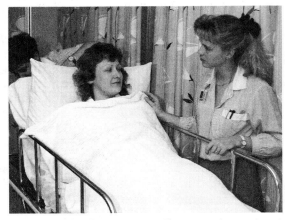

Figure 15–2. Patient counseling as an integral part of a radiation therapist's role.

Table 15–1.
Different Ways of Administering Radiotherapy

	Generating Voltage	Machine	Nature of Beam	Characteristics and Uses of Beam
External Beam				
Megavoltage	2–20 MV	Linear Accelerators	Photons (x-rays) Electrons	Sharply defined beam edge Penetrating beam Skin sparing
		Cobalt	Gamma rays	Less defined beam edge Penetrating beam Skin sparing
		Cyclotron	Particles: Neutrons Pi-mesons Protons	Experimental
Kilovoltage (orthovoltage)	200–300 kV	x-ray machine	Photons (x-rays)	Superficial lesions Not penetrating Not skin sparing
Superficial	60–140 kV	x-ray machine	Photons (x-rays)	Skin tumors

	Isotope	Main Indications
Isotopes		
Sealed Sources		
Intracavitary applicators	Previously radium now cesium (Cs-137) and iridium (Ir-192)	Gynecologic, head and neck, skin tumors
Interstitial implants (needles)		
Unsealed Sources (some examples)		
Oral	Iodine (I-131)	Thyroid
Injected	Phosphorus (P-32) Strontium (Sr-89)	Polycythaemia rubra vera Experimental for bone pain

plains the name given to treatment machines. The vast majority of patients are treated with external beam radiation, usually by megavoltage photons or electrons delivered by linear accelerators, or megavoltage gamma rays from cobalt units. Modern departments in developed countries are predominantly equipped with linear accelerators. Although installation is costly and operation requires considerable technical expertise and support, they have the advantage of allowing most

sites in the body to be treated with flexibility and sparing of normal tissue, notably sparing of the skin, with consequent reductions in the incidence and severity of acute skin reactions and late damage (Fig. 15–3). Cobalt machines produce marginally less well defined beams, and hence are inferior for high-precision therapeutic situations, but are perfectly adequate for the majority of treatments, and nearly all palliative treatments. Kilovoltage x-rays are still available in many departments, and are

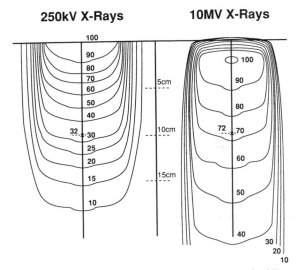

Figure 15–3. Percentage depth dose charts for kilovoltage x-rays (250 kV) and megavoltage photons (10 MV), showing depth of penetration into tissue. Compare the percentage depth dose at 10 cm and see how much less penetrating the kilovoltage beam is (32% vs. 72%).

useful to treat superficial tumors, and may be used to palliate superficial fungating, nodal, or bone disease. Modern isotope implants or intracavitary treatment occasionally are indicated for palliation. Although there is renewed interest in unsealed isotopes for the palliation of bone pain, this practice is still largely experimental.[2]

Intrinsic to the understanding of radiotherapy is the principle of the therapeutic ratio, which, as in pharmacology, is the ratio of benefits to side effects of a therapeutic intervention. An ethically based argument for the decision-making process for palliative care based on the therapeutic ratio has been proposed.[3] The side effect profile of treatment should be the minimum that is compatible with achieving its palliative aims, and should be defined in terms of palliative end points that are patient-observable. Palliative radiotherapy should be compatible with the patient's convenience, minimizing numbers of hospital visits and length of overall treatment time, so that precious remaining time away from home and family is not excessive.

DEFINITION OF AIMS OF TREATMENT

Radical

Radical therapy refers to delivery of a course of radiation with the intent of complete eradication of the tumor. To achieve this effect, a high dose, to the tolerance of the normal tissues in the irradiation volume, is required for most tumors. As the aim is cure and prolonged survival, a high level of morbidity (side effects or toxicity) may be accepted.

Palliative

Delivery of a course of palliative radiation has the intent of imposing growth restraint on a tumor or reducing or abolishing symptoms caused by the tumor (or both). When the former is the intent, a high dose may be required. However, in many palliative situations a short course, or a high-dose, single-fraction treatment may be sufficient to achieve the favorable end point desired. A lower level of morbidity should be the goal in such situations.

High-dose irradiation of tumors that are deemed incurable at presentation is often justified to achieve local control, and may be compatible with preservation of function and body image.[4] Examples include some cases of head and neck, gynecologic, breast, urologic, lung, skin, and colorectal cancers.

This area of endeavor forms a large part of the overall scope of modern radiation oncology. Much of it could be termed radical in terms of intent and dose, but in reality the outcome most often is better described as palliative. High doses in prolonged fractionation schedules may be worthwhile in these situations. Survival may be extended for months or years, and a gratifying result in terms of local control and symptom-free survival can often be obtained. In this setting, the same optimization of tumor response and normal tissue-sparing will be required as for a radical curative course of therapy.

Prophylactic

Prophylactic treatment involves the delivery of a course of radiation (in the radical context) with the intent of preventing regrowth of tumor after complete or almost complete tumor eradication by other means (*eg*, surgery or chemotherapy) when established prognostic factors predict a high probability of tumor recurrence or spread, and particularly when there is microscopic or macroscopic evidence of residual tumor. Prophylactic treatment may also be applicable to the palliative situation; treatment may be administered to prevent a predicted event related to tumor progression at a given site, for example, erosion into or compression of adjacent vessels, structures or organs, or to prevent fracture of a bone. Further validation for this role of radiotherapy is needed, there being for example some doubt as to whether it prevents pathologic fracture.

RADIATION DOSE

The SI (Systeme Internationale) unit of absorbed radiation dose is the Gray (Gy), which has replaced the more familiar units, the rad (100 rads = 1 Gy), and the Roentgen. Radiotherapists prescribe a certain number of Grays at a given defined reference point in the body (often the center of the volume, or a specified point on or below the skin surface).

FRACTIONATION

Simple comparison of the total dose in terms of the number of Grays prescribed is an error commonly made by individuals who are unfamiliar with radiation oncology. The biologic effect of radiation on tissues is a complex and incompletely understood interaction. These effects can broadly be divided into early radiation damage, which is manifested by acute side effects during and immediately after treatment, and late damage, which may not become apparent for months or years. These effects depend on the volume (how much of the body is treated), the dose delivered per

fraction (treatment session), the overall treatment time, and the type of radiation. In simple terms, the larger the volume, the lower is the dose that is tolerated. The dose per fraction has an important influence on late damage to normal tissue. Generally, for radical curative treatments, a large number of small fractions will be delivered to a small or medium-sized volume. A standard treatment regime might be 60 Gy in 30 fractions, delivered over 6 weeks with daily treatment sessions (2 Gy per fraction). When the end point is palliative, a small number of larger doses per fraction is often adequate, such as 20 Gy in five fractions delivered over 1 week in daily sessions, or alternatively, a large single fraction of 6–10 Gy. Some common palliative fractionation prescriptions are summarized in Table 15–2. For more information on radiobiology, the reader is referred to two readable and accessible reviews.[5,6]

VOLUME

If only the tumor and a margin around it are treated, this is termed involved-field treatment. If a larger area is treated or a whole region is irradiated, this may be referred to as loco-regional or wide-field treatment. It is possible to treat the whole body (TBI) or half (hemi) the body (HBI). The volume is defined by a process of treatment planning, which may require simulation (the use of a diagnostic x-ray unit specially constructed for radiotherapy planning) and computerized tomography (Fig. 15–4). For radical treatment, this is often a complicated, highly technical and precise process. For palliative care, however, this process can often be minimized to ensure as little inconvenience and discomfort to the patient as possible.

SIDE EFFECTS

There is no doubt that radiotherapy gives rise to significant side effects, although every effort is made to minimize these in the palliative

Table 15–2.
Examples of Some Commonly Used Palliative Radiotherapy Prescriptions

Total dose (Grays—Gy)	35	30	20	6–10
Dose per fraction (Gy)	2.33	3	4	6–10
Number of fractions	15	10	5	1
Overall time	21	12	5	1
Number of fractions				
per day	1	1	1	1
per week	5	5	5	1

Fraction = treatment session = visit to radiotherapy department

scenario. Side effects can be divided into two groups: those that are confined to the irradiated volume, and systemic effects. Early damage to normal tissue is summarized in Table 15–3. Most effects are transient and mild, and can be alleviated by simple remedies.

Regrettably, acute skin reactions are often referred to pejoratively as burns, when in fact they represent transient depopulation of the basal cells of the skin. Although this description is, in a sense, apt, it implies a lack of care or misadventure that is unfortunate. Severe skin reactions may occur in radical treatment, but they are rarely a significant cause of morbidity in palliative treatment. It is sometimes also feared that hair loss will occur even when the volume does not include the scalp. Counseling and education are required to dispel these myths.

Late normal tissue damage is a phenomenon related to radiation effects on slowly dividing or nondividing cell lines. Structures such as the central nervous system (particularly the spinal cord), lung, kidney, the lens of the eye, and microvasculature everywhere are especially sensitive (see Chapter 3). Late damage to normal tissue usually is not a significant problem for patients undergoing palliative therapy, as the majority do not live long enough to experience such damage. However, sound practice usually dictates that all treatment be provided within safe late normal tissue damage limits, although on occasions these constraints may be waived for short-term comfort when it is clear that survival will be very short.

INDICATIONS FOR PALLIATIVE RADIOTHERAPY

The main indications for palliative radiotherapy are summarized in Table 15–4. It is important that a radiation oncologist is consulted early on to prevent inappropriate *a priori* decisions. It is particularly unfortunate that patients are not more frequently referred, even when it is considered that a tumor is not "radiosensitive." Radiosensitivity is a radiobio-

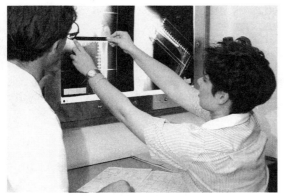

Figure 15–4. Radiotherapy treatment planning with simulator films.

Table 15–3.
Acute Side Effects of Radiotherapy

Systemic (not confined to irradiation volume)
Malaise
Nausea or vomiting
Anorexia
Fatigue

Specific (confined to irradiation volume)
Skin
  Redness
  Itching
  Breakdown
Abdomen and pelvis
  Nausea
  Vomiting
  Diarrhea
  Frequency, dysuria, hematuria (cystitis)
Head and Neck
  Dysphagia (mucositis)
  Dry mouth
  Taste alteration
Chest
  Painful dysphagia (esophagitis)
Head
  Alopecia
Bone Marrow
  Myelosuppression

logic term referring to the intrinsic response of a given cell line to radiation; radioresponsiveness is the clinical counterpart. In fact, most tumors "respond" to radiotherapy, although there is a quite marked variation in this response. For palliative end points, even the so-called "radioresistant" tumors frequently respond favorably, although often without measurable tumor regression.

When assessing patients for palliative care, one should always pose the question as to whether the disease process has been adequately treated. Oncologic treatment (radiotherapy, chemotherapy, and hormone therapy) may have a beneficial effect on palliative end points until quite late in the natural history of the disease. Retreatment with radiotherapy often may be possible for symptom control, despite previous statements about

the tolerance of normal tissues being reached with the initial radical course.

Some of the indications detailed below do not specifically address pain issues. However, cancer patients with advanced disease tend to have multiple synchronous and metachronous problems, often with overlap in time and mechanism. It is universally agreed that management of the total suffering is an essential component of comprehensive cancer care (psychosocial problems, pain, and other symptoms). It is sometimes not possible to define where pain begins and ends. Radiotherapy has a wide variety of symptomatic roles, as detailed below.

PAIN RELIEF

Bone Pain

The role of radiotherapy in the management of pain due to malignant bone metastases is unquestioned, and this indication (mainly for patients with lung, breast, and prostate primaries) constitutes at least 20% of the total number of referrals to most radiation oncology departments[7–9] (Fig. 15–5). The pathogenesis of metastatic bone pain and the mechanism of action of radiotherapy are

Table 15–4.
Indications for Palliative Radiotherapy

Pain relief
  (bone pain, nerve root and soft tissue infiltration)
Control of bleeding
  (hemoptysis, vaginal bleeding, hematuria, rectal bleeding)
Control of fungation and ulceration
Dyspnea
Oncologic emergencies
  (superior vena cava obstruction, spinal cord compression, cerebral metastases causing raised intracranial pressure)
Relief of blockage of hollow viscera
Shrinkage of tumor masses causing symptoms by virtue of site or space occupancy

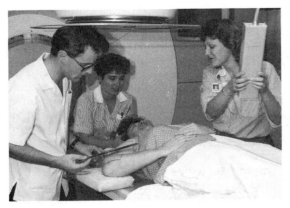

Figure 15–5. Setting up the patient in the treatment position for treatment of a bone metastasis in the right humerus.

incompletely understood. A partial or total dissociation between tumor regression and initial pain relief is suggested by similar results achieved with a very wide range of doses and fractionation schedules. Overall responses usually range between 70%–80%, independent of tumor histology. These parameters, however have a significant impact on duration of pain relief, as shown in retreatment requirements of patients in single-fraction studies.[10] The rapidity of action achieved after single-fraction local or hemibody irradiation, usually within 24 hours, is similar to that observed after pituitary ablation.[10] It has often been proposed that an effect on chemical mediators of the inflammatory response may be operative. Other proposed mechanisms include an effect on host cells that produce pain mediators or osteolytic substances, a direct effect on osteoclast activity, or disturbances of the neuronal transmission of pain.[11]

A randomized study from Tokyo emphasized patient factors rather than fractionation in achieving pain control,[12] and a retrospective study from Rome showed lower response rates for adenocarcinoma of the kidney, non-small cell lung cancer primary histologies, and limb sites of metastases. A dose response was described for total absorbed radiation dose, but not for fraction size.[13] Analysis of retrospective dose response data must, however, be viewed with caution. Higher doses for the palliation of renal cell carcinoma have been advocated elsewhere.[14] The key issues revolve around questions of what dose, fractionation, and field size are required to produce an acceptable incidence of sustained pain relief with minimal toxicity and inconvenience to patients and their families.

There has been considerable interest in the administration of large, single fractions for bone metastases. In a randomized study[15] at the Royal Marsden Hospital, a single fraction of 8 Gy was compared to a fractionated course of 30 Gy delivered in 10 daily fractions. No difference was found in the speed of onset or duration of pain relief, which was independent of the histology of the primary tumor. A subsequent study from the same group looked at 4-Gy single fractions, and suggested the need for further exploration of treatment with low-dose single fractions.[11] In a small, prospective, randomized study from Oxford, comparing 8 Gy as a single fraction to 24 Gy in six fractions, 25% of the patients required retreatment in the 8-Gy group. There was also a higher incidence of gastrointestinal side effects, but their duration was short.[16]

There is thus a growing body of evidence to show that pragmatic treatment of bone metastases with single (repeatable) fractions is safe, effective, and acceptable to patients. Crellin and co-authors have discussed the possible reasons why many radiation oncologists in the United Kingdom have been reluctant to change their prescribing patterns. They emphasize the fact that an apprenticeship training system has more influence than the published literature on practice, and discuss the difficulties of study methodology, and the lack of information on late normal tissue damage for large fractions.[8] There is wide acceptance of the justification for higher total dose fractionated courses for the prevention of pathologic fracture or vertebral fracture due to lytic metastases, particularly when there is neurologic involvement; however, there is no evidence in favor of this practice.

The use of hemibody irradiation (HBI) for bone pain is a subject of increasing interest.[17–21] This practice refers either to treatment of the upper or lower half, or both in sequence (usually separated by an interval of a few weeks). The main indications have been for widespread disease in patients with advanced multiple myeloma or prostatic carcinoma. In one comparative evaluation,[19] no difference in terms of response was noted between the two histologies, but significant toxicity is described for the doses that are widely used at present—8 Gy to lower half, and 6 Gy to the upper half. An exploration of treatment with lower doses is recommended, to reduce toxicity while retaining the high overall response rates, which are in the range of 80%. There is also considerable interest in the use of sequential hemibody irradiation as a systemic therapy for widespread disease that persists despite chemotherapy in patients with non-Hodgkins lymphoma, breast cancer, and small-cell lung cancer.[22–24] With refinements in selection, indications, technique, and fractionation, this approach shows promise, and has a small but definite place in the palliation of these, and possibly other tumors.

There has been some recent increase in interest in the idea of the systemic use of radioisotopes for bone pain.[2] It is currently regarded as suitable for comparison with HBI, but appears to have major disadvantages in terms of a later onset of pain relief at 2–4 weeks compared to 24–48 hours for HBI, and unpredictable differential isotope distribution between normal and tumor-bearing bone. Further evaluation clearly is required. Its use in combination with external beam radiotherapy is a further intriguing potential application.

Nerve Root and Soft Tissue Infiltration

Radiotherapy is often helpful in situations where tumor infiltrates directly into nerve or soft tissues, in which case it is usually administered in combination with steroids or non-steroidal anti-inflammatory drugs. Higher doses of radiation may be required in these instances than for the treatment of bone pain.

Careful planning of treatment to include the involved neurologic pathways is important. This is particularly true for head and neck tumors, which have a propensity for perineural spread, and in situations where spread into the spinal canal might be present. Cautious fractionation is required where large volumes of nervous system tissue are irradiated, such as in brachial and lumbosacral plexus invasion, where late damage to normal tissue is a particular danger. Apical lung cancers may give rise to brachial plexus invasion, or produce the classic Pancoast's syndrome, and radical irradiation may give worthwhile and sustained locoregional control and symptom relief.

The pain of pelvic recurrence of rectal adenocarcinoma is often severe and difficult to diagnose and manage. Despite some promise with preventative adjuvant radiotherapy and chemotherapy for high-risk patients,[25] it is a common clinical problem, with an incidence varying from 10%–53% in one review. Sites of recurrence include the presacral hollow (most common), anastomosis, lateral pelvic side wall, perineum, and invasion of other adjacent pelvic organs.[26] Diagnosis may be problematic owing to the distortion of pelvic anatomy after surgery, with interpretation of both computerized tomography and clinical findings difficult. Sometimes the tumor growth may be diffuse and sheet-like along tissue planes, extending into the sacral hollow and nerves. The pain mechanism may be complex, with both nociceptive (opioid-sensitive deep visceral, and anti-inflammatory sensitive deep somatic) and neurogenic (nerve damage) components. The history may be long before correct diagnosis and treatment are instituted. In some circumstances, serial serum carcinoembryonic antigen (CEA) levels and exploratory surgery may be helpful—and indeed, surgical management may be appropriate. Many recurrences are inoperable, and radiotherapy is indicated. High doses are usually administered, using three or four field plans and computer-assisted planning.[27,28] Enduring control of symptoms may be obtained, even if imaging appearances show little change. The role of hypofractionated radiotherapy has not been much explored for poor-risk patients, who are unsuitable for the protracted courses usually prescribed in this situation.

CONTROL OF BLEEDING

Hemoptysis, Vaginal Bleeding, Hematuria, Rectal Bleeding

The success of radiotherapy in controlling hemorrhage from exophytic bleeding tumors is well established. It has long been known that vaginal bleeding from cervical carcinoma may be arrested by intracavitary isotope insertion. Equally, external beam irradiation is effective either as a short palliative course, or when indicated in a high-dose, radical treatment protocol. The use of a few large fractions[29,30] is now well accepted in patients with advanced disease.

Extensive experience from Stockholm shows that hypofractionated radiotherapy (21 Gy in three fractions over 5 days) was useful in a study of 162 elderly and disabled patients with mainly advanced bladder cancer. The results achieved were similar to those with radical fractionated courses of treatment in this disease.[31] This interesting result merits further evaluation, and may be applicable to other sites and tumors.

CONTROL OF FUNGATION AND ULCERATION

Superficial tumor fungation and ulceration is a disfiguring disorder that may be associated with pain, odor, and high levels of distress. The most common of such tumors encountered in oncologic practice are breast cancer on the chest wall, fungating head and neck cancer, and both melanoma and nonmelanoma skin cancer. Most such processes respond favorably to radiotherapy. High doses may be required when warranted by the clinical situation, but a few large fractions may also be helpful for elderly patients, or those with a very poor prognosis.[32] In breast cancer,

chemotherapy and hormone therapy also have an important and effective role, either alone or in combination, for the control of chest wall disease.

DYSPNEA

The tumor most commonly responsible for shortness of breath is lung cancer, although metastases from other primary sites can, and frequently do produce respiratory symptoms. The mechanisms of dyspnea are not completely understood, are often multifactorial, and may coexist with significant levels of established chronic lung damage, most commonly chronic obstructive airways disease. Radiotherapy can provide excellent palliation for dyspnea that is due to endobronchial obstruction or extrinsic nodal compression of the bronchi, and for hemoptysis, cough, chest pain, superior vena caval obstruction, and dysphagia due to extrinsic esophageal compression. A British consensus document proposing a pragmatic treatment guide for lung cancer emphasizes that there is no evidence of benefit from early treatment of asymptomatic incurable patients, and that short courses of radiotherapy are usually as effective as are more protracted fractionated schedules when end points are palliative.[33] This view is supported by recent Medical Research Council trials in the United Kingdom, which indicate that hypofractionated regimens have a definite place in the palliation of lung cancer symptoms. In a randomized, multicenter study of 369 patients, 17 Gy in two fractions of 8.5 Gy administered one week apart gave similar results to two conventional multifractionated regimens of 30 Gy in 10 fractions or 27 Gy in 6 fractions. Hemoptysis, chest pain, and anorexia disappeared for a time in well over half the patients with these symptoms, and cough in 37%.[34] A second study will be reported shortly that indicates that similar results can be achieved even with a single fraction of 10 Gy (Bleehen, personal communication).

ONCOLOGIC EMERGENCIES

Superior Vena Caval Obstruction

The treatment of superior vena caval obstruction with radiotherapy and steroids is well established, particularly when it is associated with other features of mediastinal obstruction. The urgency of commencing treatment may have been slightly overemphasized in the past. The use of a head-up position, high-dose steroids, opioid analgesics, anxiolytics, and oxygen (if indicated) in the acute situation can often produce substantial relief pending the commencement of radiotherapy. In carefully selected cases, chemotherapy may be the initial treatment of choice, such as for patients with new small-cell lung cancer, and individuals with other rare chemosensitive tumors presenting in this manner.

Spinal Cord Compression

Metastatic spinal cord compression (see Chapters 1 and 29) is a devastating complication of malignant disease. Considerable vigilance is required to ensure early diagnosis, and the prompt institution of emergency treatment. Clinical signs and symptoms may be subtle and atypical, levels of compression may be multiple and asymmetric, and there may be mixed upper and lower motor neuron dysfunction. Vague complaints of back pain, leg weakness, shooting pains, dysesthesias, and sphincter disturbance should always be regarded seriously. Early detection and intervention appear to be more important overall in determining the functional outcome, than is tumor cell type.[35] A full clinical and radiologic assessment is essential, which may include either computerized tomography, myelography, or magnetic resonance imaging if available,[36] together with the early administration of a course of high-dose corticosteroids. Consultation with a neurosurgical service is always advisable. Results of treatment with both surgery and radiotherapy appear to be similar. Findlay has suggested a useful algorithmic approach to the problem.[37] Further work is required to identify subgroups

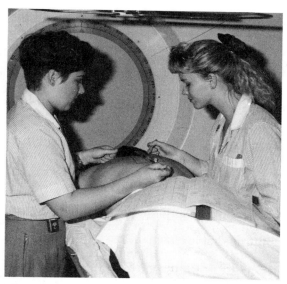

Figure 15–6. Setting up the patient in the treatment position for the treatment of dorsal spine metastases. The patient is lying prone on the treatment couch.

who may benefit from one modality rather than the other. The poor prognosis of all patients with metastatic spinal cord compression should not obscure the importance of striving to obtain the best functional result, and patients who are thought to be unsuitable for surgical intervention usually should commence a course of radiotherapy to the compression site immediately. The results for patients with evidence of established complete cord "section" who fail to respond to steroids are so poor that whether they should be subjected to treatment at all is questionable. Radiotherapy may be indicated for pain relief, however, regardless of neurologic condition (Fig. 15–6).

Cerebral Metastases Causing Raised Intracranial Pressure

Whole-brain irradiation for cerebral metastases has an important role in the palliation of this devastating complication of disseminated malignancy, although better documentation of indications and results is needed. The role of steroids in the emergency control of raised intracranial pressure is undisputed, but much remains to be understood about mechanism of action, optimal preparation, dose, and scheduling. The importance of trying to taper the dose of steroids as soon as neurologic function is stable has been emphasized.[38] There is a considerable need for more clinical research, particularly with regard to selection criteria for radiotherapy. Failure to respond to steroids, impaired level of consciousness, and neuropsychiatric dysfunction seem unfavorable prognostic factors for response to radiotherapy, whereas patients with motor deficits that have responded to steroids may have a more favorable outcome. The use of radiotherapy in the acute situation for critically increased intracranial pressure together with steroids sometimes produces impressive short-term results.

There is evidence that surgical excision for patients with solitary metastases is of value, both in terms of quality and quantity of life.[39–41] Some controversy surrounds the issue of whether higher doses of radiotherapy produce better results, either for multiple or solitary metastases, with the balance of opinion pointing toward a negative conclusion.[42,43] Trials by the Radiation Therapy Oncology Group (RTOG) in the United States have shown no difference in response or duration of response for palliation of cerebral metastases for five different regimens, ranging from 40 Gy in 20 fractions over 4 weeks, to 20 Gy in 5 fractions over 1 week.[44] A subsequent study of patients with favorable prognosis demonstrated no advantage for 50 Gy administered in 25 fractions over 5 weeks, compared to 30 Gy given in 10 fractions over 2 weeks.[45]

Several studies have addressed malignant melanoma as an entity of special interest. There are conflicting reports about the role of chemotherapy, with one study showing few long-term survivors,[46] and another with similar negative conclusions.[47] Despite suggestions that large dose-per-fraction treatment is beneficial for radiobiologic reasons, Choi and co-authors conclude that a short overall treatment time is more important.[48]

Overall, the prognosis for patients with cerebral metastases is poor. However, short palliative courses of cerebral radiotherapy should always be considered, although more information concerning prognostic selection factors is needed. Most studies focus too much on survival, whereas a greater emphasis on palliative issues seems needed. Patients with solitary metastases should have the benefit of a neurosurgical opinion.

RELIEF OF BLOCKAGE OF HOLLOW VISCERA

Any hollow organ or visceral tube may become partially or completely obstructed by the presence of tumor in its lumen or wall, or by extrinsic compression (see Chapters 13 and 29). Palliative radiotherapy may be helpful in many of these situations, although more outcome data are needed. Examples include obstruction of the bronchi, esophagus, upper aerodigestive tract, bile ducts, ureters, lymphatic channels, and blood vessels.

SHRINKAGE OF TUMOR MASSES CAUSING SYMPTOMS BY VIRTUE OF SITE OR SPACE OCCUPANCY

Most tumors can be reduced in size by a course of radiotherapy, regardless of site or histology. The important question to be posed in each case is whether a volume reduction will have a favorable effect on symptoms and consequently on quality of life. Where gains in terms of palliative end points are likely either to be small or nonexistent, it may be best not to embark on treatment. Such individual decisions may be difficult, and regrettably there is often little supporting scientific data. It may be best to withhold treatment in patients with very large tumor masses that are adjacent to critical normal tissue, especially in cases where the histology suggests poor radiosensitivity (eg, sarcoma and melanoma).

CONCLUSION

Radiotherapy is an indispensable modality in the palliation of cancer. The main indications are: pain relief (particularly bone pain); control of hemorrhage, fungation and ulceration, dyspnea, and obstruction of hollow viscera; and as a means to shrink any tumor causing problems by virtue of space occupancy. In addition, radiotherapy has an important role in the palliation of three oncologic emergencies: superior vena caval obstruction, spinal cord compression, and increased intracranial pressure caused by cerebral metastases. More pragmatic fractionation schedules are being developed that are compatible with good palliative results. The gradual acceptance of these modifications of traditional treatment techniques should give rise to shorter treatment courses with fewer hospital attendances for patient and family, with improved comfort and convenience.

A recent first Consensus Workshop in Radiation Therapy in the Treatment of Metastatic and Locally Advanced Cancer has emphasized the need for more research and large numbers in studies to resolve controversies in common management situations (American College of Radiology, personal communication). Considerable differences in patterns of care between Europe and the United States emerged. The overall trend on both sides of the Atlantic, and all around the world, appeared to be increasingly pragmatic and palliation-orientated. Better knowledge of prognostic factors to enable appropriate selection of palliative treatment regimens was recommended, although there is still substantial disagreement about when radical treatment should and should not be recommended— particularly for lung cancer.

Owing to the disappointing overall results even with aggressive management of most of the common solid tumors,[49,50] the focus of oncology has shifted in recent years. Communities and patients and their families have requested that more interest be shown in palliative care issues. Research into palliative radiotherapy methods and outcomes largely has been neglected until recently, but changes in practice are already apparent. Radiation oncologists have a duty to communicate what they have to offer patients with advanced incurable cancer, and at a time when such patients are increasingly being managed in non-oncologic settings such as hospices, or at home, it is important for their care providers to know when to consult the radiation oncologist.

REFERENCES

1. Fletcher GH: Regaud Lecture and perspectives of the history of radiotherapy. Radiother Oncol 1988;12:253.
2. Editorial: Strontium and bone pain. Lancet 1990; i 335:384.
3. Ashby MA, Stoffell B: Therapeutic ratio and defined phases: Proposal of ethical framework for palliative care. Br Med J 1991;302:1322.
4. Papillon J: The responsibility of radiologists in the preservation of breast and rectum in cancer treatment. Clin Radiol 1986;37:303.
5. Suit HD: Radiation biology: The conceptual and practical impact on radiation therapy. Radiat Res 1983; 94:10.
6. Hall EJ: Basic radiobiology. Am J Clin Oncol 1988; 11:220.
7. Coia LR, Hanks GE, Martz K et al: Practice patterns of palliative care for the United States 1984-1985. Int J Radiat Onc Biol Phys 1988;14:1261.
8. Crellin AM, Marks A, Maher EJ: Why don't British radiotherapists give single fractions of radiotherapy for bone metastases? Clin Oncol 1989;1:63.
9. Poulsen HS, Nielsen OS, Klee M et al: Palliative irradiation of bone metastases. Cancer Treat Rev 1989; 16:41.
10. Bates T: Radiotherapy for bone metastases. Clinical Oncology 1989;1:57.
11. Price P, Hoskin PJ, Easton D et al: Low dose single fraction radiotherapy in the treatment of metastatic bone pain: A pilot study. Radiother Oncol 1988;12: 297.
12. Okawa T, Kita M, Goto M et al: Randomised prospective clinical study of small, large and twice-a-day fraction radiotherapy for painful bone metastases. Radiother Oncol 1988;13:99.
13. Arcangeli G, Micheli A, Arcangeli G et al: The responsiveness of bone metastases to radiotherapy: The effect of site, histology and radiation dose on pain relief. Radiother Oncol 1989;14:95.
14. Onufrey V, Mohiuddin M: Radiation therapy in the

treatment of metastatic renal cell carcinoma. Int J Radiat Oncol Biol Phys 1985;11:2007.

15. Price P, Hoskin PJ, Easton D et al: Prospective randomized trial of single and multifraction radiotherapy schedules in the treatment of painful bony metastases. Radiother Oncol 1986;6:247.

16. Cole DJ: A randomised trial of a single treatment versus conventional fractionation in the palliative radiotherapy of painful bone metastases. Clinical Oncology 1989;1:59.

17. Qasim MM: Half body irradiation (HBI) in metastatic carcinomas. Clin Radiol 1981;32:215.

18. Salazar OM, Rubin P, Hendrickson FR et al: Single-dose half-body irradiation for palliation of multiple bone metastases from solid tumours. Cancer 1986; 58:29.

19. Hoskin PJ, Ford HT, Harmer CL: Hemibody irradiation (HBI) for metastatic bone pain in two histologically distinct groups of patients. Clinical Oncology 1989;1:67.

20. Zelefsky MJ, Scher HI, Forman JD et al: Palliative hemiskeletal irradiation for widespread metastatic prostate cancer: A comparison of single dose and fractionated regimens. Int J Radiat Onc Biol Phys 1989;17:1281.

21. Burmeister BH, Probert JC: Half body irradiation for the palliation of bone metastases. Australas Radiol 1990;34:317.

22. Urtasun RC, Belch A, Bodnar D: Hemibody radiation, an active therapeutic modality for the management of patients with small cell lung cancer. Int J Radiat Oncol Biol Phys 1983;9:1575.

23. Jullien D, Vilcoq JR, Campana F: Irradiations hemicorporelles: Resultats chez 92 patientes porteuses de cancer du sein polymetastatique traitees a l'Institut Curie. Colloque International sur la Radiotherapie dans les Pays en Developpement: Situations et Tendances. Vienne: Agence Internationale de l'Energie Atomique, 1–5 Septembre 1986.

24. Duchesne GM, Harmer CL: Hemibody irradiation in lymphomas and related malignancies. Int J Radiat Biol Phys 1985;11:2003.

25. Steele G: Combined modality therapy for rectal carcinoma: The time has come (editorial). N Engl J Med 1991;324:764.

26. Mendenhall WM, Million RR, Pfaff WW: Patterns of recurrence in adenocarcinoma of the rectum and rectosigmoid treated with surgery alone: Implications in treatment planning with adjuvant radiation therapy. Int J Radiat Oncol Biol Phys 1983;9:977.

27. Overgaard M, Overgaard J, Sell A: Dose-response relationship for radiation therapy of recurrent, residual, and primarily inoperable colorectal cancer. Radiother Oncol 1984;1:217.

28. Taylor RE, Kerr GR, Arnott SJ: External beam radiotherapy for rectal adenocarcinoma. Br J Surg 1987; 74:455.

29. Halle JS, Rosenman JG, Varia MA et al: 1000 cGy single dose palliation for advanced carcinoma of the cervix or endometrium. Int J Radiat Oncol Biol Phys 1986;12:1947.

30. Reed RC, Lowery GS, Nordstrom DG: Single high dose-large field irradiation for palliation of advanced malignancies. Int J Radiat Oncol Biol Phys 1988; 15:1243.

31. Wijkstrom H, Naslund I, Ekman P et al: Short-term radiotherapy as palliative treatment in patients with transitional cell bladder cancer. Br J Urol 1991;67:74.

32. Rostom AY, Pradhan DG, White WF: Once weekly irradiation in breast cancer. Int J Radiat Oncol Biol Phys 1987;13:551.

33. Timothy AR: Workshop on consensus guidelines for management of lung cancer. Clinical Oncology 1990;2:97.

34. Report to the Medical Research Council by its Lung Cancer Working Party: Inoperable non-small cell lung cancer (NSCLC): A Medical Research Council randomised trial of palliative radiotherapy with two fractions or ten fractions. Br J Cancer 1991;63:265.

35. Latini P, Maranzano E, Ricci S et al: Role of radiotherapy in metastatic spinal cord compression: Preliminary results from a prospective trial. Radiother Oncol 1989;15:227.

36. Williams MP, Cherryman GR, Husband JE: Magnetic resonance imaging in suspected metastatic spinal cord compression. Clin Radiol 1989;40:286.

37. Findlay GFG: Adverse effects of the management of malignant spinal cord compression. J Neurol Neurosurg Psychiatry 1984;47:761.

38. Weissman DE: Glucocorticoid treatment for brain metastases and epidural spinal cord compression: A review. J Clin Oncol 1988;6:543.

39. Sharr MM, Garfield JS: Management of intracranial metastases. Br Med J 1978;1:1535.

40. Hendrickson FR, Lee M-S, Larson M et al: The influence of surgery and radiation therapy on patients with brain metastases. Int J Radiat Oncol Biol Phys 1983;9:623.

41. Patchell RA, Tibbs PA, Walsh JW et al: A randomized trial of surgery in the treatment of single metastases to the brain. N Engl J Med 1990;322:494.

42. Sham JST, Lau WH, Tung Y: Radiotherapy of brain metastases from carcinoma of the bronchus. Clin Radiol 1989;40:193.

43. Hoskin PJ, Crow J, Ford HT: The influence of extent and local management on the outcome of radiotherapy for brain metastases. Int J Radiat Oncol Biol Phys 1990;19:111.

44. Borgelt B, Gelber R, Kramer S et al: The palliation of brain metastases: Final results of the first two studies by the Radiation Therapy Oncology Group. Int J Radiat Oncol Biol Phys 1980;6:1.
45. Kurtz JM, Gelber R, Brady LW et al: The palliation of brain metastases in a favourable patient population: A randomised clinical trial by the Radiation Therapy Oncology Group. Int J Radiat Oncol Biol Phys 1981; 7:891.
46. Retsas S, Gershuny AR: Central nervous system involvement in malignant melanoma. Cancer 1988; 61:1926.
47. Rate WR, Solin LJ, Turissi AT: Palliative radiotherapy for metastatic malignant melanoma: Brain metastases, bone metastases, and spinal cord compression. Int J Radiat Oncol Biol Phys 1988;15:859.
48. Choi KN, Withers HR, Rotman M: Metastatic melanoma in brain: Rapid treatment or large dose fractions. Cancer 1985;56:10.
49. Kearsley JH: Cytotoxic chemotherapy for common adult malignancies: "The emperor's new clothes" revisited? Br Med J 1986;293:871.
50. Braverman AS: Medical oncology in the 1990's. Lancet 1991; i 337:901.

Chapter 16

Systemic Therapy (Chemotherapy) in the Palliative Treatment of Cancer Pain

Michael R. Kurman

INTRODUCTION

It is both unfortunate and singularly illogical that in discussions concerning therapeutic options in the treatment of cancer-related pain, systemic therapy directed against the pain-producing malignancy is so infrequently mentioned. When faced with difficult patient management problems, clinicians have always been taught to "treat the underlying disease," and this valuable clinical saw is as true for the treatment of cancer-related pain as it is for any other disease condition. Unfortunately, clinicians attempting to deal with the problem of cancer pain seem sometimes to have forgotten this worthy advice. That this condition in fact prevails and is not simply a personal bias is evidenced by the content of numerous seminars, symposia, texts, monographs, reviews, and position papers dealing with cancer-related pain, almost none of which even mention, much less give appropriate emphasis to, the use of systemic antineoplastic therapy as part of the treatment of such pain. A recent review of the *Index Medicus* for the last 5 years under the headings "Pain," "Intractable Pain," and "Palliative Care" turned up only 10 articles that dealt with systemic antineoplastic treatment for cancer-related pain. In addition, the author of a recent review article on the treatment of cancer pain with systemically administered antineo-

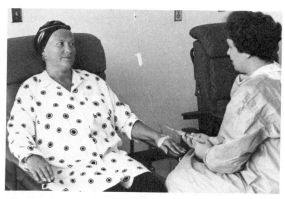

Figure 16–1. Patient with breast cancer, widely metastatic to the bone and marrow, receiving palliative chemotherapy.

plastic agents noted that searches of two computer-linked data bases, Medline and Cancerline, under the heading "Management of Pain in Cancer Patients with Hormones and Chemotherapy," turned up not a single title.[1] By the weight of this evidence, then, it would seem that in the minds of many clinicians thoughts of alleviating the pain caused by a malignancy and of eradicating the malignancy itself rarely, if ever, exist concurrently. Why and how this dichotomous way of thinking about the treatment of cancer-related pain arose is not clear. It certainly can not be because effective systemic therapy for cancer is new or novel (Fig. 16–1); such therapy has been available for over 25 years.[2] Nor can it be due to a lack of understanding regarding the manner in which malignancies cause pain, as this relationship has been understood since the days of the ancient Greeks. This view may relate to the difficulty many clinicians have regarding the often dual nature of the therapeutic process. During training, clinicians are taught to fragment their thinking about disease processes, to disassemble them to make them easier to understand and manage. Cancers, in particular, are commonly divided into those that are either curable or incurable (with the latter frequently considered synonymous with "terminal"), and ideas regarding the treatment of these two states take on a similar "either/or" aspect. No doubt because of its

frequency in patients with terminal malignancies, pain is often associated with this phase of the disease, when efforts at antineoplastic therapy have been exhausted. The treatment of pain, then (perhaps through a kind of guilt by association), becomes associated with that portion of the malignant process for which further antineoplastic therapy is futile.

What clinicians often fail to remember, however, is that pain is the symptom that most frequently brings a neoplasm to the attention of the patient and physician,[3] and is common in the earliest stages of a patient's disease, when options for antineoplastic therapy are still myriad, as well as at the end, when such choices are no longer always available. Even in those patients (admittedly, with selected malignancies) considered to have far advanced disease, dramatic and durable tumor responses, with alleviation of any coincidental tumor-causing pain, are not only possible but commonplace. In short, cancer is not two diseases, or even one disease with two clearly delineated phases, one of which is characterized by cure and the other by care, but many different diseases, each of which exists on a continuum of therapeutic options. Whether a patient is treated with systemic antineoplastic therapy, analgesics, symptomatic adjuvants, or some combination depends on the physician's knowledge of the underlying pathophysiology of the disease process and the clinical condition of the patient, not on some preconceived notion of which malignancies are curable or not curable. What needs to be kept foremost in the minds of clinicians treating patients with cancer is that despite the fact that many cancers today remain incurable, few cancers are *untreatable*, and that with properly applied antineoplastic therapy, a great deal of symptomatic palliation can be achieved.

The following pages discuss the roles of systemic treatments (pharmacologic agents such as chemotherapy and hormonal therapy, as well as surgical procedures with systemic effects) in the care of patients with cancer-related pain. Some understanding of the pharmacology and general clinical effects of available chemotherapeutic and hormonal agents will be assumed, as an in-depth discussion of these agents would be beyond the scope of this book; for a more detailed description of the action of these compounds, the reader is referred to several excellent recent reviews.[4-7] In addition to discussions of specific disease entities and therapeutic options, broader issues, such as those relating to the use of appropriate outcome measurements, cost-effectiveness, patient selection, and timing of treatment, as they apply to the use of systemic antineoplastic modalities in the treatment of cancer-related pain, will be touched on. Ultimately, however, each physician will have to rely on his or her knowledge, clinical judgment, and compassion in making the difficult decisions involved in the care and treatment of patients with cancer-related pain.

ISSUES IN PALLIATIVE SYSTEMIC ANTINEOPLASTIC THERAPY

WHO TO TREAT

Deciding which patient would be an appropriate candidate for palliative systemic antineoplastic therapy is often the most challenging in a series of difficult decisions that must be made. There are several reasons for this. First, although there are fairly extensive data on the effect that various treatments have on specific cancers, there are very few data on how a patient's clinical condition affects his or her ability to tolerate that treatment, an issue that may be more important than whether or not the patient's malignancy actually responds. Second, even if specific data were available, such information from clinical trials or the medical literature may not be pertinent in a given patient. Third, there may be psychosocial issues, such as a patient's desire for treatment (despite being advised by the physician that such treatment is ineffective and toxic) that may have to be taken into consideration. Finally, the physician will require extensive knowledge of the clinical course, pathophysiology, biology, and response rates to various systemic treatments of the underlying malignancy in order to make an informed

decision as to whether or not a particular patient is a candidate for treatment. In the final analysis, then, the physician must use his or her judgment in deciding who to treat palliatively with systemic antineoplastic therapy, and what follows can only be considered a set of imperfect guidelines.

In considering antineoplastic therapy that is strictly palliative in intent, toxicity and the ability of a particular patient to tolerate that toxicity are particularly important. Perhaps one of the best indicators of how well a patient will tolerate treatment is their performance status. The performance status is a global assessment of a patient's functional abilities, and although it is a highly subjective measure, its reliability for predicting treatment tolerance (and in many cases treatment response and even survival) has been demonstrated numerous times.[8,9] There currently are two scales used to evaluate performance status, the Eastern Cooperative Oncology Group (ECOG) Scale,[10] and the Karnofsky Scale[11] (see Chapter 30). Both are equally reliable and measure essentially the same parameters. Although scoring of the performance status depends on the patient's ability to report or the physician's ability to observe the functional capacity of the patient (eg, ability to work, to care for oneself, etc.), implicit in the performance status are all those cancer-associated factors that affect the physical status of the patient, such as weight loss, cachexia, pain, organ dysfunction, side effects of medications, and intercurrent illnesses. That these factors are reflected by performance status scores is in large part what contributes to their use as a predictive tool. A patient with an ECOG Performance Status of 3 or 4, or a Karnofsky Performance Status of less than 50, is likely to tolerate systemic antineoplastic therapy poorly, and has little chance of responding to such therapy, shifting the risk-to-benefit ratio in favor of withholding treatment. Tumor histology is a factor that is probably almost equally as important as the performance status for making decisions about who to treat with palliative antineoplastic therapy. Clearly, there are metastatic malignancies for which there is not even marginally active therapy (*eg*, renal cell carcinoma, pancreatic carcinoma). Since all systemic therapies have some side effects, in the absence of any possibility of efficacy, treatment can result *only* in side effects and a reduced quality of life for the patient. If in the investigator's opinion it is appropriate, such patients may still be recommended for entrance into clinical trials evaluating new therapies, but in the absence of access to such a trial, the risk-to-benefit ratio of currently available agents would again outweigh any decision to undertake systemic treatment. Difficulties arise when a treatment has marginal efficacy, but still has significant toxicity, such as chemotherapy for non-small-cell lung carcinoma. In these cases, it is the judgment of the physician, in conjunction with the informed wishes of the patient, that will determine if systemic therapy is appropriate.

The third factor that affects whether or not a patient is a candidate for systemic antineoplastic therapy is the patient's history of prior therapy. The chance of a malignancy responding to therapy decreases with each successive treatment. This is due not only to progression of the disease itself, with an attendant effect on the performance status, but also to progressive resistance by the tumor itself to the effects of different drugs, a phenomenon called multidrug resistance (MDR), or pleiotropic resistance.[12] Many tumors produce a membrane-bound protein (the product of the *mdr* gene) that allows the cancer cell actually to exclude many different chemotherapy compounds. Such resistant cells are frequently present at the time of diagnosis, but as a minority population of the tumor. With each successive treatment, however, there is destruction of those cells that are not resistant, and resistant cells become selected for, overgrow, and eventually become the dominant population in the tumor. At this point, further therapy usually is ineffective. In addition to the mechanism of resistance due to the product of the *mdr* gene, other mechanisms of resistance exist,[13] and the clinical effects of such resistance become more pronounced with each successive attempt at treatment.

Not only does the probability of response

decrease with each successive treatment, but the ability to tolerate treatment decreases as well. Of particular importance in this regard is bone marrow reserve, or the ability of the bone marrow stem cell population to repopulate the marrow with hematopoietic tissue after treatment. Successive chemotherapy often reduces this reserve, and a point may be reached where further cytotoxic treatment would result in complete marrow aplasia. Cumulative toxicity from antineoplastic therapy can also be manifested by reduced capacity of the lungs,[14] heart,[15] and kidneys,[16] further limiting the ability to continue treatment. Prior treatment history, then, because of its impact on both probability of response and ability to tolerate toxicity, must be factored into any equation that is used to determine whether or not a patient is a candidate for palliative systemic antineoplastic therapy.

WHEN TO TREAT

The decision of when to initiate treatment, although complex, is not as complex as the decision of whom to treat. This is because the decision on when to treat is based on readily available and objective knowledge about the disease process, as well as (at least for the individual patient) some well defined feedback from the patient about his or her clinical condition (*ie*, some symptom, such as pain, that now requires medical intervention). Of these two factors, patient requests for symptomatic relief are by far the more important. However, against the background of patient symptoms, the physician also must have knowledge of the stage and the biologic behavior of the disease in the patient in question. As an example, a patient with a cancer that often responds to systemic therapy may be highly symptomatic from a single metastatic focus. A short course of radiation, or even a surgical extirpation, coupled with analgesics, may alleviate the patient's symptoms for a prolonged period of time, sparing the patient the toxicity of systemic therapy, and allowing the clinician further treatment options in the future when the disease recurs more extensively. Prostate cancer is an excellent example of a malignancy that is highly responsive to hormonal therapy, but where early treatment of metastatic disease does not confer a survival advantage and leaves only a depleted therapeutic armamentarium when treatment for symptomatic disease is needed. The clinician, then, needs to know when to unleash the arsenal of systemic therapeutics, and when a more localized course of treatment would suffice. Often, the need for systemic treatment will be obvious, as a patient's symptoms will frequently parallel the stage of his or her malignancy. Circumspection is required, however, when a patient is symptomatic from a small tumor burden, or when a patient with a large tumor burden remains asymptomatic. In such circumstances, any urge to commence systemic treatment must be checked until the patient's clinical condition is such that maximal symptomatic relief can be expected.

WHEN TO STOP TREATMENT

Having embarked on a course of therapy, clinicians often feel compelled to "see it through," although when discussing issues in palliative therapy of cancer, such a phrase seems uniquely ridiculous. It is not clear why this situation exists, or how prevalent it truly is, but many patients continue to receive systemic antineoplastic therapy long after it has any probability of demonstrating any efficacy. Perhaps this phenomenon relates to a type of "medical inertia," such that it is harder to begin or terminate a course of treatment than it is to maintain it. Clinicians may also feel that continued therapy is desired by the patient despite decreasing efficacy and increasing toxicity. Finally, it may be difficult for a physician to admit that his or her efforts have not been successful, or to discuss such unsuccessful efforts with the patient, and so in order to avoid facing an emotionally painful experience, a potentially physically harmful one is continued. As with many of the decisions regarding the patient with cancer, there are no specific signs or symptoms that tell a physician when

further attempts at systemic antineoplastic therapy should be abandoned. Once again, the physician's judgment, knowledge of the disease and the patient, and his or her own values and feelings will guide him or her in this decision. Often, it is the patient that will ask to be removed from treatment because of inability to tolerate its associated side effects. However, if such requests are not forthcoming despite clear evidence that a patient's clinical condition is declining, then, in keeping with the dictum of *primum non nocere* (priority not to do further harm), the treating physician should seriously consider suggesting to the patient that further systemic therapy be discontinued.

COST-EFFECTIVENESS ISSUES

In an era of expanding medical technology, when our potential ability to manage illness may seem at times almost limitless, considerations of resource allocation have taken on increased importance. Whether we like to admit it or not, there is a finite amount of money that society (or even the individual, for that matter) is willing or able to expend for medical care. Cost-effectiveness analysis attempts to help in deciding how much it is appropriate to spend on medical care by measuring what various medical outcomes cost—how much medical "bang" we get for our buck. Such analysis makes no judgment about the value of any potential outcomes; such a decision is left up to those responsible for payment,[17] whether that is society or the individual. It merely determines what those outcomes cost.

Although the treatment of cancer is expensive,[18] and it is relatively easy to determine what is spent each year on its diagnosis and treatment, it is very difficult to determine what we are getting for our cancer dollars. There are very few studies that have focused on the cost-effectiveness of cancer treatment,[19,20] and most of those have looked at adjuvant therapy, not treatment in advanced disease. Intuitively, however, systemic therapy that is applied for palliative purposes results, for the vast majority of cases, in outcomes that will be restricted to small changes in the quality and/or quantity of life. When one takes into account the potential for serious toxicity inherent in much of systemic cancer treatment, it is not too difficult to develop at least a rough idea of the cost-effectiveness of a particular treatment administered to a specific patient in a given set of clinical circumstances. It should be emphasized that there is no right or wrong decision based on cost-effectiveness analysis, rather only a decision as to whether some potential result is justified by the cost, both in terms of the economic cost and the likelihood of toxicity. Such decisions will vary from patient to patient and physician to physician, based on their individual values. The concept of cost-effectiveness is presented here merely as another guide on the difficult path of clinical decision-making in the palliative care of the cancer patient.

MEASUREMENT OF RESPONSE

The issue of which criteria should be used to measure treatment response in oncology has been raging since systemic treatment first became available. Over the years, emphasis has shifted from tumor response, as determined by shrinkage of tumors measurable by physical examination or radiographic imaging, to survival, and, recently, back again to tumor response when this parameter is used under certain circumstances. Although survival remains the end point least subject to observer bias, and in most circumstances is the one most important to the physician and the patient, when discussing issues of palliation, the fact that a therapy can cause a tumor to regress (and, it is hoped, alleviate symptoms caused by the presence of that tumor) may be more important than whether or not such a therapy can have an impact on survival. To oncologists, the term "response" has a fairly clear, mathematically qualified, meaning, and a response may occur to two quantitatively different degrees[21]: a complete response represents the disappearance of all malignant disease, determined by two observations not less than 4 weeks apart; a partial response is a 50%

decrease in the sum of the products of the perpendicular diameters of all measurable lesions, determined by two observations not less than 4 weeks apart. Anything less than these two conditions is either progression (a 25% or more increase in the size of one or more measurable lesions or the appearance of new lesions), or stable disease. For the purposes of the discussion that follows, then, response will be the treatment end point emphasized as being adequate for purposes of palliation; where such treatment also has a positive effect on survival, such an effect will be noted.

TREATMENT OF SPECIFIC NEOPLASMS

INTRODUCTION

Although many malignancies today will respond to systemic treatment, the following discussion will be limited to those malignancies that are not curable in the advanced stage, but for which there is clinically relevant systemic therapy, and which often cause pain. Malignancies such as Hodgkin's disease, non-Hodgkin's lymphoma, and nonseminomatous germ cell tumors, which are curable even in advanced stages; chronic myeloid leukemia, which is not curable but rarely causes pain; and gastric, esophageal, and non-small-cell lung carcinomas, on which systemic therapy has had a marginal impact, are therefore excluded. It is hoped that the principles underlying the treatment of the following cancers will be sufficiently broad to be able to guide the practitioner when effective systemic treatment for some of the above conditions becomes available.

BREAST CANCER

Introduction

Because of the possibility of significant survival despite the presence of metastatic disease, and therefore a prolonged period of time during which a patient might be symptomatic, the palliative treatment of advanced breast cancer has assumed an expanded role in the overall treatment of this disease. Although metastatic disease, particularly to skin or lymph nodes, may be asymptomatic, the most common site of metastases (*ie*, bone) is often associated with pain. Between 40% and 60% of patients with metastatic breast cancer will have bony disease, and in many of these patients, the involved bones (vertebrae, femoral and humoral shafts, the acetabular area) are those that are most involved in motion, ambulation, and activities of daily living.[22] Moreover, several studies have shown that patients with metastatic breast cancer and bone involvement as their only site of metastatic disease have median survivals on the order of 27–29 months, during which time pain may be the chief manifestation of the disease.[23] Effective palliative treatment, then, is a legitimate and important therapeutic goal in metastatic breast cancer. Fortunately, such effective and well-tolerated systemic therapy exists today for the patient with breast cancer. A recently published text on breast cancer goes so far as to say that "undoubtedly, systemic therapy may relieve most, if not all, symptoms in patients with metastatic disease."[24] Knowing which patient will benefit from which available therapy, however, does require a brief review of the biology of metastatic breast cancer.

The Natural History of Metastatic Breast Cancer

The issues involved in the use of systemic therapy in the palliative treatment of cancer in general, as outlined in the first part of this chapter, assume particular importance when discussing patients with metastatic breast cancer because of the potentially long survival of such patients. Even patients with pulmonary metastases have median survivals on the order of 18–23 months,[25] and patients with only unilateral pleural involvement on the order of 44 months.[26] The clinician, then, will most likely have a long relationship with the patient with metastatic breast cancer, and will have

the opportunity to follow the course and progression of the disease. The importance of this cannot be overemphasized, as it is this course (in conjunction with any symptoms experienced by the patient) that should guide the therapeutic maneuvers of the physician in the palliative treatment of the patient. For the sake of simplicity, patients with metastatic breast cancer can be divided into two, somewhat broad, but clinically useful, categories: those with indolent disease or disease not immediately life-threatening, and those with rapidly progressing or extensive vital organ disease. In the former group, often characterized by bone, skin, soft-tissue, or minimal lung involvement, long disease-free intervals from the time of original diagnosis to appearance of metastatic lesions, and the postmenopausal state, the clinician has the luxury of following the patient over several weeks or months to assess the tempo of the disease and any attendant symptoms. Often, unless there is widespread bony metastatic disease, mild, nonopioid analgesics or spot radiation therapy may control symptoms adequately. As evidence generally is lacking that early systemic therapy prolongs survival in these patients, systemic therapy may be held in abeyance until less toxic or aggressive treatment modalities lose their effectiveness. Those patients whose disease is rapidly progressing, however, or who have extensive lung or liver involvement with imminent danger of vital organ compromise, should have systemic therapy initiated promptly. Knowledge of the natural history of the disease, then, is extremely important in determining the *timing* of treatment. As will be discussed below, it is important in the selection of treatment, as well.

The Estrogen Receptor

The growth dependence of certain breast cancers on the presence of circulating estrogens has been appreciated from both clinical and laboratory observations for almost 100 years.[27] Efforts to alter the endocrine milieu have resulted in responses in about one-third of otherwise unselected patients with metastatic breast cancer. However, a better understanding of the mechanism of why selected patients respond to endocrine therapy, and knowing which patients will respond in advance of therapy, has only recently been elucidated. In the early 1960s, Jensen et al discovered an estrogen-binding protein or receptor, on the surface of the cells of estrogen-sensitive tissues.[28] Since then, the estrogen receptor has been identified in many tissues, including breast cancer tumors. Other hormone-binding receptor proteins, such as for progestins and glucocorticoids, may also be present on the surface of breast cancer cells. When a particular hormone binds to its receptor, a series of biochemical signals are sent to the cell's nucleus, resulting in new RNA and protein synthesis that presumably has various physiologic effects on the cell, including the ability to maintain growth.[29] All endocrine therapies in breast cancer have as their ultimate goal disruption of this process, either by interfering with the binding of estrogen to its receptor on the breast cancer cell (by reducing the amount of circulating estrogen available for binding, or by blocking the receptor with a biochemically inactive molecule), or by affecting postbinding events. As such, since estrogen receptor-positive (ER+) cells depend on binding estrogen for their continued growth, interference with estrogen binding prevents the cell from dividing, and is the basis for the response seen after hormonal therapy in patients with ER+ breast cancer.

Subsequent studies have demonstrated that the presence of the ER correlates with other clinical characteristics of breast cancer, such as age (ER+ tumors are more common in women over the age of 50),[30] menopausal status (ER+ tumors are more common in postmenopausal patients),[31] labeling index (LI; ER+ tumors have a lower LI),[32] disease-free interval (DFI; ER+ tumors have a longer DFI),[33] and metastatic site (ER+ tumors have a lower incidence of visceral metastases).[34] Most importantly, the ER identifies those patients most likely to respond to endocrine manipulation. About one-third of unselected patients with metastatic breast cancer will respond to hormonal therapy; this number rises

to approximately 50%–60% when only ER+ patients are selected, and rises further to about 75% when both ER+ and progestin receptor-positive patients are selected.[35] Estrogen receptor-negative (ER−) patients have a response rate to hormonal therapy of only 5%–10%. Patients' ER status therefore allows the clinician to select with greater certainty those individuals who might benefit from hormonal therapy, and those who should proceed directly to chemotherapy.

Hormonal Therapy of Metastatic Breast Cancer

Before discussing specific hormonal therapies, a few general principles of endocrine therapy in breast cancer should be stated. First, because of its lower toxicity compared to cytotoxic chemotherapy, hormonal therapy should be the first therapeutic modality used in the appropriately selected patient with metastatic breast cancer. The operative phrase, however, is "in the appropriately selected patient." The most important selection criterion for the use of hormonal therapy is a positive estrogen receptor. If the ER status is unknown, its presence may be inferred by other clinical characteristics. Estrogen receptor-positive tumors are known to be associated with: long disease-free intervals; age greater than 50; menopause; slow growth of metastatic lesions; and bone and soft-tissue metastases. If these characteristics are present, there is a high likelihood that the tumor will be ER+, and a trial of hormonal therapy may be initiated. Second, relapse or progression during therapy with a particular hormonal agent does not mean a patient is refractory to hormonal therapy in general. In fact, second and even third responses may be elicited with alternative hormonal agents, although the duration of response generally diminishes with each new agent.[36] As long as a patient on hormonal therapy has not developed rapidly progressive visceral disease, a second attempt at eliciting a response with an alternative hormonal therapy should be attempted. Third, with certain specific exceptions mentioned below, in general, all hormonal agents have approximately the same response rate in patients with metastatic disease; numerous studies have failed to demonstrate convincingly the superiority of one hormonal agent over another in terms of efficacy. The selection of one therapy over another, then, should be based on toxicity profile, patient compliance, and a patient's prior history of endocrine therapy.

Oophorectomy. Surgical castration generally is recommended only for premenopausal patients, and results in a response rate of 33%; similar results may be obtained by ovarian radiation.[37] Operative mortality is generally low, and the side effects of oophorectomy are simply those of menopause: hot flashes, vaginal dryness, etc. The use of oophorectomy has declined somewhat in recent years in favor of treatment with tamoxifen, as studies have demonstrated equal effectiveness in premenopausal patients with a comparable toxicity profile.[38] Use of tamoxifen also avoids hospitalization, and the (small but significant) risks of surgery. Oophorectomy remains, however, a viable endocrine treatment in the patient who cannot, or does not wish to take oral medication, or whose compliance with such medication may be in question. Other ablative techniques, such as adrenalectomy and hypophysectomy, are rarely, if ever, performed any longer due to their high operative risk, potentially life-threatening side effects, and the advent of active second- and third-line hormonal agents and effective cytotoxic chemotherapy.

Androgens. Although they have some efficacy in the treatment of metastatic breast cancer, androgens have not been shown to be as active as other hormonal therapies.[39] To varying degrees, all have masculinizing side effects, including hirsutism, male-pattern baldness, acne, nausea, fluid retention, and weight gain. For these reasons, androgens mostly have been relegated to second- or third-line status in the hormonal therapy of breast cancer. The currently recommended androgen is fluoxymesterone (Halotestin; Upjohn, Kalamazoo, MI) administered orally in a dose of 10 mg twice daily.

Estrogens. For much of this century, estrogen therapy was the preferred mode of hormonal treatment in postmenopausal women with metastatic breast cancer. The response rate in otherwise unselected postmenopausal patients is on the order of 26%.[40] Like androgens, however, estrogens are associated with several undesirable side effects, including breast tenderness, nausea, vomiting, anorexia, vaginal bleeding, and fluid retention, and so also have been consigned to secondary roles in the treatment of metastatic disease. Currently used estrogen regimens are diethylstilbestrol 5 mg administered orally three times a day, ethinyl estradiol 1 mg orally twice daily, or Premarin (Ayerst Laboratories, New York, NY) 2.5 mg orally three times a day. One curious aspect of estrogen therapy is the estrogen withdrawal phenomenon, or secondary response, seen when the estrogen is discontinued in patients who have progressed while on estrogen.[41] For this reason, patients who progress while on estrogen therapy should be observed after discontinuing such therapy and before initiation of a new treatment.

Antiestrogens. Antiestrogens exert their effects by binding to the estrogen receptor on the surface of the breast cancer cell, thereby preventing estrogens from exerting their growth-promoting effects. Tamoxifen (Nolvadex; ICI Pharma, Wilmington, DE) is the only antiestrogen currently commercially available in the United States, although other antiestrogens are currently in the development stage. It is administered orally in a dose of 10 mg twice a day. Because of its excellent record of safety and efficacy, tamoxifen is the first-line endocrine treatment of choice in metastatic breast cancer. In otherwise unselected patients, tamoxifen has a response rate of approximately 30%, but this rises to 50% in patients who are ER+.[42] Tamoxifen has also demonstrated activity in premenopausal women with metastatic breast cancer.[43] Although this degree of efficacy may be duplicated by other hormonal treatments in breast cancer, tamoxifen's chief attraction is its safety. Side effects are for the most part limited to mild nausea and hot flashes. Tamoxifen can induce a tumor "flare," or transient worsening of metastatic disease, usually manifested by worsening bone pain or hypercalcemia in patients with bone metastases, due to its weak agonist properties (see Chapter 1). However, the flare usually passes in a few weeks, and in any event often is predictive of ultimate response.

Progestins. In physiologic doses, progestins are believed to stimulate growth of experimental breast cancers. However, in pharmacologic doses, they are clearly growth-inhibiting, in both the experimental and clinical settings. It is not clear how progestins exert their antitumoral effect, although they may alter the ability of estrogens to bind to the estrogen receptor, or even interfere with some postbinding phenomenon.[44] The two most commonly used progestins for the treatment of metastatic breast cancer are medroxyprogesterone acetate, or MPA, and megestrol acetate (Megace; Bristol-Myers Oncology Division, Evansville, IN). Megestrol acetate, in orally administered doses of 40 mg four times a day, has a response rate of approximately 30% in otherwise unselected patients,[45] but it should be noted that in several of these trials, the patients who received megestrol acetate had been pretreated by other endocrine agents. Medroxyprogesterone acetate has been reported to have response rates of approximately 25% in the recommended dose of 500 mg per day. Whether larger doses result in improved response rates has been explored in several clinical trials, the results of which are conflicting.[46] The most bothersome side effect of the progestational agents is weight gain, which occurs in about 10%–25% of patients[47]; other side effects include vaginal bleeding and nausea. Although progestins such as megestrol acetate usually are used as second-line endocrine agents, numerous studies have shown that they are equal in effectiveness to tamoxifen when used as first-line treatment.

Cytotoxic Chemotherapy

An extensive discussion of the cytotoxic therapy of breast cancer is clearly beyond the scope of this book, and the interested reader is referred to several excellent reviews.[48,49] However, because cytotoxic chemotherapy plays such an important role in the palliative therapy of metastatic breast cancer, a few points concerning its use are warranted.

1.   There is no specific time when cytotoxic therapy should be instituted. Obviously, in the patient who is ER−, or who has rapidly progressive visceral disease, cytotoxic therapy may be the first treatment of choice for metastatic disease. However, in the ER+ patient, use of cytotoxics will depend on such factors as the age and overall clinical status of the patient, predominant sites of metastases, and prior treatment history.
2.   There is no clear-cut evidence that multiagent chemotherapy consistently results in better response rates than single-agent therapy, particularly when single agents are used in doses designed to achieve toxicity equivalent to that of the combination.
3.   Several studies have demonstrated the superiority of doxorubicin-containing regimens, although the differences in response rates, time to progression, etc., usually are not statistically significant.[50] It should be remembered, however, that doxorubicin is the single most active agent in the chemotherapeutic treatment of breast carcinoma. Paradoxically, because of doxorubicin's superiority, some clinicians believe in using this agent as second-line cytotoxic chemotherapy in an effort to induce secondary responses after treatment with a nondoxorubicin-containing regimen.

Several cytotoxic chemotherapeutic regimens are presented in Table 16–1.

SMALL-CELL LUNG CARCINOMA

Introduction

Small-cell lung carcinoma (SCLC) makes up approximately 25% of all lung cancers, and therefore accounts for almost 40,000 new

Table 16–1.
Combination Chemotherapy Regimens in Metastatic Breast Cancer

Regimen	Drugs*	Doses (mg/m^2)	Frequency	Response Rate (%)	Reference
"Cooper"	CTX	100 d 1–14 po	q 4 wks	50	51
	MTX	40 d 1			
	5-FU	500 d 1			
	VCR	1 d 1			
	PRED	40 d 1–21; then taper po			
CMF	CTX	600 d 1	q 3 wks	57	52
	MTX	40 d 1			
	5-FU	600 d 1			
CAF	CTX	500 d 1	q 3 wks	82	53
	DOX	50 d 1			
	5-FU	500 d 1,8			
AV	DOX	75 d 1	q 3 wks	56	52
	VCR	1.4 d 1,8			

* CTX = cyclophosphamide; MTX = methotrexate; 5-FU = fluorouracil; VCR = vincristine; PRED = prednisone; DOX = doxorubicin.

cases of lung cancer each year in the United States.[54] Small-cell lung carcinoma is a particularly virulent malignancy, and the median survival of patients treated with supportive care only is on the order of 6–12 weeks.[55] Early studies of surgery in SCLC often resulted in median survivals not terribly different from those seen in patients treated with supportive care only, and autopsy studies have shown that essentially all patients have extensive metastatic disease at death. It is held, therefore, that SCLC, even in those patients thought to have disease limited to the thorax by clinical staging techniques, is in fact a systemic disease even at presentation.[56] For the purposes of prognosis and for analyzing data from clinical studies, SCLC has been divided into limited and extensive disease categories. Limited disease is characterized by tumor that is clinically confined to the chest, mediastinum, ipsilateral supraclavicular lymph nodes, and/or contralateral supraclavicular lymph nodes. Ipsilateral pleural effusion also is considered to represent limited disease. All other sites of metastases are defined as extensive

disease.[57] As mentioned previously, the distinction is somewhat artificial, as all patients are considered to have systemic metastases at presentation; it would appear that patients with limited-stage SCLC have micrometastases, however, whereas those with extensive-stage SCLC have metastatic disease that is clinically detectable with currently available staging techniques. The median survival for patients with limited disease is on the order of 12–18 months; for extensive disease, the figure is 9 months.[58] A small number of patients with limited stage SCLC may survive for extended periods (approximately 10%–15%), whereas virtually all patients with extensive disease are dead by 2 years.[59] As we are most concerned with the palliative treatment of SCLC, the following discussion will focus primarily on the treatment of extensive-stage disease, although many of the treatment principles and clinical trial results are applicable to limited-stage disease, as well.

At presentation, approximately 60% of patients will have extensive-stage SCLC. The sites of metastatic involvement in these pa-

Table 16–2.
Involvement of Various Sites by SCLC
at Presentation

Site	Incidence (%)
Chest	90–95
Regional lymph nodes	95
Pleura	9–10
Liver	22–32
Bone	10–38
Bone marrow	17–47
Brain	8–17

Data from Spiro (1985),[60] Comis (1987),[61] and Aisner (1988).[62]

tients are shown in Table 16–2.[60–62] Chest pain, occurring in some 40% of patients (limited and extensive stages), is the most common site of pain in patients with SCLC. Pain is often poorly localized, dull in character, may radiate to the neck or back, and may be exacerbated by cough. Although there are no figures available, given the large proportion of patients with bone, liver, and central nervous system (CNS) involvement, back, rib, and right upper quadrant pain, as well as headache, all could be expected in patients with extensive-stage SCLC. In addition to pain, patients with SCLC frequently experience other severely debilitating and disturbing symptoms, such as cough, dyspnea, hemoptysis, and weight loss.

Treatment of Small-Cell Lung Carcinoma

The treatment of choice in patients with SCLC (limited or extensive stage) is systemic chemotherapy. Although rarely curative, there are few other solid tumors in adults in which chemotherapy has had as significant an impact, both in prolonging survival and alleviating symptoms, as in SCLC. Studies carried out in the 1970s demonstrated the superiority of using combinations of drugs over single

agents, and since then a variety of regimens have been examined in patients with SCLC. These multiple regimens, however, are really only variations of three or four different combinations of agents: cyclophosphamide, doxorubicin, and vincristine[63]; cis-platinum and etoposide[64]; or some combination using three or four out of these five drugs, such as cyclophosphamide, doxorubicin, and etoposide (CAE)[65]; etoposide, vincristine, doxorubicin, and cyclophosphamide (EVAC)[66]; or cis-platinum, doxorubicin, cyclophosphamide, and etoposide (PACE).[67] These regimens, with their respective response rates and median survivals for patients with extensive-stage SCLC, are shown in Table 16–3. What is most striking about these data are the fairly high response rates, yet rather poor median survivals, regardless of regimen. Faced with such overall poor survival, the choice of a particular regimen will depend on the clinical judgment of the physician and the ability of the patient to tolerate the toxicities of a given regimen. A few general principles, however, may help to guide the practitioner:

1. Despite certain regimens demonstrating a statistically significant advantage in response rates or survival times when evaluated in a direct randomized comparison to other regimens, most of these advantages are small, and probably do not represent significant *clinical* advantages. It is for this reason that among accepted treatments, any one regimen is probably as good as another.
2. Studies in patients with extensive-stage disease have not shown impressive survival advantages for those patients who received thoracic radiation in combination with chemotherapy or prophylactic whole brain irradiation.[68] Unless there are clear indications present (documented CNS metastases, rapidly progressing superior vena cava syndrome), the use of combined chemotherapy and irradiation in patients with extensive-stage SCLC should be avoided.
3. Studies using alternating, noncross-resistant regimens have failed to

Table 16–3.
Chemotherapy Regimens for Extensive-Stage SCLC

Regimen	Drugs*	Doses (mg/m²)	Response Rate (%)	Median Survival (mos.)	Reference
CAV	CTX	1000 d 1	45	8	63
	DOX	45 d 1			
	VCR	1.4 d 1			
CAE	CTX	1000 d 1	88	10	65
	DOX	45 d 1			
	VP-16	50 d 1–5			
DDP/VP-16	DDP	60 d 1	88	10	64
	VP-16	120 d 4,6,8			
EVAC	CTX	1000 d 1	85	10	66
	VCR	1.5 d 1			
	DOX	50 d 1			
	VP-16	60 d 1–5			
PACE	DDP	20 d 1–5	NA	10	67
	DOX	45 d 1			
	CTX	800 d 1			
	VP-16	50 d 1–5			

* CTX = cyclophosphamide; DOX = doxorubicin; VCR = vincristine; VP-16 = etoposide; DDP = cis-platinum.

demonstrate an advantage for these regimens in terms of response or survival when compared to single regimens given in a repetitive fashion.[69]

4. There is some evidence that after failure of CAV, patients may have secondary responses to DDP/VP-16. The converse, however, does not appear to be true. For this reason, some clinicians favor using CAV as first-line therapy, switching to DDP/VP-16 upon progression.[70]

Finally, because of the overall poor survival, regardless of the treatment regimen in patients with extensive-stage SCLC who had high response rates, in the patient whose symptoms do not demand immediate chemotherapeutic attention, it would not be inappropriate to offer such a patient the opportunity to participate in a clinical trial of a new treatment modality.

MULTIPLE MYELOMA

Introduction

Plasma cell myeloma represents a malignant proliferation of plasma cells in the bone marrow. It is the most common malignancy of lymphatic tissue in blacks, and the second most common such malignancy in whites.[71] In 1991, it is estimated that there will be over 12,000 new cases of multiple myeloma in the United States, and 9,000 deaths.[72] Because the malignant plasma cells in the marrow may secrete local factors that activate osteoclasts,[73] osteolytic lesions and pathologic fractures are a prominent feature of plasma cell myeloma. Approximately 90% of myeloma patients have radiographic evidence of bone disease, and 75% have bone pain.[74] Although there is effective therapy for myeloma, treatment generally does not result in cure, and median survival is approximately 30 months, with less than 5%

of patients surviving 10 years.[75] Treatment, therefore, even in newly diagnosed patients, is always palliative, and like systemic palliative therapy of other tumors, a knowledge of the natural history of the disease, its tempo, and the nature of the patient's symptoms should guide the clinician's decision about when and how best to treat the patient with myeloma. The majority of patients, however, will have bone pain secondary to myelomatous bone disease at diagnosis, and will require systemic treatment early in the course of the disease. Fortunately, because a reduction in the quantity of a patient's monoclonal protein parallels a reduction in myeloma cell mass, and because bone lesions tend to be osteolytic, and therefore often easily seen on plain roentgenograms, following the patient's response to therapy is not difficult. What follows is a summary of current treatment options and results in multiple myeloma; for a more detailed review of the diagnosis, natural history, and treatment of this disease, reference is made to several excellent reviews.[76,77]

Primary Therapy

Single-agent alkylating agents such as melphalan and cyclophosphamide first were shown to possess activity in multiple myeloma as far back as 1958.[78] These agents, often used in combination with glucocorticoids (which can have response rates of 44% when used alone in myeloma[79]), remain the standard of therapy against which all new agents or combinations of agents are compared. There are several dosing regimens of melphalan/prednisone (MP) combinations used in multiple myeloma, with response rates varying between 35%–55% in previously untreated patients.[80] One such regimen combines melphalan in a dose of 8 mg/m^2 orally for 4 days and prednisone 60 mg/m^2 orally for 4 days, repeated every 3–4 weeks.[81] Therapy generally is well tolerated, even by elderly patients,[82] although careful monitoring of serum glucose levels is important in this population, and in the frankly diabetic patient, prednisone may be contraindicated.

Because there is a significant proportion of patients who do not respond to MP, regimens composed of multiple alkylating agents in combination with prednisone have been evaluated in patients with multiple myeloma. The theoretical basis for using multiple alkylating agents is the observation that patients with multiple myeloma who develop resistance to one alkylating agent may respond to an alternative alkylating agent.[83] On the assumption that patients who do not respond to MP have resistant myeloma at presentation, it is postulated that by using multiple alkylating agents, such resistance may be circumvented by the addition of another alkylating agent to the regimen. These various multidrug regimens, along with their response rates and median survivals, are shown in Table 16–4. Although multidrug regimens may have higher response rates than MP (clearly an important goal when discussing palliation), not all of these regimens have been able to prolong survival significantly beyond that which has been associated with MP treatment.

Which regimen, then, should be used as primary therapy in the patient with multiple myeloma? The answer, as is often the case with complex clinical questions, is "it depends." In the good-risk patient, with a relatively low amount of paraprotein (IgG <5 g/100 ml), normal renal function, normal serum calcium, hemoglobin >10 g/100 ml, and one or a few lytic lesions on bone roentgenogram, MP probably should be the first regimen used. The characteristics of the good-risk patient are indicative of a relatively low myeloma cell mass, due either to a long doubling time, or to a very early stage of the disease. In either case, the risk of resistant cells being present is lower than in the patient with more advanced disease, and so the good-risk patient has a reasonable likelihood of responding to MP. In the patient with more advanced disease, characterized by a large amount of paraprotein (IgG >7 g/100 ml), compromised renal function (serum creatinine >2.0 mg/100 ml), elevated serum calcium, hemoglobin <8.5 g/100 ml, and/or multiple lytic lesions on bone films, the chance of melphalan resistance may be higher, and if the clinician believes the patient would tolerate a potentially greater de-

Table 16–4.
Combination Chemotherapy Regimens in Multiple Myeloma

Regimen	Drugs*	Doses (mg/m²)	Response Rate		Reference
			Frequency	(%)	
M2	VCR	1.2 d 1			
	BCNU	20 d 1			
	CTX	400 d 1	q 5 wks	74	84
	MELPH	8 d 1–4 po			
	PRED	60 d 1–4 po			
VMCP/VCAP	VCR	1 d 1			
	MELPH	6 d 1–4 po			
	CTX	125 d 1–4 po			
	PRED	60 d 1–4 po			
			alternate q 3 wks	54	85
	VCR	1 d 1			
	CTX	125 d 1–4 po			
	DOX	30 d 1			
	PRED	60 d 1–4 po			
VMCP/VBAP	VCR	1 d 1			
	MELPH	6 d 1–4 po			
	CTX	125 d 1–4 po			
	PRED	60 d 1–4 po			
			alternate q 3 wks	54	85
	VCR	1 d 1			
	BCNU	30 d 1			
	DOX	30 d 1			
	PRED	60 d 1–4 po			

* VCR = vincristine; BCNU = carmustine; CTX = cyclophosphamide; MELPH = melphalan; PRED = prednisone; DOX = doxorubicin.

gree of toxicity, one of the multiple-alkylating agent regimens may be used first.

Management of the Responding Patient

Response in myeloma usually is defined as reduction in the amount of paraprotein by 75%, and this generally will occur in from 50%–60% of patients.[86] Such a reduction in myeloma cell mass initially occurs rapidly, then slows.[87] Once a response does occur, however, systemic therapy may be reduced in intensity, or discontinued altogether. In the patient whose paraprotein is reduced by 75% but still persists beyond the normal range,

continued therapy with MP for a total of 2 years is recommended. If a patient's initial treatment was with one of the multiple-alkylating agent regimens, the patient may then be switched to MP for the remainder of the 2-year period. In the patient whose paraprotein is decreased to the normal range, treatment for three more cycles (with whatever regimen the patient began treatment with) is recommended, after which therapy may be discontinued altogether if the response persists. Follow-up should be performed in these patients every 2–3 months, with measurement of the paraprotein each time. The median time for recurrence in these patients is 14 months,[88] and 50% will have a second reduction in paraprotein levels when retreated with the initial remission induction regimen, although usually not by 75%.

Management of the Nonresponding or Progressing Patient

Patients who fail to respond to a primary treatment regimen, or who progress while on therapy with alkylating agents, should be treated with a salvage regimen, or, if eligible, be offered entry into an investigational trial. Patients who relapse while off therapy may be retreated with the regimen to which they responded initially. The secondary regimen that has had the highest success rate is a combination of vincristine, doxorubicin, and dexamethasone (VAD), which produces responses of 65%–70% in relapsing patients, although in primarily resistant patients, the response rate is only 25%.[89] The drawback to using VAD is the fact that the vincristine and doxorubicin must be administered by constant infusion, which often requires hospitalization. An alternative salvage regimen is a combination of vincristine, carmustine (BCNU), doxorubicin, and prednisone (VBAP). In one study, patients with relapsing myeloma had a 30% response rate to this regimen, although only 7% of resistant patients responded. In general, patients with primarily resistant myeloma have a poor prognosis, and in such patients, if appropriate, opportunities for treatment with newer therapeutic modalities (bone marrow transplantation, experimental therapy with monoclonal antibodies) should be explored.

COLON CARCINOMA

Introduction

Colon carcinoma is the third most commonly occurring adult malignancy. It will affect some 112,000 individuals in the United States in 1991, and will account for 53,000 deaths.[90] Until very recently, it would not have been possible to discuss the successful use of systemic therapy in patients with metastatic colon cancer, even in a palliative sense. Several recent advances in our understanding of the biochemical modulation of fluorouracil (5-FU), however, have demonstrated that palliative therapy of metastatic colon cancer may be possible for the first time.

Treatment

The mainstay of therapy of metastatic colon cancer has always been 5-FU. Given as a bolus, 5-FU originally was thought to have a response rate of 20%. However, more recent studies, using more stringent requirements for response, have revealed a response rate on the order of only about 10%. Biochemical modulation of 5-FU with leucovorin (LV) (which, *in vitro*, has been shown to result in a tighter binding of 5-FU to its target enzyme, thymidylate synthase) has been associated with response rates on the order of 30%–40% in four out of five studies performed in the United States (Table 16–5). Only one of these studies has demonstrated a survival advantage for 5-FU/LV, and these regimens are associated with a fairly high degree of toxicity, including leukopenia, stomatitis, and diarrhea, which in one trial was associated with a treatment-related death rate of 5%. Certainly not all patients with metastatic colon cancer will be candidates for such intensive treatment, and once again, the physician's clinical judgment, in conjunction with the patient's overall clinical condition, will guide the decision-making process. Nonetheless, it seems that for the first time it is possible to treat metastatic colon carcinoma palliatively with systemic therapy with the expectation of a modicum of success.

PROSTATE CARCINOMA

Introduction

There were an estimated 100,000 new cases of prostate cancer diagnosed in the United States in 1988, with 26,000 deaths, making prostate cancer the third leading cause of cancer death

Table 16–5.
5-FU/LV in Metastatic Colon Carcinoma

Study	5-FU Dose (mg/m²)	LV Dose (mg/m²)	Frequency	Response Rate (%)	Reference
Roswell Park	600	500	Weekly	48	91
GITSG*	600	500	Weekly	30	92
NCCTG†	370	20	Daily × 5 q 4–5 wks	43	93
City of Hope	370	500	Daily × 5 q 4–5 wks	44	94
NCOG‡	400	200	Daily × 5 q 4 wks	19	95

* Gastrointestinal Tumor Study Group
† North Central Cancer Treatment Group
‡ North California Oncology Group

in men.[96] Between 40%–50% of newly diagnosed patients with prostate cancer will have advanced disease (stage D), with a median survival of approximately 2.4 years.[97] In addition, 70% of patients with clinical stage C, and 30% of patients with clinical stage B prostate cancer eventually will go on to develop pelvic lymph node or distant bony metastases. Thus, a significant proportion of patients with prostate cancer either will present with, or develop, metastatic disease, and therefore will be incurable. Moreover, because of the predilection of prostate cancer to spread to bony sites, the majority of patients with metastatic disease will have bone pain.

Natural History of Prostate Cancer

Like those breast cancers dependent on estrogens for continued growth, prostate carcinoma, which often depends on androgens for continued growth, may pursue an indolent course. Even in patients with metastatic disease, median survival may surpass 2 years, and many patients will live even longer. Early studies demonstrated that instituting systemic treatment early in the course of meta-

static disease did not affect survival,[98] and conventional medical teaching calls for withholding treatment until symptoms (usually bone pain) occur. Recently, smaller studies using a very aggressive approach to treat stage D1 prostate cancer (prostate cancer that has spread to the pelvic lymph nodes but not bone) have shown a survival advantage for early treatment, but this has yet to be confirmed on a large scale. Until such time that symptoms become very bothersome, or widespread bone metastases occurs, most patients may be managed conservatively with analgesics and/or spot radiation therapy to painful sites. In addition, since prostate cancer rarely metastasizes to vital organs (having a far greater predilection to spread to bone), the clinician usually has the luxury of observing the patient to assess the tempo of the disease and the degree of patient discomfort before instituting systemic therapy. The only exceptions to this are when there is suspected impending spinal cord compression, which will require high-dose glucocorticoids with either emergency radiation or decompressive surgery, or ureteral obstruction secondary to metastases to retroperitoneal lymph nodes, which may require either ureteral stenting or nephrostomy, the choice of which would be dictated by the degree of renal compromise and extent of disease.

When systemic therapy is required, hormonal therapy is the only real option for patients with prostate cancer. Studies of various hormonal therapies have demonstrated that 80% of patients with prostate cancer have hormone-sensitive tumors.[99] Unfortunately, there is no tissue marker akin to the estrogen receptor of breast cancer, and hence it is impossible to predict which patients will respond to hormonal therapy and which will not. However, even patients with hormone-insensitive tumors rarely have rapidly progressive disease, so that a trial of hormonal therapy is always warrented, and offers little if any risk to the patient. In addition, the appearance or worsening of metastatic disease is often heralded by a rise in a serum marker for prostate cancer, prostate-specific antigen (PSA).[100] In one study, 86% of patients whose bone scans worsened had a rise in the PSA either 3 months before, or coincident with, the appearance of new areas of metastatic disease on bone scan.[101] Therefore, clinicians will often know, even before the patient develops new symptoms, that clinical deterioration is occurring, and may choose to institute treatment at that point.

Hormonal Therapy of Prostate Cancer

All hormonal therapies in prostate cancer have one final common pathway, and that is the reduction in the amount of androgens that reach the tumor. As in breast cancer, there are several hormonal therapies available to treat metastatic prostate cancer, and the choice of one over the other will depend on several issues, such as the presence of intercurrent medical illnesses in the patient, the potential side effects of therapy, the comfort of the physician in using one treatment over another, and even the psychological state of the patient. Hormonal therapy may be highly effective in prostate cancer, and remains the mainstay of treatment for metastatic disease. Often, the response to hormonal therapy is dramatic, and most clinicians who treat meta-

static prostate cancer can recall the patient whose pain was markedly diminished within hours of orchiectomy, although it is far more common to observe such a response over several weeks or even months, as in breast cancer. Unlike breast cancer, however, there is no really effective cytotoxic chemotherapy for prostate cancer, and once a tumor demonstrates hormone unresponsiveness, median survival is only about 6 months in most series.[102,103]

Orchiectomy. Orchiectomy remains an extremely effective means of treating metastatic prostate cancer. It removes over 90% of circulating testosterone, has little morbidity, is highly cost-effective compared to other therapies for prostate cancer, and remains the treatment of choice in patients in whom compliance with medication is a problem. Some even consider orchiectomy the "gold standard" by which to measure the effectiveness of all other hormonal therapies for prostate cancer. Its major drawback is the psychological impact it has on many men, especially at a time when there are safe and effective pharmacologic hormonal alternatives. It does remain, however, a highly safe, effective, and convenient treatment for metastatic prostate carcinoma.

Estrogens. Estrogens are an effective means of achieving a "medical castration" by suppressing the secretion of luteinizing hormones from the pituitary, and thereby preventing testosterone release from the testes. Diethylstilbestrol (DES), the most commonly used estrogen, may also bind to the prostate cancer cell.[104] In a now classic trial, DES in a dose of 3 mg/day was found to be as effective as a dose of 5 mg/day in treating metastatic prostate carcinoma and in reducing serum testosterone to castration levels, without causing as many of the cardiovascular side effects seen with the higher dose.[105] Whether or not DES in a dose of 1 mg/day is as effective as the 3 mg/day dose in maintaining serum testosterone at a castration level remains controversial. There is no evidence that other estrogens (estradiol, chlorotrianisene, or TACE) have any advantages over DES. Because of their potential to cause cardiovascular events (stroke, phlebitis, myocardial infarction), estrogens probably should not be used in patients who are at increased risk for such complications, particularly given the availability of several alternatives for the treatment of prostate carcinoma today.

Gonadotropin-Releasing Hormone Agonists. Gonadotropin-releasing hormone (GnRH), also known as luteinizing hormone-releasing hormone (LHRH), is a peptide secreted by the hypothalamus that stimulates the pituitary to produce luteinizing hormones, which in turn stimulates the testes to produce testosterone. Administration of a synthetic LHRH analog initially causes a rise in production of LH and testosterone, but continued treatment causes a down-regulation of LHRH receptors on the pituitary, and ultimately causes a marked decrease of LH and testosterone synthesis. The unresponsiveness of the pituitary to LHRH is so complete after chronic administration of LHRH analogs that castration levels of testosterone usually can be achieved within a few weeks of beginning LHRH analog therapy. There are several such analogs currently available, including leuprolide (Lupron; TAP Pharmaceuticals, North Chicago, IL), goserelin (Zoladex, ICI Pharma, Wilmington, DE), and several others currently under investigation. Because they are peptides, the LHRH agonists must be given by injection, and are formulated in a depot preparation that allows for monthly administration. Because these compounds initially *increase* testosterone synthesis, in weeks following initiation of therapy, the patient may experience a worsening of bone pain, and even clinical deterioration (such as development of spinal cord compression), a phenomenon known as "flare." The true incidence of flare is generally low, on the order of 7%,[106] and can be blocked by the concurrent use of an antiandrogen (see below). Several studies have shown the LHRH agonists to be as effective as orchiectomy and DES in the treatment of metastatic prostate cancer.[107,108]

Antiandrogens. The antiandrogens block the binding of testosterone and dihydrotestosterone to the androgen receptor on the prostate cancer cell. Flutamide (Eulexin; Schering-Plough, Kenilworth, NJ), Anadron, and Casodex are nonsteroidal antiandrogens; cyproterone acetate is a steroidal antiandrogen that is related to the progestins. Only flutamide is currently approved for commercial use in the United States, and Casodex is still in clinical trials. Circulating levels of testosterone increase during administration of flutamide due to an increase in luteinizing hormone levels,[109] and these drugs generally are not used as single agents in the treatment of metastatic prostate cancer. Their greatest use has come in preventing the "flare" sometimes seen with initiation of treatment with LHRH agonists, and in the treatment approach to prostate cancer known as total androgen blockade. The main side effect of flutamide is diarrhea, which occurred in 12% of patients in one large trial.[106] Flutamide is administered orally in a dose of 250 mg three times daily.

Total Androgen Blockade. Total androgen blockade is a concept proposed by Labrie[110] as a means of preventing both testicular as well as adrenal androgens from having access to the prostate cancer cell. It consists of a combination of surgical or medical castration (eg, with an LHRH analog) to remove testicular androgens, as well as the use of an antiandrogen (such as flutamide) to prevent binding of adrenal androgens to the prostate cancer cell. The use of total androgen blockade in metastatic prostate carcinoma remains somewhat controversial, chiefly because different studies have yielded different results for survival and time to progression, and even when total androgen blockade has shown to be advantageous, the advantage generally has been small, usually on the order of a few months for both parameters.[111] For some clinicians and patients, total androgen blockade may be an attractive choice because of its theoretical advantage over monotherapy. However, it does remain controversial in terms of its scientific and clinical validity.

Treatment After Progression With Primary Hormonal Therapy. At this time, there is no reliable treatment for the patient with prostate cancer who has progressed despite primary hormonal therapy. Aminoglutethimide, administered in conjunction with hydrocortisone, can inhibit the production of several adrenal steroids, although on a clinical level it is not clear how much of this effect is due to the concurrent hydrocortisone administered with aminoglutethimide.[112] Because of their ability to suppress adrenal androgens, their salutary effect on bone pain, and their ability to provide a sense of well-being, some clinicians recommend the use of glucocorticoids alone in patients with hormone-refractory prostate cancer, particularly if the prognosis for prolonged survival is poor. Ketoconazole also can inhibit adrenal androgen production,[113] but it is not clear whether low levels of adrenal androgens can be maintained for an extended period of time. Ketoconazole, in the doses needed to suppress adrenal androgen synthesis, is also associated with gastrointestinal side effects. Estramustine (Emcyt; Pharmacia, Piscataway, NJ), a combination compound consisting of an estrogen moiety and an alkylating agent moiety, has not been shown to be more effective than DES in several European trials.[114] Finally, a comment should be made on the use of cytotoxic chemotherapy in patients with hormone-refractory prostate cancer. To date, several large trials have not demonstrated conclusive efficacy of any currently available cytotoxic agents.[115] In addition, patients with hormone-refractory prostate cancer often have extensive disease, are symptomatic with pain, anorexia, and anemia, and in general are poor candidates for aggressive cytotoxic therapy.

CONCLUSION

The palliative therapy of advanced malignancy using systemic therapy is one of the most challenging tasks the practicing physician will encounter. The successful accomplishment of this task requires that the clinician possess a broad knowledge of the natural history of the patient's disease, a thorough understanding of the physiologic effects and pharmacology of systemic treatment, an intimate knowledge of the patient's medical and psychological state, and often even requires an exploration of the physician's own values. In short, it demands that we as physicians be the very best we can be for our patients.

REFERENCES

1. Fischer DS: Hormonal and chemical therapy. Clin Oncol 1984;3:55.
2. Greenspan EM: Combination cytotoxic chemotherapy in advanced disseminated breast carcinoma. J Mt Sinai Hosp 1966;33:1.
3. Dawson DM, Fischer EG: Pain. In Holland JF, Frei E (eds): Cancer Medicine, p 1205. Philadelphia, Lea and Febiger, 1982.
4. DeVita VT, Hellman S, Rosenberg SA (eds): Cancer Principles and Practice of Oncology. Philadelphia, JB Lippincott, 1985.
5. Hellmann K, Carter SK (eds): Fundamentals of Cancer Chemotherapy. New York, McGraw-Hill, 1987.
6. Chabner B (ed): Pharmacologic Principles of Cancer Treatment. Philadelphia, WB Saunders, 1982.
7. Howell A, Dodwell DJ, Anderson H: New endocrine approaches to breast cancer. Ballieres Clin Endocrinol Metab 1990;4:67.
8. Stanley KE: Prognostic factors for survival in patients with inoperable lung cancer. JNCI 1980;65:25.
9. Cullinan SA, Moertel CG, Fleming TR et al: A comparison of three chemotherapeutic regimens in the treatment of advanced pancreatic and gastric carcinoma. JAMA 1985;253:2061.
10. Zubrod CG, Schneiderman M, Frei E et al: Appraisal of methods for the study of chemotherapy in man: Comparative therapeutic trial of nitrogen mustard and triethylene thiophosphoramide. J Chronic Dis 1960;11:7.
11. Karnofsky DA, Abelmann WH, Craver LF et al: The use of the nitrogen mustards in the palliative treatment of carcinoma. Cancer 1948;1:634.
12. Moscow JA, Cowan KH: Multidrug resistance. JNCI 1988;80:14.
13. Schimke RT: Methotrexate resistance and gene amplification. Cancer 1986;57:1912.
14. Weiss RB, Muggia FM: Cytotoxic drug-induced pulmonary disease. Am J Med 1980;68:259.
15. Schwartz RG, McKenzie WD, Alexander J et al: Congestive heart failure and left ventricular dysfunction complicating doxorubicin therapy: Seven-year experience using serial radionuclide angiocardiography. Am J Med 1987;82:1109.
16. Loehrer PJ, Einhorn LH: Cisplatin. Ann Intern Med 1984;100:704.

17. Eisenberg JM: Clinical economics: A guide to the economic analysis of clinical practices. JAMA 1989; 262:2879.

18. Brown ML: The national economic burden of cancer: An update. JNCI 1990;82:1811.

19. Goodwin PJ, Feld R, Evans WK, Pater J: Cost-effectiveness of cancer chemotherapy: An economic evaluation of a randomized trial in small-cell lung cancer. J Clin Oncol 1988;6:1537.

20. Hillner BE, Smith TJ: Efficacy and cost effectiveness of adjuvant chemotherapy in women with node-negative breast cancer. N Engl J Med 1991;324:160.

21. Miller AB, Hoogstraten B, Staquet M et al: Reporting results of cancer treatment. Cancer 1981;47:201.

22. Smith IE: Recurrent disease. In Harris JR, Hellman S, Henderson IC et al (eds): Breast Diseases, p 369. Philadelphia, JB Lippincott, 1987.

23. Valagussa P, Brambilla C, Bonadonna G: Advanced breast cancer: Are the traditional stratification parameters still of value when patients are treated with combination chemotherapy? Eur J Cancer 1979; 15:565.

24. Canellos GP: Treatment of metastases. In Harris JR, Hellman S, Henderson IC et al (eds): Breast Diseases, p 385. Philadelphia, JB Lippincott, 1987.

25. Swenerton KD, Legha SS, Smith T et al: Prognostic factors in metastatic breast cancer treated with combination chemotherapy. Cancer Res 1979;39:1552.

26. Smalley RV, Lefante J, Bartolucci A et al: A comparison of cyclophosphamide, adriamycin and 5-fluorouracil (CAF) and cyclophosphamide, methotrexate, 5-fluorouracil, vincristine and prednisone (CMFVP) in patients with advanced breast cancer. Breast Cancer Res Treat 1983;3:209.

27. Beatson GW: On the treatment of inoperable cases of carcinoma of the mamma: Suggestions for a new method of treatment with illustrative cases. Lancet 1896;ii:104.

28. Jensen EV, DeSombre ER, Jongblut PW: Estrogen receptors in hormone-responsive tissues and tumors. In Wissler RW (ed): Endogenous Factors Influencing Host Tumor Balance, p 68. Chicago, University of Chicago Press, 1967.

29. Osborne CK: Receptors. In Harris JR, Hellman S, Henderson IC et al (eds): Breast Diseases, p 210. Philadelphia, JB Lippincott, 1987.

30. Fisher ER, Redmond CK, Liu H et al: Correlation of estrogen receptor and pathologic characteristics of invasive breast cancer. Cancer 1980;45:349.

31. Allegra JC, Lippman ME, Thompson EB et al: Distribution, frequency, and quantitative analysis of estrogen, progesterone, androgen, and glucocorticoid receptors in human breast cancer. Cancer Res 1979; 39:1447.

32. Meyer JS, Rao BR, Stevens SC et al: Low incidence of estrogen receptor in breast carcinomas with rapid rates of cellular replication. Cancer 1977;40:2290.

33. McCarty KS, Barton TK, Fetter BF et al: Correlation of estrogen and progesterone receptors with histologic differentiation in mammary carcinoma. Cancer 1980;46:285.

34. Qazi R, Chuang JL, Drobyski W: Estrogen receptors and the pattern of relapse in breast cancer. Arch Intern Med 1984;144:2365.

35. Lippman ME: Steroid hormone receptors and mechanisms of growth regulation of human breast cancer. In Lippman ME, Lichter AS, Danforth DN (eds): Diagnosis and Management of Breast Cancer, p 326. Philadelphia, WB Saunders, 1988.

36. Wilson AJ: Response in breast cancer to a second hormonal therapy. Reviews of Endocrine-Related Cancer 1983;14:5.

37. Henderson IC, Canellos GP: Cancer of the breast. N Engl J Med 1980;302:17.

38. Ingle JN, Krook JE, Green SJ et al: Randomized trial of bilateral oophorectomy versus tamoxifen in premenopausal women with metastatic breast cancer. J Clin Oncol 1986;4:178.

39. Henderson MD, Buroker TR, Sanson MK et al: Response of patients with carcinoma of the breast to hormonal therapy and combination chemotherapy. Surg Gynecol Obstet 1975;141:232.

40. Santen RJ, Manni A, Harvey H et al: Endocrine treatment of breast cancer in women. Endocr Rev 1990;11:221.

41. Baker LH, Vaitkevicius VK: Reevaluation of rebound regression in disseminated carcinoma of the breast. Cancer 1972;29:1268.

42. Legha SS: Tamoxifen in the treatment of breast cancer. Ann Intern Med 1988;109:219.

43. Sawka CA, Pritchard KI, Paterson AHG et al: Role and mechanism of action of tamoxifen in premenopausal women with metastatic breast carcinoma. Cancer Res 1986;46:3152.

44. Carpenter JT: Progestational agents in the treatment of breast cancer. In Osborne CK (ed): Endocrine Therapies in Breast and Prostate Cancer, p 147. Boston, Kluwer, 1988.

45. Schacter L, Rozencweig M, Canetta R et al: Megestrol acetate: Clinical experience. Cancer Treat Rev 1989;16:49.

46. Gallagher CJ, Cairnduff F, Smith IE: High dose versus low dose medroxyprogesterone acetate: A randomized trial in advanced breast cancer. Eur J Cancer Clin Oncol 1987;23:1895.

47. Tchekmedyian NM, Tait N, Moody M et al: High-dose megestrol acetate. JAMA 1987;257:1195.

48. Henderson IC: Chemotherapy for metastatic dis-

ease. In Harris JR, Hellman S, Henderson IC et al (eds): Breast Diseases, p 428. Philadelphia, JB Lippincott, 1987.

49. Davidson NE, Lippman ME: Treatment of metastatic breast cancer. In Lippman ME, Lichter AS, Danforth DN (eds): Diagnosis and Management of Breast Cancer, p 348. Philadelphia, WB Saunders, 1988.

50. Cummings FJ, Gelman R, Horton J: Comparison of CAF versus CMFP in metastatic breast cancer: Analysis of prognostic factors. J Clin Oncol 1985; 3:932.

51. Cooper RG: Combination chemotherapy in hormone resistant breast cancer. Proceedings of the American Society of Clinical Oncology 1969;10:15.

52. Brambilla C, DeLena M, Rossi A et al: Response and survival in advanced breast cancer after two non-cross-resistant combinations. Br Med J 1976;1:801.

53. Bull J, Tormey D, Li SH et al: A randomized comparative trial of adriamycin versus methotrexate in combination drug therapy. Cancer 1978;41:1649.

54. Bergsagel D, Fell R: Small-cell lung cancer is still a problem. J Clin Oncol 1984;2:1189.

55. Viollet J, Ihde DC: Systemic therapy for small-cell lung cancer: Old themes replayed, new ones awaited. J Clin Oncol 1989;7:985.

56. Aisner J, Alberto P, Bitran J et al: Role of chemotherapy in small cell lung cancer: A Consensus Report of the International Association for the Study of Lung Cancer Workshop. Cancer Treat Rep 1983; 67:37.

57. Osterlind K, Ihde DC, Ettinger DS et al: Staging and prognostic factors in small cell carcinoma of the lung. Cancer Treat Rep 1983;67:3.

58. Seifter EJ, Ihde DC: Therapy of small cell lung cancer: A perspective on two decades of clinical research. Semin Oncol 1988;15:278.

59. Markman M: Chemotherapy with curative potential in small-cell carcinoma of the lung. Hematol Oncol Clin North Am 1988;2:375.

60. Spiro SG: Symptoms and diagnostic techniques. Clin Oncol 1985;4:59.

61. Comis RL: Chemotherapy of small cell lung cancer. Principles and Practices of Oncology Updates 1987;1:1.

62. Aisner J: Chemotherapy for small-cell carcinoma of the lung. In Bitran JD, Golomb HM, Little AG et al (eds): Lung Cancer: A Comprehensive Treatise, p 307. Orlando, FL, Grune and Stratton, 1988.

63. Comis RL: Clinical trials of cyclophosphamide, etoposide, and vincristine in the treatment of small-cell lung cancer. Semin Oncol 1986;13 (Suppl 3):40.

64. Sierocki JS, Hilaris BS, Hopfen S et al: Cis-dichlorodiamineplatinum and VP-16-213: An active regimen for small cell carcinoma of the lung. Cancer Treat Rep 1979;63:1593.

65. Aisner J, Whitacre M, Van Echo DA et al: Combination chemotherapy for small cell carcinoma of the lung: Continuous versus alternating non-cross-resistant combination. Cancer Treat Rep 1982;66:221.

66. Jackson DV, Zeckan PJ, Caldwell RD et al: VP-16-213 in combination chemotherapy with chest irradiation for small-cell lung cancer: A randomized trial of the Piedmont Oncology Association. J Clin Oncol 1984; 2:1343.

67. Aisner J, Whitacre M, Abrams J et al: Doxorubicin, cyclophosphamide, etoposide and platinum, doxorubicin, cyclophosphamide, and etoposide for small-cell carcinoma of the lung. Semin Oncol 1986;13 (Suppl 3):54.

68. Turisi AT: Combined modality treatment of limited small cell lung cancer. Advances in Oncology 1988; 4:17.

69. Elliot JA, Osterlind K, Hansen HH: Cyclic alternating "non-cross-resistant" chemotherapy in the management of small cell anaplastic carcinoma of the lung. Cancer Treat Rev 1984;11:103.

70. Natale R: Alternating chemotherapy for small-cell lung cancer. Advances in Oncology 1988;4:26.

71. Pottern LM, Blattner WA: Etiology and epidemiology of multiple myeloma and related disorders. In Wiernik PH, Canellos GP, Kyle RA et al (eds): Neoplastic Diseases of the Blood, p 529. New York, Churchill Livingstone, 1985.

72. Silverberg E, Boring CC, Squires TS: Cancer Statistics. CA 1990;40:19.

73. Mundy GR, Bertolini DR: Bone destruction and hypercalcemia in plasma cell myeloma. Semin Oncol 1986;13:291.

74. Alexanina R: Diagnosis and management of multiple myeloma. In Wiernik PH, Canellos GP, Kyle RA et al (eds): Neoplastic Diseases of the Blood, p 413. New York, Churchill Livingstone, 1985.

75. Bergsagel DE: Controversies in the treatment of plasma cell myeloma. Postgrad Med J 1985;61:109.

76. Osserman EF, Merlini G, Butler VP: Multiple myeloma and related plasma cell dyscrasias. JAMA 1987;258:2930.

77. McIntyre, OR: Current concepts in cancer: Multiple myeloma. N Engl J Med 1979;301:193.

78. Blokhin N, Larionov LF, Perevodchikova NI et al: Clinical experience with sarcolysin in neoplastic disease. Ann NY Acad Sci 1958;68:1128.

79. McIntyre OR, Pajak TF, Kyle RA et al: Response rates and survival in myeloma patients receiving prednisone alone. Med Pediatr Oncol 1985;13:239.

80. Sporn JR, McIntyre OR: Chemotherapy of previously untreated multiple myeloma patients: An analysis of recent treatment results. Semin Oncol 1986;13:318.

81. Salmon SE, Hamt A, Bonnet JD et al: Alternating combination chemotherapy and levamisole improves survival in multiple myeloma: A SWOG study. J Clin Oncol 1983;1:453.

82. Cohen HJ, Bartolucci A: Age and the treatment of multiple myeloma. Am J Med 1985;79:316.

83. Bersagel DE, Cowan DH, Hasselback R: Plasma cell myeloma: Response of melphalan-resistant patients to high dose cyclophosphamide. Can Med Assoc J 1972;107:851.

84. Oken MM, Tsiatis A, Abramson N et al: Comparison of standard MP with intensive VBMCP therapy for the treatment of multiple myeloma. Proceedings of the American Society of Clinical Oncology 1984;3:270.

85. Alexanina R, Dreicer R: Chemotherapy for multiple myeloma. Cancer 1984;53:583.

86. Bergsagel DE: Plasma cell myeloma. In Williams WJ, Beutler E, Erslev AJ et al (eds): Hematology, p 1078. New York, McGraw-Hill, 1983.

87. Durie BGM, Salmon SE: Staging, kinetics and flow cytometry of multiple myeloma. In Wiernik PH, Canellos GP, Kyle RA et al (eds): Neoplastic Diseases of the Blood, p 513. New York, Churchill Livingstone, 1985.

88. Alexanina R, Salmon SE, Gutterman J: Chemoimmunotherapy for multiple myeloma. Cancer 1981;47:1923.

89. Kyle RA, Greipp PR, Gertz MA: Treatment of refractory multiple myeloma and considerations for future therapy. Semin Oncol 1986;13:326.

90. Boring CC, Squires TS, Tong T: Cancer statistics, 1991. CA 1991;41:19.

91. Petrelli N, Herrera L, Rustum Y et al: A prospective randomized trial of 5-fluorouracil versus 5-fluorouracil and high-dose leucovorin versus 5-fluorouracil and methotrexate in previously untreated patients with advanced colorectal carcinoma. J Clin Oncol 1987;5:1559.

92. Pitrelli N, Douglass HO, Herrera L et al: The modulation of fluorouracil with leucovorin in metastatic colorectal carcinoma: A prospective randomized phase III trial. J Clin Oncol 1989;7:1419.

93. Poon MA, O'Connell MJ, Moertel CG et al: Biochemical modulation of fluorouracil: Evidence of significant improvement of survival and quality of life in patients with advanced colorectal carcinoma. J Clin Oncol 1989;7:1407.

94. Doroshow JH, Multhauf P, Leung L et al: Prospective randomized comparison of fluorouracil versus fluorouracil and high-dose continuous infusion leucovorin calcium for the treatment of advanced measurable colorectal cancer in patients previously unexposed to chemotherapy. J Clin Oncol 1990;8:491.

95. Vone FH, Friedman MA, Wittlinger PS et al: Treatment of patients with advanced colorectal carcinomas with fluorouracil alone, high-dose leucovorin plus fluorouracil, or sequential methotrexate, fluorouracil, and leucovorin: A randomized trial of the Northern California Oncology Group. J Clin Oncol 1989;7:1427.

96. Gittes RF: Carcinoma of the prostate. N Engl J Med 1991;324:236.

97. Javadpour N: Endocrine therapy of disseminated prostatic cancer. In Javadpour N (ed): Principles and Management of Urologic Cancer, p 409. Baltimore, Williams and Wilkins, 1983.

98. Blackard CE: The Veteran's Administration Cooperative Urological Research Group studies of carcinoma of the prostate: A review. Cancer Chemotherapy Reports 1975;59:225.

99. Murphy GP: National survey of prostatic cancer. J Urol 1982;127:928.

100. Stamey TA, Yang N, Hay AR et al: Prostate specific antigen as a serum marker for adenocarcinoma of the prostate. N Engl J Med 1987;317:910.

101. Cooper EH, Armitage TG, Robinson MRG et al: Prostatic specific antigen and the prediction of prognosis in metastatic prostatic cancer. Cancer 1990;66:1025.

102. Eisenberger MA, Blumenstein B, Scardino P et al: Evaluation of chemotherapy in endocrine-resistant prostate cancer patients with measurable versus bone disease only: The SWOG experience. Proceedings of the American Society of Clinical Oncology 9:596, 1990.

103. Eisenberger MA, Bezerdjian L, Kalash S: A critical assessment of the role of chemotherapy for endocrine-resistant prostatic carcinoma. Urol Clin North Am 1987;14:695.

104. Eaton CL, Griffiths K: The role of endocrine therapy in prostatic cancer. Ballieres Clin Endocrinol Metab 1990;4:85.

105. Byar DB: The VACURG's studies of cancer of the prostate Cancer 1973;32:1126.

106. The Leuprolide Study Group: Leuprolide versus diethylstilbestrol for metastatic prostate cancer. N Engl J Med 1984;311:1281.

107. Keuppens F, Denis L, Smith P et al: Zoladex and flutamide versus bilateral orchiectomy. Cancer 1990;66:1045.

108. Turkes AO, Peeling WB, Griffiths K: Treatment of patients with advanced cancer of the prostate: Phase III trial, zoladex against castration: A study of the British Prostate group. J Steroid Biochem 1987;27:543.

109. Balzano S, Cappa M, Migliari R et al: The effect of flutamide on basal and ACTH-stimulated plasma

levels of adrenal androgens in patients with advanced prostate cancer. J Endocrinol Invest 1988; 11:693.

110. Labrie F, Dupont A, Cusan L et al: Combination therapy with castration and flutamide: Today's treatment of choice for prostate cancer. J Steroid Biochem 1989;33:817.

111. Crawford DE, Eisenberger MA, McLeod DG et al: A controlled trial of leuprolide with and without flutamide in prostatic carcinoma. N Engl J Med 1989;321:419.

112. Harnett PR, Raghavan D, Caterson I et al: Amino-glutethimide in advanced prostatic carcinoma. Br J Urol 1987;59:323.

113. Trump DL, Havlin KH, Messing EM et al: High-dose ketoconazole in advanced hormone-refractory prostate cancer: Endocrinologic and clinical effects. J Clin Oncol 1989;7:1093.

114. Hoisaeter PA, Bakke A: Estramustine phosphate (Emcyt): Experimental and clinical studies in Europe. Semin Oncol 1983;10 (Suppl 3):27.

115. Eisenberger MA, Keddedy P, Abrams J: How effective is cytotoxic chemotherapy for disseminated prostatic carcinoma? Oncology 1987;1:59.

Chapter 17

Therapeutic Decision-Making for Invasive Procedures

Richard B. Patt

Subhash Jain

PERSPECTIVES

So-called "anesthetic procedures" (local anesthetic blocks, chemical neurolysis, intraspinal opioids) play an important role in the management of cancer pain.[1,2] Like other similar interventions they should be regarded neither as a panacea nor as treatment to be instituted in isolation. Rather, they are best regarded as a component of a therapeutic matrix that includes antitumor therapy, various pharmacologic strategies, neurosurgical and neuroaugmentative procedures, and behavioral and psychiatric approaches. This matrix of complementary interventions, when applied together in an individualized fashion by a compassionate, knowledgeable, and committed team of health care providers, permits extremely effective management of cancer pain. This complementary, as opposed to primary, role of anesthetic interventions is all the more apparent when viewed against the larger construct of palliative care, a philosophy of care that endeavors to control the protean symptoms of terminal illness including pain with quality of life as the end point.[3]

Individuals with advanced disease are often debilitated and physically, psychologically, and emotionally overwhelmed by their prognosis and symptoms. On this basis, every intervention, no matter how minor, must be weighed carefully against its cost in terms of inconvenience, recuperative time, energy, and cooperation demanded of the patient as well as the potentially devastating impact of a poor outcome. Every effort should be made to select a therapeutic option with a high likelihood of success that is not too demanding on patients' limited resources. In this regard, many anesthetic procedures can be viewed as preferable to many neurosurgical procedures which, with the exception of percutaneous cordotomy and some others, are very demanding of the critically ill, preterminal patient. Patients may occasionally be too unwell to receive treatment in a traditional setting, in which case a personal decision must be made by the treating anesthesiologist if it is appropriate to render treatment at the bedside[4] or whether some other therapeutic option may be more appropriate.

RISK VERSUS BENEFIT

The control of pain in patients with cancer remains a challenging endeavor for many reasons, including the heterogeneity of the physiologic and psychosocial manifestations of cancer, and the variable nature of pain, suffering, and therapeutic response. Many modalities have been employed in attempts to control or palliate patient suffering. All treatment with the potential to provide benefit, however, has associated risks. A most basic premise of therapeutics that is particularly applicable to the care of patients with cancer is that the simplest and least hazardous intervention that is associated with a reasonable likelihood of achieving the desired results ought to be applied first. The merits of oral pharmacotherapy for the control of cancer symptoms have been summarized in Chapter 6 and detailed in Chapters 7–12. Although more than 70% of patients with moderate to severe pain will achieve adequate control of their symptoms with carefully instituted pharmacologic management, up to 30% of patients may require alternate treatment.[5,6,7] The array of available alternate treatment modalities includes various neurosurgical and nerve blocking procedures, electrical stimulation, and physical and psychological measures. Although treatment algorithms have been proposed (Fig. 17–1),[8,9] decision-making regarding invasive procedures is an inexact science, and doubtless will remain so until better-controlled comparative studies have been carried out.

Each potentially useful therapeutic modality is associated with a risk-to-benefit ratio that is, to some extent, inherent in the procedure itself. In large part, however, this relationship of potential risk and benefit must be determined anew in the context of a host of factors that relate to the individual patient under consideration at a given time. These factors include the nature and severity of the symptoms, response to previous interventions, the level to which the symptoms interfere with the various dimensions of the patient's life, the status of the underlying disease, the patient's functional and psychosocial status, and patient preference. Practitioner factors include specialty interest, level of experience, bias, and access to consultants and specialized facilities. To complicate matters further, the dynamic nature of cancer and its tendency toward relentless progression insure that a calculation of the risk-to-benefit ratio for a given set of interventions must be reformulated over time. Finally, the determination of risk and benefit for a particular therapeutic option must be weighed against those of other available treatments.

RECENT ADVANCES

Neural blockade (peripheral, sympathetic, epidural, subarachnoid, regional opioid) is among the various methods that historically have been applied successfully to manage intractable pain. The discovery of the hollow needle by Rynd (1845) and its use in humans by Wood (1855)[10] (artfully recounted by Mather[11]) can be considered as perhaps the most important clinical advance in drug delivery systems. This development made possible the parenteral administration of opioids and other analgesics, as well as the local administration of substances intended to interrupt pain pathways. The histories of neural blockade, neurolytic blockade, and intraspinal opioid analgesia are amply annotated by Fink,[12] Swerdlow,[13] and Benedetti,[14] respectively. Suffice it to say here that the introduction of

(*text continues on page 279*)

Footnotes for Pain Treatment Flow Chart

1. Treat patient's pain according to indications. Monitor for recurrence of cancer.

2. Evaluate patient for anti-tumor therapy, or changes in current anti-tumor therapy.

3. The patients' treatment is selected to match their level of pain, not the etiology of the disease.

4. First try a nonsteroidal anti-inflammatory drug. Most of these drugs have ceiling effects indicating that increasing dosage will not provide additional analgesia after ceiling dose is reached. If customary dosages fail to provide adequate analgesia, try switching drugs or adding an opiate.

5. Start with titration of an opiate/nonsteroidal combination drug (eg, codeine/aspirin). The physician must be aware of reaching unacceptable side effects before analgesia occurs with these drugs. If pain continues at the maximum tolerable dose, switch to a potent opiate.

6. Administer a potent opiate. Titrate upward until dose has been reached for appropriate analgesic effects, or unacceptable-side effects occur. For a patient who is not currently receiving opiates, one may try an opiate/nonsteroidal combination drug (eg, codeine/aspirin) for a brief period—typically this will only be for one or two days—to see if this will provide adequate pain control.

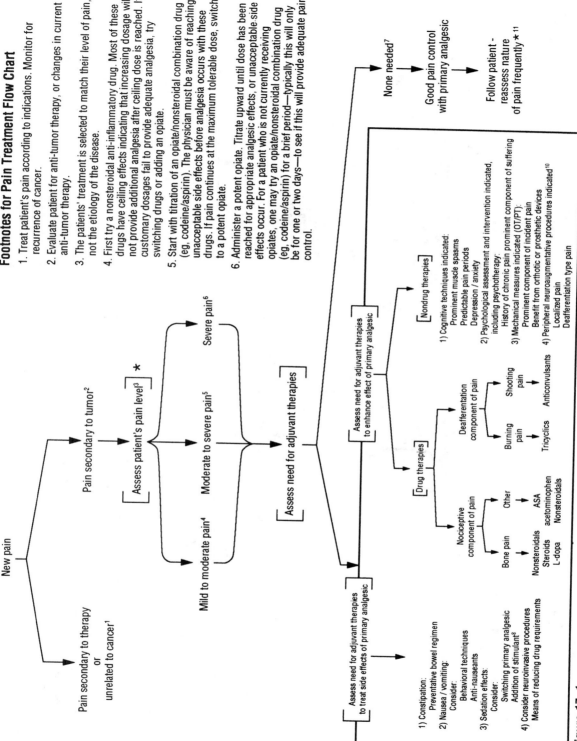

Figure 17–1.

(Continued)

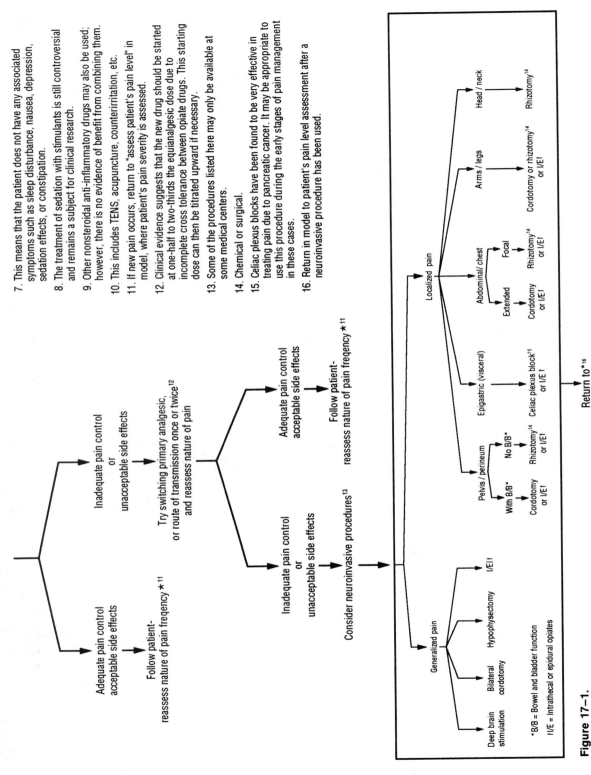

7. This means that the patient does not have any associated symptoms such as sleep disturbance, nausea, depression, sedation effects, or constipation.

8. The treatment of sedation with stimulants is still controversial and remains a subject for clinical research.

9. Other nonsteroidal anti-inflammatory drugs may also be used; however, there is no evidence of benefit from combining them.

10. This includes TENS, acupuncture, counterirritation, etc.

11. If new pain occurs, return to "assess patient's pain level" in model, where patient's pain severity is assessed.

12. Clinical evidence suggests that the new drug should be started at one-half to two-thirds the equianalgesic dose due to incomplete cross tolerance between opiate drugs. This starting dose can then be titrated upward if necessary.

13. Some of the procedures listed here may only be available at some medical centers.

14. Chemical or surgical.

15. Celiac plexus blocks have been found to be very effective in treating pain due to pancreatic cancer. It may be appropriate to use this procedure during the early stages of pain management in these cases.

16. Return in model to patient's pain level assessment after a neuroinvasive procedure has been used.

Figure 17–1.

cocaine (Köller), other local anesthetics, alcohol, and phenol (the latter popularized by Dogliotti, Maher, and others) serves as the basis for the current practice of neurolytic blockade. Although neither the basic methods of chemical blockade nor the useful pharmacologic agents have undergone marked change over the intervening years, new techniques have been developed, and standard techniques have been modified. These are detailed in the text (Chapters 18–22), and include novel approaches to the celiac axis, the introduction of intraspinal opioids and blockade of the hypogastric plexus and ganglion impar, pituitary adenolysis, and increased use of radiologic guidance. Despite an overall reliance on the same time-tested tools for neurolysis, important advances have taken place in our regard for the role of these procedures within the context of other related developments. Contemporary applications of these techniques represent advances insofar as: 1) increased experience and the availability of additional alternatives permit more sophisticated decision-making with regard to screening patients and selecting the optimal procedure; (2) the appreciation of the concept of "total pain"[15] and recognition that suffering is multiply determined have promoted an integration of anesthetic care into a multi-disciplinary matrix; and (3) there has been an upsurge of interest and an increase in the dissemination of knowledge, number of skilled practitioners, and patient contacts.

THERAPEUTIC GOALS

Careful assessment (see Chapters 1–5) remains the foundation for therapeutic decision-making. The likelihood of successful treatment hinges on careful consideration of all the elements gleaned from this assessment, with particular regard for shared goals and expectations that are realistic and specific. Most treatment is geared toward enhancing quality of life, a condition that is multiply determined and depends on a great deal more than the simple absence or presence of pain. Overall function and other symptoms must be taken into account, and, when considering pain management options, their respective effects on these other determinants of quality of life must be appraised. In general, treatment is geared toward both reducing (rarely eliminating) pain and restoring function. Thus, pharmacologic management that results in undue sedation or intractable nausea is undesirable, even if pain is reduced. By the same token, an invasive procedure that results in bladder or muscle paresis in an individual who otherwise is highly functional yields an inappropriate outcome, even if pain is diminished. Since, by and large, the side effects of pharmacotherapy are reversible and treatment is relatively undemanding, every effort should be made first to control pain with analgesic medications, with the aim of reducing pain without adversely affecting functional status. If dose-limiting side effects prevent these goals from being met, trials of administering other drugs to reverse side effects should be instituted (see Chapter 12). If comfort and function still cannot be mutually maintained, and palliative radiotherapy or chemotherapy (see Chapters 15 and 16) are impractical, consideration should then be given to invasive procedures.

SELECTION OF NERVE BLOCKS

In considering the range of invasive procedures that are available to manage pain, the

Figure 17–1. A proposed treatment algorithm for the management of cancer pain. Schema recommends treatment responses for pain of varying severity and types, drawing on the entire armamentarium of interventions at the pain specialist's disposal. Algorithms of this type have not been rigorously tested. Due to the factors cited in the text, at best, such algorithms only approximate the complex decision-making that must be applied on an individualized basis according to the specific needs of each patient. Reproduced with permission, Cleeland CS, Rotondi A, Brechner T et al: A model for the treatment of cancer pain. J Pain Symptom Management 1986;1:209.

relative likelihood of relief and of side effects must be balanced. Considerations related to the pain *per se* include its etiology, mechanism, location, severity/urgency, and the presence or absence of concomitant pain elsewhere. Considerations related to the patient and practitioner have already been mentioned. In general, nerve blocks are most applicable for pain that is (1) well characterized, (2) well localized, (3) somatic or visceral in origin and (4) that does not comprise a component of a pain syndrome characterized by multifocal aches and pains.

Patients with vague complaints are prone to be ill-served by treatment with nerve blocks simply because their clinical presentation may increase the difficulty of selecting the proper procedure. In addition, patients who "feel bad all over," or who volunteer that "I can't describe it, it just hurts" may be experiencing a symptom complex defined not just by nociceptive elements but by spiritual, psychological, social and/or economic malaise, in which case no amount of morphine or nerve ablation will enhance their sense of well-being. Depression, anxiety, and other psychological disorders occur in a high proportion of patients with cancer, even independent of symptoms (see Chapter 14).[16] Careful screening should be conducted early on to identify psychosocial disturbances, many of which are potentially reversible with counseling and medications. Nevertheless, the importance of pain management should not be minimized because of psychological problems since inadequate pain control is an important factor predisposing to psychological disturbances and suicide.[17,18]

With regard to its distribution, pain may be well localized or, more commonly, generalized or located in more than one site.[19] Most nerve blocks are relatively efficacious for pain that is well localized, but when extended to provide analgesic coverage for pain that is extensively distributed are more prone to failure, or of greater concern are associated with increased risks of undesirable neurologic deficit. There are, however, a few exceptions to this general dictum. Sympathetic blockade (stellate ganglion, celiac, lumbar sympathetic, and hypogastric block) often provides topo-

graphic analgesia that is ample for the visceral or sympathetically mediated pain syndromes, most of which are relatively diffuse. Epidural neurolysis, although currently performed in a limited number of centers, can often be successfully employed to manage broadly based pain without inducing unwanted neurologic deficit, although this is certainly a risk. Finally, although its availability is even more restricted, transnasal alcohol neurolysis of the pituitary gland is applicable for widely disseminated bony metastatic pain.

Pain that is due to somatic or visceral injury is more likely to respond beneficially to neural blockade than is neuropathic pain, an adage that holds true for most ablative procedures as well as for treatment with opioid analgesics.[20] Neurolytic blocks need not be summarily excluded in the management of intractable neuropathic pain, but should be preceded by careful trials of local anesthetic blocks to determine the likelihood of efficacy.

Surveys of patients with advanced cancer have determined that pain is usually present in more than one body part simultaneously.[21] Patients may complain of one predominant source of pain only to find that when it is eliminated by a nerve block or some other procedure, other previously secondary complaints increase in severity. Nevertheless, even in patients with multiple sources of pain, a localized procedure that reduces the most severe complaint is sometimes of value, permitting control of the secondary symptoms with conservative means.

Multiple other considerations apply to selecting a nerve block. The role of local anesthetic injections in the performance of diagnostic and prognostic blocks is discussed in Chapter 18. With regard to therapeutic procedures, local anesthetic blocks, so widely used in the management of pain of nonmalignant origin, play a more limited role in the treatment of cancer pain. A local anesthetic or steroid injection (see Chapter 18), administered either as a single shot, in series, or through a catheter, serially or as an infusion, may be considered for pain that is of a reflex or inflammatory nature or is not expected to persist. Local anesthetic injections have a potential therapeutic role in the management of painful nononcologic syndromes that occur in patients with cancer such as herpes zoster and pain following thoractomy, mastectomy, and radical neck dissection (see Chapter 3). Finally, local anesthetic blocks, administered either in a series or continuously via a catheter have a potential role in the "pain emergency" to provide respite from pain and distress so that a more accurate assessment and long-term plan can be formulated.

Neurolytic blocks are more appropriate for pain that is due to documented tissue injury and that is expected to persist. Neurolytic blocks, especially in the periphery (see Chapter 21), are associated with a risk of neuritis and deafferentation pain, and in this regard, the severity and intractability of the pain together with predicted life expectancy help determine whether a neurolytic block is warranted. The likelihood of inducing unwanted physiologic alterations must be considered together with the predicted impact of such changes on the patient. For example, motor weakness is a concern when a mixed nerve is injected, as is incontinence when a subarachnoid block is performed at lower levels. The relative importance of these concerns depends on many aspects of the patient's overall status. For example, motor changes are more likely to be well accepted when a limb has already been rendered useless by tumor invasion or severe pain, or when a patient is already bed-bound due to some other condition. Likewise, incontinence is not truly an issue when normal bowel and bladder continuity have already been surgically or mechanically diverted by colostomy or catheterization. Finally, the selection of a nerve block is guided by technical feasability. Factors that must be considered here include the practitioner's experience and abilities, the availability of proper facilities including specialized tables, needles, and radiologic equipment and whether the proposed procedure is anatomically possible.

INTRASPINAL OPIOIDS

The popularization and recent addition of intraspinal opioids to the pain specialist's armamentarium has extended therapeutic options dramatically (see Chapter 18). Among the main advantages of intraspinal opioid therapy are its reversibility and the availability of simple screening measures to determine the likelihood of efficacy. This latter attribute distinguishes this approach from neurolytic blockade, in which the diagnostic/prognostic results of local anesthetic injections only roughly approximate the ultimate therapeutic results. Intraspinal opioid therapy is more likely to be effective when brisk responsivity to opioids already has been demonstrated, but treatment has been limited by systemic side effects. Intraspinal opioid therapy generally is more appropriate when pains are multiple or widely distributed. Pain in the trunk or below is often amenable to lumbar administration, whereas more rostral pain may require higher catheter placement or even intraventricular administration. Despite persistent controversy surrounding selection of the most desirable route of administration, drug, schedule, and delivery system, guidelines are proposed in Chapter 18.

OTHER OPTIONS

Percutaneous cordotomy (see Chapter 26) is an important option for intractable pain that is unilateral and restricted to the lower part of the body. Its applicability is greatest for pain below the waist or trunk, and decreases as the height that must be covered increases. It should be pursued only cautiously in patients with pulmonary disease due to the risk of nocturnal respiratory failure. Pituitary ablation (see Chapter 26), when available, has a role in patients with widely disseminated pains, especially when pain is of bony metastatic origin, and in patients with primary tumors that are hormonally responsive (breast, prostate). The role of electrical stimulation remains controversial. Percutaneous stimulation with transdermal electrical neural stimulation (TENS) is relatively innocuous, but rarely provides durable relief.[22] Spinal stimulation has not emerged as an important option for patients with cancer pain.[23] Despite considerable experience accumulated mostly in a few centers, stimulation of deep brain structures (see Chapter 26) is currently regarded as an experimental modality. Stimulation of areas that are rich in opioid receptors (periaqueductal gray) has been shown to be effective for somatic pain syndromes,[24] whereas thalamic stimulation may be effective for neuropathic pain.[25]

INTRACTABLE PAIN

In a small proportion of cases, comfort and function cannot be maintained mutually at optimal levels. In general, when this difficult choice is encountered, patients and families will elect comfort at the expense of moderate decrement in function, since the latter often is expected to fail as disease progresses. Nevertheless, these issues must be prioritized carefully on an individual basis. Some patients will opt for comfort over function, a circumstance that is particularly likely if function has already deteriorated or a prior episode of uncontrolled pain has intensified the anticipation and memory of pain. Other patients exhibit higher pain thresholds, and will tolerate higher levels of pain, particularly when a patient's identity is highly equated with his or her functional role. These factors all need to be taken into account when assessing the risk–benefit ratio of various treatment options. Throughout, the health care provider must provide appropriately balanced therapy, even in the presence of severe distress.

REFERENCES

1. Cousins MJ: Anesthetic approaches in cancer pain. In Foley KM, Bonica JJ, Ventafridda V: Advances in Pain Research and Therapy, vol 16. New York, Raven Press, 1990, pp 249.
2. Bonica JJ: Treatment of cancer pain: Current status and future needs. Seminars in Anesthesia 1985;9:589.
3. Ventafridda V: Continuing care: A major issue in cancer pain management. Pain 1989;36:137.
4. Patt RB: Interventional analgesia: Epidural and subarachnoid therapy. Am J Hospice Care 1989;6:18.
5. Ventafridda V, Tambutini M, Carceni A: A validation study of the WHO method for cancer pain relief. Cancer 1987;59:850.
6. Toscani F, Carini M: The implementation of the WHO guidelines for the treatment of advanced cancer pain in a district general hospital in Italy. Pain Clinic 1989;3:37.
7. Takeda F: Preliminary report from Japan on results of field testing of WHO draft interim guidelines for relief of cancer pain. Pain Clin 1:83, 1986.
8. Cleeland CS, Rotondi A, Brechner T et al: A model for the treatment of cancer pain. J Pain Symptom Management 1986;1:209.
9. Ferrer-Brechner T: Neurolytic blocks for cancer pain. In Abrams S (ed): Cancer Pain, Boston, Kluwer Academic, 1988, p 111.
10. Wood A: New method of treating neuralgia by the direct application of opiates to the painful points. Edinburgh Med Sci J 1855;82:265.
11. Mather LE: Novel methods of drug delivery. In Bond MR, Charlton JE, Woolf CJ (eds): Proceedings of the VI World Congress on Pain. Amsterdam, Elsevier, 1991, p 159.
12. Fink BR: History of neural blockade. In Cousins MJ, Bridenbaugh PO (eds): Neural Blockade, 2nd ed. Philadelphia, JB Lippincott, 1988, p 3.
13. Swerdlow M: The history of neurolytic blockade. In Racz GB (ed): Techniques of Neurolysis. Boston, Kluwer Academic, 1989, p 1.
14. Benedetti C: Intraspinal analgesia: An historical overview. Acta Anaesthesiol Scand 1987;85:17.
15. Saunders C: The management of terminal illness. London, London Hospital Medical Publications, 1967.
16. Derogatis LR, Morrow GR, Fetting J et al: The prevalence of psychiatric disorders among cancer patients. JAMA 1983;249:751.
17. Holland J: Managing depression in the patient with cancer. Ca—A Cancer Journal for Clinicians 1987; 37:366.
18. Foley KM: The relationship of pain and symptom management to patient requests for physician-assisted suicide. J Pain Symptom Management 1991 6:289.
19. Twycross RG, Lack SA: Therapeutics in Terminal Cancer. Edinburgh, Churchill Livingstone, 1986, p 9.
20. Portenoy R: The nature of opioid responsiveness and its implications for neuropathic pain: New hypothesis derived from studies of opioid infusions. Pain 1990; 43:273.
21. Twycross RG: Relief of pain. In Saunders CM (ed): The Management of Terminal Disease. Chicago, Yearbook Publishers, 1978, p 65.
22. Ventafridda V, Sganzerla EP, Fochi C et al. Transcutaneous nerve stimulation in cancer pain. In Bonica JJ, Ventafridda V (eds): Advances in Pain Research and

Therapy, vol 2, New York, Raven Press, 1979, pp 509.
23. Patt R: Pain control in oncology. In Rubin P (ed): Clinical Oncology Syllabus: A Multidisciplinary Approach for Medical Students and Physicians. Philadelphia, WB Saunders, 1991.

24. Young RF, Brechner T: Electrical stimulation of the brain for relief of intractable pain due to cancer. Cancer 1986;57:1266.
25. Hosobuchi Y: Subcortical electrical stimulation control of intractable pain: Report of 122 cases. J Neurosurg 1986;64:543.

Chapter 18

Intraspinal Opioid Therapy

Steven D. Waldman   L. Douglas Kennedy

David W. Leak   Richard B. Patt

INTRODUCTION

The introduction and evolution of intraspinal opioid therapy has dramatically altered contemporary cancer pain management over a remarkably short period of time. Intraspinal opioid therapy is the logical outgrowth of the discovery of opioid receptors (1971) and their isolation in the brain (1973) and spinal cord (1976). Researchers investigating applications for intraspinal opioids first reported analgesia in laboratory animals in 1976, and for human subjects in 1979 (see reference for detailed historical account).[1]

Rapid, relatively widespread acceptance of intraspinal opioid therapy contrasts with the characteristic pattern for clinical applications of new scientific findings, that is, new developments in medicine tend to require long periods of time and extensive, controlled clinical trials before they are applied on a large scale. One certain explanation for this phenomenon is that restrictions usually applicable to the introduction of a new drug or device are less rigorously applied when a familiar drug is used for a new purpose or by a different route. The April 12th, 1982 issue of the Food and Drug Administration (FDA) *Bulletin* has clarified the FDA's favorable position on physician prescription of FDA-approved drugs for unlabeled uses.[2] Nevertheless, the rapidity with which clinical experience and acceptance has accrued over a less than 12-year period serves as indirect testimony to the efficacy and favorable risk-to-benefit ratio of intraspinal opioid therapy. This is particularly true for patients with refractory cancer pain, as will be discussed below.

RATIONALE FOR USE

Historically, patients with cancer pain served as the first human subjects for treatment with intraspinal opioids, and continue to be the primary target population. The chronic administration of intraspinal opioids in noncancer pain only recently has been the subject of serious investigation, and remains controversial.[3-7] Although most patients with cancer pain can achieve adequate comfort with the application of standard pharmacologic interventions (see Chapters 6–11),[8,9] a significant proportion of patients (10%–30%) will require alternate therapies because of persistent pain or medication-induced side effects.[10]

Intractable cancer pain served as the initial focus of treatment with intraspinal opioids in part from the frustration born of the need to resort to potentially hazardous, invasive, and irreversible neurodestructive procedures that require special training, skills, and careful patient selection (see Chapters 20–24 and 26). It is notable that some investigators have observed a decline in frequency of neuroablative procedures performed to palliate intractable cancer pain coincident with the rise in popularity of intraspinal opioid therapy.[11,12] In contrast to neurolytic blocks and neurosurgery, intraspinal opioid therapy produces reversible analgesia that is more likely to be effective for multiple pains or for pain that is bilateral or crosses the midline. Most patients with symptomatic cancer have or will develop pain in multiple sites.[13] Intraspinal opioid therapy is most efficacious for somatic and visceral pain,[14,15] and that these mechanisms frequently underlie the pain of cancer is another factor favoring cancer patients as candidates for treatment. Finally, cancer patients are ideal recipients of therapy because of the favorable risk-to-benefit ratio that exists in the treatment of terminally ill patients, as well as the accuracy and ease in prognosticating successful treatment by screening with temporary noninvasive percutaneous catheters (see "Screening," below). This methodology is a relatively safe, reproducible way to predict successful outcome before proceeding to implantation of a long-term delivery system.

DEFINITIONS

Cousins, Cherry, and Gourlay recently called for a more precise use of terminology,[16] and probably in no other area is this consideration more critical. "Opioid" is a broad term, but one that is precisely defined, and for this reason its use is preferred. It refers to the entire range of exogenous drugs with morphine-like properties (ie, agents that exhibit agonist properties at opioid receptors), including naturally occurring derivatives of opium, newer semisynthetic and wholly synthetic compounds, as well as endogenous peptides with agonist properties.[16] "Opiate" refers specifically to opium derivatives and some semisynthetic congeners, and its use is declining since it technically does not include newer synthetic drugs or drugs with partial agonist effects.[17] It has been recommended that the term "narcotics" (Greek *narco* = "deaden") be abandoned since its meaning is vague, and its use raises not just medical considerations but legal and social implications.[17,18] "Central nervous system" (CNS) is a general term that includes the brain and spinal cord. "Neuraxial" is defined as the axial, unpaired part of the central nervous system (spinal cord and brain stem), but not the paired structures (both hemispheres and telencephalon). "Spinal" is a broad term meaning "relating to the vertebral column," and "intraspinal" a more precise term defined as "within the vertebral canal or spinal fluid." The two intraspinal routes commonly used are epidural (peridural) and subarachnoid (intrathecal).[19] Except when it is specifically pertinent to differentiate between routes, the term "intraspinal opioid therapy" will be used here to refer generically to epidural and intrathecal administration. The term "regional opioid analgesia" has been used in a similar manner, but also includes perineural injections outside the CNS.[20]

The administration of *local anesthetics* into the epidural and subarachnoid space for the management of pain has a long and rich heritage. Epidural and spinal anesthesia have assumed an important, growing role in the management of acute pain associated with labor, surgery, surgical recovery, and trauma, but only occasionally have been used to manage chronic cancer pain.[21] Pain relief associated with local anesthetics administered by the epidural or subarachnoid route is nonspecific and is accompanied by motor weakness, sensory anesthesia, and interference with sympathetic function. These latter features make continuous epidural or intrathecal *anesthesia* generally inappropriate for chronic use in the home care or hospice environment. In contrast, the hallmark and main advantage of epidural and intrathecal *opioid analgesia* is its selectivity: motor, sensory, and sympathetic systems are unaffected.[22,23] Although preparation and education of health care professionals and family members is required for their maintenance, these modalities are well suited for the home-based management of chronic cancer pain.[24–26]

It should be noted that experience is accruing with techniques for providing more potent intraspinal *analgesia* using combinations of opioids and dilute (subanesthetic) concentrations of local anesthetics (see "Management of Tolerance") in selected patients.

MECHANISM OF ACTION

The mechanism of action of intraspinal and supraspinal opioids appears to be generally consistent with Melzack and Wall's "Gate Control Theory of Pain."[27] A number of components, both peripheral and supraspinal, converge on a central processing or summation center (dorsal horn of the spinal cord), resulting in modulation of afferent impulses conveying noxious stimuli. Various means of suppressing afferent nociceptive input have been explored over the last two decades, including centrally administered opioids, the neuraxial administration of other peptides, and CNS stimulation (see Chapter 26). Intraspinal opioids are believed to modulate input from high-threshold, small-diameter afferents, and/or to act through a postsynaptic effect at second-order neurons.[23,28]

Intraspinal opioid analgesia involves the delivery of minute quantities of drug (relative to systemic opioid requirements) in close proximity to their sites of action in the spinal cord.[29] Analgesia is often superior to that achieved when opioids are administered by other routes,[10,30–32] presumably because higher drug concentrations are achieved locally at spinal opioid receptor sites.[33,34] Since the absolute amount of drug administered is less than that with traditional routes, side effects are minimized.[7,10,32] It is postulated that saturation of rostral opioid receptor sites may be responsible for some opioid-mediated side effects, effects that may be minimized by intraspinal administration. Sites for rostral opioid receptors include the brain (limbic system, periaqueductal gray, thalamus) and brainstem. Opioid receptor agonism at these sites results in activation of descending inhibitory tracts with suppression of nociceptive input at the spinal cord level. Electrophysiologic studies have confirmed such activity (*eg*, in the bulbospinal system[28]). Side effects mediated by the activation of rostral receptors include sedation (brain), as well as nausea, vomiting, and respiratory depression (primarily brain-stem).[20]

The site of action for nociceptive modulation or suppression in the spinal cord is predominantly in the dorsal horn. The highest concentration of opioid receptors is located in Rexed's laminae numbers II and III (substantia gelatinosa).[22,29] These opioid receptors are located both presynaptically in primary afferent neurons, and postsynaptically in second-order afferent neurons.[35] Opioid receptor agonism at these sites results in a change in either 1) neuronal membrane hyperexcitability and depolarization (mu and delta receptor-mediated), with resultant refractoriness to further excitation[36]; or 2) inhibition of neurotransmitter release.[37] The end result is local inhibition of nociceptive transmission, probably through mediation at the level of ion channels.[29,38]

PHYSICOCHEMICAL CLINICAL CORRELATES

Many factors determine clinical efficacy for intraspinal opioid therapy, including patient characteristics (age, height, weight, configuration of the spinal column), route (epidural, intrathecal, intraventricular), technique of injection (direction and type of needle, rate and turbulence of injection), characteristics of the cerebrospinal fluid (CSF) and constituent neurologic structures (CSF density, baricity, volume, circulation, host receptor system, local chemical milieu), and the physical and chemical properties of the drug that is injected.[33] Physical and chemical properties of the drug (density, volume, concentration, pKa, oil : water partition coefficient, molecular weight, protein binding) influence the onset, duration of action, and migration away from the primary site of delivery.[18,33]

Receptors are protein moieties located within the bilipid membrane of cell walls. Many of the pharmacokinetic and pharmacodynamic properties of intraspinal opioids can be explained by the influence of their relative lipid solubilities on receptor binding and systemic uptake. Sufentanil, with an oil : water partition coefficient of 1,778, can be regarded as the prototype for the lipophilic opioids. Morphine, with a coefficient of 1.42, can be regarded as the prototype of the hydrophilic opioids, with other agents occupying intermediate positions (see Table 18-1). Highly lipophilic drugs (*eg*, sufentanil) are associated with a more rapid onset of peak effect (5 to 15 minutes) when administered in the epidural space than are the more hydrophilic agents (*eg*, morphine), which may take up to 1 hour to produce peak analgesia.[39] Lipophilicity also accounts for suggestions of low rostral concentrations of epidurally administered sufentanil[40] and similar drugs,[33] and may explain the apparent decreased side effect profile of the lipophilic agents relative to their more hydrophilic counterparts.[22,41] Lipophilicity has not only been suggested to account for reductions in rostrally mediated side effects (nausea, vomiting, late respiratory depression), but also forms the basis for the potential *early* respiratory depressant effect observed for the more lipophilic agents that are rapidly absorbed into the systemic circulation and distributed rostrally through the blood stream. As noted, there seems to be relatively insignificant rostral spread via the CSF with sufen-

tanil.[39,40] An alternate view proposes that the difference in side effect profile (if it indeed exists) among agents of varying lipophilicity may not be related to rostral redistribution but is simply due to the more evanescent effects of the more lipid-soluble drugs (Yaksh TL: written communication, October 1991). As a result of morphine's relative hydrophilicity, receptor saturation is delayed, accounting for its longer onset of peak action (30–60 minutes), and efflux from the spinal cord is slowed, accounting for its longer duration of action (12–24 hours).[42] Delayed uptake from intrathecal and epidural depots results in a "reservoir" effect[43] and cephalad migration of drug within the CSF.[42,44] Rostral spread to brain-stem centers correlates with the occurrence of *late* respiratory side effects.[22,41] Delayed respiratory depression is the main impediment to the more liberal use of intraspinal opioids in acute care settings for labor and postsurgical pain. Delayed respiratory depression has been reported up to 12–14 hours after the administration of a single dose of epidural or subarachnoid morphine to opioid-naive patients, but occurs rarely if at all in patients taking opioids chronically (see "Side Effects," below).[20]

Although lipid solubility seems to have the greatest influence on pharmacodynamics, other properties of the opioids contribute as well. Molecular weight correlates inversely with ease of passage across the dura.[45] In contrast to systemic administration, protein binding plays only a minor role in the distribution of intraspinal opioids, since the protein content of the CSF is low.[20] Protein content is not distributed uniformly, however, and Cousins and Mather have suggested that as a result, potency may be increased with more rostral injections.[22] Volume of distribution and metabolism probably are relatively unimportant in determining clinical activity.[20]

Opioid receptor characteristics also play an important role in determining clinical efficacy. Three distinct classes of opioid receptors, mu, sigma, and kappa, have been well characterized,[46,47] and evidence for two other opioid receptors, delta[48] and epsilon,[49] and subsets of the kappa and mu receptor (mu-1

Table 18–1.
Some Properties of Some Opioids for Intraspinal Use

Drug	Lipid Solubility	Average Effective Dose* (mg/70 kg body weight)			Onset/Peak/Duration (epidural—min)		
		IV	EPI	IT	O	P	D
Morphine	1.42	10	5–10	0.1–0.5	20–35	30–60	8–22 hr
Diamorphine	1.7	5–10	5–10	1	5–10	30–60	6–12 hr
Meperidine	38.8	100	25–50	35–70	15–20	20	7–10 hr
Methadone	116	10	4–5	—	10–15	20–30	7–9 hr
Alfentanil	131	0.5–1	0.5–1	—	5	15	1.5 hr
Hydromorphone	—	1–2	1–1.5	—	10–20	20–30	6–19 hr
Fentanyl	813	0.1	0.1	—	4–6	10–20	2–3 hr
Lofentanil	1,450	0.002	0.005	—	20–30	50	5–10 hr
Sufentanil	1,778	0.02	0.05	—	5	10	4–6 hr
Buprenorphine	—	0.3	0.15–0.3	—	5–10	30–60	4–10 hr

* IV = intravenous; EPI = epidural; IT = intrathecal.

and mu-2) has been described.[46,50,51] Most clinical and experimental data relate to the mu receptor, and, to a lesser extent, delta and kappa receptors. Mu and delta receptors are associated with robust, dose-dependent suppression of thermal, chemical, and mechanical nociceptive input.[28,42] Agents with predominantly agonist effects at the mu receptor include morphine, meperidine, fentanyl, sufentanil, and hydromorphone. Meperidine, although not generally favored in cancer pain management, is unique in that when administered intrathecally in high doses it acts as a local anesthetic, a property that has been studied in surgical and laboring patients,[20,52] but has not yet been exploited in patients with cancer pain. Limited experience with the predominantly delta agonist DADL (D-ala²-D-leu⁵-enkephalin) has demonstrated considerable antinociceptive activity in animals and man (see "Tolerance," below).[53,54] Kappa receptors, at least experimentally, appear to be associated with a ceiling effect with respect to their ability to suppress some types of nociceptive stimuli when activated. Kappa agonists butorphanol and nalbuphine are reported to provide significant clinical analgesia for some types of pain in humans (see "Opioid Agonist/Antagonists as Analgesics," below).[28,55,56] Specificity has been observed for both the type of pain affected and side effects, relative to which type of receptor is activated. This may account for the relatively segmental analgesia seen with intraspinal infusions of the lipophilic opioids, and might explain the "distant" effect sometimes observed with the more hydrophilic opioids. An example of the latter effect can be found in reports of successful treatment of head and neck cancer pain with the lumbar and cervicothoracic epidural administration of morphine sulfate.[57] Specificity for the type of pain that is most responsive to intraspinal opioids has been observed clinically, although few controlled studies have been carried out. Complete blockade of nociception and reflex response, as seen with local anesthetic blockade, does not occur. Acute, sharp "incidental" breakthrough or surgical pain (so-called "first pain," usually associated with rapid transmission along the myelinated A-delta fibers/neospinothalamic tract) is relieved less readily by intraspinal opi-

Table 18–2.
The Likelihood* of Various Types of Pain to Respond to Treatment with Intraspinal Opioids

Continuous somatic pain
Continuous visceral pain
Intermittent somatic pain
Intermittent visceral pain
Neuropathic pain
Cutaneous, ulcer and fistula

From Arner S, Arner B: Differential effects of epidural morphine in the treatment of cancer related pain. Acta Anaesthesiol Scand 1985;29:32.
* From most to least likely

oids. Dull, constant pain (so-called "slow" or "second" pain, associated with C fiber transmission/neospinothalamic tract) is more amenable.[18] Arner and Arner[14] reported on the use of epidural morphine in the management of 55 patients with cancer pain that was refractory to systemically administered opioids. The results of their study suggested a progressive order for likelihood of response to epidurally administered morphine by type of pain (see Table 18–2) (from most to least likely to respond): 1) continuous somatic pain; 2) continuous visceral pain; 3) intermittent somatic pain; 4) intermittent visceral pain; 5) neurogenic pain; and 6) cutaneous ulcer and fistula. This work is supported by a study of patients with postoperative pain that was relieved with epidural morphine but in whom experimental cutaneous pain induced by heat and electrical stimulation was unaffected.[58] These results notwithstanding, patients with so-called "opioid-resistant" pain syndromes still should be considered candidates for (relatively) noninvasive trials of intraspinal opioid therapy, since a proportion will achieve satisfactory pain relief. This is highlighted in a small study of patients with demonstrated tolerance to high oral doses of opioids,[59] and a larger study of patients with radiating neuropathic pain.[32]

SIDE EFFECTS AND THEIR MANAGEMENT

As is stressed below, relative to their opioid-naive counterparts, dose-limiting side effects are rare in cancer patients who have been exposed chronically to systemic opioids.[20,22] Potential side effects of intraspinal opioids that occur with clinically significant frequency include respiratory depression, gastrointestinal hypomotility, inhibition of micturition, nausea, vomiting, pruritus, and sedation.[60] DeCastro and colleagues[20] list a multitude of other side effects that occur much more rarely or have been reported anecdotally, but of which the clinician should be aware. These include dysphoria, hypothermia, oliguria, failure of ejaculation, headache, erythema, agitation, miosis, muscle weakness, hallucinations, catatonia, abdominal spasm, diarrhea, shivering, hypotension, abstinence syndrome, and (in a patient with intracranial hypertension) seizure.[61] Treatment of side effects generally is symptomatic, but when persistent or severe they usually can be countered with intravenous or intramuscular naloxone, often with preservation of analgesia.[62,63]

RESPIRATORY DEPRESSION

Of all potential complications, the risk of respiratory depression generates the most clinical concern. Respiratory depression may be an early (less than 2 hours from initial administration) or late phenomenon (4–24 hours after administration).[64–67] Activity at both the mu and delta receptors has been demonstrated to be associated with both types of respiratory depression.[28,68] Kappa receptor activation may not be associated with significant respiratory depression.[69] Unfortunately, a pure kappa agonist with reliable analgesic properties is not available, but future development of such an agent may help reduce the potential for clinically important respiratory depression.[28,69] The administration of combinations of opioid receptor agonists is

Table 18–3.
Respiratory Depression: Predisposing Factors

Opioid naiveté
Accidental overdosage
Absence of severe pain
Advanced age
Debility
Coexisting pulmonary disease
Sleep apnea
Coadministration of other central nervous system depressant drugs
Coadministration of opioid analgesics by alternate routes

an additional strategy that has been used to reduce side effects (see "Summary," below).

Management

Factors that predispose to respiratory depression (see Table 18–3) include accidental overdosage, an absence of severe pain, advanced age or debility, coexisting pulmonary disease, sleep apnea, the coadministration of opioid analgesics by alternate routes, and opioid naiveté.[20] As noted, respiratory depression is significantly more likely to occur in opioid-naive patients, and there are few or no reports of late respiratory depression in patients previously maintained on systemic opioids for even short periods. Reversal of respiratory depression can be accomplished with the administration of a mu antagonist (naloxone) or the kappa agonist/mu antagonist, nalbuphine.[62,70–74] Oral naltrexone administered (prophylactically) in surgical patients reduces pruritus, nausea, and somnolence, but may be associated with a decrement in analgesia.[75] That these agents must be administered cautiously and in small increments is supported by reports of cardiogenic shock, irreversible ventricular fibrillation, and pulmonary edema associated with the acute reversal of systemic and intraspinal opioids.[71,76–78] A recent report of the successful reversal of respiratory depression by the replacement of aspirated CSF with normal saline suggests another intriguing therapeutic approach.[79]

GASTROINTESTINAL DYSFUNCTION—CONSTIPATION

Gastrointestinal function and constipation are of particular concern in the cancer patient (see Chapters 12, 13, and 30). Systemic opioids delay gastric emptying and decrease lower gastrointestinal tract motility, presumably by their action on opioid receptors located in the gut. Experimental work suggests that intrathecal morphine does not decrease peristalsis,[18,35] but systematic studies in humans have not been reported.[18] Clinically, gastrointestinal motility seems to be preserved much better with intraspinal versus systemic opioids, but may be affected adversely as dosage is increased. Studies in postoperative patients, however, do confirm that postoperative ileus persists for a longer period when pain is treated with epidural morphine as opposed to bupivacaine.[80]

Management

Constipation in the patient with cancer frequently is multifactorial. Reversible causes should be identified and treated, and, in addition, a prophylactic symptomatic approach using a sliding-scale laxative regimen should be adopted (see Chapters 12, 13, and 30). The tendency toward less constipation with intraspinal opioids provides a rationale for a transition from systemic to intraspinal therapy when intractable constipation complicates management with systemic opioids.[81]

GASTROINTESTINAL DYSFUNCTION—NAUSEA AND VOMITING

Epidural morphine has been observed to reduce gastric emptying and small intestinal transit in volunteers.[82] The incidence of nausea and vomiting associated with the administration of intraspinal opioids may range from as high as 25%–30% in opioid-naive subjects, but is infrequent in patients with prior chronic exposure to opioids. As with nausea and vomiting induced by oral opioids (see Chapter 9), these effects generally resolve rapidly with continued administration.[1,83] Nausea and vomiting are believed to be related to activity at the chemoreceptor trigger zone and vomiting center. That the vestibular system is often involved as well is suggested by an increased incidence of nausea and vomiting in ambulatory versus bed-bound patients.[84]

Management

Nausea and vomiting may be reversed with the administration of nalbuphine or naloxone (see above), but this usually is unnecessary as symptoms generally will recede with time. If symptoms persist, patients may benefit from a trial of a more lipophilic agent, or should be treated symptomatically with standard antiemetics, such as metoclopramide, a phenothiazine, a butyrophenone, or hydroxyzine (see Chapters 12, 13, and 30).[20] In a double-blind, placebo-controlled study specifically targeting patients receiving epidural morphine (after surgery), transdermal scopolamine was shown to be more effective than both placebo and combinations of metoclopramide and droperidol.[85]

URINARY SYMPTOMS

Intraspinally administered morphine may be associated with naloxone-reversible urinary retention predominantly due to decreased detrusor muscle tone and detrusor–urethral sphincter dyssynergia.[22,86,87] Such effects on the urinary tract appear to be mediated by mu and delta, but not kappa receptors.[88] Urinary retention has not been reported after intraventricular administration of morphine, suggesting that a spinally mediated mechanism is responsible. Despite incidences of 20%–40%[89] and higher in male patients after initial dosing of intraspinal opioids, retention is rarely observed in (opioid-tolerant) cancer patients.

Management

Tolerance to this effect often develops after 24 to 48 hours of continued treatment, during which time treatment with the administration of small doses of an opioid antagonist[89] or intermittent bladder catheterization may be undertaken. Alternate approaches include conversion to treatment with a more lipid-soluble opioid (especially methadone, which has been observed actually to increase detrusor tone, or buprenorphine, which seems to have little or no effect), or a trial of oral phenoxybenzamine.[90–93]

PRURITUS

This side effect is highly disturbing to patients. Although extremely common in opioid-naive subjects, especially after intrathecal administration, it is fortunately extremely uncommon in cancer patients. Treatment with diphenhydramine, antihistamines, opioid antagonists,[74] and droperidol have been recommended, but all such interventions yield mixed results.[20,22]

INFECTIOUS COMPLICATIONS

Serious infection has not emerged as a common sequela to intraspinal opioid therapy administered either by percutaneous or implanted catheters.[94] Superficial infection at the catheter exit site may occur in as many as 6% of cases, however,[20] and serves as one of the rationales for the use of tunneled catheters. By increasing the distance between the catheter exit site and the spinal region, the incidence of serious central nervous system infections should be reduced with such systems, although this advantage has not been demonstrated clearly. Recently, a commercially available Silastic epidural catheter (Du Pen Epidural Catheter with VitaCuff, Davol, Inc., Salt Lake City, Utah) has incorporated a silver-impregnated cuff near the exit site to impede infection further, with encouraging preliminary results.[95]

Infection may occur at the catheter exit site, along the superficial or deep catheter track, or within the epidural or intrathecal space.[96] Undetected and untreated, such infection may progress to abscess formation within the epidural space and subsequent vascular compromise and neurologic deficit.[97] In 339 cancer patients with surgically implanted, externalized Silastic epidural catheters (over 32,000 days of use), Du Pen noted 24 exit site or superficial track infections, 6 deep track, and 14 epidural infections, all of which were successfully managed conservatively, without surgical intervention. Exit site and superficial track infection resolved with topical care (povidine iodine or antibiotic ointment) and/or systemic antibiotics. Deep track and epidural infections resolved with antibiotic therapy and catheter removal. Patients with deep infections who were treated with antibiotics alone experienced recurrent infection. The incidence of infection seemed unrelated to duration of treatment. Epidural infections were associated mostly with contamination from skin flora. Contamination from the injectate, and, in three cases, hematogenous spread of systemic infection were implicated as well.

Exit site and superficial catheter track infections are associated with local inflammation and/or drainage, and in some cases with inflammatory changes extending to the catheter's Dacron cuff. Deep catheter track infections are associated with inflammatory changes along the catheter track proximal to the cuff, and may be associated with epidural infection. Epidural space infection is associated with constant, nonspecific back pain, pain on injection, fluid collection near the proximal incision, and reduced analgesia. None of the patients in Du Pen's series demonstrated meningismus, leukocytosis, fever, or neurologic abnormalities.[97]

The overall results of Du Pen's series are comparable to those from studies investigating the rate of infection in similar devices placed for vascular access. Results emphasize the importance of good local skin care, observation of filtered, aseptic administration, and vigilant assessment. Infectious disease and/or neurosurgical consultation is indicated in all cases of suspected infection. Evidence suggests that superficial infections can be managed successfully with topical treatment, whereas deeper infections require catheter removal and systemic antibiotic therapy. In the latter cases, serial magnetic resonance imaging will help determine resolution, following which, if indicated, a catheter can be replaced.

ANAPHYLAXIS

Despite a high incidence of patients with so-called "morphine allergy," true allergic reactions to morphine and its congeners are rare (see Chapters 9 and 12).[98] Such histories usually are more consistent with the occurrence of an unpleasant side effect. A single, well documented case of a life-threatening anaphylactic reaction to the administration of epidural fentanyl has been described.[99] True hypersensitivity to fentanyl (with positive skin testing), or indeed to any epidurally administered drug, is an extremely rare event. The subject of this report (and first author) was an anesthesiologist, and this first-person narrative makes fascinating reading.

MISINJECTIONS

Various substances have been injected accidentally through epidural and intrathecal catheters, including thiopental, methohexital, diazepam, pancuronium, gallamine, potassium chloride, magnesium sulfate, ephedrine, ranitidine, cephazolin, paraldehyde, total parenteral nutrition solutions, hypertonic contrast medium, hypertonic saline, and collodion.[100] Most cases have occurred with the injection of dilute solutions, and have resulted in self-limited back pain and spasm, although severe permanent neurologic injury has occurred in several cases.[100] Prevention of such incidents by applying special care in affixing distinct labels to intraspinal catheters, lines, and infusion devices, occlusion of accessory ports, and reducing the proximity of ports by thoughtful routing cannot be overemphasized. Various interventions have been undertaken once an incident has occurred, including the injection of epidural steroids, dilution with epidural saline, and aspiration and dilution via an intrathecal catheter (for catheter-related complications, refer to Chapter 24).

THERAPEUTICS

INDICATIONS AND CONTRAINDICATIONS

Acute Pain

Spinal opioids may be useful acutely for temporary palliation of symptoms in patients receiving antineoplastic treatment that is anticipated ultimately to provide long-term relief of pain. Treatment may be useful transiently to allow patients with severe movement-related pain to undergo diagnostic or therapeutic procedures.[101] This is true for patients who need to remain immobile for radiotherapy that is administered in fractionated doses over days or weeks, and for patients receiving chemotherapy, which usually is associated with pain relief that accrues slowly over time as tumor mass is reduced (see Chapters 15 and 16). Finally, the acute administration of intraspinal opioids may be useful for the management of these and other "pain emergencies" (pathologic fracture, nerve invasion) that cannot readily be controlled with other modalities.

Chronic Pain

As with neural blockade and neurosurgery, the most accepted indication for chronic therapy with intraspinal opioids is pain that is controlled inadequately despite aggressive efforts at systemic pharmacologic management, due either to persistent pain or intractable side effects.[18,31] This recommendation recognizes that more traditional pharmacologic modalities are associated with a more favorable risk-to-benefit ratio than relatively more invasive treatment, and that the benefits of the former should be exhausted before applying the lat-

ter. In the case of intraspinal opioid therapy, this general principle is open to challenge on two counts: 1) in the context of the entire spectrum of treatment modalities available to render pain control in this population, some authorities still consider intraspinal opioid therapy "conservative and noninvasive"[102]; and 2) on the basis that when its implementation is delayed, treatment may be relatively ineffective in patients who have been exposed to very high doses of systemic opioids,[103–106] and when instituted early, may be especially efficacious in relatively opioid-naive subjects.[107] This is an important area for further research. In contrast to neural blockade and neurosurgery, intraspinal opioid therapy more often provides effective relief of generalized pain as well as pain that is bilateral or midline, particularly when located in the trunk or lower limbs.[18,108,109]

Proper patient selection is critical if intraspinal opioids are to be used successfully to treat cancer pain, and requires that numerous factors be considered in the screening of patients.[110] Absolute contraindications include significant bleeding diathesis, anticoagulation therapy, and/or major anatomic abnormalities that would preclude proper catheter and system placement. These include localized infection, systemic sepsis, or localized tumor invasion that prevent safe access to the spinal canal. Behavioral dysfunction (severe debilitation, mental obtundation, and/or major psychiatric disturbances) may interfere with patients' ability to assess the nociceptive component of pain and to care properly for an externalized catheter, and as such are poor prognostic factors. Adequate support systems are essential to obtain, prepare, and administer intraspinal opioids.[24,25,111] When these do not exist, the anesthesiologist or neurosurgeon can play a pivotal role in their institution.

Pediatrics

Intraspinal opioid therapy has a well established role in the management of acute postoperative pain in children, although very little experience has been documented for chronic administration (Fig. 18–1A,B).[107,112,113]

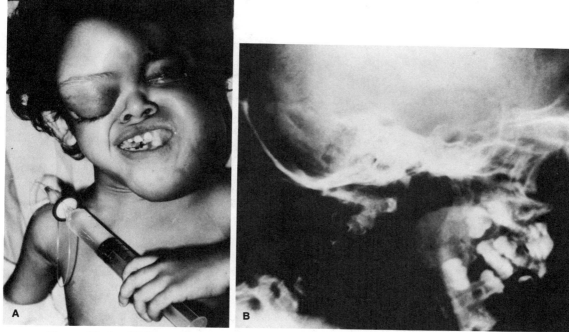

Figure 18–1. **(A)** Four-year-old boy with bilateral retinoblastoma. Pain was effectively palliated for 4 months with meperidine and droperidol administered via percutaneously placed cervical epidural catheter. **(B)** Radiograph of same patient obtained during placement. Note epidural needle at C6–7 interspace. Catheter tip has been advanced in proximity to foramen magnum. Courtesy, Ricardo Plancarte, MD, National Cancer Institute, Mexico City, Mexico.

SCREENING

Before commencing chronic therapy, it is necessary to determine that the pain syndrome is amenable to treatment with intraspinal opioids. In general, prior demonstration of systemic opioid responsivity is a good prognostic sign. Included in this group of patients are those who have achieved good analgesia with conventional systemic opioid therapy but in whom treatment has been frustrated by the development of undesirable opioid-mediated side effects and/or the development of significant tolerance. Despite a high degree of interindividual variability, it has been observed that continuous or intermittent somatic pain and visceral pain are most responsive to intraspinal opioid therapy, whereas cutaneous and neuropathic pain are most in-

tractable[14,106] (see Table 18–2), although a proportion of patients will respond satisfactorily regardless of the underlying mechanism of pain (see above, "Physicochemical Clinical Correlates"). Causes for inadequate relief have been summarized by Coombs[114] (Table 18–4).

The institution of intraspinal opioid therapy requires participation of an anesthesiologist or a neurosurgeon familiar with techniques of screening, implantation, and maintenance, as well as a home care system that is adaptable and innovative.[24–26,111] Anesthesiologists have assumed a major role in the institution of intraspinal opioid therapy, often including the (minor) surgical placement of indwelling delivery systems. Enthusiasm of patients treated with these modalities, as well as that of their primary care providers, oncolo-

Table 18–4.
Potential Causes of Failure of Intraspinal
Opioid Analgesia

- Neuropathic pain
- Incident pain
- Failure of delivery system
- Inadequate dose
- Incorrect prescription
- Tolerance
- Obstructed CSF mechanics (*ie*, epidural tumor)
- Psychoemotional decompensation

Modified from Coombs DW: Intraspinal narcotics for
intractable cancer pain. In Abrams S (ed): Cancer
Pain, p 82, Boston, Kluwer, 1989.

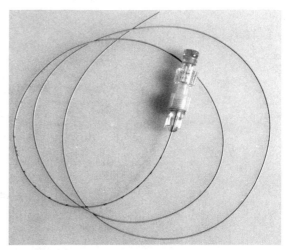

Figure 18–3. Standard (type I) percutaneous lumbar
epidural catheter used for screening purposes.

gists, and nurses has resulted in a substantial
increase in the visibility of anesthesiologists
in the role of pain specialists (Fig. 18–2).

Screening generally can be accomplished
on an inpatient or outpatient basis by observing the patient's response to morphine or a
similar agent administered through a temporary percutaneously inserted epidural catheter or via single epidural injection (Figs. 18–3
and 18–4).[31] As a rule, patients who have been
exposed chronically to oral opioids exhibit a
sufficient degree of opioid tolerance to obviate

the side effects of intraspinal opioid therapy
(see "Side Effects," above), making outpatient
screening a safe practice in most patients, although other authorities prefer screening to
take place on an inpatient basis.[111]

Before consideration of screening, a diagnosis of the pain problem and the magnitude
of oncologic disease are determined to the extent that is both practical and possible. It
should be determined that appropriate efforts

```
7-20-89

     A call from Dr. Patt:  the dose of intrathecal Morphine is 1
mg. q 12 hours, may be increased cautiously  from there.   Family
knows how to do it.

WST/ls

8-4-89

     Patient has marvelous pain control with 1 cc. of intrathecal
Morphine once a day.  It's truly amazing.  I'll  be able  to get
back to trying some chemotherapy.
```

Figure 18–2. Note from referring medical oncologist describing postoperative course of
patient with breast carcinoma and spinal metastases after insertion of intrathecal port. Before
surgery, patient had been receiving 200–300 mg intravenous morphine daily, and was obtunded
and bed-bound. After surgery, mental status cleared and patient ambulated with assistance.

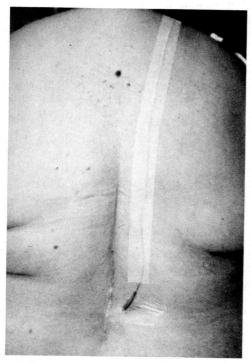

Figure 18–4. Standard percutaneously placed temporary epidural catheter for trial of intraspinal opioid analgesia. Note that catheter has been placed in the midlumbar region by a paramedian approach. Further reinforcement with additional paper tape and benzoin is required to reduce the likelihood that the catheter will be dislodged.

have been made to optimize more conservative therapy. As noted above, not all oncologic pain problems are palliated adequately by the application of intraspinal opioid therapy. Therefore, before implantation of a long-term delivery system, it is essential that clinical efficacy be verified with a percutaneous trial. This may be accomplished using an intermittent bolus technique, in which case adequacy of relief ideally is confirmed by at least two separate injections, spaced far enough apart in time to allow recovery from the prior injection.[110] When a continuous infusion method is used for screening, the demonstration of significant analgesia during a 24- to 48-hour treatment period is recommended.[115] As a rule

of thumb, the magnitude of relief obtained should exceed 50% of the preinjection pain level, and a duration of action of at least twice the normal half-life of the agent used should be observed (ie, 8–12 hours in the case of intraspinally administered morphine).[115] Residual pain relief after discontinuation of a continuous infusion method should also be present, and should be consistent with the elimination half-life of the agent used. It is preferable that test injections mimic the definitive therapy that is planned, since side effects and analgesic effects of epidural versus subarachnoid administration may not be identical, even when patients serve as their own controls.

ROUTES OF ADMINISTRATION

The field of CNS opioid therapy is sufficiently new that guidelines for administration and selection of route, drug, and protocol still are emerging (Table 18–5). Controlled studies are lacking. Epidural and subarachnoid administration of opioids produce analgesia by similar mechanisms,[22] and evidence is lacking for important distinctions in efficacy between

Table 18–5.
Decision-Making: Neuroaxial Opioids for
Cancer Pain

Selection of drug
  Morphine versus a more lipophilic opioid
  Opioid alone versus opioid + local anesthetic
Selection of route
  Epidural versus intrathecal versus intraventricular
Selection of catheter
  Percutaneous/externalized versus tunneled catheter
  If tunneled catheter is selected, externalized hub
    versus subcutaneous port versus totally implanted
    subcutaneous pump
Selection of schedule/means of administration
  Intermittent bolus versus continuous infusion ±
    patient-controlled anesthesia
  Self-administration versus external portable pump
    versus totally implanted pump

Table 18–6.
Potential Advantages of Epidural and
Intrathecal Placement

Epidural
- Reduced risk of postdural puncture headache and chronic CSF leak.
- Dura acts as barrier to infection. If infection occurs, it is more likely to be limited to epidural abscess (as opposed to meningitis).
- Permits greater flexibility in selection of drugs. Lipophilic agents and local anesthetics can be used more safely and successfully.
- Side effects tend to be less common and less intense.
- Permits greater flexibility in selection of site. Rostral placement may be combined with a lipophilic opioid for more segmental analgesia.
- Risk of neurologic injury probably is reduced.
- Margin of safety may be increased in the case of accidental overdose.

Intrathecal
- Technically easier to locate the intrathecal space reliably.
- Less risk of catheter obstruction from epidural fibrosis or metastases.
- Less likelihood of pain on injection.
- Analgesia is often more intense, rapid in onset and longer in duration.
- Lower doses (and volume) of opioid are required to produce analgesia (about 1:10 in the case of morphine). When long-term use is likely, doses associated with predominantly spinal (as opposed to systemic) effects can be used longer.
- Absence of risk from migration since catheter already is intrathecal.

---

routes. Nevertheless, the route selected has important clinical implications, and numerous important factors must be considered (Table 18–6). Ultimately, the selection of route, hardware, drug, dosage, and mode of administration must be individualized to the patient's unique circumstances (see Table 18–5).

Epidural Versus Subarachnoid Administration

Global clinical experience is greatest with epidural morphine administered by means of a lumbar epidural catheter, an approach that provides a generally dependable means of access to the central nervous system. The risk of postdural puncture headache is reduced, and, should infection occur, epidural abscess is more likely than meningitis since the dura acts as a barrier to leptomeningeal infection. At least theoretically, there is greater risk of catheter dysfunction secondary to epidural tumor deposits and fibrosis than when the subarachnoid route is used. In fact, in laboratory animals, the rapid formation of a fibrous sheath surrounding the tip of indwelling epidural catheters, and subsequent interference with drug distribution has been observed routinely.[116]

Administered either by the epidural or subarachnoid route, the equianalgesic opioid dose is a fraction of that required for the subcutaneous, intramuscular, or intravenous administration (see Fig. 18–2).[10,32,117] The epidural route requires about a 10-fold increase in opioid dose relative to subarachnoid administration, because the dura acts as a barrier to the transfer of drug into the CSF and to receptor sites in the spinal cord. This factor recommends subarachnoid administration for long-term use (greater than 3 to 6 months), since once tolerance develops, the higher epidural doses can result in increased systemic side effects. Passage across the dura may account for slight increases in latency of onset and slight reductions in duration of action, when compared to subarachnoid administration. The epidural route, however, does permit greater flexibility in drug selection: substitution of a lipid-soluble opioid or the addition of a local anesthetic have more predictable results than when the subarachnoid route is used. Localization of the epidural space requires greater skill than does subarachnoid puncture, especially in the presence of osteoarthritis, metastatic tumor, or orthopedic hardware.

Selection of the epidural route more readily permits catheter placement at a rostral dermatome level, which may be desirable for the administration of lipid-soluble opioids in close proximity to the receptors corresponding to a more cephalic site of pain (see Fig. 18–1A,B), as in the case of superior sulcus lung tumors. When a large-bore Silastic catheter and radiologic guidance is used, however, the catheter tip often can be threaded as far cephalad as necessary by either route (Fig. 18–5).[118] Easy passage, however, may be impeded by the presence of epidural metastases or severe osteoarthritis. An intraprocedural epidurogram (Fig. 18–6A,B) and test doses of local anesthetic are recommended to verify epidural placement. Although there have been anecdotal reports of rostral analgesia from morphine administered in the lumbar region,[57,107,119] the treatment of more cephalic pain is facilitated by catheter implantation at thoracic or cervical levels.[57,113,120,121] (see Fig. 18–1A,B).

Infection is uncommon with epidural placement, whether the catheter hub is internalized or externalized (see "Infectious Complications," above). For chronic use, subarachnoid placement requires that the drug portal be internalized, either by means of an internalized infusion pump or portal (see "Selection of Implantable Drug Delivery Systems," below), to minimize the likelihood of meningitis.

Intraventricular/Cisternal (Intracerebroventricular) Administration

Increasing experience with small doses of morphine administered through Ommaya reservoirs suggests that this is an effective and practical method of relieving pain in selected patients. This modality is often effective in the setting of intractable tolerance to intraspinal opioid administration, and, in one study, patients exposed to both modalities consistently rated intraventricular administration higher with respect to quality of pain relief.[122] Access to the ventricular system usually is through a coronal burr hole made under local anesthesia (Figs. 18–7 and 18–8). An alternative technique involving passage of a percutaneous catheter through a 14-gauge Touhy needle into the cisterna magna also has been described.[123] The goal of most practitioners is ongoing outpatient administration by a family member or visiting nurse.[102,124–126]

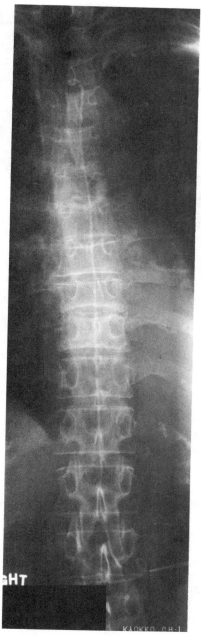

Figure 18–5. Anteroposterior radiograph demonstrating radiopaque DuPen catheter (Davol, Inc.) inserted at L1–2 and threaded cephalad to T2. Courtesy, Stuart DuPen, Seattle, Washington.

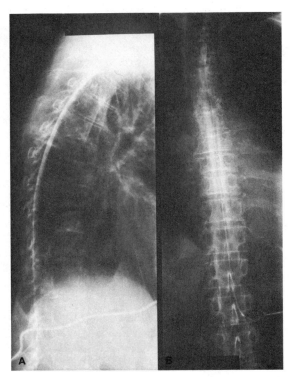

Figure 18–6. (A,B) Anteroposterior and lateral epidurograms. Courtesy, Stuart DuPen, Seattle, Washington.

The quality of analgesia is excellent in most cases, and apparently is unaffected by the site of pain. The majority of treatment has been rendered for patients with cervicofacial pain, because more conservative or traditional techniques frequently prove inadequate (see Chapter 26).[127] Other candidates include patients with cervicobrachial pain, bilateral or midline pain, or unremitting pain in any body part that persists despite trials of more conservative measures. A trial of lumbar or cisternal morphine generally precedes implantation.[124,126] Optimum life expectancy is on the order of about 6 months. Premature initiation increases risks of sepsis, tolerance, and respiratory depression. In imminently preterminal patients, tolerance may already exist, which, together with a high incidence of mental confusion, complicates management.[124,125]

Various hardware, drug preparations, and dosing schedules have been devised. Doses of morphine between 0.2 mg and 4 mg are used most commonly, and duration of analgesia averages 24 hours after a single dose.[125,126] Minor side effects similar to those associated with the administration of intraspinal opioids (see "Side Effects and Their Management," above) have been reported. Dose-related respiratory depression and infection, potentially serious sequelae, are extremely rare in published series.[125,128]

SELECTION OF AGENT

Preservatives

Despite an absence of exhaustive histopathologic surveys, there has been an intuitive reluctance to infuse preservative-containing preparations of analgesics intraspinally. Preservative-free morphine is available commercially for intraspinal use, or can be manufactured by a pharmacist (see Appendix C), and other drugs are available in preservative-free preparations. Multiple-dose vials contain preservatives and should not be used. DuPen[129] has reported a case of the accidental use of epidural morphine containing phenol and formaldehyde. The patient experienced burning pain on injection and eventually disorientation and confusion. An epidurogram revealed new nonspecific filling defects. Despite chronic administration, however, no sensory or motor deficits were observed. Citing the high cost of chronic administration of preservative-free morphine, Du Pen recommends the use of Tubex (Wyeth Laboratories, Philadelphia, PA) morphine, a preparation containing low concentrations of chlorobutanol, a chloroform derivative. Administration of this product in 57,087 injections over 15,023 days of catheter use[118] has resulted in no neurologic abnormalities.

Hydrophilic Agents: Morphine

A wide variety of opioid and nonopioid substances (see "Tolerance," below) have been administered intraspinally to produce clini-

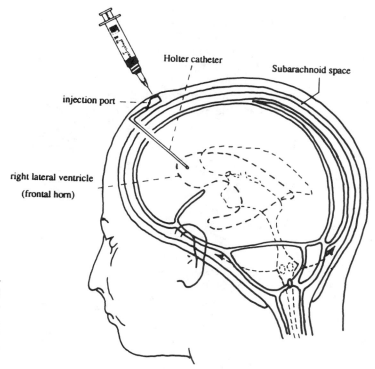

Figure 18–7. Schematic representation of intracerebroventricular opioid administration. Reprinted with permission from De Castro J, Meynadier J, Zenz M: Regional Opioid Analgesia p 402. Dordrecht, Kluwer Academic, 1991.

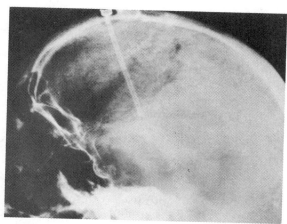

Figure 18–8. Lateral radiograph demonstrating an implanted intracerebroventricular catheter and subcutaneous port. Reprinted with permission from De-Castro J, Meynadier J, Zenz M: Regional Opioid Analgesia p 402. Dordrecht, Kluwer Academic, 1991.

cally useful analgesia. As the most commonly administered intraspinal drug for the control of chronic cancer pain, morphine is the most useful standard for comparison. As a rule, peak analgesic effects are obtained within 30–60 minutes of administration, and a duration of 6–24 hours can be anticipated from a single dose. Single doses of between 2.5–5.0 mg and 0.1–0.5 mg are used most commonly in opioid-naive subjects, administered by the epidural and intrathecal routes, respectively. Significantly higher doses may be required to manage chronic cancer pain in the relatively opioid-tolerant patient. Relatively high levels of morphine can be detected in the CSF for a prolonged period after administration,[41,42,44] and may account for the nature of observed side effects (see "Side Effects," above), especially in opioid-naive patients. In a review of published reports of 107 cancer patients being treated chronically with intrathecal morphine,

Ventafridda et al[130] noted a dose range of between 0.5–85 mg daily, with a single patient receiving 150 mg/day. Epidural doses ranged from 1–240 mg in 306 cases, although a separate report documents a single case of a patient receiving 540 mg of epidural morphine daily by the end of 1 year's treatment. Tolerance occurs in a variable proportion of patients, and appears to be related more to the duration of prior morphine therapy than to the actual dose of morphine.[131] It is possible that when epidural doses are driven so high, the advantages of intraspinal therapy (enhanced analgesia with decreased side effects) may be lost because of high plasma levels, and alternate therapy might be considered in such cases.

Baricity. Except when combined with an anesthetic agent, intrathecal morphine is administered most often as an isobaric solution. Preliminary studies in cancer patients suggest that when hyperbaric solutions of morphine (7% dextrose) are used, rostral redistribution is reduced.[132] The onset and density of analgesia did not appear to differ, but duration of analgesia was prolonged (24–30 vs. 12–24 hours), and side effects may be reduced for hyperbaric versus isobaric injections, especially when patients are nursed in the head-up position.

Lipophilic Agents: Sufentanil and Fentanyl

Sufentanil is the prototype of the lipophilic opioids. Characteristically, analgesia is observed within a few minutes of epidural injection, peaks at 10 minutes, and is sustained for 2–5 hours. The optimal dose in opioid-naive patients seems to be 50 μg diluted in 10 ml of saline.[20] Due to its lipophilicity, analgesia has a more regional, segmental nature, and catheter placement near the area of the cord corresponding to the site of pain is required. It has been proposed that the administration of a large volume of dilute drug is essential for a good effect, although Boersma has reported excellent long-term analgesia in cancer patients with the administration of an undiluted infusion.[133] In the case of fentanyl, larger volumes of diluent have been observed to result in a more rapid onset and longer duration of analgesia.[134] The addition of epinephrine 1:200,000 to epidural sufentanil has been shown to intensify the segmental nature of analgesia, as well as its duration.[135] For epidural fentanyl (50–100 μg diluted in saline), analgesia is noted within about 5 minutes, peaks at 10–20 minutes, and is sustained for 2–3 hours. Administered epidurally, high doses of fentanyl and sufentanil are required to produce analgesia relative to an equianalgesic dose of morphine. This factor, combined with the potential for rapid venous uptake, warrant increased vigilance for early side effects, particularly in opioid-naive patients. The incidence of delayed side effects is minimal or nil.[22,41,136] In one study of the pharmacokinetics of lumbar epidural fentanyl, high concentrations of fentanyl in the lumbar CSF were observed, together with low concentrations in the cervical CSF and bloodstream. In the same study, intravenous doses of fentanyl produced negligible CSF levels of drug.[34]

The chronic administration of intrathecal sufentanil and fentanyl has not been reported as of this writing. Fentanyl 50 μg was administered intrathecally as a supplement to spinal anesthesia in a pilot double-blind study of perioperative patients.[137] One patient experienced respiratory and subsequent cardiac arrest 1 hour after administration. Trends toward periodic breathing, pruritus, and sedation were noted, suggesting clinically significant rostral spread at least in opioid-naive subjects. The blinded addition of 20 and 40 μg of fentanyl to spinal anesthesia in another group of perioperative patients resulted in a doubling of the duration of postoperative analgesia.[138] Although pruritus was noted in most patients, no serious side effects were observed. A third pilot study evaluating the addition of 10 μg of fentanyl to spinal anesthesia was unable to discern differences between the study group and controls, except when fentanyl was combined with epinephrine.[139]

Alfentanil does not appear to be a very suitable sole agent for chronic administration, although there has been some preliminary work in the setting of acute pain. Alfentanil is a mu agonist that is less lipid-soluble, and, when administered epidurally, less potent than fentanyl. In doses of 0.15–0.30 mg/kg, analgesia is rapid in onset (about 5 minutes) but of short duration (90–100 minutes).[140]

Opioid Analgesics of Intermediate Lipophilicity

Most of the experience with these agents relates to their use in acute pain populations. General pharmacodynamic information is presented here, along with data pertaining to chronic use.

Epidural methadone, administered in 4-mg boluses every 8 hours, provides a rapid onset of good relief for postoperative pain.[90] Its lower incidence of urinary (and respiratory) disturbances compared to epidural morphine suggests a role in chronic management in the unusual circumstance of the cancer patient with urinary symptoms referable to the administration of intraspinal opioids.[91] Methadone's long plasma half-life and potential for clinically important accumulation warrants caution when considering chronic administration. The use of epidural methadone as the sole means of management for two patients with diffuse bone pain from multiple myeloma has been reported anecdotally as being efficacious, without side effects, and relatively free of tolerance.[141]

Epidural hydromorphone, administered in 1.5-mg boluses, is associated with rapid onset of relief from postoperative pain, with a duration ranging from 6 to 19 hours.[142,143] Coombs et al[144] reported on the successful management of a patient with pelvic cancer pain with the continuous administration of intrathecal hydromorphone (2.4–10 mg/day) for a period of months. Subsequent increases in pain were managed in this patient with the addition of intrathecal clonidine.

Meperidine has already been mentioned (see "Physicochemical Clinical Correlates," above) as having local anesthetic effects when administered intrathecally. Epidural meperidine administered in bolus doses of 20–50 mg for postoperative pain is associated with a rel-atively rapid onset and peak effect of analgesia (15–20 minutes) lasting 3–6 hours or longer.[20,145] Potential problems related to the accumulation of normeperidine, a metabolite associated with CNS toxicity, particularly in patients with renal and hepatic dysfunction, limit the desirability of chronic administration.[146]

Epidural diamorphine (heroin) has been used to manage both acute[147] and chronic cancer pain,[59] although not extensively. After administration, diamorphine is rapidly de-acetylated into morphine and monoacetyl-morphine, and is about as potent and slightly more lipophilic than morphine (1.5 vs. 1.7). As a result, after epidural administration, relatively higher systemic levels are achieved for diamorphine, but the duration and depth of analgesia are similar to those of epidural morphine.[20] Delayed respiratory depression has not been reported. Administered intrathecally in comparable doses, the depth and duration of analgesia seem to be superior for diamorphine when compared to morphine.[20]

Endogenous Opioids: Synthetic Beta-Endorphin

Although because it does not cross the blood–brain barrier, pain relief does not occur for intravenous administration, synthetically prepared beta-endorphin (the body's most potent endogenous opioid) has been demonstrated to possess analgesic properties when administered intraventricularly[148] and intraspinally[149–151] in cancer patients. Profound analgesia results just a few minutes after injection, and often persists for days. One investigator has suggested that pretreatment with intrathecal beta-endorphin renders subjects more sensitive to the subsequent administration of other analgesics.[149] Transient psychological disturbances have been observed after administration, but other side effects were less prominent than with intrathecal morphine administration.

Preliminary work with inhibitors of endogenous enkephalinase (an enzyme that degrades endogenous peptides) has been reported in animals and humans, suggesting another important area for research (see "Future Developments in Intraspinal Analgesia," below).

Opioid Agonist/Antagonists as Analgesics

Buprenorphine is an agonist/antagonist agent that is relatively lipophilic (3.96), and has been used in a wide spectrum of settings, including the management of chronic cancer pain.[152,153] Administered epidurally (0.15–0.3 mg), analgesia is noted within 5–10 minutes, peaks within 30–60 minutes, and lasts 4–10 hours.[20] Side effects are similar to those observed for other agents, but are less problematic than with epidural morphine.[152] Late respiratory depression does not occur, although early respiratory depression may be somewhat greater than that seen with morphine because of greater systemic absorption.[153] Unwanted agonist effects are not readily reversed with naloxone, and, as with other agonist/antagonist agents, there is a ceiling dose above which further analgesia cannot be achieved. Nalbuphine, butorphanol, and pentazocine have all been used for the management of acute pain with some success. None of these agents has any demonstrated properties recommending their use for the management of chronic cancer pain, and, in particular, pentazocine should be avoided due to its propensity to produce psychomimetic side effects.[20]

ADMINISTRATION BY CONTINUOUS INFUSION VERSUS INTERMITTENT BOLUS

Each technique has its advantages and disadvantages (see Table 18–7), but most authorities favor the use of infusions when adequate resources are available. The main advantage of treatment with a continuous infusion is maintenance of stable therapeutic CSF levels of drug, resulting in fewer episodes of pain and toxicity.[154] In contrast, bolus doses are more likely to produce transiently high plasma levels of drug and cephalad diffusion.[20] Reductions in dose requirements have

Table 18–7.
Continuous Infusion versus Intermittent Bolus Administration

Potential Advantages of Continuous Infusion
- More consistent level of analgesia
- Reduced side effects
- Reduced dosage requirements
- Reduced nursing care
- Reduced patient/family anxiety
- Reduced handling of catheter/infection
- Delayed development of tolerance
- More facile use of short-acting agents
- Potential for addition of patient-controlled analgesia

Potential Disadvantages of Continuous Infusion
- Expense of infusion devices
- Limited availability of infusion devices
- Availability of trained personnel to service pumps and monitor care
- Potential for device malfunction
- Potential for errors in prescribing and refilling infusion device
- Potential for overtreatment, undertreatment, and unrecognized breakthrough pain

been observed, and tolerance may be delayed with continuous infusion techniques (see "Tolerance," below). In the case of catheter migration, attendant side effects may occur more gradually, providing a warning period when treatment is being rendered by an infusion. A further advantage is that continuous administration uses a more "closed" system, and less frequent handling of the catheter system may reduce infection risks. The use of an infusion device in the home may cause some initial anxiety, but when proper orientation, education, and support are instituted, concerns about the patient's and family's competence to administer intermittent injections are allayed. Families are often relieved to be able to depend on a mechanical device and back-up support personnel. Some continuous systems may be supplemented by the addition of patient-controlled analgesia (PCA), which has considerable advantages in selected patients (see "Patient-Controlled Analgesia," below).

The greatest disadvantage of continuous infusion techniques relates to the costs of obtaining and maintaining infusion devices. In developing nations, the technology is unavailable and/or unaffordable (see Chapter 27). The use of a relatively inexpensive disposable portable infusion device (Travenol Infusor, Travenol Inc., Deerfield, IL) has been described,[155] and may be useful in such settings. Some communities initially may be reluctant to accept the heightened level of nursing care required for the provision of safe intraspinal infusion therapy.

Patient-Controlled Analgesia

The provision of on-demand boluses as a supplement to a continuous background infusion of drug is simply an adaptation of standard oral pharmacotherapy for cancer pain using a sustained-release basal analgesic and the as-needed administration of "rescue" doses (see Chapters 6–9). The limitations of therapy include practical ones related to community resources (see "Administration by Continuous Infusion Versus Intermittent Bolus," above) and patient considerations (see below).

Cancer is associated with a variety of losses, including progressive loss of control. Patient-controlled analgesia is ideally suited as a measure to insure return of some degree of control over the environment. At the same time, instituting PCA addresses one of patients' greatest fears: uncontrolled pain.

Patient-controlled analgesia, however, is not appropriate for all patients. Patients and their family members often are overwhelmed by the technical aspects of their care. They may not welcome the additional responsibility of self-medication. These objections often can be overcome by thorough teaching. Nevertheless, the health care team must be sensitive to patients with a more passive style who prefer to surrender control, and in whom the addition of PCA may contribute to preexisting anxiety. Also, patients with a history of drug-seeking behavior frequently are excluded from treatment. Patients must understand the concept and technique of PCA in order to use it effectively. Patients with cognitive deficits, whether due to age, cerebral metastases, psychiatric disturbances, or drug intoxication are not suitable candidates for treatment with PCA. So-called "spouse-controlled analgesia" (SCA), and even "parent-assisted PCA" has been advocated for patients unable to use PCA to its full advantage because of physiologic or psychologic limitations. Successful SCA requires careful screening, teaching, and frequent reassessment. As with other significant medical interventions, PCA should not be used unless proper supervision from a family member and/or visiting health professional is provided. It is essential that a member of the health care team be available around-the-clock to respond to mechanical problems that sometimes occur with any technologic or pump-based therapy.

Since most patients report some degree of constant pain, PCA usually is administered as a supplement to rather than as a substitute for a continuous background infusion of drug. Combining continuous infusion and PCA features eliminates the need for frequent bolus administration, as well as awakening to administer boluses.

Physician-ordered parameters for continuous plus PCA treatment include 1) drug concentration, 2) background infusion rate, 3) bolus dose, and 4) lockout interval. The lockout interval refers to the minimum interval between doses, the time period during which the system is refractory to additional patient requests. In addition, if an effort is being made to titrate analgesia, orders might include a schedule for upward or downward increases in dosing.

Drug selection and regimens for drug administration vary considerably in the literature, due in part to relative inexperience with PCA, drug tolerance, and variations in patient response. The background infusion rate should be adjusted to provide adequate analgesia with a minimum of sedation. The bolus dose should be adjusted to provide supplemental analgesia to counter spontaneous exacerbations of pain (breakthrough pain), as well as to minimize predictable episodes of pain that correlate with increased activity (incident pain). Lockout interval is chosen based on predictions of peak effects on pain and ventilation. One acceptable regi-

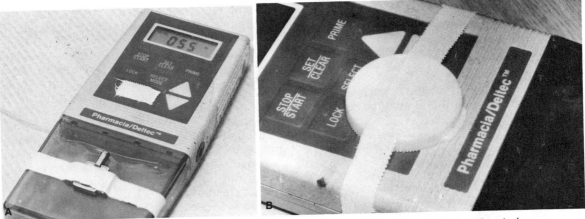

Figure 18–9. **(A)** Portable continuous infusion device with patient-controlled analgesia feature modified by patient to permit easy nocturnal location of demand button. **(B)** Same device, modified by patient with taped medicine cap to retard easy access to bolus to prevent accidental overdose.

men uses epidural or intrathecal morphine, and calls for an initial bolus dose of 25% of the hourly dose with an initial lockout interval of between 30 and 60 minutes. These parameters are then adjusted according to the patient's response to treatment. Treatment with continuous epidural infusions of lipophilic opioids (fentanyl and sufentanil) is particularly well suited to the addition of PCA due to the more rapid onset of relief that usually occurs.

We have observed two phenomena that may produce difficulties when portable pumps are used, and on the basis of our experience with an ingenious patient have proposed simple solutions.[156] One involves the placement of a strip of adhesive tape over the bolus button, at least for nocturnal use, to facilitate locating the proper control in the dark (Fig. 18–9A). The second involves the potential for patients to self-administer bolus accidentally or to over-administer boluses if they should become confused, a scenario that could further compound confusion. The solution involves simply taping the cap from a medicine vial over the bolus button during the day, so that accessing it requires greater intent (see Fig. 18–9B).

SELECTION OF IMPLANTABLE DRUG DELIVERY SYSTEMS

Waldman and Coombs have recommended a system for classifying the six basic types of implantable drug delivery systems (IDDS) (see Table 18–8) that serves as a useful reference.[101,157] The pain specialist's thorough understanding of each system's unique profile of advantages and disadvantages is essential for optimal selection and use.

Anesthesiologists are most familiar with the type I system, which consists of a simple percutaneous catheter, essentially identical to that routinely used for obstetrical and surgical pain control (see Figs. 18–3, 18–4).[158] The type II system (Fig. 18–10) is identical with the exception that the catheter is tunneled subcutaneously (Fig. 18–11A,B).[109,118] Its administration hub remains externalized. The type III system consists of a totally implantable injection port attached to a type II catheter that is tunneled subcutaneously in its entirety (Figs. 18–11A,B and 18–12). The type IV system substitutes a totally implantable mechanically activated pump for the portal of the type II system; the result is a totally implantable patient-controlled analgesia device (Fig. 18–

Table 18–8.
A Classification of Implantable Drug Delivery
Systems (IDDS)*

Type I	Percutaneous epidural or intrathecal catheter (taped)
Type II	Percutaneous epidural or subarachnoid catheter with a portion of the catheter tunneled subcutaneously from entrance site
Type IIA	Standard epidural catheter partially tunneled (usually) at beside using another epidural needle or intracatheter
Type IIB	Silastic epidural catheter more completely tunneled through paraspinal incision in O.R. setting
Type III	Totally implanted epidural or intrathecal catheter attached to subcutaneous injection port
Type IV	Totally implanted epidural or intrathecal catheter attached to implanted manually activated pump (PCA)
Type V	Totally implanted epidural or intrathecal catheter attached to implanted infusion pump (constant rate)
Type VI	Totally implanted epidural or intrathecal catheter attached to implanted infusion pump (computer programmable)

* Modified from Waldman SD, Coombs DW: Selection of implantable narcotic delivery systems. Anesth Analg 1989;68:377.

allows a broad spectrum of delivery rates and modes, including preprogrammed bolus injections.

A variety of factors enter into the complex decision of properly selecting the ideal IDDS. First, preimplantation screening with a percutaneous catheter (see "Screening," above) should suggest the likelihood of an adequate therapeutic response. Economic factors play an important role in the selection of a delivery system, but unfortunately have received little scholarly attention. The costs of the intended delivery system, surgical and hospital fees, drugs, disposable supplies, and home care nursing must all be considered. The cost of sophisticated nonreusable implantable devices (hardware alone) ranges between $6,000 and $8,000, and is difficult to justify for use in an imminently preterminal patient. A preliminary study comparing partially implanted versus fully implanted systems suggests that despite a greater "up front" cost, at about 3 months after the initial implant, savings begin to be realized with the fully implanted system due to reduced needs for drug, disposables, and home care.[159]

Type I Percutaneous Catheter

The type I percutaneous catheter (see Figs. 18–3 and 18–4) has gained wide acceptance for the short-term administration of intraspinal opioids and/or local anesthetics for the relief of acute obstetric, intraoperative, and

13A,B). The type V system (Figs. 18–14 and 18–15) is a totally implantable, nonprogrammable (fixed-rate), continuous infusion pump (Infusaid Model 400 pump, Infusaid Inc., Norwood, MA) connected to a type II catheter. The type VI (SynchroMed Infusion system, Medtronic, Minneapolis, MN) (Figs. 18–16 and 18–17) is a further modification of the type V system that incorporates external programmability via a lap-top computer (Fig. 18–18) and telemetry (Fig. 18–19). The programmable feature of the type VI system

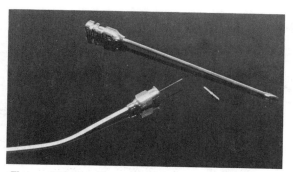

Figure 18–10. Type II Silastic intraspinal catheter with guide wire and 14-gauge epidural needle.

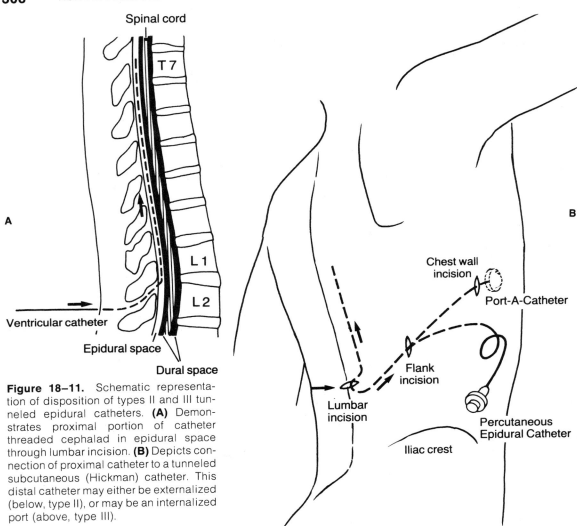

Figure 18–11. Schematic representation of disposition of types II and III tunneled epidural catheters. **(A)** Demonstrates proximal portion of catheter threaded cephalad in epidural space through lumbar incision. **(B)** Depicts connection of proximal catheter to a tunneled subcutaneous (Hickman) catheter. This distal catheter may either be externalized (below, type II), or may be an internalized port (above, type III).

postsurgical pain.[158] In cancer pain management the type I catheter is used for preimplantation screening as well as to control acute pain (see "Screening" and "Acute Pain," above). A further important use is in imminently preterminal patients (life expectancy less than 4 weeks) who are unfit even for minor surgery.[160] In either case, consideration should be given to the use of a wire-reinforced catheter (Fig. 18–20), which has the advantages of greater durability, radiopacity, and less risk of shearing during repeated passage

through the epidural needle that occasionally is needed to facilitate cephalad placement.[161]

Chronic use of the type I system is limited by increased risks of catheter migration and CNS infection.[109] Erythema and seropurulent drainage commonly is observed at catheter exit sites within 7 days of percutaneous placement. Infection is most likely to occur initially at the catheter exit site, which in this case is in close proximity to the spine, resulting in enhanced risks of a superficial skin infection that will progress to epidural abscess or men-

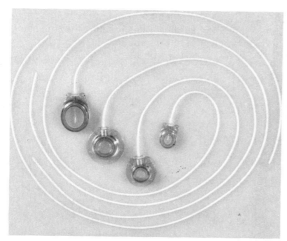

Figure 18–12. Assortment of type III systems consisting of implantable ports and Silastic intraspinal catheters.

ingitis. Although the prolonged use of the type I catheter has been reported to be reliable and safe,[162] most authorities believe its use should be limited to the acute care setting because of the more favorable risk-to-benefit ratio associated with the use of the type II system.[101]

Type II Subcutaneously Tunneled Catheter

Superior catheter fixation, probable reduced risks of CNS infection, and the relative ease of tunneling make this system more desirable than the type I system for patients with a life expectancy of weeks or months. Two alternate systems have been devised for catheter placement. The simplest involves the placement of a standard or wire-reinforced epidural catheter. The catheter is threaded through the needle into the epidural space. Before the needle's removal, a small incision is made through the skin and subcutaneous tissue at the site where the needle enters the back, after which the catheter is tunneled toward the flank in one or more passes using another epidural needle or venous cannula as a tunneling device (Fig. 18–21).[163,164] This technique involves a minimum of stress and risk

to the patient, and can be performed at the bedside, although some authorities recommend the use of an operating room.[10] Potential disadvantages are that the relatively fragile epidural catheter cannot readily be threaded very far cephalad, and may migrate or become obstructed over time.

A modified technique[118] involves an initial surgical incision in the lumbar region and introduction of a 16-gauge Silastic catheter through a 14-gauge epidural needle from a paramedian approach (see Figs. 18–10, 18–11A,B, and 18–22). If the incision is carried through the superficial and deep lumbar fascia, the paravertebral muscles can be pushed aside, and the catheter can be tunneled deeply and fixed firmly to the tough periosteal fascia, further assuring its immobility. A separate Silastic catheter is then tunneled from the flank and is sutured to the epidural catheter over a stainless steel connector (Fig. 18–23). This technique involves moderately greater skill and experience, is more invasive, and is associated with greater stress to the patient. Sterile operating room facilities, including an electrocautery and fluoroscope are required (Fig. 18–24). There are increased acute risks of superficial and deep bleeding, kinking, leakage, and acute infection. With good technique, however, these risks are low. Monitored anesthesia care or general anesthesia and a single intravenous dose of antibiotics are recommended.

Silastic, long used for Hickman and Broviac catheters, is extremely biocompatible, and the large-caliber tubing makes migration and obstruction less likely (see Fig. 18–10). Using radiologic control, the catheter tip often can be threaded as far cephalad as is required (see Figs. 18–5, 18–24). One manufacturer (Davol Inc., Salt Lake City, Utah) provides a kit that comes complete with a disposable tunneling device and all other items required for insertion.[118] The distal catheter is fitted with a Dacron cuff that adheres to the subcutaneous tissue and further discourages displacement. The recent addition of a silver-impregnated cuff is intended further to prevent infection. With the exception of the sutures used to bridge the two catheters, all other suture ma-

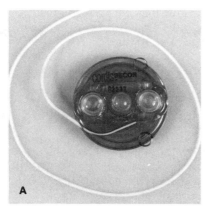

Figure 18–13. **(A)** Type IV fully implantable (patient-controlled) infusion device and Silastic catheter. **(B)** Illustrates means of replenishing reservoir and (patient-controlled) pump operation.

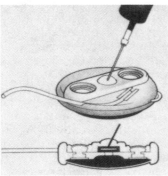
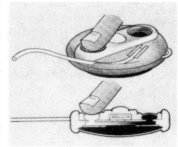
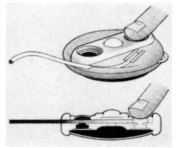

B   1. The reservoir is filled via a self-sealing dome

2. Press button 1 and a single dose is transferred to the delivery button

3. Press button 2 and, whilst button 1 is filling, a single bolus is delivered

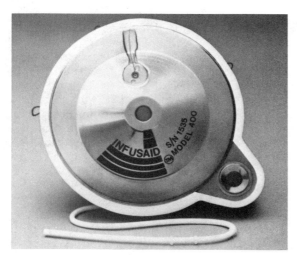

Figure 18–14. Type V fully implantable intraspinal infusion device with Silastic catheter and sideport, Infusaid model 400 by Shiley.

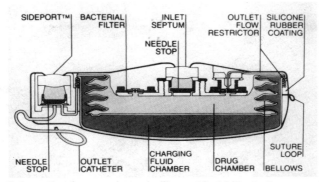

Figure 18–15. Schematic of pump shown in Figure 18–14 illustrating pumping mechanism.

terial is absorbable so that the catheter can later be removed if necessary. In fit patients the procedure can be performed on an ambulatory basis, but a short hospital stay is often necessary. Transient peri-incisional pain is expected.

Type III Totally Implantable Reservoir/Port

This system consists of a subcutaneously tunneled Silastic catheter attached to a stainless steel-backed silicone port (see Figs. 18–11A,B and 18–12).[43,107,165,166] The silicone dome re-

seals after puncture with an atraumatic Huber needle, and is designed to withstand over 1,000 punctures without leakage. Injection is somewhat more difficult to accomplish than with the type I and II systems, but can be taught readily, or alternatively a portable infusion pump can be attached.

MEDTRONIC SYNCHROMED® INFUSION PUMP

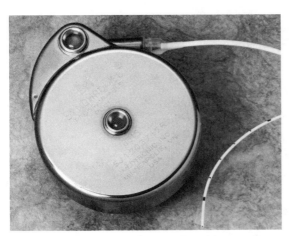

Figure 18–16. Type VI fully implantable, computer-programmable intraspinal infusion device, Model 8611-H Synchromed pump by Medtronics.

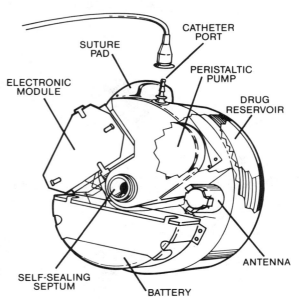

Figure 18–17. Schematic of pump illustrated in Figure 18–16 demonstrating pumping mechanism.

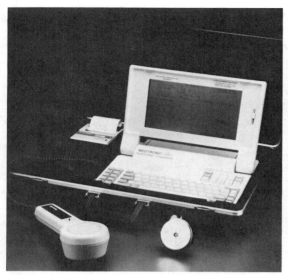

Figure 18–18. Portable lap-top computer used with Synchromed pump.

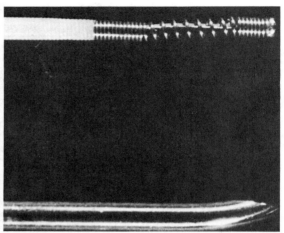

Figure 18–20. Racz epidural catheter: consists of a stainless steel spiral coated with fluoropolymer along its entire length up to near the tip. The tip is blunt, and spirals are spread. Within the catheter's lumen is a stainless steel supporting straight wire that is welded at each end. The flexible tip is designed to reduce the potential for nerve injury, and the body design is intended to reduce the potential for kinking, shearing, and false-negative aspiration tests. The blunt margins of the accompanying 17-gauge epidural needle are designed to reduce the likelihood of shearing catheters, and as a result it can be moved in and out more freely. Courtesy, Gabor Racz, MD, Lubbock, Texas

A type III system often is selected for use in patients with life expectancies ranging from months to years. It is an acceptable means for administering drugs into the subarachnoid space, since it is completely internalized. Once established, the risk of infection and

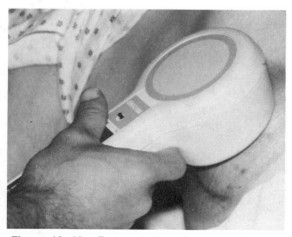

Figure 18–19. Demonstration of process of reprogramming type VI pump using microcircuitry-driven telemetry.

catheter malfunction should be lower than with the type I and II systems. Implantation technique is similar to that described above for the Silastic type II catheter, except that a small pocket is made distally using an electrocautery device. Removal or revision requires a surgical incision.

Type IV Totally Implantable Mechanically Activated Pump

Poletti and colleagues devised one of the earliest totally implantable systems for patient-activated drug delivery.[167] This system consisted of an implantable sterile blood bag, and a hydrocephalus shunt valve and spinal catheter attached in series. The valve could be activated by the patient to affect self-administration of a precalculated bolus of opioid. This

Figure 18–21. Process of subcutaneous tunneling of a type I epidural catheter performed at patient's bedside using two epidural needles. The tip of the right-sided (midline) needle has been withdrawn from the epidural space. A small nick has been made with a scalpel at the needle's entrance site. After the administration of subcutaneous local anesthetic, the left-sided needle is passed toward the midline nick, so that after the first needle is removed, the catheter can be threaded laterally through the tip of the second needle.

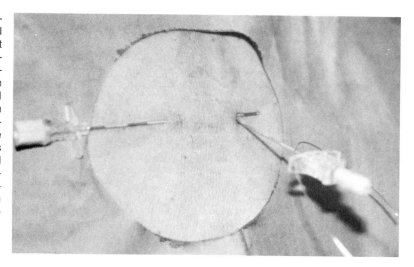

concept was modified by Cordis, Miami, FL. Their device is a totally implantable reservoir that is accessed percutaneously by pressure on a septum on the surface of the device (see Fig. 18–13A,B). A set of buttons on the pump's surface activates a mechanical valve system when they are pressed in proper sequence.[101,167] The type IV system has poten-

tially less risk of infection than types I–III, and, as with type III, subarachnoid delivery is possible. The greatest advantage of the system is that, as with any PCA device, the patient can titrate drug dosage based on symptoms, and can pretreat symptoms before periods of increased activity. This system is not currently available in the United States,

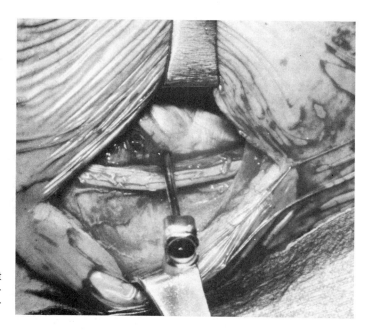

Figure 18–22. Intraoperative placement of 14-gauge epidural needle for implantation of a Du Pen (Davol, Inc.) Silastic intraspinal catheter.

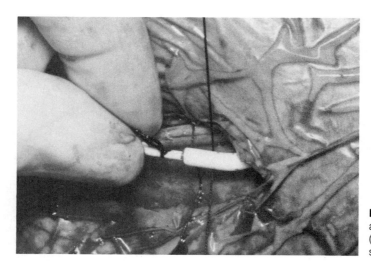

Figure 18–23. Demonstrates means of affixing proximal (intraspinal) and distal (Hickman) Silastic catheters together over stainless steel pin.

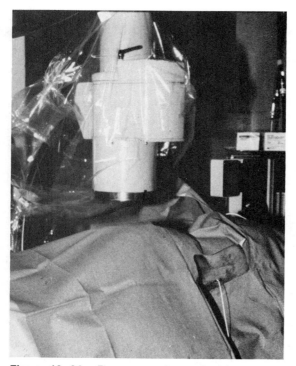

Figure 18–24. Fluoroscopy is required intraoperatively to verify placement and integrity of intraspinal catheter.

although FDA approval is pending for a device that functions similarly (written communication, April 1992, Pudenz-Schulte Medical Corp., Goleta, CA).

Type V Totally Implantable System

This totally implantable system also is used for patients with a life expectancy of months or years. Its reservoir needs to be refilled infrequently, making this an ideal system for highly functional individuals who desire to minimize reminders of their illness and the intrusion of home health care, portable pumps, and the like. These systems are also beneficial when nonmedical family support systems are inadequate. In contrast to the type IV system, this system provides a constant infusion of drug, obviating the need for patients to self-administer boluses, an advantage in confused or debilitated patients.

The prototype system, Shiley's Infusaid pump (Norwood, MA),[3,7,31,117,168,169] was developed originally for transarterial hepatic chemotherapy. The pump, similar in size to a hockey puck, is implanted into the subcutaneous tissue of the abdominal wall and is connected to a tunneled Silastic epidural or subarachnoid catheter (see Fig. 18–14). The pump contains two chambers (see Fig. 18–15) separated from each other by a diaphragm, one containing Freon and another serving as a drug reservoir (capacity 47 ml). Filling the drug reservoir displaces the adjacent diaphragm and compresses the Freon in the companion chamber. The Freon then gradually expands at a consistent, predictable rate, and the corresponding pressure on the diaphragm results in a continuous fixed outflow of drug from the reservoir (2–4 ml/day). The drug reservoir has a 50-ml capacity, and is refilled percutaneously by a physician usually every 14 to 21 days (Fig. 18–25). Alterations in dosage are accomplished by replenishing the reservoir with drug of an appropriate concentration or by bolus administration into a separate port. The main disadvantage of this system, aside from its cost, is that the rate of administration cannot readily be altered in response to varying requirements for analgesia.

Type VI Totally Implantable Programmable Infusion Pump

The type VI totally implantable programmable infusion pump (see Fig. 18–16)[7,170] physically resembles the type V system and is implanted with the same relative ease.[101] The same ad-

vantages cited for the type V system apply, but, in addition, the drug delivery rate can be altered readily (0.025–0.9 ml/hour). Further, alternate modes of delivery can be used that permit alterations in diurnal versus nocturnal flow and the administration of preprogrammed boluses. An "upfront" investment for the purchase of a special lap-top computer is required (see Fig. 18–18). Alterations in drug delivery are accomplished by entering the parameters into the computer and placing a hand-held wand against the skin overlying the pump (see Fig. 18–19). A further important investigational application of this device is for the infusion of intrathecal baclofen for treatment of intractable spasticity.[171]

TROUBLESHOOTING

FAILURE OF ANALGESIA

Despite the numerous potential advantages of intraspinal opioid therapy, treatment is not without problems. A variety of clinically challenging scenarios exist. The management of pain coincident with injection is addressed in Table 18–9. One of the most common problems is that of a patient who has been evaluated properly and screened, has undergone

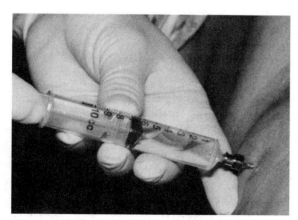

Figure 18–25. Process of replenishing the reservoir of a subcutaneously implanted type V or VI system.

Table 18–9.
Management of Pain on Epidural Injection*

- Withdraw catheter 1 cm (if possible).
- Decrease volume of injection (and increase concentration).
- Administer drug slowly.
- Precede injection with small volume 1% lidocaine.
- Consider repositioning catheter.
- Consider intrathecal placement.

Note: may consider radiologic evaluation of epidural/intrathecal space at any stage to elucidate nature of problem.
* Adapted from De Castro J, Meynadier J, Zenz M: Regional Opioid Analgesia, p 386. Dordrecht, Kluwer Academic, 1991.

implantation, and has been well maintained on intraspinal opioids with adequate analgesia, but presents some time later with increasing pain. How does one proceed? A natural tendency is to assume the development of tolerance, and to respond by increasing the amount of drug delivered. Although this often is ultimately a correct and effective approach, intervention should be individualized and predicated on a careful history and examination. The differential diagnosis includes the provision of an incorrect prescription, failure to load the pump properly, pump malfunction,[170] disconnection, obstruction, or migration of the catheter system,[172] new pain foci, and the development of tolerance. Data obtained should be supplemented by communication with the family, primary care physician, oncologist, and home nursing and pharmacy service.

After the above assessment has been undertaken to exclude the presence of a new lesion or new, potentially correctable underlying pathology, an examination of the infusion system is performed. This process can be accomplished by applying a simple, logical approach that involves working from the periphery of the system centrally, and includes: 1) examination of the drug prescription and confirmation of its accuracy; 2) examination of the infusion device and verification that the program and prescription are correct; proper battery function should be confirmed and it should be verified that the volume and reservoir correspond with the expected and actual volume of drug delivered; 3) examination of external portions of the system for kinking, and to confirm that the drug actually is exiting the pump tubing; and 4) examination of the tunneled portion of the catheter to detect kinks or rents in the tubing and/or evidence of infection or subcutaneous drug deposition. In the absence of demonstrable defects in the integrity of the delivery system, the injection of a local anesthetic test dose and/or radiopaque contrast medium should be performed. The results of these studies provide more definitive data regarding the system's integrity, and help diagnose catheter migration into unintended locations or diminished drug delivery due to tumor or the deposition of fibrous tissue around the catheter tip's outlet. These events can be documented further with magnetic resonance imaging and/or postmyelographic computed tomography scanning. Magnetic resonance imaging is relatively contraindicated in patients with a type VI infusion device (externally, telemetrically programmable delivery pump or Synchromed [Medtronic Inc., Minneapolis, MN] pump), due to the potential for damage to the computer chip contained in the pump and of program alterations. In this setting, a myelogram performed after injection of contrast medium through the access port and subsequent computed tomography is recommended.

TOLERANCE

Once problems related to the integrity of the delivery system and demonstrable new underlying pathology (physical and psychological) have been excluded, then the most likely explanation for increased pain is that of inadequate dosage relative to the patient's nociceptive input. In the past, loss of analgesia had been assumed to be related rather uniformly to the development of tolerance. More recently, it has been accepted that loss of analgesia is related more frequently to undetected progression of cancer and increased tissue damage.[9] Nevertheless, tolerance certainly remains an important causal factor. Strictly defined, tolerance refers to "the power of resisting the action of a drug or taking a drug continuously or in large doses without injurious effects."[19] Tolerance usually does not develop equally to all effects of a drug at the same rate, and, fortunately, tolerance to a drug's undesirable effects also occurs (see "Side Effects," above).[17]

Tolerance is a pharmacodynamic event thought to be related to so-called "receptor down-regulation," that is, an uncoupling or inactivation of some receptors resulting in a decrease in the receptor reserve.[28,173] Down-regulation is characterized by continued agonist stimulation of receptors, resulting in a state of desensitization (also referred to as refractoriness) such that the effect that follows continued or subsequent exposure to the same dose of the drug is diminished.[17] As noted, the development of tolerance is relatively unpredictable. There are reports of patients with chronic cancer pain who have been treated effectively for many months with a stable dose of opioid.[18,174,175] Consistent reports from different sources suggest that tolerance is, at least to some extent, 1) time-dependent, 2) concentration-dependent, and 3) receptor-selective.[28,176–179]

MANAGEMENT OF TOLERANCE

Prophylaxis

The emergence of true, pharmacodynamically based tolerance can be managed in a number of ways, although none is entirely satisfactory. One approach is that of prophylaxis. It has been suggested that tolerance appears to be less troublesome when intraspinal opioids are administered by continuous infusion as opposed to intermittent boluses,[1,3,31,180] although this has not been demonstrated convincingly. It has also been suggested that the use of a more potent opioid such as sufentanil may result in less rapid down-regulation of receptors.[28,177,181]

Nonopioid Substances: Clonidine and Others

Once tolerance occurs, other spinal antinociceptive modulating systems theoretically could be used, either transiently to "rest" and "recruit" receptors, or chronically as an alternative or supplement to opioid therapy. A variety of disparate substances have been administered intraspinally in efforts to obtain safe, reliable analgesia. Even encouraging reports warrant cautious interpretation, since animal and human studies of toxicology and efficacy are inadequate in many cases.

The alpha-2 adrenergic agonist clonidine is perhaps the best studied of these agents. Successful management of both cancer and postoperative pain has been reported with the administration of epidural and intrathecal clonidine.[182–184] Clonidine appears to produce spinally mediated antinociception by its action on postsynaptic receptors within the dorsal horn, activating descending noradrenergic inhibitory systems.[185] Analgesia is reversible with alpha antagonist agents, but is not affected by naloxone. Hypotension is the main potential adverse effect. When used in combination with opioids, opioid-mediated respiratory depression may be potentiated, especially in opioid-naive patients. Administration appears to be free of local toxicity.[186] Reporting on 52 patients with chronic cancer pain, Glynn and colleagues observed persistently adequate analgesia in 20 patients, with a low incidence of side effects,[184] and Eisenach and colleagues treated patients successfully with intrathecal clonidine and morphine for up to 5 months.[182] It has been suggested that intraspinal clonidine may have a particularly important role in the management of opioid-resistant neuropathic pain syndromes. Preliminary evaluations of two other alpha adrenergic agonists, tzantidine and dexmedetomidine, are currently underway.

Droperidol appears to be a safe and effective adjunct to intraspinal opioid therapy. Animal experiments have demonstrated that intrathecal morphine analgesia is prolonged and potentiated by the addition of droperidol, and that tolerance is delayed.[187] The pooled results of clinical series suggest that the addition of 2.5 mg of droperidol to epidural or intrathecal morphine may potentiate analgesia, reduce a range of side effects (nausea, vomiting, pruritus, urine retention, hypotension), and delay tolerance, although sedative effects may occur as well.[188,189]

Chrubasik[190,191] has reported that somatostatin, an endogenous neuropeptide, injected intrathecally, epidurally, and within the ventricular system produces analgesia equal to that of intrathecal morphine in patients with postoperative and cancer pain. Based on these findings, the administration of somatostatin represents another potential means to limit or manage tolerance, although expense and suggestions of local neurotoxicity are barriers to more widespread trials.[20,192] By the same token, intrathecal salmon calcitonin, while probably ineffective as a sole analgesic agent, used in conjunction with morphine permits reductions in doses of the latter drug.[20,193] There is currently an insufficient base of animal research to recommend the routine clinical use of intrathecal or epidural calcitonin.[194]

Stein and Brechner[195] administered epidural norepinephrine (50–250 μg) combined with morphine in a tolerant patient, and consequently were able to reduce the dose of opioid by 50% without altering analgesia. Russell and Chang have demonstrated in rats that alternating the administration of relatively receptor-specific agents (morphine = predominantly mu; DADL = predominantly delta) modifies tolerance favorably.[196] Anecdotal reports describing analgesia in morphine-tolerant patients administered intrathecal DADL (D-ala^2-D-leu^5-enkephalin), a synthetic enkephalin analogue, also have appeared in the literature.[197,198] Other substances with potential antinociceptive activity at the level of the neuroaxis include ketamine,[199] midazolam,[200] baclofen,[201] an injectable form of aspirin (lysine-acetylsalicylate), and various alpha adrenergic adenosine analogues.[20]

Cross-tolerance refers to a phenomenon whereby tolerance to one drug induces tolerance to another. The issue of cross-tolerance among the various subsets of opioid receptors and different receptor systems is an important one. There is some evidence for an absence of complete cross-tolerance,[23,196,202] but further research is required to determine the extent to which this is true.

An alternative strategy for reversing tolerance or slowing its development involves the administration of epidural local anesthetics. Local anesthetic may be substituted for opioids to provide an opioid-free interval (so-called "drug holiday"), during which receptor activity may revert toward normal, once again rendering the patient opioid-sensitive.[15] This strategy should be used only in a closely supervised setting to monitor for adverse sequelae of opioid withdrawal (abstinence syndrome) and the administration of local an-

esthetics (hypotension). Alternatively, dilute concentrations of local anesthetic (0.012%– 0.25% bupivacaine) can be added to the opioid infusion. Such combinations commonly are used successfully for the management of acute pain, and have well established safety profiles in the acute care setting. DuPen has demonstrated the safety of combining the administration of epidural morphine and dilute bupivacaine in the home.[203] In a series of 105 patients treated with epidural morphine, 7.5% (eight patients) required further analgesia with bupivacaine for new bone or nerve pain. In addition to epidural morphine, these patients received epidural bupivacaine 0.125%–0.5% with epinephrine administered at 6 ml/hour. Clinically significant hypotension did not occur, and a number of patients remained ambulatory. Patients should be well hydrated and should be restricted to bed rest during the initial stages of therapy. Such combination therapy may minimize the adverse side effects from each type of agent,[18] and may be particularly efficacious for sharp, incidental pain due, for example, to a pathologic fracture or a neurogenic process.

Finally, animal evidence for synergistic effects after the administration of combinations of opioids with distinct receptor affinities[204] or an opioid and alpha agonist[205] suggest combining such agents as a further means of reducing or countering tolerance.

OPIOID WITHDRAWAL
(Abstinence Syndrome)

The abrupt conversion from the administration of systemic to intraspinal opioids may result in opioid withdrawal, with its classic signs and symptoms.[206] These include lacrimation, rhinorrhea, mydriasis, diaphoresis, pilomotor erection, restlessness, irritability, tremor, nausea, vomiting, diarrhea, and abdominal cramping.[17] Episodes of heightened pain, pulmonary edema, and cardiovascular collapse have been reported in such patients.[35,207] The development of this syndrome presumably is due to reductions in the total dose of drug that is administered and the consequent delivery of reduced quantities of opioid to rostral central nervous system sites. The administration of an opioid antagonist or agonist–antagonist drug to an opioid-dependent patient, systemically or at the neuraxial level, can also induce profound withdrawal and even shock.[22,208] Prevention of this syndrome is essential and is facilitated by tapering systemic opioids, and, should they be indicated, cautious introduction of drugs with antagonist properties. Guidelines for these procedures have been published.[209]

TREATMENT PROTOCOLS

A variety of protocols have been used relatively successfully to institute and maintain intraspinal opioid analgesia, although controlled comparisons are lacking. No single treatment protocol can be recommended for uniform use in all patients. When analgesia is difficult to maintain, the following recommendations have proven useful in clinical practice: 1) The maximum hourly rate for epidural administration generally should not exceed 10 to 15 ml, whereas the volume administered intrathecally over 24 hours should not exceed approximately 10% of a given patient's calculated cerebrospinal fluid volume.[6] 2) Once these maximal rates have been achieved, if dose augmentation is still required the concentration of the opioid may be increased two- to four-fold, and the rate correspondingly decreased 25%–50% from the previous rate. 3) Boluses of 10%–25% of the previous 24-hour requirement then can be provided while the rate of continuous infusion is increased by 10%–25% increments. This method is preferred when breakthrough pain is severe and regaining control is a high priority. For milder exacerbations of pain, simple increases in the rate of continuous infusion by 10%–25% are sufficient. Limitations on the maximum

amount of opioid that can be delivered readily relate to the commercial availability of sufficiently concentrated preparations of the drug. Often it will be necessary to use made-to-order formulations specially prepared by a trained pharmacist from powdered opioid base, in which case the only limits relate to the solubility of the particular opioid. Morphine can be concentrated readily to 50 mg/ml, and hydromorphone to about 200 mg/ml (see Appendix C). Chronic infusions of high concentrations of morphine have not been associated with neurotoxicity or CNS lesions.[210] Maximum daily doses encountered in the literature range from 60–480 mg of epidural morphine,[211] and up to 150 mg of intrathecal morphine.[130]

SUMMARY

Careful assessment will help determine the relative contribution of each of the factors potentially responsible for loss of analgesia during previously reliable intraspinal opioid therapy. Evaluation should include the system's integrity and the patient's physiologic and psychological status. Subsequent management must be highly individualized.

Psychological and emotional adjustments to progressive cancer, disability, and impending death may modify subjective reports of pain and must be addressed. Increased complaints of pain may signal the need for counseling and/or treatment with psychotropic agents, including antidepressants and sleep-restoring medications. The onset of new pathology (bowel obstruction, pathologic fracture, spinal cord compression) should be identified, and, when appropriate, managed with alternate palliative interventions (radiation therapy, surgery, steroids, etc). Neuropathic pain often is resistant to intraspinal opioid therapy, but may be managed effectively with oral adjuvants (antidepressants, anticonvulsants, sodium channel blockers) or local anesthetic blockade. Intermittent regional blocks and/or the addition of a local anesthetic to the intraspinal opioid infusion may be particularly efficacious when symptoms are sympathetically maintained. Incident pain often can be managed effectively by supplementing the continuous intraspinal opioid infusion with oral opioids. Depending on the system that is in use, patient-controlled analgesia or the addition of a preprogrammed bolus schedule may be useful. As clinical experience with new agents and methods of administration accrues, more defined roles for these interventions can be anticipated.

FUTURE DEVELOPMENTS IN INTRASPINAL ANALGESIA

Future advances in the treatment of intractable cancer pain will focus implicitly on the maintenance of adequate analgesia with preservation of function. Intraspinal opioid therapy is well suited to play an important role in achieving this paradigm. Areas in which new developments are in progress and/or can be anticipated include:

1. Technical improvement in delivery systems.
2. Increased understanding of the neuropharmacology involved in central nervous system modulation and processing of pain.
3. Improved clinical application/integration between these modulating systems.
4. Enhanced ability to match delivery system with drugs to correspond better with patients' individualized needs.
5. Application of a multidisciplinary approach to cancer pain management to integrate better the plethora of available treatment options.

The addition of a patient-controlled analgesia feature to drug delivery systems confers enhanced flexibility and control (see Chapter 11). This feature is available for systems that use external pumps and a few prototype internalized systems. The most sophisticated delivery system, the type VI system (internalized programmable pump, *ie,* Synchromed by Medtronics) offers the capability of continuous infusion, but supplementation with intermittent boluses is limited to predetermined intervals, and hence the system is not truly patient-controlled. Treatment of patients with unscheduled incident or breakthrough pain will be facilitated by the development of a portable, hand-held system that would allow the patient to administer a bolus (patient-controlled analgesia) with a predetermined lockout interval. Figures 18–26A and B illustrate a device that is currently near completion of FDA approval that operates by a similar mechanism as does the Type V system, but due to

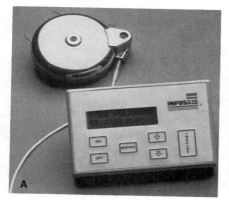
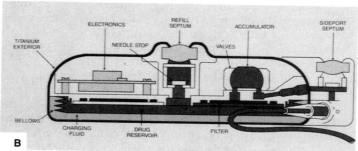

Figure 18–26. New implantable device for the administration of intraspinal opioids, FDA approval pending at this time. The pump and programmer **(A)** are illustrated along with a schematic view of its interior **(B)**.

the addition of a hand-held, patient-operated programmer, permits supervised alterations in flow at the bedside.

Work to characterize better the opioid and other modulating systems in the spinal cord is in progress, and promises to have important clinical implications. Receptor systems with purported, but as yet incompletely understood influences on pain modulation include those related to the action of $GABA_B$ alpha-2 adrenergic substances, neuropeptide-Y, cholinergic agents, adenosine, and NMDA-glutamate. The nociceptive-modulating activity of these substances, as well as the potential for synergistic action at their sites of action, are being investigated.[28,35] Considerable work is also required to characterize better the various subsets of opioid receptors. It is anticipated that in the future more receptor-specific compounds will be identified that, when administered, may produce analgesia that is totally free of side effects.[16] Combination therapy with currently available agents is another therapeutic strategy that may improve efficacy, such as in opioid and local anesthetic combinations or the use of a predominantly mu agonist (morphine) with a kappa agonist (butorphanol or nalbuphine).[28,212,213] It has been postulated that specific receptors may mediate distinct types of pain, another intriguing possibility. For example, Sanders and Gintzler[213a] propose that the kappa receptor is the predominant receptor involved in mediating pain associated with the third trimester of pregnancy, in which case the development of a more potent kappa agonist may make profound analgesia without respiratory depression possible (increased clinical efficacy).[16,214] Likewise, animal work suggests that the intrathecal administration of nalbuphine may preferentially relieve visceral pain.[215] The various means that have been suggested to have a potential role in slowing or arresting tolerance (see above) need further elucidation and confirmation from workers in both the clinical and basic sciences. Endogenous opioids are known to be degraded by enzymes, termed enkephalinases. Work with exogenous inhibitors of enkephalinase (thiorphan and bestatin) in both animals and hu-

mans has been described, and suggests another important area for research.[216,217] The use of drugs that influence other types of modulating systems to control tolerance is also open for study.[28,183]

CONCLUSION

Cancer pain can be managed adequately in the majority of patients with oral analgesics, provided they are prescribed in a systematic, thoughtful fashion. A proportion of patients, however, will not achieve adequate comfort, usually due to dose-limiting side effects. Neuroablative techniques are effective in some patients, but produce irreversible effects, and are associated with risks of loss of function and independence. Although in its current stage of development intraspinal opioid therapy cannot be regarded as a panacea, it provides an important therapeutic alternative. The process is reversible, and allows for a trial screening period before implantation of a semipermanent device. A great deal of flexibility exists in the selection of drug, route, and delivery system.

Understanding of the neuropharmacology pertaining to the modulation of high-threshold, small-diameter afferent fibers has advanced greatly in the past two decades due to the work of Yaksh and others (see References). Work is under way to characterize opioid receptors further, as well as to determine the role of other receptor systems in the modulation of nociception. Continued cooperation among basic scientists, clinicians, and industry, and progression from laboratory to clinical trials, promise the likelihood of major advances that will permit more certain control of intractable cancer pain over the next decade. Basic scientists are challenged with establishing therapeutic ratios for various agents and developing better clinical models,[28] whereas clinician researchers must institute well controlled human studies to supplant the anecdotal and retrospective reports that are more common today. A more rapid and meaningful application to cancer pain management promises to ensue.

REFERENCES

1. Benedetti C: Intraspinal analgesia: An historical overview. Acta Anaesthesiol Scand 1987;85:17.
2. Unlabeled Use of FDA Approved Drugs. US FDA Drug Bulletin, p 12. Washington, DC, U.S. Food and Drug Administration, 1982.
3. Coombs DW, Saunders RL, Harbaugh R et al: Relief of continuous chronic pain by intraspinal narcotics infusion via an implanted reservoir. JAMA 1983; 250:2336.
4. Jacobson L, Chabal C, Brody MC: Relief of persistent postamputation stump and phantom limb pain with intrathecal fentanyl. Pain 1989;37:317.
5. Murphy TM, Hinds S, Cherry D: Intraspinal narcotics: Non-malignant pain. Acta Anesthesiol Scand 1987;31 (Suppl):75.
6. Leak WD, Kennedy LD, Graef W: Clinical experience with implantable, programmable pumps: The Medtronic Synchromed pump. Clinical Journal of Pain 1991;7:44.
7. Penn RD, Paice JA: Chronic intrathecal morphine for intractable pain. J Neurosurg 1987;67:182.
8. World Health Organization: Cancer Pain Relief. Geneva, World Health Organization, 1986.
9. Portenoy R: Practical aspects of pain control in the patient with cancer. CA 1988;38:327.
10. Malone BT, Beye R, Walker J: Management of pain in the terminally ill by administration of epidural narcotics. Cancer 1985;55:438.
11. Waldman SD: The role of spinal opioids in the management of cancer pain. Journal of Pain and Symptom Management 1990;5:163.
12. Cherry DA, Gourlay GK: The spinal administration of opioids in the treatment of acute and chronic pain: Bolus doses, continuous infusion, intraventricular administration and implanted drug delivery systems. Palliative Medicine 1987;1:89.
13. Twycross RG, Lack SA: Therapeutics in Terminal Cancer, p 9. Edinburgh, Churchill Livingstone, 1986.
14. Arner S, Arner B: Differential effects of epidural morphine in the treatment of cancer related pain. Acta Anaesthesiol Scand 1985;29:32.
15. Coombs DW: Intraspinal narcotics for intractable cancer pain. In Abrams S (ed): Cancer Pain, p 82. Boston, Kluwer, 1989.
16. Mather LE: Pharmacology of opioids. Med J Aust 1986;144:424.
17. Jaffe JH, Martin WR: The Opioid analgesics and antagonists. In Gillman AG, Rall TW, Nies AS et al (eds): The Pharmacological Basis of Therapeutics, 8th ed. New York, Pergamon Press, 1990.
18. Cousins MJ, Cherry DA, Gourlay GK: Acute and chronic pain: Use of spinal opioids. In Cousins MJ, Bridenbaugh PO (eds): Neural Blockade, 2nd ed, p 955. Philadelphia, JB Lippincott, 1988.
19. Stedman's Medical Dictionary, 25th ed. Baltimore, Williams and Wilkins, 1990.
20. De Castro J, Meynadier J, Zenz M: Regional Opioid Analgesia. Dordrecht, Kluwer Academic, 1991.
21. Pilon RN, Baker AR: Chronic pain control by means of an epidural catheter. Cancer 1976;37:903.
22. Cousins MJ, Mather LE: Intrathecal and epidural administration of opioids. Anesthesiology 1984; 61:276.
23. Yaksh TL: Spinal opiates: A review of their effect on spinal function with an emphasis on pain processing. Acta Anaesthesiol Scand 1987;31 (Suppl 85):25.
24. Smith DE: Spinal opioids in the home and hospice setting. Journal of Pain and Symptom Management 1990;5:175.
25. Boersma FP, Buist AB, Thie J: Epidural pain treatment in the northern Netherlands: Organizational and treatment aspects. Acta Anaesthesiol Belg 1987; 38:213.
26. Crawford ME, Andersen HB, Augustenborg G et al: Pain treatment on outpatient basis using extradural opiates: Danish multicenter study comprising 105 patients. Pain 1983;16:41.
27. Melzack R, Wall PD: Pain mechanisms: A new theory. Science 1965;150:971.
28. Sosnowski M, Yaksh TL: Spinal administration of receptor-selective drugs as analgesics: New horizons. Journal of Pain and Symptom Management 1990;5:204.
29. Snyder SH: Opiate receptors in the brain. N Engl J Med 1977;296:266.
30. Zenz M: Epidural opiates for the treatment of cancer pain. Recent Results Cancer Res 1984;89:107.
31. Shetter AG, Hadley MH, Wilkinson E: Administration of intraspinal morphine sulfate for the treatment of intractable cancer pain. Neurosurgery 1986; 18:740.
32. Vainio A, Tigerstedt: Opioid treatment for radiating cancer pain: Oral administration vs. epidural techniques. Acta Anaesthesiol Scand 1988;32:179.
33. Payne R: CSF distribution of opioids in animals and man. Acta Anaesthesiol Scand 1987;31 (Suppl 85):38.
34. Gourlay GK, Murphy TM, Plummer JL et al: Pharmacokinetics of fentanyl in lumbar and cervical CSF following lumbar epidural and intravenous administration. Pain 1989;38:253.
35. Yaksh TL, Noueihed R: The physiology and pharmacology of spinal opioids. Annu Rev Pharmacol Toxicol 1985;25:433.
36. Zieglgansberger W: Opiate actions on mammalian spinal neurons. Int Rev Neurobiol 1984;25:243.

37. Werz MA, McDonald RL: Dynorphin reduces calcium-dependent action potential duration by decreasing voltage-dependent calcium conductance. Neurosci Lett 1984;46:185.

38. Zieglgansberger W: Opiate actions on mammalian spinal neurons. Int Rev Neurobiol 1984;25:243.

39. Klepper ID, Sherrill DL, Boetger CL et al: Analgesia and respiratory effects of extradural sufentanil in volunteers, and the influence of adrenaline as an adjuvant. Br J Anesth 1987;59:1147.

40. Hansdottir V, Hedner T, Woestenborghs R et al: The CSF and plasma pharmacokinetics of sufentanil after intrathecal administration. Anesthesiology 1991; 74:264.

41. Gourlay GK, Cherry BA, Cousins MJ: Cephalad migration of morphine CSF following lumbar epidural administration in patients with cancer pain. Pain 1985;23:317.

42. Max MB, Inturrisi CE, Kaiko RF et al: Epidural and intrathecal opiates: Cerebral spinal fluid and plasma profiles in patients with chronic cancer pain. Clin Pharmacol Ther 1985;38:631.

43. Madrid JL, Fatela LV, Lobato RD et al: Intrathecal therapy: Rationale, technique, clinical results. Acta Anaesthesiol Scand 1987;31 (Suppl 85):60.

44. Payne R, Inturissi CE: CSF distribution of morphine, methadone and sucrose after intrathecal injection. Life Sci 1985;37:1137.

45. Moore AR, Bullingham RES, McQuay CW et al: Dural permeability to narcotics: In vitro determination and application to extradural administration. Br J Anaesth 1982;54:1117.

46. Martin WR, Eades CG, Thompson JA et al: The effects of morphine and nalorphine-like drugs in the nondependent and morphine dependent chronic spinal dog. J Pharmacol Exp Ther 1976;197:517.

47. Sabbe MB, Yaksh TL: Pharmacology of spinal opioids. Journal of Pain and Symptom Management 1990;5:191.

48. Lord JAH, Waterfield AA, Hughes J et al: Endogenous opioid peptides: Multiple agonists and receptors. Nature 1977;267:495.

49. Schulz RE, Wuster M, Herz A: A pharmacologic characterization of the epsilon-receptor. J Pharmacol Exp Ther 1981;216:604.

50. Pasternak GW, Childers SR, Snyder SH: Opiate analgesia: Evidence for mediation by a subpopulation of opiate receptors. Science 1980;208:514.

51. Attali B, Gouarderes C, Mazarguil H et al: Differential interaction of opiates to multiple "kappa" binding sites in the guinea pig lumbosacral spinal cord. Life Sci 1982;31:1371.

52. Johnson MD, Hurley RJ, Gilbertson LI et al: Continuous microcatheter spinal anesthesia with subarachnoid meperidine for labor and delivery. Anesth Analg 1990;70:658.

53. Tung AS, Yaksh TL: In vivo evidence for multiple opiate receptors mediating analgesia in the rat spinal cord. Brain Res 1982;247:75.

54. Onofrio BN, Yaksh TL: Intrathecal delta-receptor ligand produces analgesia in man. Lancet 1983;i: 1386.

55. Schmauss C, Yaksh TL: In vivo studies on spinal opioid receptor systems mediating antinociceptive: Pharmacological profile suggesting differential association of mu, delta, and kappa receptors with visceral chemical and cutaneous thermal stimuli in the rat. J Pharmacol Exp Ther 1984;228:1.

56. Tyers MD: A classification of opioid receptors that mediate antinociception. Br J Pharmacol 1980;69: 503.

57. DuPen SL: Management of maxillofacial cancer pain with epidural narcotic analgesia. Anesthesiology 1989;71 (Suppl):A740.

58. Eriksson MBE, Lindahl S, Nyquist JK: Experimental cutaneous pain thresholds and tolerance in clinical analgesia with epidural morphine. Acta Anaesthesiol Scand 1982;26:654.

59. Fisher AP, Simpson D, Hanna M: A role for epidural opioid in opioid-insensitive pain? Pain Clinic 1987; 1:233.

60. Ventafridda V, Spoldi E, Caraceni A et al: Intraspinal morphine for cancer pain. Acta Anaesthesiol Scand 1987;31 (Suppl 85):47.

61. Arai T, Dote K, Senda T et al: Convulsion after epidural injection in a patient with increased intracranial pressure. Pain Clin 1987;3:195.

62. Korbon GA, James DJ, Verlander JM et al: Intramuscular naloxone reverses the side effects of epidural morphine while preserving analgesia. Reg Anesth 1985;10:16.

63. Rawal N, Schott U, Dahlstrom B: Influence of naloxone infusion on analgesia and respiratory depression following epidural morphine. Anesthesiology 1986;64:194.

64. Baskoff JD, Watson RL, Muldoon SM: Respiratory arrest after intrathecal morphine. Anesthesiology 1980;53:12.

65. Davies GK, Tolhurst-Cleaver CL, James TL: CNS depression from intrathecal morphine. Anesthesiology 1980;52:280.

66. Glynn CJ, Mather, LE, Cousins, MJ et al: Spinal narcotics and respiratory depression. Lancet 1979; i:356.

67. Christensen V: Respiratory depression after extradural morphine. Br J Anesth 1980;52:841.

68. Pazos A, Florez J: Interaction of naloxone with m and d agonists on the respiration of rats. Eur J Pharmacol 1983;87:309.

69. Abboud TK, Moore M, Zhu J et al: Epidural butorphanol or morphine for the relief of post cesarean section pain, ventilatory responses to carbon dioxide. Anesth Analg 1987;66:887.

70. Latasch L, Probst S, Dudziak R: Reversal by nalbuphine of respiratory depression caused by fentanil. Anesth Analg 1984;63:814.

71. Baise A, McMichan JC, Nugent M et al: Nalbuphine produces side effects while reversing narcotic induced respiratory depression. Anesth Analg 1986;65 (Suppl):S19.

72. Hammond JE: Reversal of opioid associated late onset respiratory depression by nalbuphine hydrochloride. Lancet 1984;ii:1208.

73. Schmauss C, Doherty C, Yaksh TL: The analgesic effects of an intrathecally administered partial opiate agonist, nalbuphine hydrochloride. Eur J Pharmacol 1983;86:1.

74. Wakefield RD, Mesaros M: Reversal of pruritus secondary to epidural morphine with a narcotic agonist/antagonist nalbuphine (Nubaine). Anesthesiology 1985;63 (Suppl):A255.

75. Abboud TK, Lee K, Zhu J et al: Prophylactic oral naltrexone with intrathecal morphine for Cesarean section: Effects on adverse reactions and analgesia. Anesth Analg 1990;71:367.

76. Taff RH: Pulmonary edema following an naloxone administration in a patient without heart disease. Anesthesiology 1983;59:576.

77. Prough BS, Roy R, Bumgarner J et al: Acute pulmonary edema in healthy teenagers following conservative doses of intravenous naloxone. Anesthesiology 1984;60:485.

78. DesMarteau JK, Cassot AL: Acute pulmonary edema resulting from nalbuphine reversal of fentanyl-induced respiratory depression. Anesthesiology 1986;65:237.

79. Kaiser KG, Bainton CR: Treatment of intrathecal morphine overdose by aspiration of cerebrospinal fluid. Anesth Analg 1987;66:475.

80. Sundberg TT, Wattwil M, Garvill JE et al: Effects of epidural bupivacaine and epidural morphine on bowel function and pain after hysterectomy. Acta Anaesthesiol Scand 1989;33:181.

81. Patt R, Jain S: Long term management of a patient with perineal pain secondary to rectal cancer. Journal of Pain and Symptom Management 1990;5:127.

82. Thorn T, Tanhhoj H, Jarnerot G: Epidural morphine delays gastric emptying time and small intestinal transit in volunteers. Acta Anaesthesiol Scand 1989;33:174.

83. Watson RL, Rayburn RL, Muldoon SM et al: The mechanism of action and utility of epidurally administered morphine. In Wain HJ (ed): Treatment of Pain. New York, Aaronson, 1982.

84. Calvey TN: Side effect problems of the mu and kappa agonists in clinical use. Update in Opioids 1987;1:803.

85. Loper KA, Ready LB, Dorman BH: Prophylactic transdermal scopolamine patches reduce nausea in postoperative patients receiving epidural morphine. Anesth Analg 1989;68:144.

86. Rawal N, Mollefors K, Axelsson K et al: An experimental study of urodynamic effects of epidural morphine and of naloxone reversal. Anesth Analg 1983; 62:641.

87. Dray A: Epidural opiates and urinary retention: New models provide new insights. Anesthesiology 1988; 68:323.

88. Durant PAC, Yaksh TL: Drug effects on urinary bladder tone during spinal morphine-induced inhibition of the micturition reflex in unanesthetized rats. Anesthesiology 1988;68:325.

89. Rawal N, Mollefors K, Axelsson K et al: Naloxone reversal of urinary retention after epidural morphine. Lancet 1981;ii:1411.

90. Evron S, Samueloff A, Simon A et al: Urinary function during epidural analgesia with methadone and morphine in post-cesarean section patients. Pain 1985;23:135.

91. Drenger B, Magora F, Evron S et al: The action of intrathecal morphine and methadone on lower urinary tract in dog. J Urol 1986;135:852.

92. Drenger B, Pikarsky AJ, Magora F: Urodynamic studies after intrathecal fentanyl and buprenorphine in the dog. Anesthesiology 1987;67 (Suppl):A240.

93. Evron S, Magora E, Sadovsky E: Prevention of urinary retention with phenoxybenzamine during epidural morphine. Br Med J 1984;288:190.

94. Nickels JH, Poulos JG, Chaouki K: Risks of infection from short-term epidural catheter use. Reg Anesth 1989;14:88.

95. Wright BD: The use of an attachable silver impregnated cuff on chronically implanted epidural catheters for infection prophylaxis. Regional Anesthesia 1990;15 (Suppl):38.

96. Du Pen SL, Peterson DG, Williams A et al: Infection during chronic epidural catheterization: Diagnosis and treatment. Anesthesiology 1990;73:905.

97. Vandam LD: Complications of epidural and spinal anesthesia. In Orkin FK, Cooperman LH (eds): Complications in Anesthesiology, p 75. Philadelphia, JB Lippincott, 1983.

98. Fisher MM: The diagnosis of acute anaphylactoid reactions to drugs. Anaesthesia Intensive Care 1981;9:234.

99. Zucker-Pinchoff B, Ramanathan S: Anaphylactic reaction to epidural fentanyl. Anesthesiology 1989; 71:599.

100. Kopacz DJ, Slover RB: Accidental epidural cephazolin injection: Safeguards for patient controlled analgesia. Anesthesiology 1990;72:944.
101. Waldman SD, Coombs DW: Selection of implantable narcotic delivery systems. Anesth Analg 1989;68:377.
102. Lazorthes J, Verdie JC, Bastide R et al: Spinal versus intraventricular chronic opiate administration with implantable drug delivery devices for cancer pain. Appl Neurophysiol 1985;48:234.
103. Moulin DE, Max M, Kaiko RF et al: The analgesic efficacy of intrathecal D-ala²-D-leu⁵-enkephalin in cancer patients with chronic pain. Pain 1985;23:213.
104. Payne R: Role of epidural and intrathecal narcotics and peptides in the management of cancer pain. Med Clin North Am 1987;71:313.
105. Tanelian DL, Cousins MJ: Failure of epidural opioid to control cancer pain in a patient previously treated with massive doses of intravenous opioid. Pain 1989;36:359.
106. Chabal C, Buckley FP, Jacobson L et al: Long-term epidural morphine in the treatment of cancer pain. Pain Clin 1989;3:19.
107. Madrid JL, Fatela LV, Alcorta J et al: Intermittent intrathecal morphine by means of an implantable reservoir: A survey of 100 cases. Journal of Pain and Symptom Management 1988;3:67.
108. Hamar O, Csomor S, Kazy Z et al: Epidural morphine analgesia by means of a subcutaneously tunneled catheter in patients with gynecologic cancer. Anesth Analg 1986;65:531.
109. Wang JK: Intrathecal morphine for intractable pain secondary to cancer of the pelvic organs. Pain 1985;21:99.
110. Waldman SD, Feldstein GS, Allen ML: Selection of patients for implantable intraspinal narcotic delivery systems. Anesth Analg 1986;65:883-885.
111. Turnage G, Clark L, Wild L: Spinal opioids: A nursing perspective. Journal of Pain and Symptom Management 1990;5:154.
112. McIlvaine WB: Spinal opioids for the pediatric patient. Journal of Pain and Symptom Management 1990;5:183.
113. Plancarte R, Patt R: Intractable upper body pain in a pediatric patient relieved with cervical epidural opioid administration. Journal of Pain and Symptom Management 1991;6:98.
114. Coombs DW: Intraspinal narcotics for intractable cancer pain. In Abram S (ed): Cancer Pain, p 82. Boston, Kluwer, 1989.
115. Coombs DW, Saunders RL, Gaylor LM: Epidural narcotic infusion reservoir: Implantation techniques and efficacy. Anesthesiology 1982;56:469.
116. Edwards WT, DeGirolami U, Burney RG et al: Histo-
117. Krames ES, Gershow J, Glassberg A et al: Continuous infusion of spinally administered narcotics for the relief of pain due to malignant disorders. Cancer 1985;56:696.
118. Du Pen SL, Peterson DG, Bogosian AC et al: A new permanent exteriorized epidural catheter for narcotic self-administration to control cancer pain. Cancer 1987;59:986.
119. Sullivan SP, Cherry DA: Pain from an invasive facial tumor relieved by lumbar epidural morphine. Anesth Analg 1987;66:777.
120. Waldman SD, Cronen MC: Thoracic epidural morphine in the palliation of chest wall pain secondary to relapsing polychondritis. Journal of Pain and Symptom Management 1989;4:60.
121. Waldman SD, Feldstein G, Allen ML et al: Cervical epidural implantable narcotic delivery systems in the management of upper body cancer pain. Anesth Analg 1987;66:780.
122. Roquefeuil B, Benezech J, Blanchet P et al: Intraventricular administration of morphine in patients with neoplastic intractable pain. Surg Neurol 1984;21:155.
123. Schoeffler PF, Haberer JP, Monteillard CM et al: Morphine injections in the cisterna magna for intractable pain in cancer patients. Anesthesiology 1987;67(Suppl):A246.
124. Lobato RD, Madrid JL, Fatela LV et al: Intraventricular morphine for control of pain in terminal cancer patients. J Neurosurg 1983;59:627.
125. Lenzi A, Galli G, Gandolfini M et al: Intraventricular morphine in paraneoplastic painful syndrome of the cervicofacial region: Experience in 38 cases. Neurosurgery 1985;17:6.
126. Obbens EAMT, Stratton-Hill C, Leavens ME et al: Intraventricular morphine administration for control of chronic cancer pain. Pain 1987;28:61.
127. Patt R: Neurosurgical interventions for pain problems. Anesthesiology Clinics of North America 1987;5:609.
128. Black P: Neurosurgical management of cancer pain. Semin Oncol 1985;12:438.
129. DuPen SL, Ramsey D, Chin S: Chronic epidural morphine and preservative-induced injury. Anesthesiology 1987;67:987.
130. Ventafridda V, Spoldi E, Caraceni A et al: Intraspinal morphine for cancer pain. Acta Anaesthesiol Scand 1987;31: (Suppl 85):47.
131. Pfeifer BL, Sernaker HL, Ter Horst UM et al: Cross tolerance between systemic and epidural morphine in cancer patients. Pain 1989;39:181.
132. Caute B, Monsarrat B, Gouardes C et al: CSF morphine levels after lumbar intrathecal administration

of isobaric and hyperbaric solutions for cancer pain. Pain 1988;32:141.

133. Boersma FP, Heykants J, ten Kate A et al: Sufentanil concentrations in the human spinal cord after long term epidural infusion. Pain Clin (in press).

134. Birnbach DJ, Johnson MD, Arcario T et al: Effect of diluent volume on analgesia produced by epidural fentanyl. Anesth Analg 1989;68:808.

135. Klepper ID, Sherrill DL, Boetger CL et al: Analgesic and respiratory effects of epidural sufentanil in volunteers and the influence of adrenaline as an adjuvant. Br J Anaesth 1987;59:1147.

136. Lam AM, Knill RL, Thompson WR et al: Epidural fentanyl does not cause delayed respiratory depression. Canadian Anaesthesia Society Journal 1983;30 (Suppl):S78.

137. Celleno D, Capogna G, Dardes N et al: Ventilatory effects of subarachnoid fentanyl. Reg Anesth 1988; 13 (Suppl):29.

138. Bohannon TW, Estes MD: Evaluation of subarachnoid fentanyl for postoperative analgesia. Anesthesiology 1987;67 (Suppl):A237.

139. Nomura MK, Mokriski BK, Malinow AM: Effect of epinephrine on intrathecal fentanyl analgesia. Reg Anesth 1989;14 (Suppl):25.

140. Chauvin M, Salbaing J, Perrin D et al: Clinical assessment and plasma pharmacokinetics associated with intramuscular or extradural alfentanil. Br J Anaesth 1985;57:886.

141. Shir Y, Yehuda DB, Polliack A et al: Prolonged continuous epidural methadone analgesia in the treatment of back and pelvic pain due to multiple myeloma. Pain Clin 1987;1:255.

142. Dougherty TB, Baysinger CL, Henenberger JC et al: Epidural hydromorphine with and without epinephrine for post-operative analgesia after cesarean delivery. Anesth Analg 1989;68:318.

143. Henderson SK, Matthew EB, Cohen H et al: Epidural hydromorphone: A double blind comparison with intramuscular hydromorphone for postcesarean section analgesia. Anesthesiology 1987;66:646.

144. Coombs DW, Saunders RL, Fratkin JD et al: Continuous intrathecal hydromorphone and clonidine for intractable cancer pain. J Neurosurgery 1986;64:890.

145. Glynn CJ, Mather LE, Cousins MJ et al: Peridural meperidine in humans: Analgesic response, pharmacokinetics and transmission into CSF. Anesthesiology 1981;55:520.

146. Kaiko RF, Foley KM, Grabinski PY et al: Central nervous system excitatory effects of meperidine in cancer patients. Ann Neurol 1983;13:180.

147. Wheatley RG, Somerville ID, Jones JG: The effect of diamorphine administered epidurally or with a patient-controlled analgesia system on long-term postoperative oxygenation. Eur J Anaesthesiol 1989; 6:64.

148. Hosobuchi Y, Li Chi: The analgesic activity of human B-endorphin in man. Commun Psychopharmacol 1978;2:33.

149. Van de Woerd A, Oyama T, Trouwborst A et al: Intrathecal B-endorphin treatment in man with intractable cancer pain. Pain Clin 1985;1:99.

150. Oyama T, Jin T, Murkawa T: Analgesic effect of continuous intrathecal beta-endorphin in cancer patients. Pain Clin 1985;1:93.

151. Oyama T, Fukushi S, Jin T: Epidural b-endorphin in treatment of pain. Canadian Anaesth Society Journal 1982;29:24.

152. Carl P, Crawford ME, Ravlo O et al: Longterm treatment with epidural opioids. Anaesthesia 1986;41:32.

153. Pasqualucci V, Tantucci C, Paoletti F et al: Buprenorphine vs morphine via the epidural route: A controlled comparative clinical study of respiratory effects and analgesic activity. Pain 1987;29:273.

154. Oyama T, Murkawa T, Baba S et al: Continuous vs bolus epidural morphine. Acta Anaesthesiol Scand 1987;21 (Suppl 85):77.

155. Wermeling DP, Foster TS, Record KE et al: Drug delivery for intractable cancer pain. Cancer 1987; 60:875.

156. Patt R, Loughner J: Problems and innovations in home-based patient controlled analgesia with epidural opioids. Anesthesiology 1990;72:215.

157. Waldman SD: Implantable drug delivery systems: Practical considerations. Journal of Pain and Symptom Management 1990;5:169.

158. Covino BG, Scott DB: Handbook of Epidural Anaesthesia and Analgesia. Orlando, FL, Grune and Stratton, 1985.

159. Bedder MD, Burchiel KJ, Larson A: Cost analysis of two implantable narcotic delivery systems. Journal of Pain and Symptom Management 1991;6:368.

160. Patt R: Letter to the editor. American Journal of Hospice Care 1989;6:18.

161. Racz GB, Sabonghy M, Gintautas J et al: Intractable pain therapy using a new epidural catheter. JAMA 1982;248:646.

162. Downing JE, Busch EH, Stedman PM: Epidural morphine delivered by a percutaneous epidural catheter for outpatient treatment of cancer pain. Anesth Analg 1988;67:1159.

163. Campailla A: Fixation of extradural catheters. Br J Anaesth 1985;57:1043.

164. Parker OE: Epidural narcotic use for outpatient pain treatment. Anesth Analg 1989;69:408.

165. Cousins M, Gourlay G, Cherry D: A technique for the insertion of an implantable portal system for the long-term epidural administration of opioids in the treatment of cancer pain. Anaesthesia Intensive Care 1985;13:145.

166. Andersen HB, Kjaregard J, Eriksen J: Subcutaneously implanted injection system for epidural ad-

ministration. Acta Anaesthesiol Scand 1986;30: 473.

167. Poletti CB, Cohen AL, Todd DP et al: Cancer pain relieved by long-term epidural morphine with a permanent indwelling system for self-administration. J Neurosurg 1981;56:581.

168. Gestin Y: A totally implantable multi-dose pump allowing cancer patients intrathecal access for the self-administration of morphine at home: A follow-up of 30 cases. Anaesthetist 1987;36:391.

169. Onofrio BM, Yaksh TL, Arnold PG: Continuous low-dose intrathecal morphine administration in the treatment of chronic pain of malignant origin. Mayo Clin Proc 1981;56:516.

170. Penn RD, Paice JA, Gottschalk W et al: Cancer pain relief using chronic morphine infusions: Early experience with a programmable implanted drug pump. J Neurosurg 1984;61:302.

171. Penn RD, Kroin JS: Long-term intrathecal baclofen infusion for the treatment of spasticity. J Neurosurg 1987;66:181.

172. Hirsch LF, Thanki A, Nowak T: Sudden loss of pain control with morphine pump due to catheter migration. Neurosurgery 1985;17:965.

173. Rogers NF, El-Fakahany EE: Morphine induced opioid receptor down regulation detected in intact adult rat brain cells. Eur J Pharmacol 1986;124:221.

174. Onofrio BM, Yaksh TL, Arnold PG: Continuous low dose intrathecal morphine administration in the treatment of chronic pain of malignant origin. Mayo Clin Proc 1981;56:516.

175. Richelson E: Spinal opioid administration for chronic pain: A major advance in therapy. Mayo Clin Proc 1981;56:523.

176. Wiesenfeld Z, Gustafsson LL: Continuous intrathecal administration of morphine via osmotic mini-pump in the rat. Brain Res 1982;247:195.

177. Stevens CW, Yaksh TL: Potency of spinal antinociceptive agents is inversely related to magnitude of tolerance after continuous infusion. J Pharmacol Exp Ther 1989;250:1.

178. Stevens CW, Monaski MS, Yaksh TL: Spinal infusion of opiate and alpha$_2$ agonists in rats; tolerance and cross tolerance studies. J Pharmacol Exp Ther 1988;244:63.

179. Russel RD, Chang KJ: Alternated delta and mu receptor activation: A stratagem for limiting opioid tolerance. Pain 1989;36:381.

180. Pasqualucci V: Advances in the management of cardiac pain. In Benedetti C, Chapman RC, Moricca G (eds): Advances in Pain Research and Therapy, vol XX, p 7. New York, Raven Press, 1990.

181. Sosnowski M, Stevens CW, Yaksh TL: Comparison of magnitude of tolerance development observed after continuous spinal intrathecal infusions in rats. Reg Anesth 1989;14:76.

182. Eisenach JC, Rauck RL, Buzzanell C et al: Epidural clonidine analgesia for intractable cancer pain: Phase I. Anesthesiology 1989;71:647.

183. Coombs DW, Saunders RL, LaChance D et al: Intrathecal morphine tolerance: Use of intrathecal clonidine, DADL and intravenous morphine. Anesthesiology;1985;62:358.

184. Glynn CJ, Jamous A, Dawson D et al: The role of epidural clonidine in the treatment of patients with intractable pain. Pain 1987;4 (Suppl):45.

185. Yaksh TL, Reddy SV: Studies in the primate on the analgesic effects associated with intrathecal actions of opiates, alpha-adrenergic agonists and baclofen. Anesthesiology 1981;54:451.

186. Coombs DW, Allen C, Meier FA et al: Chronic intraspinal clonidine in sheep. Reg Anesth 1984; 9:47.

187. Kim KC, Stoelting RK: Effect of droperidol on the duration of analgesia and development of tolerance to intrathecal morphine. Anesthesiology 1980;35 (Suppl):S219.

188. Naji P, Farschtschian M, Wilder-Smith O et al: Epidural droperidol and morphine for postoperative pain. Anesth Analg 1990;70:583.

189. Bach V, Carl P, Ravlo ME et al: Potentiation of epidural opioids with epidural droperidol. Anaesthesia 1986;41:1116.

190. Chrubasik J, Meynadier J, Blond S et al: Somatostatin, a potent analgesic. Lancet 1984;ii:1208.

191. Intrathecal somatostatin in terminally ill patients: A report of two cases. Pain 1985;23:9.

192. Gaumann DM, Yaksh TL, Post C et al: Intrathecal somatostatin in cat and mouse studies on pain, motor behavior and histopathology. Anesth Analg 1989;68:623.

193. Fiore CE, Castorina F, Malatino LS et al: Antalgic activity of calcitonin: Effectiveness of the epidural and subarachnoid routes in man. Int J Clin Pharmacol Res 1983;3:257.

194. Eisenach JC: Demonstrating safety of subarachnoid calcitonin: Patients or animals. Anesth Analg 1988; 67:298.

195. Stein C, Brechner T: Epidural morphine tolerance: Use of norepinephrine. Clinical Journal of Pain 1987;2:267.

196. Russell RD, Chang KJ: Alternated delta and mu receptor activation: A strategy for limiting opioid tolerance. Pain 1989;36:381.

197. Krames ES, Wilkie DJ, Gershow J: Intrathecal D-ala^2-D-leu^5-enkephalin (DADL) restores analgesia in a patient analgetically tolerant to intrathecal morphine sulfate. Pain 1986;24:205.

198. Onofrio BM, Yaksh TL: Intrathecal delta-receptor ligand produces analgesia in man. Lancet 1983; ii:1386.

199. Naguib M, Adu-Gyamfi Y, Absood GH et al: Epi-

dural ketamine for postoperative analgesia. Anesth Analg 1988;67:798.

200. Cripps TP, Goodchild CS: Intrathecal midazolam and the stress response to upper abdominal surgery. Br J Anaesth 1986;58:1324.

201. Wilson PR, Yaksh TL: Baclofen is anti-nociceptive in the spinal intrathecal space of animals. Eur J Pharmacol 1978;51:323.

202. Coombs DW: Effect of spinal adrenergic analgesia on opioid resistant pain. Acta Anaesthesiol Scand 1989;91:37.

203. Du Pen SL: After epidural narcotics: What next? Anesth Analg 1987;66 (Suppl):S46.

204. Omote K, Nakagawa I, Kitahata LM et al: The anti-nociceptive role of mu and delta opiate receptors and their interactions in the spinal dorsal horn of cats. Anesth Analg 1989;68 (Suppl):S215.

205. Omote K, Nakagawa I, Kitahata LM et al: Spinal delta but not mu opiate receptors appear to interact with noradrenergic systems in the cat's spinal dorsal horn. Anesth Analg 1989;68 (Suppl):S216.

206. Messahel FM, Tomlin PJ: Narcotic withdrawal syndrome after intrathecal administration of morphine. Br Med J 1981;283:471.

207. Delander GE, Takemori AE: Spinal antagonism of tolerance and dependence induced by systemically administered morphine. Eur J Pharmacol 1983;94:35.

208. Christensen FR, Anderson LW: An adverse reaction to extradural buprenorphine. Br J Anaesth 1982;54:476.

209. Dubner R: Principles of analgesia use in the treatment of acute and chronic cancer pain: A concise guide to medical practice, 2nd ed. Skokie, IL: American Pain Society, 1989.

210. Yaksh TL, Onofrio BM: Retrospective consideration of the doses of morphine given intrathecally by chronic infusion in 163 patients by 19 physicians. Pain 1987;31:211.

211. Arner S, Rawal N, Gustafsson LL: Clinical experience of long-term treatment with epidural and intrathecal opioids: A nationwide survey. Acta Anaesthesiol Scand 1988;32:253.

212. Naulty JS, Labove P, Datta S et al: Epidural butorphanol/fentanyl for postcesarean delivery analgesia. Anesthesiology 1987;67 (Suppl):A463.

213. Henderson SK, Cohen H: Nalbuphine augmentation of analgesia and reversal of side effects following epidural hydromorphone. Anesthesiology 1986;65:216.

213a. Sanders HW, Gintzler AR: Spinal cord mediation of the opioid analgesia of pregnancy. Brain Research 1987;408:389.

214. Sanders HW, Portoghese PS, Gintzler AR: Spinal kappa opiate receptor involvement in the analgesia of pregnancy: Effects of intrathecal norbinaltorphimine, a kappa selective antagonist. Brain Res 1988;474:343.

215. Schmauss C, Doherty C, Yaksh TL: The analgesic effects of an intrathecally administered partial opiate agonist, nalbuphine hydrochloride. Eur J Pharmacol 1983;86:1.

216. Reisine T: Pharmacology of pain. Presented at Reflex Sympathetic Dystrophy: Current Strategies in Diagnosis and Treatment Conference, May 3–4, 1991, Thomas Jefferson University, Philadelphia, PA.

217. Meynadier J, Gros C, Lecomte JM et al: Analgesic effectiveness of intrathecal inhibitors of enkephalinase and aminopeptidase in man. Anesth Analg 1987;66 (Suppl):S117.

Chapter **19**

Local Anesthetic Blockade

P. Prithvi Raj

INTRODUCTION

A substantial number of cancer patients benefit dramatically from techniques such as local nerve blocks,[1] which modulate neural responses to noxious stimuli. Although such techniques are not generally a long-term solution, they are useful for the immediate relief of regional pain originating in nerves and muscles, provide a temporary alternative for the alleviation of pain that has not been treated successfully with other techniques, and are useful in developing a plan of action during routine testing or when simpler blocks fail to provide guidelines on how to proceed with treatment. For the cancer patient, local anesthetic nerve blocks have the potential to fulfill diagnostic, prognostic, and therapeutic roles in the management of pain.

DIAGNOSTIC LOCAL ANESTHETIC BLOCKADE

Diagnostic nerve blocks may be used to ascertain the specific pain pathway by which a presumed nociceptive input mediates pain, and to aid in the differential diagnosis of the source of pain. Information as to the nociceptive component of pain can provide accurate detail about one or more aspects of the cancer patient's pain; however, it should be evaluated within the context of a detailed physical and psychological work-up. The results of nerve blocks should not be used as a basis for interpretations of whether pain is organic or not, nor should they be used to confirm the presence or absence of psychological aberrations in the pattern of pain behavior.[2]

Diagnostic nerve blocks are intended 1) to identify the anatomic source of pain, 2) to determine the visceral or somatic origin of thoracoabdominal pain, and 3) to determine whether peripheral pain is of sympathetic or somatic etiology.

ANATOMIC SOURCE OF PAIN

When injected directly into superficial sites of pain or tenderness, local anesthetic blocks can be used to diagnose definitively the tissue source of pain. Trigger points and soft-tissue sites of pain can be identified fairly easily in patients with cancer pain.[3] In addition, the injection of local anesthetic blocks into deep-sited joint structures allows pain to be localized to tissues within or around the joint itself, or to adjacent structures mimicking articular pain.

VISCERAL VERSUS SOMATIC PAIN

Local anesthetic blocks can be useful in determining whether pain is of somatic or visceral origin. For instance, in many cases of truncal pain involving the chest, abdomen, or pelvis, the body wall may be overlooked as a source of pain; diagnostic injections into rib cartilages, nerve, or soft tissues often provide effective pain relief, thus verifying the presence of a parietal process. Celiac plexus or splanchnic blocks can be used to identify visceral sources of epigastric or poorly defined lower chest pains, whereas somatic blocks such as paravertebral nerve root block or intercostal block are useful in the assessment of the origin of abdominal pain. Cervicothoracic sympathetic blockade effectively addresses chest pain of visceral origin, and intercostal blocks result in improvement of pain originating in the chest wall.

Since somatic and visceral nociceptive fibers converge on the same dorsal horn neuron, the recommended procedure is to carry out both somatic and visceral blocks, noting efficacy and duration of analgesia. When feasible, it is also advisable to administer at least one placebo injection before the blocks, to compare placebo response to that of the diagnostic blocks.

SYMPATHETIC VERSUS SOMATIC PERIPHERAL PAIN

Diagnostic nerve blocks also can be useful in identifying a sympathetic mechanism of pain in nonvisceral structures. For this purpose, sympathetic nerve blocks can be administered at sites such as the cervicothoracic sympathetic chain, splanchnic nerves, celiac plexus, and lumbar sympathetic chain, where sympathetic fibers are separate from somatic fibers. Although a positive response to local anesthetic sympathetic block indicates a significant contribution by sympathetic mechanisms to pain, it does not necessarily predict a long-term successful outcome for procedures that alter sympathetic function. In some cases, intravenous (IV) regional sympathetic block may be a more acceptable diagnostic alternative to the patient.

Since it is difficult to produce somatic blocks without inducing at least some degree of sympathetic block, it is advisable to carry out sympathetic block first. Relatively pure somatic blocks may result from injection of trigger points, painful scars, neuromas, and other localized disease, as well as individual branches of nerves.

Another method of examining pain pathways and the central and peripheral components of pain is that of a differential nerve block study,[4] which can be performed on any mixed nerve containing A-alpha, beta, delta, and C fibers and at any site, including the brachial and lumbosacral plexuses, major peripheral nerves, and subarachnoid and epidural regions. This technique differentially blocks sympathetic and somatic fibers, and is applicable for patients who have pain in the lower extremities, low back, lower abdomen, or pelvis.

The differential spinal block is based on findings that the stimulation of a mixed peripheral nerve produces a compound action

Table 19–1.
General Classification of Mixed Peripheral Nerve Fibers*

Fiber	Diameter (μm)	Conduction Velocity (m/sec)	Function Sensory	Motor
A fiber	2–20	6–120	Muscle tendon and spindle	Skeletal muscle and spindle control
Alpha	10–20	60–120	Vibration	
Beta	5–15	30–80	Deep pressure, touch	
Gamma	3–7	10–50		
Delta	2–5	6–30	Prickling pain, cold, warmth	
C fiber	0.5–2	0.5–2	Crude touch, pressure, aching pain, cold, warmth	Sympathetic

From Raj PP, Ramamurthy S: Differential nerve block studies. In Raj PP (ed): Practical Management of Pain p 174. Chicago, Year Book, 1986.

potential that changes with the varying distances of the stimulating electrode.[5] Since A-alpha, beta, and delta fibers can be separated at a suitable distance, peripheral nerve fibers have been classified into A, B, and C fibers (see Table 19–1), which have varying levels of sensitivity to different local anesthetics and concentrations of anesthetics.[6] Sharp pain is associated with A fiber activation, whereas dull, burning pain is associated with C fibers (see Chapter 1). It has been established that preganglionic autonomic fibers (B fibers) are most susceptible to local anesthetics, with C fibers less susceptible and A-delta fibers least susceptible.[7,8]

Four techniques of differential block may be used: antegrade spinal, retrograde spinal, differential epidural or differential brachial, or lumbosacral plexus block. In the standard antegrade spinal procedure, four different solutions of procaine are injected into the subarachnoid space at the L3–4 interspace, after the administration of placebo solution. Evidence of sympathetic block with complete pain relief without loss of pinprick sensation confirms an underlying sympathetic mechanism. If pain relief is not achieved despite loss

of pinprick sensation, or if there is no sensory loss, motor block is obtained through an additional injection. Absence of pain relief despite complete sensory loss and motor block over the affected area indicates that the cause of pain is proximal to the site of block. The most important finding resulting from such a study is that a peripheral procedure such as surgery or nerve block is unlikely to be successful.[4]

With the retrograde spinal block, a concentrated local anesthetic is injected intrathecally, and the position of the patient is adjusted to achieve sensory and motor block at the T10 or T6 level. Failure to achieve relief of pain despite sensory and motor blockade indicates an etiology proximal to the site of block, eliminating peripheral procedures such as surgery and nerve blocks as possible therapies. Pain relief indicates a sympathetic or somatic mechanism, which is further evaluated an hour later. Pain relief that persists despite the return of sensation indicates that a sympathetic mechanism is responsible for the patient's symptoms, whereas the return of pain with the reappearance of sensation allows a diagnosis of an underlying somatic mechanism.

Differential epidural blocks reduce the risk

of postdural puncture headache, and the option of inserting a catheter[9,10] permits the patient to assume a more comfortable position during the procedure. Antegrade and retrograde evaluations have been performed.[10] In the latter, 20 ml of a 3% solution of 2-chloroprocaine is injected through an epidural needle or after placement of an epidural catheter. The rapid onset of action of 2-chloroprocaine allows quick assessment, with C, A-delta, and A-alpha fiber function able to be evaluated within 1 hour. The rapid disappearance of the anesthetic effects of 2-chloroprocaine due to elimination by plasma cholinesterase facilitates the patient's return to normal physiologic status.

Differential brachial or lumbosacral plexus block also can be performed to delineate pain mechanisms. The site selected should allow all branches of the plexuses to be blocked above the suspected peripheral pathology. The recommended procedure is to start with an injection of saline (placebo), then to administer 40 ml of 0.25% lidocaine after 30 minutes, followed by 40 ml 0.5% lidocaine and 1% lidocaine at 30-minute intervals if pain is not relieved. Retrograde evaluation of plexus block after one injection of 40 ml 1.5% lidocaine also can be attempted. Typical dosages of local anesthetics for differential studies are shown in Table 19–2.

PROGNOSTIC LOCAL ANESTHETIC BLOCKADE

A frequent use of local anesthetic blocks is as a predictor of the efficacy of ablative procedures such as rhizotomy, gasserian ganglion ablation, celiac plexus neurolysis, or sympathectomy (see Chapters 20–24, and 26). In such cases a single or prolonged local anesthetic nerve block can be administered to allow the patient to experience the neurologic changes that are likely to accompany a more definitive, enduring procedure,[11–13] and to allow the patient and physician to decide whether or not to proceed with a neurolytic block or neurosurgical procedure. Although the immediate numbness resulting from a prognostic block may be welcomed by the patient, prolonged numbness resulting from surgical ablation may over time develop into a chronic deafferentation syndrome followed by dysesthesia, which may be as distressing as the original symptoms (see Chapters 1, 3, 21, and 26).

It is important to note that although prognostic blocks may be helpful in arriving at decisions for surgery or neurolytic blocks, reliance on their results does not guarantee long-term pain relief.[14,15] However, since a lack of response to local anesthetic blocks reliably predicts failure, it is still worthwhile to perform predictive blocks when a more permanent procedure is being considered.

THERAPEUTIC LOCAL ANESTHETIC BLOCKADE

The rationale for the use of therapeutic local anesthetic nerve blocks in cancer patients is the reliability with which they interrupt sensory and nociceptive pathways, effectively blocking the A-delta, beta, and unmyelinated C-delta fibers, effects that, depending on the nature of the nerve block, may be produced without clinically significant impairment of motor function.[16] Such blocks can result in prolonged pain relief that outlasts the pharmacologic action of the drug, which may be due to a reversal of physiologic changes that accompany some forms of chronic pain.[17]

Therapeutically, local anesthetic nerve blocks are effective in treating sympathetically mediated pain syndromes such as causalgia and reflex sympathetic dystrophy, myofascial pain, neuropathic conditions, and severe acute pain such as that experienced with acute herpes zoster. Local anesthetic blocks also may be used effectively as a crisis management tool to provide temporary relief of incapacitating pain. In addition, therapeutic nerve blocks of local anesthetics and steroids have applications in the management of acute herpes zoster and postherpetic neuralgia.[18] Recommended drugs, applications, and doses are listed in Table 19–3.

Table 19–2.
Dosage of Local Anesthetics for Differential Studies*

Agents	Spinal		Epidural		Brachial Plexus	
	Antegrade VC†	Retrograde VC	Antegrade VC	Retrograde VC	Antegrade VC	Retrograde VC
Procaine	5 ml saline 5 ml 0.25% 5 ml 0.5% 5 ml 1.0% (in some cases may need 2 ml of 5%)	2 ml 5%		5 ml cervical 10 ml thoracic 20 ml lumbar 30 ml caudal		
Lidocaine	—	2 ml 5%	saline 0.25% 0.5% 1.0% 2.0%	2%	40 ml saline 40 ml 0.25% 40 ml 0.51% 40 ml 1.0%	40 ml 1.5%
2-chloro-3.0% procaine	—			3%	saline 40 ml 1% 40 ml 2% 40 ml 3%	40 ml

* From Raj PP, Ramamurthy S: Differential nerve block studies. In Raj PP (ed): Practical
Management of Pain, p 177. Chicago, Year Book, 1986.
† VC, volume concentration.

REFLEX SYMPATHETIC DYSTROPHY AND CAUSALGIA

Reflex sympathetic dystrophy and causalgia are the two common pain syndromes representing overactivity of the peripheral sympathetic nervous system involving the somatic structures (see Chapters 1 and 22).[19,20] Reflex sympathetic dystrophy is the more prevalent disorder, and can be triggered in cancer patients by tumor spread, pathologic fracture, radiation, surgery, or neurolytic therapy.

It is well established that relief of both syndromes can be achieved with stellate ganglion blocks in the upper extremities and lumbar sympathetic blocks in the lower extremities.[21,22] However, although nerve block therapy may be quite successful in treating reflex sympathetic dystrophy occurring in cancer patients after surgery, a greater number of blocks may be required for treatment than is usually required to treat cases occurring after trauma. Causalgia sometimes can be successfully treated with nerve block therapy, but often requires surgical sympathectomy.[19]

True causalgia occurs after injury to a major nerve trunk or its branches. The neural structures most often involved include the median nerve, medial cord of the brachial plexus, or the tibial division of the sciatic nerve. Although adequate therapy with chemical or surgical sympathectomy can result in permanent relief in the early course of the disease, treatment often is less successful in the later stages.

Intravenous regional administration of guanethidine has been shown to be as effective as local anesthetic block for treating reflex sympathetic dystrophy of nonmalignant origin.[23] Although it has been demonstrated that

(text continues on page 336)

Table 19–3.
Clinical Profile of Local Anesthetic Agents

Agent	Concentration (%)	Clinical Use	Onset	Usual Duration (h)	Recommended Maximum Single Dose (mg)	Comments	pH of Plain Solutions*
Amides							
Lidocaine	0.5 –1.0	Infiltration	Fast	1.0–2.0	300	Most versatile agent	6.5
	0.25–0.5	i.v. Regional			500+ epinephrine		
	1.0 –1.5	Peripheral nerve blocks	Fast	1.0–3.0	500+ epinephrine		
	1.5 –2.0	Epidural	Fast	1.0–2.0	500+ epinephrine		
	4	Topical	Moderate	0.5–1.0	500+ epinephrine		
	5	Spinal	Fast	0.5–1.5	100		
Prilocaine	0.5 –1.0	Infiltration	Fast	1.0–2.0	600	Least toxic amide agent	4.5
	0.25–0.5	i.v. Regional			600		
	1.5 –2.0	Peripheral nerve blocks	Fast	1.5–3.0	600	Methemoglobnemia occurs usually above 600 mg	
Mepivacaine	2.0 –3.0	Epidural	Fast	1.0–3.0	400	Duration of plain solutions longer than lidocaine without epinephrine. Useful when epinephrine is contraindicated.	4.5
	0.5 –1.0	Infiltration	Fast	1.5–3.0	500+ epinephrine		
	1.0 –1.5	Peripheral nerve blocks	Fast	2.0–3.0			
	1.5 –2.0	Epidural	Fast	1.5–3.0			
	4.0	Spinal	Fast	1.0–1.5	100		
Bupivacaine	0.25	Infiltration	Fast	2.0–4.0	175	Lower concentrations provide differential sensory/motor block. Ventricular arrhythmias and sudden cardiovascular collapse reported following rapid i.v. injection.	4.5–6
					225+ epinephrine		
	0.25–0.5	Peripheral nerve blocks	Slow	4.0–12.0	225+ epinephrine		
	0.25–0.5	Obstetrical epidural	Moderate	2.0–4.0	225+ epinephrine		
	0.5 –0.75	Surgical epidural	Moderate	2.0–5.0	225+ epinephrine		
	0.5 –0.75	Spinal	Fast	2.0–4.0	20		
Etidocaine	0.5	Infiltration	Fast	2.0–4.0	300	Profound motor block useful for surgical anesthesia but not for obstetrical analgesia.	4.5
					400+ epinephrine		
	0.5 –1.0	Peripheral	Fast	3.0–12.0	400+		

Agent	Concentration (%)	Clinical Use	Onset	Duration (min)	Maximum Dose (mg)	With epinephrine	Comments	pH
Dibucaine	1.0 –1.5	Surgical epidural	Fast	2.0–4.0		epinephrine 400+ epinephrine	Recommended only for spinal and topical use	5 –6.5
	0.25–0.5 hyperbaric	Spinal	Fast	2.0–4.0	10			
	0.00067 hypobaric	Spinal	Fast	2.0–4.0	10			
	1.0	Topical	Slow	30–60	50			
Esters								
Procaine	1.0	Infiltration	Fast	30–60	1000		Used mainly for infiltration and differential spinal blocks. Allergic potential after repeated use	2.7–4
	1.0 –2.0	Peripheral nerve blocks	Slow	30–60	1000			
	2.0	Epidural	Slow	30–60	1000			
	10.0	Spinal	Moderate	30–60	200			
Chloroprocaine	1.0	Infiltration	Fast	30–60	800	1000+ epinephrine	Intrathecal injection may be associated with sensory/motor deficits.	
	2.0	Peripheral nerve block	Fast	30–60		1000+ epinephrine		
	2.0 –3.0	Epidural	Fast	30–60		1000+ epinephrine		
Tetracaine	0.5	Spinal	Fast	2.0–4.0	20		Use is primarily limited to spinal and topical anesthesia.	4.5–6.5
	2.0	Topical	Slow	30–60	20			
Cocaine	4.0–10.0	Topical	Slow	30–60	150		Topical use only. Addictive, causes vasoconstriction. CNS toxicity initially features marked excitation ("Fight and Flight" Response). May cause cardiac arrhythmias owing to sympathetic stimulation.	
Benzocaine	Up to 20	Topical	Slow	30–60	200		Useful only for topical anesthesia.	

*Note: Epinephrine-containing solutions have a pH 1 to 1.5 units lower than plain solutions.
Reproduced with permission from Covino BG: Clinical pharmacology of local anesthetic agents. In Cousins MJ, Bridenbaugh PO (eds): Neural Blockade, 2nd ed. Philadelphia, JB Lippincott, 1988, p 112–113.

patients experiencing transient relief from sympathetic blocks often get longer relief with IV regional guanethidine block, these patients nevertheless are not likely to experience long-term or permanent relief from this procedure.[24] Continuous epidural or brachial plexus blocks carried out for several days may produce permanent relief of the burning pain and hyperpathia of "causalgia" associated with damage by tumor to the brachial or femoral plexus. If these procedures prove unsuccessful, neurolytic or surgical sympathectomy may provide alternative treatments.

MYOFASCIAL PAIN

Cancer patients often develop myofascial pain secondary to somatic or visceral pain from tumor spread (see Chapter 1). Trigger-point injections can be very effective in overall pain management. The objective of this therapeutic measure is to decrease pain to tolerable levels, improve function, and prevent permanent disability. Techniques such as muscle relaxation, spray-and-stretch techniques or trigger-point injection, exercise programs, and stimulation analgesia are often used.

Myofascial trigger-point injection of local anesthetics is a simple, commonly used pain management procedure, which, by producing physicochemical interruption of reflex pathways almost at the source of the nociceptive process, effectively relieves pain.

Trigger-point injection is a useful technique when a few trigger points are present and the muscle is unable to stretch because of excessive pain or its sequelae. Localization of the trigger point can be achieved with flat palpation by feeling the tight band within the muscle and rolling it back and forth between the fingers (Fig. 19–1). The trigger point will be the most sensitive spot in the band. Keeping the trigger point fixed between the fingers, the needle is inserted perpendicularly to the skin and advanced to the required depth of the trigger point. When the patient reports

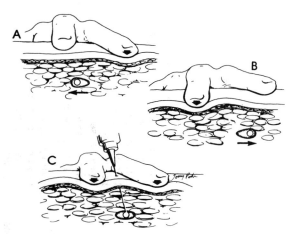

Figure 19–1. Method of palpating and fixing an isolated trigger point in muscle with two fingers before inserting the needle tip into the trigger area for injection. **(A)** Fixation of the trigger point by proximal finger. **(B)** Fixation of the trigger point by distal finger. **(C)** Needle within trigger point.

the worst pain, the trigger point usually will be impaled.

Although dry needling of trigger points may be efficacious, more effective therapy may be achieved by injection of a local anesthetic; in addition, postinjection pain may occur after dry needling.[25] Saline has been reported to be effective in pain relief,[26] although other investigators advocate the use of procaine.[27] My preference is a mixture of 0.5% etidocaine and 0.375% bupivacaine, which produces a long-lasting effect without systemic toxicity or myotoxicity, and better relief than dry needling, saline, or lidocaine.

A mixture of corticosteroid and local anesthetic has been advocated for trigger-point injections for patients with soft-tissue inflammation or postinjection soreness of muscles.[27] For this procedure, I have found dexamethasone (4 mg/10 ml of local anesthetic solution), mixed with bupivacaine and etidocaine, useful in not producing untoward sequelae. After trigger-point injections, stretch is important[25,28]; vapocoolant spray or heat also may be applied during stretching of the muscle to full length. The most common combination of techniques includes stretch-and-spray, trigger-point injection, and transcutaneous nerve stimulation therapy.

The earlier a patient is treated, the more effective and longer-lasting treatment will be. Injections repeated every several days for a week or two may be effective; however, a series of six injections at weekly intervals with other associated therapy usually is required for chronic trigger-point pain.

NEUROPATHIC PAIN

Invasion or compression of intraspinal nerve roots, brachial and femoral plexus, or major peripheral nerves can be a source of severe pain in cancer patients. Inflammation appears to play a major role in the production of pain: mechanical compression by tumor produces local irritation of nerve roots, which then become edematous and elaborate nociceptive/algesic substances. Epidural injections of local anesthetic–steroid mixtures are useful in treatment of lumbosacral and cervical radiculopathy, perhaps due to reduction of the inflammatory response of affected nerve roots.[29] With this technique, 80 mg of methylprednisolone acetate or 50 mg of triamcinolone diacetate is suspended in 10 ml of 0.25% or 0.125% bupivacaine, and is injected slowly into the epidural space. Patchy degenerative changes, although without neurologic deficit, have been observed in nerves treated with methylprednisolone acetate,[30] whereas triamcinolone diacetate has been shown to cause only minimal localized mononuclear cell meningeal infiltration, which apparently is of no clinical significance.[31] After the first injection, a catheter can be introduced to inject a second dose of the steroid–local anesthetic mixture, if needed to reach the appropriate nerve root. Patients are reevaluated in 2 weeks, at which time another injection can be repeated.

Similar injections of steroid–local anesthetic mixture can be used to treat pain caused by tumor invasion at the site of plexus involvement: brachial plexus via brachial plexus blockade, Pancoast tumors involving the proximal portion of the plexus via interscalene or subclavian perivascular blocks, tumor invasion closer to the axilla via infraclavicular or axillary block, and pelvic tumor invading the femoral plexus via a paravertebral approach to the femoral plexus, or psoas compartment block.[32]

ACUTE HERPES ZOSTER AND POSTHERPETIC NEURALGIA

Acute herpes zoster and postherpetic neuralgia are common in cancer patients (see Chapter 3); early and complete resolution of the acute condition often can prevent the development of postherpetic neuralgia. Usual methods of treatment include drug therapy, nerve blocks, psychosocial interventions, physical measures, and surgery. Nerve blocks used to treat these two disorders include local infiltration, somatic nerve blocks, sympathetic nerve blocks, and epidural blocks.

Local Infiltration

Epstein achieved excellent results in resolving the acute pain of herpes zoster (approaching a 100% success rate), and was able to achieve a reduction in the development of postherpetic neuralgia to 2% by injecting 0.2% triamcinolone in normal saline subcutaneously into areas of eruption and sites of pain and itching.[33,34] I have had similar results with this technique, which offers the benefits of simplicity, cost-effectiveness, and a fairly predictable response to treatment. However, no block technique reliably prevents postherpetic neuralgia in a high proportion of older patients.[35]

Somatic Nerve Blocks

Somatic nerve blocks, including brachial plexus, paravertebral, intercostal, and sciatic blocks, have been found to be of only limited

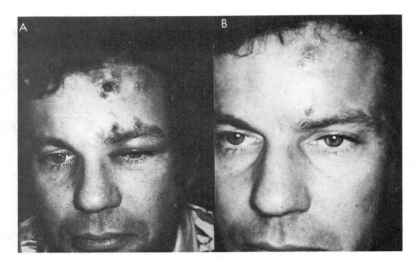

Figure 19–2. **(A)** Acute herpes zoster of the left eye and forehead before treatment with intralesional injection of local anesthetic and steroid and left stellate ganglion block. **(B)** Appearance 3 days later. Note clearing of the eye and lesions of the forehead.

value in treating acute herpes zoster; they are not in the least efficacious in treating postherpetic neuralgia.

Sympathetic Nerve Blocks

Sympathetic blockade often can alleviate the pain of acute herpes zoster (Fig. 19–2). Although the evidence for its effectiveness in treating postherpetic neuralgia is less clear-cut, it may prevent the development of this disorder, which suggests that it probably should be used as early as possible.[36] Trigeminal herpes zoster has been successfully treated with a bupivacaine block of the ipsilateral stellate ganglion,[37] and other studies have successfully treated herpes zoster with one or two sympathetic blocks.[38] Another researcher has linked the success rate with sympathetic blockade to the proximity of administration after onset of the disease (*ie*, almost 100% success if performed within 2 to 3 weeks after onset), with a subsequent decrease in responsiveness thereafter.[39] It is certain that patients must be treated within the first 2 to 3 weeks

of the disease in order to achieve the most favorable outcome.

Epidural Blocks

Acute herpes zoster also has been treated successfully with epidural local anesthetic blockade, without the subsequent development of postherpetic neuralgia[40]; however, objective, controlled studies to confirm the efficacy of neural blockade in postherpetic neuralgia in older patients have not been reported.[35]

CRISIS MANAGEMENT

Continuous local anesthetic blockade can provide complete analgesia for the temporary control of severe, intractable pain in cancer patients. Such therapy allows patients at least a brief respite from opioid analgesics, and provides an opportunity for reversal of the tolerance to opioids that chronic patients develop.

Infusion Technique

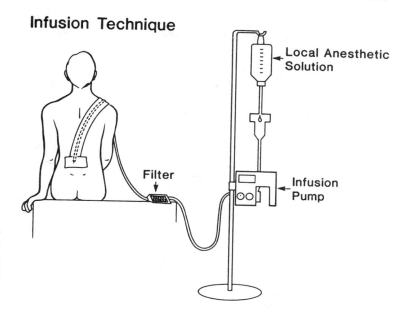

Figure 19–3. Diagram showing arrangement used for continuous epidural analgesia. Reproduced with permission from Raj PP: Handbook of Regional Anesthesia p 104. New York, Churchill Livingstone, 1985.

Good analgesia can be achieved with the continuous infusion of 0.125% bupivacaine. A wide margin of safety at dosages up to 30 mg/hour has been demonstrated in normal patients.[41] A significant decrease in bupivacaine total clearance with increasing alpha-1-acid glycoprotein concentrations also has been reported.[42] A typical arrangement used for continuous epidural analgesia is shown in Figure 19–3.

SUMMARY

Local anesthetic blocks have a definite and important role to play in the alleviation of pain for cancer patients. When skillfully administered, they are among the most effective methods of relieving pain. However, despite their long use, some pain specialists remain skeptical about their efficacy.

Certainly, therapies such as oral analgesics, psychotropics, and nonsteroidal anti-inflammatory drugs should be considered as first-line therapies in the management of pain for cancer patients. However, if insufficient pain relief is achieved with analgesic agents or adverse side effects are noted—or if temporary relief of severe pain is needed—local anesthetic blocks often are successful in a substantial number of patients.

REFERENCES

1. Abram SE: The role of nonneurolytic nerve blocks in the management of cancer pain. In Abram SE (ed): Cancer Pain, p 67. Boston, Kluwer Academic, 1989.
2. Boas RA, Cousins MJ: Diagnostic neural blocks. In Cousins MJ, Bridenbaugh PO, eds. Neural Blockade, p 885. Philadelphia: JB Lippincott, 1986.
3. Porges P: Local anesthetics in the treatment of cancer pain. Recent Results Cancer Res 1984;89:127.
4. Raj PP, Ramamurthy S: Differential nerve bock studies. In Raj PP (ed): Practical Management of Pain, p 173. Chicago, Year Book, 1986.

5. Gasser HS, Erlanger J: Role of fiber size in establishment of nerve block by pressure or cocaine. Am J Physiol 1929;88:581.
6. Nathan PW, Sears TA: Some factors concerned in differential nerve block by local anesthetics. J Physiol (London) 1961;157:565.
7. Gentry WD, Newman MC, Goldner JL et al: Relation between graduated spinal block technique and MMPI for diagnosis and prognosis of chronic low back pain. Spine 1977;2:210.
8. McCollum DE, Stephen CR: Use of graduated spinal anesthesia in the differential diagnosis of pain of the back and lower extremities. South Med J 1964;57:410.
9. Raj PP: Sympathetic pain mechanisms and management. Presented at the Second Annual Meeting of the American Society of Anesthesiologists, March 10–11, 1977, Hollywood, FL.
10. Raj PP: Case history 2: Nesacaine for retrograde differential epidural blocking: Nesacaine (chloroprocaine hydrochloride). In Finster M, (ed): Case Studies in Obstetrical and Surgical Regional Anesthesia, p 8. New York, Pennwalt Corp., 1979.
11. Bonica JJ: Management of Pain. Philadelphia, Lea & Febiger, 1953.
12. Bonica JJ: Clinical Applications of Diagnostic and Therapeutic Nerve Blocks. Springfield, IL, Charles C Thomas, 1959.
13. Bonica JJ: Current role of nerve blocks in the diagnosis and therapy of pain. In Bonica JJ (ed): Advances in Neurology, vol 4, p 445. New York, Raven Press, 1974.
14. Tasker R: Deafferentation and causalgia. In Bonica JJ (ed): Advances in Pain Research and Treatment, p 305. New York, Raven Press, 1980.
15. Loeser JD: Dorsal rhizotomy for the relief of chronic pain. J Neurosurg 1972;36:745.
16. Bonica JJ: Management of pain with regional analgesia. Postgrad Med 1984;60:897.
17. Brena SF: Nerve blocks and chronic pain states—an update: Clinical indications. Postgrad Med 1985;78:77.
18. Mayne GE, Brown M, Arnold P et al: Pain of herpes zoster and postherpetic neuralgia. In Raj PP (ed): Practical Management of Pain, p 345. Chicago, Year Book, 1986.
19. Bonica JJ: Causalgia and other reflex sympathetic dystrophies. In Bonica JJ, Liebeskind JC, Albe-Fessard D (eds): Advances in Pain Research and Therapy, vol 3, p 141. New York, Raven Press, 1979.
20. Mitchell SW, Morehouse GR, Keen WW: Gunshot Wounds and Other Injuries of the Nerves. Philadelphia, JB Lippincott, 1964.
21. Bonica JJ: Sympathetic Nerve Blocks for Pain Diagnosis and Therapy. New York, Breon Laboratories, 1984.
22. Leriche R: La Chirurgie de la Douleur: Paris, Masson et Cie., 1949.
23. Boneli S, Conoscente F, Movilla PG et al: Regional intravenous guanethidine vs stellate block in reflex sympathetic dystrophies: A randomized trial. Pain 1983;16:279.
24. Abram SE, Kettler RD, Reynolds AC et al: Potential advantage of IV regional guanethidine over sympathetic blocks. ASRA Abstracts 1986;11:85.
25. Kraus H: Clinical Treatment of Back and Neck Pain. New York, McGraw-Hill, 1970.
26. Sola AE, Kuitert JH: Myofascial trigger point pain in the neck and shoulder girdle. Northwest Medicine 1955;54:980.
27. Travell J, Simons DG: Myofascial Pain and Dysfunction: The Trigger Point Manual. Baltimore, Williams & Wilkins, 1983.
28. Zohn DA, Mennell JM: Musculoskeletal Pain: Diagnosis and Physical Treatment, p 126. Boston, Little Brown, 1976.
29. Benzon HT: Epidural steroids for low back pain and lumbosacral radiculopathy. Pain 1986;24:277.
30. Wood KM, Arguelles J, Norenberg MD: Degenerative lesions in rat sciatic nerves after local injection of methylprednisolone in sterile aqueous suspension. Reg Anaesth 1980;5:13.
31. Delaney TJ, Rowlingson JC, Caron H et al: The effects of steroids on nerves and meninges. Anesth Analg 1980;59:610.
32. Chayen D, Nathan H, Chayen M: The psoas compartment block. Anesthesiology 1976;45:95.
33. Epstein E: Triamcinolone-procaine in the treatment of zoster and postzoster neuralgia. California Medicine 1971;115:6.
34. Epstein E: Treatment of herpes zoster and postzoster neuralgia by subcutaneous injection of triamcinolone. International Journal of Dermatology 1981;20.
35. Loeser JD: Herpes zoster and postherpetic neuralgia. Pain 1986;25:149.
36. Murphy T: Herpes zoster. In Advances and Update in Pain Therapy. ASA Annual Meeting, October 25, 1982, p 40, Philadelphia: JB Lippincott.
37. Olson ER, Ivy HB: Stellate block for trigeminal herpes zoster (letter). Arch Ophthalmol 1980;98:1656.
38. Rosenak SS: Paravertebral block for the treatment of herpes zoster. NY State J Med 1956;56:2684.
39. Winnie AP: The patient with herpetic neuralgia. In Moya F, Gion H (eds): Postgraduate Seminar in Anesthesiology (program syllabus), p 165. Postgraduate Seminar in Anesthesiology, Miami Beach, FL, 1983.

40. Perkins HM, Hanlon PR: Epidural injection of local anesthetic and steroids for relief of pain secondary to herpes zoster. Arch Surg 1978;113:253.

41. Denson DD, Raj PP, Saldahna F, et al: Perineural infusions of bupivacaine for prolonged analgesia: Pharmacokinetic considerations. Int J Clin Pharmacol Ther Toxicol 1983;21:591.

42. Raj PP, Denson PP: Prolonged analgesia technique. In Raj PP (ed): Practical Management of Pain, p 687. Chicago, Year Book, 1986.

Chapter 20

Neurolysis: Pharmacology and Drug Selection

Sampson Lipton

INTRODUCTION

More than 4 million people die from cancer annually. Three to four
times as many individuals suffer from the disease, and about 70% of
patients with advanced disease experience significant pain (see Chapter
17). Pain is most often associated with tumor invasion, but about 30%
is due to related nonmalignant causes, such as treatment, concurrent
disease, debility, and psychological factors. Each component contributing to the global suffering of the patient requires management. Pain
tends to worsen as disease progresses, and as a result, treatment must
be dynamic. Multiple sites of pains are common. Various types of pain
may develop, such as pain that is sympathetically maintained or of
central origin (see Chapters 1, 3, and 10). These entities do not generally
respond favorably to the treatment discussed here, and adjuvant drugs
or other treatment will be required.

Neurolysis at different anatomic levels has specific indications and
disadvantages that are discussed by each chapter author in relation to
their particular chapter (see Chapters 21–23). This author believes that
neurolytic methods in the subarachnoid space are only indicated in
cancer patients with pain that is unresponsive to more conservative
measures, and then only when all possible measures are instituted
to ensure that the injection is made at the intended site. Important
precautions include positioning the patient carefully, checking the dose
and spinal level, and administering the lytic substance in small divided

increments interrupted by careful neurologic assessment. Although it is not used uniformly for intraspinal neurolysis, the use of an image intensifier and water-soluble radiopaque contrast (see Chapter 24) is recommended by this author. Similar radiologic precautions should be observed for all neurolytic procedures, except for superficial ones, such as injection into a stump neuroma. It should be recalled that 1) even with strict attention to regional anatomy, the needle may be located incorrectly; and 2) sharp needles tend to move easily even when the utmost care is exercised to ensure their immobility. The author has been involved as a consultant in a number of medico-legal cases involving the administration of neurolytic drugs, and invariably radiologic control has not been used.

HISTORY

NEUROLYTIC AGENTS

A surprisingly large number of different agents have been used to produce neurolysis in the past 120 years, including distilled water,[1] hot saline,[2] hypertonic cold saline,[3] serapin (pitcher plant distillate),[4-6] ammonium salt solutions,[5,6] silver nitrate,[2,7] chloroform,[2] osmic acid,[8-12] phenol,[7,13,14] alcohol,[15-18] esters of alcohol,[15] guaicol (2 methoxyphenol),[15] glycerin,[15,19] chlorocresol,[20,21], and ricin.[22] This list is by no means complete, but it includes the agents that have withstood the test of time and are still used in contemporary practice.

EARLY USE

Some of the early the practitioners did not know the effect of the substances they were injecting. Initially they apparently were used as counter-irritants, and were injected subcutaneously over or into painful areas, but some produced true neurolysis. The results were encouraging. A recent comprehensive history of neurolytic block by Swerdlow is recommended reading.[23] Some of the more important substances are discussed below.

Osmic Acid

Luton[1] appears to have used irritant substances injected into painful areas as a method of achieving pain relief. He used silver nitrate, saline, and hypertonic saline. In particular, he mentions injecting over the sciatic nerve. Osmic acid was introduced by Neuber,[8] and its use was subsequently adopted by others.[9-12] He used 1% osmic acid by hypodermic injection to treat various types of neuralgias with good results. The number of injections used was large, on the order of 6 to 20 in a single patient. Jacoby[9] used 0.5–1.0 ml per patient of an aqueous solution of osmic acid. This method produced unwanted and untoward effects, and the writing of the period cautions that injection should occur near, but not into the substance of the sciatic nerve. Patients appeared willing to accept pain during treatment and sometimes paralysis afterward, particularly when they had experienced long periods of severe neuralgia beforehand. The treatment of the day was not sophisticated.

In the era preceding the therapeutic use of anticonvulsants, trigeminal neuralgia was one of the most persistent and difficult neuralgias to treat. In the succeeding years, much effort was devoted to developing and using neurolytic drugs for this application. Initially, osmic acid,[8-12] formaldehyde,[13] alcohol,[2,15-17] and phenol[2,18] were injected into the peripheral branches of the trigeminal nerve at the various superficial foramina. As might be expected, the effects of these blocks were relatively transient, and soon Pitres and Verger,[16] followed by others, were using alcohol on the trigeminal divisions administered by deep injections. Cushing[23] wrote extensively on blocking the trigeminal ganglion and its branches, noting that Hartel was the first to block the gasserian ganglion directly. Trigeminal neuralgia was treated by alcohol injection from 1902 onward.[16,24-27]

Alcohol

Based on anecdotal information suggesting that complications could be reduced when less concentrated solutions of neurolytic agents were used, Pitres and Vaillard[15] carried out investigations on the effects of alcohol applied to the sciatic nerves of guinea pigs. Paralysis and anesthesia occurred with 85% alcohol, and lesser damage was observed when weaker concentrations were used. Physicians began treating neuralgias of various types with alcohol neurolytic block, but time elapsed before it was used for cancer pain on any regular basis.[27-29] Dogliotti[30] used absolute alcohol intrathecally, and suggested that it would be useful in cancer pain. Putnam and Hampton[13] used alcohol for symptomatic oral cancer, but preferred phenol. Mixtures of cocaine and phenol (one part cocaine, two parts phenol) were used by Braun.[31] This was soluble in alcohol but was not used as an injection. A 5% solution of olive oil was favored because it was relatively less irritating to tissue. Mixtures with benzyl alcohol were used to prolong local anesthetic action.[32,33] It was only later realized that this prolonged duration of action was due to nerve destruction, when Duncan and Jarvis demonstrated that 10% benzyl alcohol destroys all small nerve fibers.[34]

Phenol

In general terms, alcohol was preferred to phenol and other agents until about 1950, but its popularity began to wane after Mandl's[35] consideration of using phenol for lumbar sympathetic block. Later he and others[36] reported on the use of phenol for this purpose. Maher[14] first used phenol solutions for subarachnoid neurolysis. Phenol dissolves readily in water up to a concentration of 6.7%, and thereafter remains insoluble until the concentration of phenol is raised to a sufficiently high level that the water becomes soluble in the phenol. Because of these limitations, Maher[7,14,20] used glycerin or myodil (ethyl iodophenylundeclate) as the solvent. Maher described not only subarachnoid phenol injection, but epidural and subdural injection, as well.[7,37] He also advocated the use of silver nitrate[7]: ". . . when the initial phenol injections do not give adequate relief, the phenol and silver nitrate solution can be used at resistant sites after a few days." Maher believed that the silver nitrate acted as a mordant, helping to "fix"

the phenol to resistant or perhaps sheltered nerve roots. In this author's experience, silver nitrate produces a meningeal reaction of variable severity, and as a result its use is not recommended.

Chlorocresol

Maher introduced this phenol derivative (parachlormetacresol)[20,21] in an effort to find a substance that ". . . would have a selective action on continuous-pain fibres and yet be able to penetrate inflamed tissue or growth around the nerve roots." He used chlorocresol with glycerin in a 1:50 solution in doses of 0.75 ml. Administered in this fashion, fewer nerve roots are affected than when phenol is injected, and Maher advocated injections of adjacent segments after 3 weeks. He concluded that the effects of chlorocresol were more reliable than those of phenol, but take time to develop. Its use requires experience and careful judgment, since the warmth, numbness, and tingling[21] characteristically experienced by the patient immediately after phenol is injected does not occur, and the dermatomes affected are not easily distinguished. It may be valuable when phenol has partially failed and a stronger effect is needed.

Patient Position During Intrathecal Injections. The specific gravity of each of these solutions is one of their most important features, especially when they are being considered for subarachnoid injection. Phenol mixed in glycerin or myodil (or equivalent modern water-soluble radiopaque mediums) is hyperbaric with respect to cerebrospinal fluid (CSF), and as a result, the patient must be positioned on the painful side for dural puncture and then tilted further posteriorly so that the posterior sensory nerve root is dependent (see Chapter 23). The patient lies on a longitudinally tilting table with the affected nerve roots at the lowest level of the spinal theca. Since alcohol is hypobaric with respect to the CSF, the opposite position is adopted: the patient is positioned with the painful side uppermost, and, after dural puncture is performed, is tilted anteriorly so that the posterior sensory roots transmitting pain are uppermost. The table again is tilted longitudinally, but this time so that the point at which the targeted nerve rootlets enter the spinal cord is at the highest point of the spinal theca. The use of pillows, rolled towels, and an operating room-type table that "breaks" are useful adjuncts to obtaining the desired posture. Characteristically, assuming and maintaining the anatomically correct position is more distressing and painful to the patient than is the actual injection. Careful observation of these guidelines is more important when alcohol is used as it "flashes away" to the high point of the theca as it is injected. Phenol in contrast medium is also fairly mobile within the theca. Phenol in glycerin is highly viscid and moves slowly, but it does "creep," and the patient should be positioned so that the neurolytic solution does not spread toward vulnerable, nontargeted nerve roots.

Maher used phenol solutions for the control of chronic cancer pain. It was also used to produce destruction of anterior nerve roots for the control of spasticity.[38,39] The concentration used has varied considerably. Whereas most investigators recommend 5%–6% phenol, Kelly and Gautier-Smith[38] used 10%, and this author has used up to 25%. When administered intrathecally, these concentrated phenol solutions flow past the posterior sensory root before reaching the anterior root, and thus a band of anesthesia usually is produced. The use of modern catheter techniques might prevent this disadvantage nowadays, and recently has been reported.[40]

Phenol gradually has supplanted alcohol as the agent of choice for many indications because it is more controllable within the subarachnoid space, and because of an impression that neuritis is less frequent after peripheral nerve injections.[41]

Glycerin USP (Glycerol)

In 1963, Jefferson[42] reported on the use of a phenol–glycerin mixture injected under radiologic guidance into Meckel's cave (the trigeminal cistern) for trigeminal neuralgia. Although not entirely free of the drawbacks associated with alcohol injection (anesthesia, sensory deficit), the results of this method were reasonably satisfactory, and it was well received. The injection is made into the trigeminal cistern with the patient seated. In this technique glycerin is the carrying agent, and phenol is the effector substance. More recently Hakanson[19,43] has used glycerol alone to produce neurolysis and pain relief. The clinically useful neurolytic capabilities of glycerol for this application were discovered serendipitously. Glycerol was injected for another purpose during gamma-ray radiation of the gasserian ganglion for trigeminal neuralgia, and pain relief was noted. Ischia[44] recently reviewed the course of 112 patients treated in this manner (mean follow-up of 3.5 years). At 1 month, 92% of patients reported complete relief of pain. At the end of the follow-up, 71.4% still had complete pain relief. Abnormal facial sensations were reported in 44%, mild hypoesthesia in 32%, paresthesia in 19%, and dysesthesia in 3%. The corneal reflex was partially or completely affected in 8%. Of note is an absence of reports of anesthesia dolorosa, diplopia, and neuroparalytic keratitis. This method is currently in vogue due to the lack of serious complications. Its effectiveness seems to be related to accurate placement of the needle tip within the trigeminal cistern, ensuring that the subsequent injection of glycerol does not spill over to neighboring brain structures, and maintenance of the seated position after injection. About one-third of patients report recurrence of pain within a year of treatment.

Ammonium Sulfate

Ammonium salts[4-6] enjoyed frequent use as neurolytic agents for a time, although their use is uncommon today. Their purported benefit, particularly for subcostal blocks, was an absence of neuritis. Miller et al[45] stated that 60% (28/47) of treatments with 10% ammonium sulfate produced complete or nearly complete (excellent) relief of pain, which persisted for more than 20 days after 22 treatments, and for more than 90 days after 7 treatments. In his series, post-block neuritis did not occur. Charlton,[46] however, mentions unremitting neuritis as a hazard. When used intrathecally the results were not always benign: motor effects were observed,[5,6] as was urinary incontinence of 1–2 days' duration. In the technique originally advocated by Judovitch et al,[5,47] a 6% solution (60 mg/ml) of either ammonium chloride or ammonium sulfate was used in doses of 200–400 mg that, before injection, was diluted with CSF by barbotage. Insufficient dilution was implicated in the production of adverse effects secondary to nonselective injury to nerve fibers. The technique was later amended by the substitution of a reduced amount of ammonium salt (200 mg) diluted in a fixed volume of CSF (50 ml). It is thus obvious that ammonium salts can cause nerve damage, particularly when more concentrated solutions are used. A case of paraplegia was documented after the intrathecal injection of 8% ammonium sulfate and procaine,[48] and subsequent autopsy revealed nerve damage similar to that which would be expected after phenol or alcohol injection. In a series of patients treated with injections to the peroneal nerve, motor changes were absent when a 10% solution of ammonium chloride was used, versus 15%, which produced foot drop.[49] Wood[50] has suggested that ". . . for a short term effect a 10% solution of the sulfate salt is as reliable as alcohol and phenol, with possibly less complication."

Subarachnoid Infusion of Saline

This has not been a popular method of pain relief, although it still occasionally is used.[51] Introduced in 1967[52] by Hitchcock, it was based on work showing that local cooling of nerve fibers produces a reversible conduction block. The original technique involved removal of large volumes of CSF, followed by replacement with large volumes of iced isotonic saline.[52] Observations that thawing isotonic saline usually produces a hypertonic supernatant led to the development of Hitchcock's more widely accepted modified technique, which substitutes normothermic hypertonic (12%–15%) saline for infusion, and does not involve removal of significant volumes of CSF.[51] General anesthesia is used to alleviate the severe pain that follows injection

and to allow for prolonged (30-minute) recovery. Lumbar injection frequently is followed by fasciculations, piloerection, venostasis, and cyanosis of the lower limbs. Tachypnea and hypertension are common responses, and blood pressure control with potent antihypertensives is essential to limit morbidity.[51] Respiratory arrest may occur, and resources for cardiopulmonary resuscitation must be available.

In a series reported by Hitchcock,[52] treatment produced good initial results in 79%–93% of 116 patients. Late success was 38% and 25% after 1 and 3 months, respectively. A survey by the National Spinal Cord Injury Registry[53] reported on the incidence of adverse reactions in 2,105 patients treated with either normothermic hypertonic saline or iced isotonic saline injection. Two hundred and twenty-three patients (10.6%) suffered adverse symptoms, of which muscle spasm, alterations in blood pressure, and seizure activity were most prominent. Significant morbidity, primarily paraplegia or quadriplegia, was noted in 22 patients (1.03%), and 2 patients succumbed to myocardial infarction. A single case of pulmonary edema has been reported after the instillation of iced saline.[54]

The mechanisms of pain relief are still unclear. Postmortem studies of patients treated with iced saline infusion showed several small areas of peripheral demyelination of the spinal cord and brain-stem.[55] Temporary conduction blockade has been proposed to explain the effects of cold saline, and an osmolar gradient of chloride affecting C fibers has been suggested as the mechanism for pain relief with hypertonic saline.[52,56]

Cryoprobe Therapy

Lloyd[57] developed an apparatus that uses the cooling effect produced by the expansion of nitrous oxide (Joule–Thompson effect) to lower the temperature of the tip of a 15-gauge needle to about −75°C. This has been used to produce pain relief by freezing neural tissue, the architecture of which consequently is disrupted. One of the main advantages of cryotherapy is that regeneration of the disrupted nerve characteristically occurs in an orderly manner, and the incidence of subsequent neuritis and neuralgia is lower than with other (chemical) forms of nerve destruction. The freezing process produces minimal effects on the endoneurium, and as a result, connective tissue elements of nerve fibers have a well defined pathway along which to regrow. Cryotherapy produces a tiny lesion, and hence effects will be poor unless the tip is located directly on the targeted nerve. It is thus best used on easily accessible peripheral nerves. As the duration of benefit is relatively short, a series of treatments is often necessary. It has a definite but limited place in neurolysis.

Thermally Generated Radiofrequency Lesioning

See Chapter 26.

PHARMACOLOGY OF NEUROLYTICS

ETHYL ALCOHOL

Ethyl alcohol is the second compound in the alcohol series, and is commonly used for medical purposes. When used in appropriate concentrations (about 75%) it is an antimicrobial of low potency, but it is unsuitable for use as a sterilizing agent because it is not sporicidal.[58] Alcohol is rapidly absorbed from the stomach, small intestine, colon, and as a vapor from the lungs. When alcohol is injected subcutaneously, its rate of absorption depends on the quantity injected and the blood supply of the site, particularly since alcohol induces local vasoconstriction. When large volumes of alcohol are used for celiac plexus block, however, it spreads widely and absorption is characteristically rapid. Thompson et al measured alcohol blood levels in patients after celiac block (50 ml of 50% ethanol) (see Chapter 22), and found a peak level of 21 mg/100 ml, 20% of the legal definition of intoxication.[59] In a similar study, Jain and colleagues noted either the presence of euphoria or the characteristic odor of alcohol on the breath of patients within 15 minutes of the procedure, and a mean blood level of alcohol of 30 mg/100 ml at 30 minutes.[60]

Direct contact between alcohol and protoplasm produces dehydration and precipitation, a process that underlies the mechanism of nerve injury (see below). It is irritating when applied to the mucosa, but does not affect intact skin. Injection into the superficial tissues induces pain and later anesthesia of the region. When a percutaneous injection is made sufficiently close to nerves, nerve degeneration occurs, and later tissue irritation (neuritis) may develop. The incidence of alcoholic neuritis after peripheral nerve block is probably about 15%, although figures of 10%–60% have been quoted.

Ethyl alcohol is commercially available in ampules of 1 and 5 ml as a colorless solution that can be injected readily through small-bore needles. Depending on the site of injection and the concentration of alcohol, its administration is accompanied by a variable degree of discomfort that, at its extreme, is excruciating, though transient. It generally is used undiluted (absolute or 100% alcohol) for peripheral or subarachnoid block, in which case exposure to the atmosphere is avoided to prevent dilution by absorbed moisture, or in 50% concentrations for sympathetic block.

Direct injection of a sufficient quantity of concentrated alcohol into a nerve produces conduction blockade, the effects of which depend on the nature of the nerve that is blocked. Blockade of a sensory nerve produces anesthesia or hypoesthesia of the sensory field, muscle paralysis or paresis results from injection of a motor nerve, and both results occur when a mixed nerve is injected. These effects generally are not permanent in peripheral nerves, and, over time, recovery to greater or lesser degree is the rule. Alcohol produces a depolarizing block of nerve fibers[61] that may be reversible when low concentrations, which preferentially affect small fibers, are used. This effect is produced by most anesthetic and neurolytic agents by alteration of the transport of sodium and potassium ions across the myelin sheath.[62] When high concentrations are used, nerve tissue is destroyed (see below). Since alcohol diffuses more rapidly through biologic tissue than phenol, its effects cannot be confined as easily to small areas.

Interactions

Side effects have been reported after alcohol injection in patients receiving disulfiram-type drugs (Antabuse; Ayerst, New York, NY), which inhibit aldehyde dehydrogenase.[63,64] Umeda and Arai[63] reported a transient episode of flushing, sweating, dizziness, vomiting, and marked hypotension after alcohol celiac plexus block in a patient taking Moxolactam (Eli Lilly & Co., Indianapolis, IN). Drugs with the potential to induce this type of interaction include the beta-lactam antibiotics (including Moxalactam), metronidazole (Flagyl; Searle, Chicago, IL), chloramphenicol (Chlormycetin; Parke-Davis, Morris Plains, NJ), tolbutamide (Orinase; Upjohn, Kalamazoo, MI), and chlorpropamide (Diabinese; Pfizer Laboratories, New York, NY). Of greatest concern is the administration of alcohol to patients with a history of alcoholism who are undergoing maintenance treatment with disulfiram (Antabuse).[63]

Alcohol has multiple effects on the central nervous system (CNS). It is a general anesthetic and has a depressant effect on the CNS, producing apparent central stimulation due to the release of inhibition by a depressive action on the CNS inhibitory centers. The effects of alcohol on the CNS are proportional to the concentration of alcohol in the blood.

Cross-tolerance between alcohol and other drugs may be due to hepatic microsomal enzyme activity, which is increased in regular alcohol users, or to pharmacodynamic tolerance in the CNS. Pharmacodynamic tolerance is probably the cause of the cross-tolerance to general anesthetics seen in chronic alcoholics. When blood alcohol levels are high, the effects of other CNS depressants are additive.[65]

Pathology

When injected near or into a large nerve such as the sciatic nerve, alcohol produces either a reversible conduction block or a permanent block followed by degeneration and possible regeneration, depending on the extent of injury and fibrosis. Despite the fact that the intent of intrathecal injection is to create a lesion restricted to the targeted nerve roots (rhizolysis), both the roots and the cord itself may be affected. Since the course of events that takes place when nerve structures are damaged is similar for both alcohol and phenol, the following discussion applies to both these agents, and probably to all agents that cause chemical nerve damage.

Nerve Degeneration. Damage to nerve cells and fibers produces degeneration and/or death of the nerve cell. If the extent of degeneration is limited it may be followed by regeneration. When damage affects the cell body the changes that result are classified as primary degeneration; when the axon is affected, the changes are classified as secondary degeneration.

Primary degeneration: Injury can be caused by many agents, including chemical trauma, which is the particular concern here. Chromatolysis occurs in the cell body with disappearance of Nissl bodies, which spreads in a centripetal fashion. The cell and nucleus swell, after rupture the nucleus is extruded, neurofibrils become fragmented, and eventually the neurofibrillary system disappears. The quantity of neuroglial cells increases, and they envelop the nerve cell and replace it. When the cell body is destroyed regeneration does not follow, but if the cell body remains, regeneration occurs in reverse order to the degeneration.

Secondary degeneration: Secondary degeneration is due to injury of the axon and is also referred to as "Wallerian" degeneration. A lesion placed at a distance from the cell body results in degeneration up to the nearest node of Ranvier. The whole of the peripheral axis of the nerve degenerates, which is manifest as fragmentation and disappearance of the axon. Neurofibrils become tortuous, the myelin sheath breaks up into globules, and eventually there is total disappearance of neural elements except for an empty neurolemmal sheath. If the cell body is close to the point of axonal damage, it too may undergo a similar process.

Regeneration: Regeneration does not occur if the cell body is destroyed. Otherwise, the beginning of regeneration is marked by an increase in neurofibrils, which spread from the proximal end of the axon along its previous track. This pathway is maintained by a proliferation of neurolemmal cells, which are essential for the regeneration of nerve fibers. Since regeneration of nerve fibers can occur only in the presence of neurolemma cells, and, as these are absent in the CNS, regeneration generally does not occur in the CNS. Neurolemmal cells can, however, grow into the spinal axis from peripheral nerves, but this growth is limited.

Axons regenerate at 1.0–1.5 mm per day. Problems may arise during regeneration when growing neurofibrils have to advance through scar tissue and this is only partially achieved. Many fibrils lose their way and form multiple small hair-like structures at their ends that are highly responsive to catecholamines and vibration. Over time, these changes may contribute to the development of neuropathic pain (see Chapters 1, 3, and 10).[66] Byrne,[67] in an early paper, mentions that ". . . injection of 80% alcohol into the sciatic nerve caused marked paralysis of the limb and intense axonal phenomena as well as interstitial changes within the related ganglia. Injections of 60% alcohol especially when made just under the sheath and not too deeply into the nerve, only caused transitory and almost imperceptible disturbances of motor function, but at the same time caused marked axonal reaction phenomena." The changes described are reminiscent of those detailed in reports of the effects of osmic acid.[8–12] At autopsy, Gallagher[17] examined changes in the spinal cords of 12 patients who had undergone treatment with subarachnoid alcohol injection for cancer pain. He reported the alcohol injection produced minimal gross changes. Slight to moderate meningeal congestion was observed in four subjects. Histologic changes were found in the spinal cords of all subjects, and ranged from slight defects in the myelin sheaths to extensive degeneration with reparative fibrosis. The nerve roots were always affected, and in cases where time had elapsed after the injection of alcohol, the root was replaced with Schwann cells. Spinal ganglia were affected in four patients in whom the alcohol injection was performed more than 60 days before autopsy. Changes in the spinal cord *per se* were of two types. One type of injury probably was due to direct contact between alcohol and the substance of the cord. This type of injury appeared early, and in one subject, the cord showed a shallow zone of demyelination at the level of injection. The other type of injury was characterized by Wallerian degeneration in the lateral dorsal funiculus and in Lissauer's tract.

It would appear that alcohol produces controlled nerve damage with a tendency to subsequent neuritis when injected into or near nerves. With subarachnoid injections, there may be a direct effect on the surface of the spinal cord, probably due to the strong solutions that are used clinically. Gerberschagen[68] points out that hypobaric alcohol acts mainly on the 8 to 12 fila radicularia that compose the dorsal root as it enters the dorsal horn. The alcohol has to reach these fila, which anatomically may be a few segments above the exit of the root they form (see Chapter 23).

PHENOL

Phenol is bacteriostatic in dilute solution (0.2%), bactericidal in a 1% solution, and fungicidal over 1.3%. It is more effective in aqueous solution or in saline than when dissolved in glycerin or lipids, and its activity is reduced in alkaline media and at low temperatures. It is diffusible, penetrates tissues including the skin, and denatures protein. If a 5% solution remains in contact with tissue, penetration continues, and for this reason, persistent contact with the skin can produce extensive necrosis. When applied to nervous tissue, its depolarizing anesthetic action results in a characteristic sensation of tingling, warmth, and local anesthesia in the region subserved by the affected nerve. If contact with tissue is persistent, sufficient quantities of the drug may reach the circulation and produce depressant effects (see below).

Phenol first stimulates, then depresses the CNS, and, in humans, the stimulation phase is brief. Systemically absorbed drug depresses the circulation markedly and can induce hypotension, mainly due to a direct toxic action on the myocardium and small blood vessels. It is a powerful antipyretic. It is excreted mostly through the kidney (80%), either unchanged or conjugated with glucuronic acid or sulfuric acid. The remaining 20% is oxidized to hydroquinone, pyrocatechol, or is oxidized completely.

Phenol is soluble in water to a maximum ratio of 1:15, and as a result, at room temperature a concentration of 6.7% cannot be exceeded for aqueous phenol. More concentrated solutions can be obtained by adding small amounts of glycerin. Over time, oxidation can occur with the production of quinones, which color the stored phenol solution pink. Shelf life is said to exceed 1 year when preparations are refrigerated and not exposed to light. Generally, hospital pharmacists prepare solutions to order. Alternatively, 1.0-g amounts can be sterilized, maintained in 20-ml ampules, and any required concentration can be manufactured by the clinician[50] by the addition of the necessary amount of water, saline, glycerin, or contrast media. This author believes it is preferable to have the solutions manufactured by trained pharmacists beforehand to minimize the likelihood of error.

Controlled spread of the phenol in biologic tissue is important to optimize control of the neurolytic lesion, but, unfortunately, insufficient research in this area permits only limited conclusions. Solutions in water diffuse most actively, followed by mixtures with the modern water-soluble radiopaque contrast media that dissolve phenol freely, then solutions in glycerin that extrude their phenol slowly, and finally solutions in myodil. Myodil is a contrast medium that is no longer commercially available except to a few algologists with personal residual supplies. Five per cent phenol in myodil is said to be equivalent to 0.1% phenol in water[69], whereas others[70] state that phenol in glycerin is more effective than phenol in myodil. This author recommends that aqueous phenol should be avoided inside the theca. In practice, in equivalent strengths, phenol in myodil produces less profound effects than phenol in glycerin. Thus, phenol in myodil 1:15 is roughly equivalent to phenol 1:20 in glycerin. In the epidural space, 6% aqueous phenol can be administered at any level through an epidural catheter,[71] as long as its position has been verified carefully in advance. Subdural injection (see Chapter 23) is more difficult, but is possible,[37] especially in the cervical region. A particular feature of this method is that the disposition of the injected solution (the author used radiopaque phenol in myodil in those he performed) should be observed with an image intensifier. As the injection proceeds, contrast medium should be observed to move upward bilaterally in the subdural plane and out along the nerve roots. The bilateral distribution is affected to some extent by gravity, in that the spread of the contrast solution is greater on the dependent side. This method is useful for the management of bilateral pain in the cervical region.

Reactions

Other than as a neurolytic, there are few contemporary therapeutic uses for phenol. Its original value was as an antiseptic, but its use for this purpose has been superseded by modern substances. It is still used in dermatologic and anorectal preparations, in mouth washes, and as an antipruritic. Aqueous solutions of more than 2% should not be used near the skin for reasons mentioned previously. The fatal absorbed dose for adults is 8–15 g, which is usually followed by death within 24 hours, or occasionally much later. If it has been absorbed through the skin it can be removed with 50% alcohol, glycerin vegetable oils, sodium bicarbonate, or even water.[58] Phenol has a greater affinity for vascular than neural tissue,[72] and intravascular injections must be avoided. Charlton[46] has suggested this as a possible explanation for some of the complications of phenol blocks, suggesting that untoward results may stem from damage and infarction to blood vessels rather than direct neural injury.

Pathology

A multitude of investigators have reported on the effects of phenol[7,14,18,37,50,68–78] on human and animal tissue. Early observations of an association between the application of phenol to neural tissue and the prolonged relief of pain in the absence of complete anesthesia led investigators to postulate a selective action on the smaller nerve fibers carrying pain sensation (C fibers).[73,79] Small myelinated fibers were thought to be more susceptible than large myelinated fibers. The slower A fibers were thought to be the most susceptible of the myelinated fibers, and these were believed to be blocked before activity attributable to C-fiber transmission (in the compound action potential) was abolished, despite the fact that the C fibers still were shown to be more susceptible than the largest myelinated fibers. One explanation for the apparent differential blockade that was advanced related to the role of the nodes of Ranvier. Since conduction block occurs only when more than one node is affected, and the nodes are further apart in larger myelinated axons, it was suggested that when contact with phenol is restricted to a small portion of nerve, the smaller nerve might be blocked more effectively because more nodes are involved. Similarly, since blockade of unmyelinated nerves is independent of effects on the nodes (which are absent), a short blocked zone of an unmyelinated fiber might permit the passage of impulses less readily than would myelinated fibers, and thus the observed differences might be due to blocking a short length of nerve. This thesis was tested experimentally, and was found to be incorrect, as large fibers were still more resistant.

Examination of the pathologic changes occurring in the spinal cord after phenol block helped resolve the problem of which nerve fibers are destroyed, and whether this occurred on any preferential or selective basis.

Berry and Olszewski[74] found that all sizes of fibers were affected, that the damaged zone was well demarcated. They could demonstrate no intermediate zone in which the small fibers were affected selectively. The lesions were more severe in the dorsal than in the ventral roots, and predominated on the dependent side during phenol treatment where the phenol was thought to have pooled. In the spinal cord there was ascending degeneration of the corresponding fasciculus gracilis in one case, and in another marked demyelination in the treated dorsal roots that was less severe in the corresponding ventral roots. There were minimal changes in the opposite dorsal and ventral roots at the same level. The only differential feature was that the outer part of the roots was severely damaged but the central core was spared. These results did not support the theory that phenol acted only on small nerve fibers.

Using a cat model, Stewart and Lourie[75] also concluded that subarachnoid phenol (in pantopaque) does not selectively destroy the smaller fibers in the roots or cord. They found that the overall degree of destruction was related to the concentration of phenol–pantopaque used. Similar results were obtained by Smith[76] in postmortem studies of 19 patients who had undergone intrathecal injections of phenol solutions for relief of neoplastic pain. She determined that ". . . the phenol caused degeneration of both large and small fibers and acted on the fibers in the nerve roots and not on the ganglia or spinal cord. Posterior root degeneration was found in all the cases. . . . No excessive pathological reactions to the injections were found, with the exception of one patient receiving silver nitrate in phenol in glycerin where meningitis and death resulted."

Nathan and Sears[79] examined the susceptibility of nerve fibers to analgesics, and stated in their conclusions that it is usually believed that analgesics block nerve fibers according to their size, the smaller before the large. This is so, but only when one considers together fibers having the same mode of impulse conduction. One cannot compare A, B, and C fibers as though they form a continuous series; they conduct the nerve impulse in different fashions. This paper gave an explanation as to why clinically there appeared to be a differential block of nerve fibers. Differential block does occur when anesthetic solutions are applied to nerve fibers in low concentrations, or in experiments when nerve fibers are bathed in solutions with a low sodium concentration. Differential block also occurs when low concentrations of phenol act as a local anesthetic. In more concentrated solutions, however, it and the other local anesthetics produce blockade of all types of fibers. In the concentrations used clinically to manage cancer pain, intrathecal phenol destroys all nerve fibers with which it comes into contact in an indiscriminate fashion. The concentration tends to fall as the phenol penetrates more deeply, and as a result, some nerve fibers survive, but no particular size is selected preferentially. If the phenol solution does not completely surround the nerve root but is only in contact with a segment of the root, then this portion is affected, and all or some of its constituent fibers are destroyed. This explains pathologic and electromyographic findings. In their later work, Nathan and Sears concluded that ". . . the explanation of therapeutic success must be a quantitative not a qualitative one; the pain is stopped not by destroying certain fibers preferentially, but by destroying an adequate number of fibers. . ."[69]

CHOICE OF NEUROLYTIC DRUG AND METHOD OF APPLICATION

In the course of this book, different authorities advocate alternate methods of solving a particular chronic pain problem using neurolytic methods. Each will have his or her own ideas on drug selection and procedure. This author does not wish to make statements that may conflict. In this context, only suggestions are indicated, since, over time, all specialists develop their own preferences and methods that are safe in their hands. What can be offered is mostly common sense, developed partly by experience and partly by fear. Make no mistake about it: the use of neurolytic drugs

is dangerous, and more medico-legal confrontations are due to problems in this field of analgesia than in the rest of anesthesia. Charlton[46] wrote a very apt and cogent summary of important general considerations, including:

1. Swerdlow's paper[80] on medico-legal aspects is necessary reading for those carrying out neurolytic blocks.
2. Careful selection of patients, preparation of equipment, immaculate technique, and observation before and after the block are necessary.
3. A careful examination pre- and post-block with sound record-keeping is important. A claimed complication may have pre-existed or only been aggravated, not caused.
4. Once injected the effects do not wear off. Use small volumes and the lowest concentration of neurolytic agent that will be effective.
5. A block can always be repeated; better to give too little than too much.
6. Know the side effects of the given technique to enable a proper clinical decision.

To which I add three of my own:

7. Make sure the patient and the relatives know the possibilities for complications or failure.
8. Use radiologic guidance when appropriate.
9. Use intrathecal neurolytics only on inoperable cancer patients.

CHOICE OF NEUROLYTIC

Many important details need to be observed, including positioning of the patient, checking the correct side to be blocked, and ensuring that the correct neurolytic in its correct strength is available. These and many other conditions need to be met before a neurolytic block is performed, but are discussed in separate chapters. Some indication will be given on which neurolytic substances are best for particular blocks, as well as some details of particular dangers this author has encountered.

There are only two neurolytics that are in

common use, alcohol and phenol. Others used occasionally include ammonium chloride, chlorocresol, and cryotherapy. Their attributes already have been discussed.

Alcohol

This drug is used in high concentrations and often in large volumes. That it may damage blood vessels should be borne in mind. Some of its clinical uses include the following.

The Trigeminal Nerve and Its Branches. There are occasions in cancer affecting the head when this nerve or its branches needs to be blocked (see Chapters 1 and 21). In these cases, alcohol is the drug of choice, even though in contemporary practice it is rarely used for trigeminal neuralgia, except in minimal quantities.[70] The author has encountered one problem after repeated infraorbital block that deserves mention. An infraorbital nerve block with alcohol was planned for a patient with multiple sclerosis and well localized trigeminal neuralgia. The same procedure had been performed uneventfully many times over the previous 7 years. On this occasion, despite ease of performance and successful analgesia, a portion of skin sloughed in the nasal fold, presumably due to damage of the vasculature from repeated alcohol injections. When one searches carefully, the literature mentions this possibility.[81] There were no medico-legal repercussions in this case.

Celiac Plexus Block. Another problem arose in the course of repeated celiac plexus block for chronic pancreatitis, but could occur in cancer pain management. One of the potential dangers of the standard technique for celiac block is the vulnerability of the artery of Adamkiewitz, which supplies a major portion of the mid- to low thoracic spinal cord. Usually this artery arises from the midthoracic aorta and enters the spinal cord somewhat more distally, but it can have a tortuous path, in which case it is vulnerable in the lumbar region. If this artery is obliterated, paraplegia results, and did in the case in question. An image intensifier and contrast medium were used, and demonstrated that no direct injec-

tion into the subarachnoid space occurred, so presumably this result was due to repeated damage to the artery. The value of the image intensifier here is obvious, as in its absence, an accidental subarachnoid injection could have been implicated. This case resulted in litigation.

Splanchnic Block. This alternative to celiac plexus is said to have advantages in selected cases.[82] One must always remember, however, that the techniques described here and in other references do not, in actual practice, always proceed so smoothly, as is illustrated here. A patient with severe abdominal pain from metastatic cancer had undergone several celiac plexus blocks without persistent relief from pain. It was elected to perform bilateral splanchnic blocks with alcohol. An image intensifier and separate preparations of water-soluble contrast medium and alcohol were used. Injection was performed on one side without problems. On the contralateral side, contrast was observed spreading upward during a check for needle position. Contrast continued to move upward despite altering the needle position, and was observed to continue to track along the aorta, eventually reaching the arch. The procedure on this side was abandoned.

Intrathecal. There are a number of potential problems when blocking nerve roots intrathecally:

1. In the lumbar region, the patient should be positioned so that the solution does not flow over the second sacral nerve root, which contains most of the fibers governing bladder function. Similarly, in the cervical region, the outflow to the phrenic nerve (C 3–5) should be avoided.
2. There is one problem that is particularly likely to occur in patients with superior sulcus lung tumors. These tumors often extend directly into the epidural and/or subarachnoid space. The author has provided treatment for two such patients that resulted in unwanted neurologic injury. One patient was affected at the upper thoracic level, and the second at the midthoracic level. When puncture was

made in the first patient at the second thoracic interspace, CSF was obtained, and 1.0 ml of phenol in glycerin was injected in divided doses. A Brown–Séquard syndrome followed very rapidly. At postmortem, a double ring of tumor tissue was found within the subarachnoid space. The spinal puncture had been made between them, CSF was obtained, but the injected phenol in glycerin, being viscid, could not escape, and the resulting pressure produced paraparesis. Since then, we have instituted CSF pressure measurements to verify free flow of CSF from above and below the puncture site. If flow is not completely free in both directions, the procedure is delayed for further investigation. In the second patient, free flow was observed in one direction but not completely in the other, but it was thought safe to use 1.0 ml of alcohol, because of its fluidity. Paraparesis developed that was in the process of clearing when the patient died (pain free) from her malignancy. Thus, flow should be completely free in both directions before intrathecal injection.

3. Access for spinal puncture at the midthoracic region may be difficult due to the marked imbrication of the dorsal spines in this region (see Chapter 23). A paramedian approach may be successful, or a lower or higher thoracic puncture can be made, and, after positioning the patient carefully, alcohol can be flowed up or down, respectively, to the required site.

Phenol

Phenol can be used in most of the blocks already mentioned.

The Trigeminal Nerve and Its Branches. Whereas phenol in glycerin has been used to control the pain of trigeminal neuralgia,[42] it often does not produce sufficiently dense anesthesia when cranial nerves need to be destroyed, particularly if they are sheltered by tumor tissue. This procedure is best undertaken with absolute alcohol. The foramen ovale can be approached almost as if with direct vision using an image intensifier as an adjunct.[83]

Celiac Plexus Block. Phenol can be used to treat abdominal pain of neoplastic origin without the degree of pain associated with the corresponding injection of 50% alcohol. There is no difference in the results, as these depend on whether the loose tissue around the aorta where the plexus lies is infiltrated with tumor. Fluoroscopy or computed tomography scanning may be used[82] to verify that the needles are positioned correctly.

Splanchnic Block. Phenol can be used here, but there is no great advantage over using alcohol. If alcohol spreads to the intercostal nerves, the incidence of neuritis will be higher, but one of the advantages of this approach is that the injected solutions are separated from the intercostal nerves.

Intrathecal. Phenol in glycerin is this author's choice for carrying out neurolysis in the subarachnoid space. Being viscid, it is relatively slow-moving and does not spread as quickly as alcohol. The solution also releases its phenol slowly over a short but valuable time (about 10 minutes), and it is possible to alter the patient's position during the first 5 minutes of the procedure before effects are permanent. The great disadvantage of this technique is that the patient must be positioned with the painful side down. Patients may find it difficult to maintain this position during the procedure, and in fact usually alter it by "creeping" into a more comfortable position. The author performs most intrathecal phenol blocks with the patient anesthetized. This is simple to do: more than one spinal needle is inserted and the dose spread over these to provide better coverage. The level can be checked by placing a small bolus of 0.1 ml of contrast medium through the uppermost and the lowermost needles, using the image intensifier to observe the flow pattern, and altering the table tilt to make corrections if they are necessary.

When a spinal needle is inserted for an injection of hyperbaric phenol with the patient lying on his or her side, it should be placed either 1) at the center of the theca, posteriorly, or 2) below this level (*ie*, nearer the lowest nerve root). In either case, the injected phenol runs along the inside of the dura and reaches the dependent nerve root, or is injected directly on to it. If the spinal needle enters the dura near the uppermost nerve root, it will be deeper than in 1), and injected phenol may drip onto the spinal cord, or, in the lower lumbar region, onto the cauda equina. This may be the cause of unexpected complications post-block, as untargeted nerve roots may be affected.

Ammonium Sulfate

There are conflicting reports on this drug. It is said to cause less neuritis when used subcostally, and this might be an appropriate situation for its use.

Cryoprobe

Although this is an excellent method for producing reversible, semipermanent neural blockade in patients with nonmalignant pain, there are few occasions for its use in cancer pain. Its disadvantages in this setting relate to its impermanence and the need to place the freezing tip onto the nerve with the utmost accuracy. Even when using its built-in nerve stimulator, this is difficult. Complications are rare, and the affected nerves appear to regenerate without complications. It is useful when repeated small and superficial nerve blocks are indicated.

CONCLUSION

There is only one final remark that needs to be made. Neurolytic blocks are only as safe as the person performing them, but if proper care is taken, they are a boon and provide unique advantages to the cancer patient with pain that is otherwise intractable.

REFERENCES

1. Luton A: Archives general de medecin. 1863.
2. Hauck L: The treatment of neuralgias with injections of alcohol. St Louis Med Rev 1906;54:505.
3. Hitchcock E: Hypothermic subarachnoid irrigation for intractable pain. Lancet 1967;1:1133
4. Judovich BD: Relief of pain. Med J Rec 1935;141:583.
5. Bates W, Judovich BD: Intractable pain. Anesthesiology 1942;3:663.
6. Stewart WB, Judovich BD, Hughes J et al: Ammonium chloride in the relief of pain. Am J Physiol 1940;129:474.
7. Maher RM: Neurone selection in relief of pain: Further experiences with intrathecal injections. Lancet 1957;1:16.
8. Neuber G: Ueber osmiumsaure-injectionen bei periphare neuralgien. Med Chir Central Blat 1884;19:230.
9. Jacoby WJ: The use of osmic acid in peripheral neuralgias. New York Medical Journal 1885;42:123.
10. Eulenberg: Die osmiumsaure-behandlung bei peripharen neuralgien. Berliner Klinische Wochenschrift 1884:99.
11. Merces J: Osmic acid in sciatica. Lancet 1885:58.
12. Fraenkel E: Ueber parenchymatose ueberosmiumsaure-injectionen. Berliner Klinische Wochenschrift 1884:234.
13. Putnam TJ, Hampton AO: The technique of injection into the gasserian ganglion under roentgenographic control. Archives of Neurology and Psychiatry 1936;35:92.
14. Maher RM: Relief of pain in incurable cancer. Lancet 1955;i:18.
15. Pitres A, Vaillard: Des nevrites provoquees par le contact de L'alcool pur oe dilue avec les nerfs vivants. Compte Rendu Soc Biol 1888;5:550.
16. Pitres JA, Verger TPH: Memorrio et bulletin de medecine et chirurgie de Bordeaux. 1902:91.
17. Gallagher HA, Yonezawa T, Hay RC et al: Subarachnoid alcohol block: 2. Histologic changes in the central nervous system. Am J Pathol 1961;38:679.
18. Wood KM: The use of phenol as a neurolytic agent: A review. Pain 1978;5:205.
19. Hakansson S: Retrogasserian glycerol injection as a treatment of tic douloureax. Adv Pain Res Ther 1983;5:927.
20. Maher RM: Intrathecal chlorocresol in the treatment of pain in cancer. Lancet 1963;i:965.
21. Swerdlow M: An assessment of intrathecal chlorocresol. In Proceedings of the 4th European Congress on Anaesthesiology, p 34. Amsterdam, Elsevier, 1974.
22. Pubols LM, Foglesong ME: Acute and chronic effects of the neurolytic agent ricin on dorsal root ganglia, spinal cord, and nerves. J Comp Neurol 1988;275:271.
23. Swerdlow M: The history of neurolytic block. In Racz GB (ed): Techniques of Neurolysis, p 1. Boston, Kluwer Academic, 1989.
24. Cushing H: The role of deep alcohol injections in the treatments of trigeminal neuralgia. JAMA 1920;75:441.

25. Patrick HJ: The treatment of trifacial neuralgia by means of deep injections of alcohol. JAMA 1907; 49:1567.

26. Harris W: The alcohol injection treatment for neuralgia and spasm. Lancet 1909:1311.

27. Hartel F: Die behandlung der trigeminusneuralgia mit intracraniellen alcoholeinspritzungen. Deutsch Z Chir 1914;126:429.

28. Brissaud, Sicard, Tanon: Dangers des injections d'alcool dans la nerf sciatique au cours des neuralgies sciatiques. Rev Neurol 1907;15:633.

29. Swetlow GI, Weingarten B: Alcohol nerve block for pain in malignant disease. Med J Rec 1926;123:728.

30. Dogliotti AM: Nouvelle methode therapeutique pours les algies peripheriques: Injection d'alcool dans l'espace arachnoidien. Rev Neurol 1931;11:485.

31. Braun H: Local Anesthesia, its Scientific Basis and Practical Use. London, Kimpton, 1914.

32. Yeomans FC, Gorsch RV, Mathesheimer JL: Bebacol in the treatment of pruritus ani: Preliminary report. Med J and Rec 1928;127:19.

33. Steinberg N: Recent advances in the treatment of rectal diseases by injection methods in ambulatory patients: Pruritis ani. N Engl J Med 1936;215:1019.

34. Duncan D, Jarvis WH: A comparison of the actions on nerve fibers of certain anesthetic mixtures and substances in oil. Anesthesiology 1943;4:465.

35. Mandl F: Paravertebral Block. New York, Grune and Stratton, 1947.

36. Boyd AM, Ratcliffe AH, Jepson RP: Intermittent claudication: A clinical study. J Bone Joint Surg 1949; 31B:325.

37. Maher RM, Mehta M: Spinal (intrathecal) and extradural analgesia. In: Lipton S (ed): Persistent Pain, vol 1, p 61. London, New York, Grune and Stratton, 1977.

38. Kelley RE, Gautier-Smith PC: Intrathecal phenol in the treatment of reflex spasms and spasticity. Lancet 1959;ii:1102.

39. Nathan PW: Intrathecal phenol to relieve spasticity in paraplegia. Lancet 1959;ii:1099.

40. Szalados J, Patt R: Management of a patient with displaced orthopedic hardware. Journal of Pain and Symptom Management 1991 (in press).

41. Adriani J: In Labat G (ed): Regional Anesthesia, 2nd ed. Philadelphia, WB Saunders, 1967.

42. Jefferson A: Trigeminal root and ganglion injections using phenol in glycerin for the relief of trigeminal neuralgia. J Neurol Neurosurg Psychiatry 1963;26:345.

43. Hakanson S: Trigeminal neuralgia treated by the injection of glycerol into the trigeminal cistern. Neurosurgery 1981;9:638.

44. Ischia S, Luzzani A, Polati E: Retrogasserian glycerol

45. Miller RD, Johnston RR, Hosobuchi Y: Treatment of intercostal neuralgia with 10% ammonium sulfate. J Thorac Surg 1975;69:476.

46. Charlton JE: Current views on the use of nerve blocking in chronic pain. In Swerdlow M (ed): Therapy of Pain, 2nd ed, p 133. Lancaster, MTP Press, 1986.

47. Judovich BD, Bates W, Bishop K: Intraspinal ammonium salts for the intractable pain of malignancy. Anesthesiology 1944;5:341.

48. Guttman SA, Pardee I: Spinal cord level syndrome following intrathecal ammonium sulfate and procaine hydrochloride: A case report with autopsy findings. Anesthesiology 1944;5:347.

49. Davies JI, Stewart PB, Fink HP: Prolonged sensory block using ammonium salts. Anesthesiology 1967;28:244.

50. Wood KM: Peripheral nerve and root chemical lesions. In Wall PD, Melzack R (eds): Textbook of Pain, 2nd ed, p 768. Edinburgh, Churchill Livingstone, 1989.

51. Hitchcock E: Subarachnoid saline infusion. In Morley TP (ed): Current Controversies in Neurosurgery, p 515. Philadelphia, WB Saunders, 1976.

52. Hitchcock E: Hypothermic subarachnoid irrigation for intractable pain. Lancet 1967;i:1133.

53. Lucas JT, Ducker TB, Perot PL: Adverse reactions to intrathecal saline for control of pain. J Neurosurg 1975;42:55.

54. Thompson GE: Pulmonary edema complicating intrathecal hypertonic saline injection for intractable pain. Anesthesiology 1971;35:425.

55. Lloyd JW: Treatment of intractable pain with cerebrospinal fluid barbotage. In Morley TP (ed): Current Controversies in Neurosurgery, p 520. Philadelphia, WB Saunders, 1976.

56. King JS, Jewett DL, Sundberg HR: Differential blockade of cat dorsal root C fibers by various chloride solutions. J Neurosurg 1972;36:569.

57. Lloyd JW, Barnard JDW, Glynn CJ: Cryoanalgesia: A new approach to pain relief. Lancet 1976;ii:932.

58. Harvey SC: Antiseptics and disinfectants; fungicides; ectoparasiticides. In: Goodman LS, Gilman A (eds): The Pharmacological Basis of Therapeutics, 5th ed, p 987. New York, Macmillan, 1975.

59. Lubenow TR, Ivankovicj AD: Serum alcohol, CPK and amylase levels following celiac plexus block with alcohol. Reg Anaesth 1988;13 (Suppl):S64

60. Jain S, Hirsh R, Shah N et al: Blood ethanol levels following celiac plexus block with 50% ethanol. Anesth Analg 1989;68 (Suppl):S135.

61. Armstrong CM, Binstock L: The effects of several

alcohols on the properties of the squid giant axon. J Gen Physiol 1964;48:265.

62. Posternack J, Arnold E: Action de l'anelectrotonus et d'une solution hypersodique sur la conduction dans un nerf narcotise. J Physiol Paris 1954;46:502.

63. Umeda S, Arai T: Disulfiram-like reaction to moxalactam after celiac plexus alcohol block. Anesth Analg 1985;64:377.

64. Lyness WH: Pharmacology of neurolytic agents. In: Racz GB (ed): Techniques of Neurolysis, p 13. Boston, Kluwer Academic, 1989.

65. Hug CC: Characteristics and theories related to acute and chronic tolerance development. In Mule SJ, Brill H (eds): Chemical and Biological Aspects of Drug Dependence, p 307. Cleveland, CRC Press, 1972.

66. Ochoa JL, Torebjork E, Marchettini P et al: Mechanisms of neuropathic pain: Cumulative observations, new experiments, and further speculation. In Fields HL, Dubner R, Cervero F (eds): Advances in Pain Research and Therapy, vol 9, p 431. New York, Raven Press, 1985.

67. Byrne J: The mechanism of referred pain, hyperalgesia (causalgia) and of alcoholic injections for the relief of neuralgia. J Nerv Ment Dis 1921;53;6;433.

68. Gerberschagen HU: Neurolysis: Subarachnoid neurolytic blockade. Acta Anaesthesiol Belg 1981;1:45.

69. Nathan PW, Sears TA, Smith MC: Effects of phenol solutions on nerve roots of cat: Electrophysiological and histological study. J Neurol Sci 1965;2:7.

70. Greitz T, Lindblom U: Selective nerve root blocking with phenol under myelographic control. Invest Radiol 1966;1:257.

71. Racz BR, Heavner J, Haynsworth R: Repeat epidural phenol injections in chronic pain and spasticity. In Racz GB (ed): Techniques of Neurolysis, p 193. Boston, Kluwer Academic, 1989.

72. Nour-Eldin F: Preliminary report: Uptake of phenol by vascular and brain tissue. Microvasc Res 1970; 2:224.

73. Iggo A, Walsh EG: Selective block of small fibers in the spinal roots by phenol. Brain 1960;83:701.

74. Berry K, Olszewski J: Pathology of intrathecal phenol in man. Neurology 1963;13:152.

75. Stewart AW, Lourie H: An experimental evaluation of the effects of subarachnoid injection of phenol-pantopaque in cats: A histological study. J Neurosurg 1963;20:64.

76. Smith MC: Histological findings following intrathecal injections of phenol solutions for relief of pain. Br J Anaesth 1964;36:387.

77. Fusfeld RD: Electromyographic findings after phenol block. Arch Phys Med Rehabil 1968;49:217.

78. Brattstrom M, Moritz U, Svantesson G: Electromyographic studies of peripheral nerve block with phenol. Scand J Rehabil Med 1970;2:17.

79. Nathan PW, Sears TA: The susceptibility of nerve fibers to analgesics. Anaesthesia 1963;18;467.

80. Swerdlow M: Medicolegal aspects of complications following pain relieving blocks. Pain 1982;13:321.

81. Swerdlow M: Complications of neurolytic blockade. In Cousins M, Bridenbaugh PO (eds): Neural Blockade, p 549. Philadelphia, JB Lippincott, 1980.

82. Moore DC, Bush WH, Burnett LL: Celiac plexus block: A roentgenographic, anatomic study of technique and spread of solution in patients and corpses. Anesth Analg 1981;60:369.

83. Delfino U: An advance in trigeminal therapy. In Lipton S, Miles J (eds): Persistent Pain, vol 4, p 145. London, New York, Grune and Stratton, 1983.

Chapter 21

Peripheral Neurolysis and the Management of Cancer Pain

Richard B. Patt

INTRODUCTION

Although most cases of cancer pain can be controlled adequately by pharmacologic means (see Chapters 6–12), chemical neurolysis still has an established role in the management of intractable pain.[1,2] Most reports presenting data on large series of patients focus on neurolysis performed at the level of the neuraxis or sympathetic chain (see Chapters 22 and 23). Peripheral neurolysis is described primarily in isolated case reports and a few small series. Despite suggestions by some authorities that peripheral neurolysis has little or no clinical value,[3,4] when applied selectively for patients with oncologic pain, these procedures have a definite and important, though circumscribed, therapeutic role. Bonica and others subscribe to this point of view, as well.[2,5,6] Unfortunately, no controlled clinical trials have been reported, and, as noted, published series are few and often lacking in detail. Nevertheless, taken together, general references, case reports, and clinical series suggest an important role in cancer pain management. These published reports, together with our personal experience, will be described here.

LOCAL ANESTHETIC VERSUS NEUROLYTIC BLOCKADE

Local anesthetic blockade of the peripheral nerves (see Chapter 19) is well described in various texts,[2,5,7,8] and since the actual techniques of needle placement usually do not vary for local anesthetic versus neurolytic block, with a few exceptions they are not discussed in detail here. The important differences between local anesthetic and lytic blocks of the peripheral nerves lie in their 1) respective indications, 2) potential complications, 3) relative necessity for careful preliminary diagnostic and prognostic blocks, and 4) relative need for precise localization, often necessitating radiologic guidance for the latter.[9]

Since pain due to cancer is most often (but not always) constant and unremitting, the relief afforded by the injection of local anesthetics and even steroids is, in most cases, inadequate as a long-term therapeutic measure. The main exception, and contraindication to neurolysis of any type, is cancer pain that is expected to improve as a consequence of treatment of the underlying malignancy, in which case serial or continuous injections of local anesthetic and/or steroid may be indicated as therapeutic measures (see Chapter 19). Other conditions in which local anesthetic injections have a potential therapeutic role in the cancer patient include "pain emergencies," sympathetically maintained pain (see Chapters 1 and 22), muscle spasm (see Chapter 1), and nonmalignant causes of pain in the cancer patient (see Chapter 3).

Despite a limited therapeutic role in patients with cancer pain, local anesthetic injections do play a pivotal role as preliminary measures to determine the probable efficacy, safety, and acceptability of neurolytic blocks, especially when performed in the periphery (see Chapter 19). As diagnostic blocks, they are used as an aid to determine the origin of the pain syndrome and the neural pathways involved in its transmission. As prognostic blocks, local anesthetic injections assist in predicting patient response to more prolonged blockade (see Chapter 19). Although, at least in the short term, the results of these procedures often have good predictive value of therapeutic response and patient acceptance, their reliability is still incomplete.

GENERAL CONSIDERATIONS

As with other components of the nervous system, prolonged interruption of function in the

Table 21–1.
Indications for Peripheral Neurolysis

Patient Characteristics
- Limited life expectancy (up to about 12 months)
- Tolerance of effects achieved with prognostic block
- Valid informed consent

Pain Characteristics
- Pain is severe
- Pain is expected to persist
- Pain cannot be modified by less invasive measures
- Pain is well localized
- Pain is of somatic origin
- Pain is relieved with prognostic local anesthetic block
- Absence of undesirable deficits after local anesthetic block

periphery necessarily involves the creation of a lesion by chemical, thermal, cryogenic, or surgical means. As with interruption at other levels of the nervous system, most experience is with the percutaneous injection of alcohol or phenol (see Chapters 20 and 22–24).

Objections to the more liberal use of neurolytics in the periphery include concerns about 1) impermanence, 2) neuritis and deafferentation pain, 3) sensory overlap, 4) potential for motor deficit when mixed nerves are injected, and 5) unintentional damage to nontargeted tissue. The impact of each of these potential problems can be minimized by careful patient selection and attention to technique.

PATIENT SELECTION

The important features of patient selection are listed in Table 21–1, and include 1) a limited life expectancy; 2) pain that is severe, expected to persist, and cannot be modified by less invasive measures; and 3) pain that is amenable to peripheral neurolysis (localized, somatic pain).

The significance of impermanence of effect, a feature common to most neuroablative procedures,[10,11] is minimized by limiting the selection of patients to those in whom life expectancy is unlikely to exceed the duration of pain relief, and by recognizing that in the event that effects are more short-lived than anticipated, the procedure can be repeated at the same site or more proximally.

Similarly, problems related to postinjection dysesthesia are minimized by screening for patients who are likely to succumb to their primary disease before the development of these sequelae, and in whom the original pain is so severe that, by comparison, dysesthesias are unlikely to be troublesome.

The provision of neurolytic blockade in patients with chronic nonmalignant pain is controversial. Some authorities contend that, with proper informed consent, this is an acceptable practice in carefully selected patients with pain that is otherwise intractable.

The potential for overlap of sensory fields, when taken into account during the stage of diagnostic/prognostic local anesthetic blockade, is not a barrier to the success of the subsequent therapeutic nerve block. The selection of the definitive neurolytic procedure simply is guided by the results of the prognostic (local anesthetic) block.

Similarly, the potential for motor weakness and disturbances in autonomic function can be assessed in advance with local anesthetic blockade. Blockade of a purely sensory peripheral nerve will not result in motor deficit. Thorough assessment identifies patients in whom a degree of motor weakness will be well tolerated—for example, patients already confined to bed, patients with preexisting motor deficit, and those with pain sufficiently severe to render the involved limb already useless.

Finally, the potential for damage to nontargeted tissue is of concern with any destructive procedure, but in general is less likely to occur for peripheral blocks than when central or deep sympathetic blocks are undertaken, particularly when localization is facilitated by electrical stimulation, radiographic guidance, and/or test doses of local anesthetic.

TECHNICAL ASPECTS

A careful review and thorough knowledge of the pertinent anatomy form the basis for the other important technical aspects of peripheral neurolytic blockade. These include careful selection of the procedure, with consideration of blocking neighboring nerves, attention to the position of the patient, proper selection of drug and drug dosage, and verification of needle placement by aspiration, test doses with local anesthetic, electrical stimulation,[12-14] and/or the judicious use of radiologic guidance.[9]

The reasons for the limited duration of analgesia that is often observed are uncertain, but it has been postulated to be related to the creation of an incomplete lesion of the targeted nerve.[15] Whereas local anesthetic injected in the general vicinity of a nerve trunk may diffuse through neighboring soft tissue and still result in effective neural blockade, neurolytic drugs spread worse in biologic tissue than do local anesthetics,[16] and as a result must be deposited directly on to the nerve for the best effect. To avoid complications, the volume and the concentration of the injected neurolytic must be carefully limited. Controlled comparisons between different concentrations and volumes of neurolytic agents have not been carried out, and it also may be that incomplete lesions and consequent impermanence are influenced by these factors as well. Most early investigators have used either absolute alcohol or 5%–7% phenol. In an effort to maximize the likelihood of a good result, our group and others usually use either absolute alcohol or higher than usual concentrations of phenol (10%–12%), while still subscribing to traditional volume limits.[17-21] A maximum of 6.7% phenol can be dissolved in water at room temperature, but the addition of small amounts of glycerin increases its solubility (see Chapter 20). Other authorities have expressed concern that the use of higher concentrations of phenol might predispose to vascular injury.[22] It is sufficiently common for the initial results of a neurolytic block to be transient; and it is our policy to forewarn patients to expect that the procedure will need repetition at least once. In most clinical series a large proportion, usually more than half the patients, receive more than one block.

It has also been suggested that incomplete lesions may lead to the development of post-treatment neuritis,[15,16] further emphasizing the need for careful localization, and careful selection of a drug, dosage, and volume that will maximize the lesion without causing unwanted deficit or injury to neighboring tissue. An association between the creation of incomplete or inaccurate lesions and subsequent neuritis is supported indirectly by the work of Roviaro and colleagues,[23] who injected three neighboring intercostal nerves with 6% phenol in glycerin (1 ml per segment) under direct vision at thoracotomy. Of 32 patients treated, neither neuritis nor deafferentation pain were reported at 1-year follow-up, a finding that is in marked contrast to results following percutaneous neurolytic intercostal blocks.[7]

Accurate localization and subsequent immobilization of the needle is critical to success. Most nerve blocks are performed percutaneously, without the benefit afforded by direct vision, and as such, information about needle placement is inferred from indirect evidence gathered from multiple sources. A thorough knowledge of the pertinent regional anatomy supplemented by a preprocedural review help to make the best use of surface, vascular, and deep bony landmarks. Paresthesia is usually a sensitive guide to the proximity of the investigating needle to the targeted nerve, but is subject to differences in technique and interpretation. If paresthesia is to be relied on, the patient must be coached in advance, and maintained in a cooperative, lucid state; the technique must be slow and deliberate, with careful maintenance of verbal contact throughout. Localization can be facilitated further by electrical stimulation and radiographic guidance, with observation of the spread of contrast medium. These adjuncts are particularly useful when anatomy has been altered by tumor invasion, surgery, and radiotherapy. Unfortunately, it is often difficult to elicit the aid of a qualified radiologist (see Fig. 21–1A,B), and a comprehensive text on roentgenographic aids to needle placement is not yet available. Although the above techniques are useful, a preneurolytic test dose of local anesthetic should be regarded as essential both to exclude aberrant placement to guard against possible injury, and as a further confirmation of correct placement. Clearing

the injecting needle with air or saline after the administration of the neurolytic agent is a further measure that may help avoid skin slough and tissue injury from drug spilled on tissue during withdrawal of the needle.

SELECTION OF AGENT

Alcohol and phenol are the only agents commonly used for producing chemical neurolysis in contemporary practice, although ammonium sulfate and chlorocresol occasionally are advocated. These agents, along with the histopathologic sequelae of their use, are discussed in detail in Chapters 20 and 23. Compared to sympathetic and central sites,[16] peripheral neurolysis is unique in that neuritis and dysesthesias follow treatment in a variable proportion of cases, quoted as ranging between 2%–28%.[16,24] The incidence of neuritis after peripheral neurolysis with alcohol is widely held to be higher than when phenol is used,[2,25] although this finding has not been documented in controlled studies.

The perineural injection of alcohol is followed immediately by severe burning pain along the targeted nerve's distribution, which lasts only about a minute before giving way to a warm, numb sensation. Pain on injection may be blunted, indeed often eliminated, by the prior injection of a local anesthetic. Some authors recommend against the injection of a local anesthetic and neurolytic drug in succession because of theoretical concerns about dilution of the latter, and because pain on injection serves to help confirm needle placement.[7] The policy we and others[26] have adopted is always to precede the injection of any neurolytic drug with an injection of local anesthetic, both to optimize comfort and primarily as a "test dose" to exclude aberrant needle placement and the likelihood of irreversible side effects. This practice has been advocated since as far back as 1920 ("The injection of alcohol without the part being previously anesthetized by a local anesthetic, should not be practiced, for the patient's feelings should always be considered."[26]), and allowing a brief interval to pass between injections is likely to pre-

> **A** FLUOROSCOPY:
>
> Fluoroscopy was performed for nerve root block. Three films were taken during the procedure.
>
> **B** CELIAC NERVE PLEXUS LOCALIZATION, CT OF ABDOMEN
>
> 22 gauge needles were placed into the left para-aortic and right aorto-intercaval region under CT guidance by Dr. Patt of Anesthesiology. These were placed approximately at the level of the celiac access takeoff from the abdominal aorta. This procedure was done with the patient in the prone position from paravertebral approaches bilaterally. Approximately 20% contrast was used to verify position of these needles. The patient subsequently had alcohol injected through these needle placements by Dr. Patt. The needles were then withdrawn. The patient tolerated the procedure well without complication. No definite evidence of pneumothorax was demonstrated by CT. The patient received 100 cc. of Omnipaque 300 intravenously prior to placement of the 22 gauge spinal needles.

Figure 21–1. Examples of reports rendered when radiologic studies are used as adjuncts to nerve blocks. Reports exemplified by **A** are all too common. The report in **B** represents a more appropriate example.

vent dilution, if indeed it is an issue at all. Some burning or pain is still likely, but is well tolerated when patients are forewarned. Extreme care must be taken to brace the needle to avoid movement when syringes are changed. The injection of phenol also may be accompanied by discomfort, but is more often associated with a sensation of warmth and numbness.

Alcohol (see Chapters 20 and 23) is commercially available in 1-ml and 5-ml ampules as a colorless solution that can be injected readily through small-bore needles, and that is hypobaric with respect to cerebrospinal fluid (CSF), although specific gravity is not of concern in the periphery because injection takes place into a nonfluid medium. In the periphery, alcohol generally is used undiluted (100% or absolute alcohol). If left exposed to the atmosphere, highly concentrated alcohol will be diluted by absorbed moisture. Dener-

vation and pain relief sometimes accrue over a few days after injection.

Injectable phenol requires preparation by a pharmacist (see Appendix C). Various concentrations of phenol, ranging from 3%–15%, prepared with saline, water, glycerin, and different radiologic dyes have been advocated. Phenol is relatively insoluble in water, and at room temperature, concentrations in excess of 6.7% cannot be obtained without the addition of glycerin. Phenol mixed in glycerin is hyperbaric with respect to CSF, but is so viscid that even when warmed, injection is difficult through needles smaller in caliber than 20 gauge. Shelf life is said to exceed 1 year when preparations are refrigerated and not exposed to light. A biphasic action has been observed clinically, characterized by an initial local anesthetic effect producing subjective warmth and numbness that gives way to chronic denervation. It is our impression that the hypalgesia that follows phenol injection generally is not as dense as that after alcohol. Quality and extent of analgesia may fade slightly within the first 24 hours of administration.

Although some authors have suggested that alcohol and phenol essentially are interchangeable, due to the contention that neuritis is more likely to follow injections of alcohol, phenol generally is preferred for peripheral injections. Our policy is to use phenol when a peripheral injection is indicated in patients with a moderate or indeterminate life expectancy, thus theoretically minimizing the chance of neuritis. Our clinical impression is that alcohol produces more intense nerve destruction and blockade than phenol, and for this reason we continue to use alcohol for peripheral nerve blocks in patients with predictably short life expectancies. Further, we (and others[27]) use alcohol for injections of the cranial nerves, independent of life expectancy. Bonica noted an absence of neuritis after cranial nerve and subarachnoid injections in 157 and 110 patients, respectively,[16] an observation consistent with our experience.

Although less commonly applied, other alternatives for interrupting nerve transmission warrant discussion. Surgical interruption of peripheral nerves (see Chapter 26) is rarely performed, in part because referral patterns tend to direct patients to anesthesiologists who are facile with percutaneous techniques, and also because surgery is generally more invasive. Glycerol, noted only serendipitously to have neurolytic properties (see Chapters 20 and 26), is used to treat idiopathic trigeminal neuralgia,[28] and is being investigated for efficacy in peripheral blocks, but its use is complicated by its high viscosity. Butyl-amino-benzoate (butamben) is a substance that recently has been reported to have neurolytic characteristics, and is expected to be a subject of further research.[29–32] Cryoanalgesia has its proponents,[33] but results have been disappointing, despite theoretical advantages of producing reversible injury. Results are often transient, probes are bulky, and the technique requires exquisitely precise placement, often necessitating the creation of lesions under direct vision. Cryoanalgesia probably

should be reserved for patients with longer life expectancies, in whom it is essential to minimize the likelihood of neuritis. In contrast, thermal ablation by means of radiofrequency coagulation (see Chapter 26) has numerous potential advantages over injection techniques, and is increasing in popularity. Probes are superior to those used for cryogenic lesioning, and the discrete, controllable lesion that results avoids the uncertainties associated with the spread of injected solutions. A radiofrequency lesion is produced within seconds, so great care must be taken to assure that the probe is positioned properly. Unfortunately, equipment is costly, and anesthesiologists are less likely than neurosurgeons to be trained in this technique.

HEAD AND NECK

GENERAL CONSIDERATIONS

Neoplastic head and neck pain remains a therapeutic challenge,[34] particularly if radiotherapy has proven ineffective or has already been maximized. Conventional analgesic therapy may prove inadequate because of the erosive nature of many tumors, and the area's rich innervation. Further, physiologic splinting, ordinarily an important protective reflex, is often ineffective in cases of craniocervical pain because pain is aggravated by relatively involuntary motion produced by swallowing, eating, coughing, talking, and other movements of the head. Despite overlapping contributions from cranial nerves V, VII, IX, X, and the upper cervical nerves, pain relief often can be obtained with carefully planned nerve blocks. Treatment success may be affected adversely by anatomic distortion induced by previous surgery or radiotherapy, and the potential for tumor invasion or radiation fibrosis to reduce contact between the neurolytic and targeted nervous tissue, a so-called "sheltering" effect. Typically, there is considerable overlap among the sensory fields of neighboring nerves, a variable that is further subject to interindividual differences. For this reason, as well as the influence of the cranial nerves

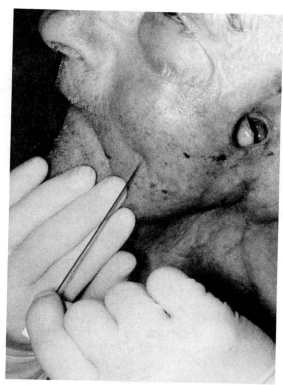

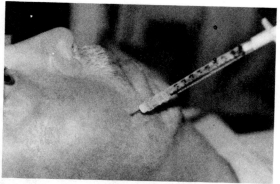

Figure 21–3. Outward appearance of 3.5-inch, 20-gauge needle correctly placed for gasserian ganglion injection in patient with base of the skull metastases secondary to lung cancer. Facial droop is a preexisting deficit.

Figure 21–2. Patient with invasive squamous cell tumor, status postsurgical resection and radiotherapy. Location of tumor, likelihood of further extension, and anatomic derangements suggested treatment with gasserian ganglion block, as opposed to blockade of a smaller branch of the fifth nerve.

on swallowing and control of breathing, neurolytic blocks should be preceded by diagnostic/prognostic local anesthetic injections. Despite these considerations, blockade of the cranial and/or upper cervical nerves is of great value in selected patients.

Blockade of the trigeminal nerve within the foramen ovale at the base of the skull or of its branches may be sufficient treatment for localized pain (Figs. 21–2 to 21–5). Lysis of the second division (maxillary nerve) or third division (mandibular nerve) usually is performed by the extraoral route, most commonly with absolute alcohol. Mandibular block is indicated for pain involving the jaw and anterior two-thirds of the tongue. Maxil-

lary block is indicated for pain involving the middle third of the face (*ie*, the maxilla, cheek, nasal cavity, hard palate, and tonsilar fossa). Alcohol block of the mandibular nerve occasionally has been associated with localized gangrene and skin slough,[7] presumably due to vascular thrombosis. A similar case of slough after one of several supraorbital alcohol nerve blocks has occurred in a patient with multiple sclerosis (Lipton S, personal communication, September 1991). Blockade of the first division (opthalmic nerve) is well described in the older literature,[8] but is rarely used in contemporary practice. If tumor progression is anticipated (see Fig. 21–2), it is preferable to extend the field of analgesia prophylactically by blocking the gasserian ganglion in its entirety.[27] Gasserian ganglion injection also is considered for pain in the distribution of the second or third division when tumor growth or postsurgical changes prohibit access to the maxillary or mandibular nerve. When pain extends cervically or to the angle of the jaw, supplementary paravertebral blockade of the second or third cervical nerve root may be necessary for more complete relief of pain.[35] Blockade of the smaller branches of the trigeminal nerve has been described,[16] and may be undertaken for well localized pain in a confined distribution, particularly due to an

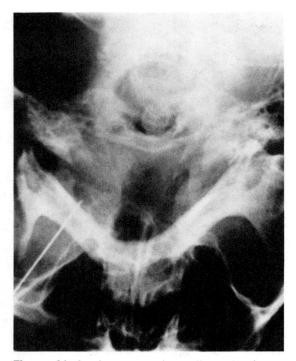

Figure 21–4. Anteroposterior radiograph of gas-serian ganglion block demonstrating needle tip impinging on foramen ovale. Initial placement at the entrance of the canal resulted in a mandibular paresthesia, signifying need to advance needle slightly further, as demonstrated here, where a maxillary paresthesia resulted.

ence with swallowing mechanisms and protective airway reflexes.[16,27] When available, radiofrequency coagulation is the preferred means of lesion generation. Blockade of the superior laryngeal nerves has been described for laryngeal pain of tabetic, tuberculous, and malignant origin.[5,21,37]

Intractable hiccups (singultus) also is amenable to nerve block therapy. Unilateral phrenic nerve block has been used under these circumstances with excellent results,[16] although conservative measures[38] should be exhausted first. Before performing a neurolytic phrenic nerve block, the results of a prognostic block with local anesthetic are evaluated to assure that ventilatory function will not be compromised by a more lasting procedure. Resuscitation equipment should be immediately available.

When intractable craniocervical pain is not amenable to nerve block therapy, intraspinal opioid therapy (see Chapter 18) by means of an implanted cervical epidural catheter,[39] or intraventricular opioid therapy, may be considered.[40] Numerous neurosurgical proce-

endophytic lesion that is more likely to erode than spread, or when anatomic distortion precludes access to the parent nerves.

In cases of pain that are less well localized or are concentrated near the base of the tongue, pharynx, or throat, blockade of the ninth or tenth cranial nerve may be required to achieve more complete relief.[5,36] The sensory field of the glossopharyngeal nerve includes the nasopharynx, eustachian tube, soft palate, uvula, tonsil, base of the tongue, and part of the external auditory canal. The vagus nerve subserves the larynx and contributes fibers to the ear, external auditory canal, and tympanic membrane. Bilateral destruction of the glossopharyngeal and vagus nerves is not recommended because of potential interfer-

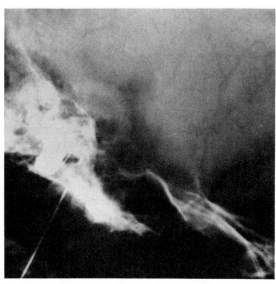

Figure 21–5. Lateral radiograph of gasserian ganglion block illustrating needle tip near clivus, partially obscured by dental fillings.

dures have been devised to manage rostral pain (see Chapter 26), but are of limited practical value because of their invasive nature and high morbidity and mortality.[10]

CLINICAL EXPERIENCE

In 1951, Bonica provided a moderately detailed description of a series of 70 patients with head and neck pain of oncologic origin treated with neurolysis of the peripheral and cranial nerves.[41] Forty-four (62.9%) patients achieved complete relief of pain, 22 (31.4%) moderate relief, and in 4 (5.7%) pain relief was slight or absent. These results are comparable to those published in an earlier series by Grant.[42] Complications of a "serious" and "not serious" nature occurred in 4 (5.7%) and 22 (30%) patients, respectively, and in all cases were predictable: corneal ulceration in a small proportion of patients after trigeminal blocks, unilateral masticatory paresis in a larger proportion of patients after mandibular block, and 1 case of unilateral dysphagia after glossopharyngeal block. Of note is that in addition to blockade of the cranial nerve trunks and their major branches, Bonica's series included patients treated with blockade of the smaller peripheral branches (ie, supraorbital, orbital, infraorbital, sphenopalatine, dental, lingual, inferior alveolar, and superior laryngeal nerves), often administered in a combined fashion. In another study, McEwen et al[43] reported achieving good or fair relief in 70% of cancer patients treated with gasserian ganglion block. The potential advantages of radiofrequency thermocoagulation already have been mentioned. Siegfried and Broggi have reported achieving lasting comfort in about 50% of 20 patients treated with percutaneous thermal ablation of the trigeminal ganglion.[44] The same authors[45] reported their results in two patients treated with thermal ablation of the glossopharyngeal nerve. Although one patient underwent a repeat procedure at 6 months for recurrence of pain, and the other had temporary dysphagia and permanent 12th nerve palsy, long-term results ultimately were gratifying. Using an anterior approach,

Pagura et al[46] reported good to excellent results in 15 cancer patients treated with thermocoagulation of the glossopharyngeal nerve. Treatment was supplemented by trigeminal thermoablation in eight patients because of overlapping pain, and other than transient vagal stimulation, no adverse effects were encountered.

UPPER EXTREMITY

GENERAL CONSIDERATIONS

Although most patients gratefully exchange unremitting pain for numbness, iatrogenic loss of motor strength must be avoided carefully so as not to compound further the other inevitable losses associated with the experience of cancer. Since in therapeutically useful strengths, alcohol and phenol produce indiscriminate destruction of neural tissue, nerves that transmit motor impulses to the limbs should not be targeted for injection unless movement already is compromised and the limb is nonfunctional or minimally functional. A useless limb may result either from neurologic dysfunction secondary to tumor invasion, radiation, or surgical fibrosis, or from forced immobilization and splinting from severe pain. All neurolytic procedures that have the potential to relieve upper extremity pain are associated with some degree of risk for weakness of the limb. Carefully performed, cervical subarachnoid injections of phenol or alcohol (see Chapters 20 and 23) are most likely to relieve pain without affecting motor function (because the drug is deposited preferentially on to sensory rootlets), and should be considered for patients with brachialgia and unimpaired function. Paravertebral block is applicable for very localized pain, and even then, because of sensory overlap, multiple nerves usually need to be blocked, and some degree of motor dysfunction should be anticipated. Radiologic guidance is strongly recommended for neurolytic paravertebral block, as well as the careful observation of the effects of preneurolytic test doses of local anesthetic, and fractionated administration to avoid sub-arachnoid or epidural spread.

The brachial plexus has a high proportion of motor fibers, and is therefore an example of a nerve bundle not to be injected unless motor strength is already deficient, as in some cases of Pancoast tumor, or unless the arm already is rendered useless by intractable pain, as in the case of pathologic fracture.

Relatively little experience has been reported with neurolytic block of the more peripheral nerves of the upper limb for carcinomatous pain. Our experience with neurolytic suprascapular block is reported here, and the results and relevance of peripheral neurolysis for spasticity are discussed near the end of the chapter.

CLINICAL EXPERIENCE

Bonica[5] describes the treatment of "several" cancer patients who presented with pain and edema sufficient to render their involved upper limb useless. After having observed good preliminary results with tetracaine injections, the brachial plexus was infiltrated with 20 ml of 95% alcohol, resulting in paralysis but relief of pain until death (duration unspecified). He also mentions having achieved pain relief of 3.5 weeks' to 3.5 months' duration with injections of 5% aqueous phenol in the vicinity of the brachial plexus. Kaplan et al[47] reported on a single, but well documented case of phenol brachial plexus block performed in a patient with recurrent sarcoma involving the humeral head. After a successful prognostic local anesthetic block, 12.5 ml of 6% phenol in water was injected by the supraclavicular route, resulting in a significant, but incomplete level of pain relief. Residual pain was managed by supplementary paravertebral phenol blocks of C5 and C6, and later, in response to increased tumor growth, T1–3 paravertebral blocks (0.5–1.0 ml 6% aqueous phenol/segment). In a report of a single case, Neill achieved excellent palliation of pain secondary to a pathologic fracture of the humerus in a man with multiple myeloma with two successive intrascalene injections of 20 ml of 50% alcohol.[48] In a report

of five cases, Mullin et al used an intrascalene injection of 3% aqueous phenol to manage the pain of Pancoast's syndrome.[49] Excellent short-term relief of pain was obtained in all patients, and was sustained for up to 7 months in three patients, but only at the expense of relatively frequent repetition at 3- to 6-week intervals. Neurologic sequelae were not observed, suggesting that dilute phenol, although its effects are short in duration, may be relatively safe in patients with normal motor function.

Paravertebral injections of C5–T1 may be effective, and an approach to anesthetizing multiple spinal nerves through a single skin wheal has been described.[5]

In response to concerns about reports of inadequate or short-lived analgesia after lytic brachial plexus block,[49] our group elected treatment with a higher concentration of phenol than has been reported previously.[17] Four patients underwent brachial plexus block with 10–20 ml 10%–12% aqueous phenol mixed with 20% glycerin to maintain the phenol's solubility in water. The resulting solution is only mildly viscid, and is readily injected through a 20- or 22-gauge needle. Three patients had pain and muscle weakness secondary to tumor invasion of the apex of the lung and brachial plexus, and one patient with breast cancer had painful metastases to the cervical spine. Pain had persisted in the latter patient despite two cervical subarachnoid neurolytic blocks. One patient had a pathologic fracture of the humerus as well, and all four patients had a useless limb from either neurologic involvement or intractable pain.

An axillary approach was used in all patients (Fig. 21–6), and was supplemented in one patient with a repeat block by the intrascalene approach. A paresthesia or positive response to electrical nerve stimulation was relied on for verification of needle placement in all but the most recent case, which was conducted under fluoroscopy through a catheter. Good to excellent pain relief was obtained in all patients until death occurred at 12 weeks in two patients, 8 weeks in one patient, and 5 weeks in another. No unexpected complications occurred. Increased motor weak-

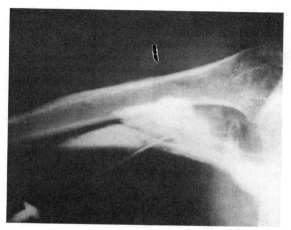

Figure 21–6. Anterior–posterior radiograph demonstrating contrast medium within the axillary brachial plexus compartment.

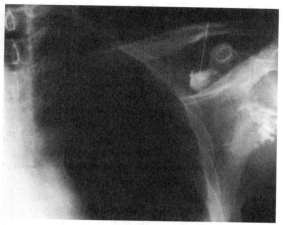

Figure 21–8. Anteroposterior radiograph of chest demonstrating correct needle placement for suprascapular nerve block. Note characteristic configuration of contrast medium near suprascapular notch.

ness was observed in all cases, but was well tolerated. Interestingly, in three of the four cases, relief of pain was not immediately forthcoming, but accrued gradually over several days.

An additional patient with shoulder and upper arm pain was referred for brachial plexus block, but was found to have excellent upper limb strength. After a diagnostic/prognostic local anesthetic block, she instead was treated with a 4-ml injection of 10% phenol in the vicinity of the suprascapular nerve, which was localized with a nerve stimulator. No loss

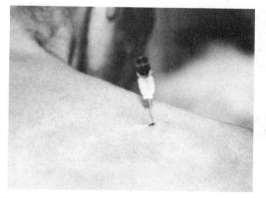

Figure 21–7. Final placement of 3.5-inch, 22-gauge needle for neurolytic suprascapular block.

of motor power occurred, and she had excellent pain relief until her death 8 weeks later. Another preterminal patient with shoulder pain secondary to multiple myeloma received a suprascapular block with 4 ml of absolute alcohol, which resulted in moderate relief of pain without complications until his death 4 weeks later. A final patient (see Figs. 21–7 and 21–8) who initially refused radiation therapy for a periscapular soft tissue mass secondary to lung cancer experienced good pain relief of 4 weeks' duration after a phenol suprascapular block (5 ml of 10% phenol). Pain gradually returned, and the patient was persuaded to undergo radiotherapy, which provided pain relief that persisted until his death.

THORACIC AND ABDOMINAL WALL

GENERAL CONSIDERATIONS

Pain originating in the thoracic wall, abdominal wall, or parietal peritoneum can be treated with multiple intercostal[15,21,50,51] and paravertebral blocks.[16,52] Except after pneumonectomy, the risk of pneumothorax exists for blocks performed in the thoracic region, although when proper technique is observed it should occur infrequently. For example, in a series of 50,097 intercostal blocks performed in 4,333 patients, pneumothorax was detected in only 4 patients (0.092%).[51] Although other studies have documented higher incidences of pneumothorax, the cited report of Moore (in which 85% of these procedures were performed by supervised residents) suggests that low incidences of complications can be obtained. Whereas the use of radiologic guidance has been reported for intercostal block,[15] (Fig. 21–9) "walking the needle off" the rib and the presence of a paresthesia usually are relied on as guides for placement. Localized bony pain associated with rib metastases also may respond to local infiltration around the bone with steroids, a technique that has produced good response in our hands and others, and which is repeatable.[53] Using the transverse process as a bony landmark, paravertebral block of the somatic nerve may be performed as it emerges from the intravertebral foramen.[54] Radiologic guidance is strongly recommended for neurolytic paravertebral block, as well as the careful observation of the effects of preneurolytic test doses of local anesthetic, and fractionated administration to avoid subarachnoid, epidural, or intrapleural spread, all of which have been documented.[55]

CLINICAL EXPERIENCE

Doyle[50,56] reported on a series of 46 patients treated in a hospice with multiple phenol intercostal blocks. He used 1.0–1.5 ml 5% phenol "in oil" per segment, and obtained total relief of pain for a mean duration of 3 weeks (range, 1–6 weeks). Radiologic guidance was not used, and no complications occurred. That additional caution is advisable when blocking the intercostal nerves of patients who have undergone complicated lung resection is suggested by a case report of a patient with adhesions who experienced acute bronchospasm after an unintentional presumed intrabronchial or intrapulmonary injection of small amount (0.5 ml) of 8% phenol in saline.[57]

Bonica mentions favorable results subsequent to the paravertebral injection of 1 ml alcohol per involved segment in patients with abdominal and chest wall pain secondary to

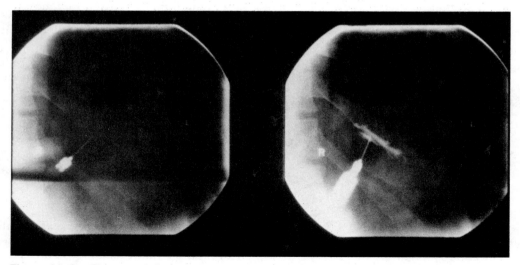

Figure 21–9. Figure on left demonstrates characteristic anteroposterior radiologic view of needle and syringe positioned correctly for intercostal block. Figure on the right demonstrates the spread of contrast medium along the lower border of the rib, verifying placement. (Courtesy P. Prithvi Raj, M.D.)

vertebral, paravertebral, and visceral neo-plasms associated with peritoneal invasion.[16] In an anecdotal report, Vernon[52] noted good relief of back pain of metastatic origin and no untoward effects after paravertebral injection of alcohol in two patients, although little detail was provided.

A report by Mehta and Ranger,[58] suppos-edly of blocks of the individual branches of the lumbar plexus in 103 patients with abdominal pain of unknown etiology, is mentioned be-cause it raises the question of whether block-ade of the peripheral nerves within the ab-dominal wall might be feasible. The authors describe having blocked the iliohypogastric (65), ilio-inguinal (10), and upper and lower intercostal (28) nerves within the rectus sheath with 2–3 ml of aqueous phenol. De-spite their use of a primitive nerve stimulator in some cases, however, their description sug-gests that trigger-point injections (see below) rather than true peripheral blocks actually may have been administered. Follow-up at 3 weeks revealed complete and partial relief of pain in 58% and 32% of patients, respectively, with no recurrence in 70% of respondents at 3-year follow-up.

PERINEUM AND LOWER EXTREMITIES

GENERAL CONSIDERATIONS

Treatment of intractable perineal and lower limb pain is problematic because pain is often bilateral or midline in distribution, and the relevant neuroanatomy predisposes to risks of muscular paresis and incontinence when neurolytic techniques are applied. When bowel and bladder function are not of concern because of preexisting dysfunction and/or sur-gical diversions, neurolytic subarachnoid sad-dle block (see Chapters 20 and 23) is a sim-ple and effective procedure that should be strongly considered. Decision-making is more difficult in the continent, ambulatory patient with intractable pain. Although neurolytic subarachnoid and epidural block can be per-formed in the thoracic region relatively safely,

these techniques are hazardous when per-formed in the lumbosacral region, even with careful attention to technique (see Chapters 20 and 23).

Recently, blocks of the hypogastric plexus and ganglion impar (see Chapter 22) have been introduced,[59,60] and can be considered as options for pelvic or rectal pain that is sympa-thetically mediated. Diagnostic local anes-thetic block is strongly recommended before neurolysis to "map out" the nerves that should be targeted for therapeutic blockade.

The sacral roots are accessed readily as they emerge from the posterior plate of the sacrum, and injections here may relieve pel-vic, rectal, and lower extremity pain. Selective sacral root block is preferable to spinal injec-tions in this region in patients with normal urinary and bowel function, as carefully exe-cuted nerve blocks here will not affect conti-nence.[61] A single sacral nerve, most often one of the third[62] or sometimes fourth sacral nerves,[63] usually exerts a dominant influence on bladder musculature, and as a result, blockade of the nondominant nerves, based on trials of local anesthetic injections, has little urodynamic effect. We have found radiologic guidance to be a useful adjunct to sacral nerve block. Whereas the foramina frequently are not well visualized on anteroposterior views, needle penetration of the posterior sacral plate is readily apparent on lateral views.

Neurolytic injections of other peripheral nerves subserving the lower extremity some-times are attempted, but generally only after local anesthetic injection has confirmed that reduction in pain is possible without un-wanted decrement in motor function.

CLINICAL EXPERIENCE

Robertson[61] described a series of nine patients with intractable perineal pain secondary to carcinoma of the rectum whom he treated with sacral nerve root block. After successful local anesthetic block, he performed injections of 2.5 ml 6.66% aqueous phenol at the S4 fora-men on the side of predominant pain. Satis-factory analgesia was obtained in all cases, and persisted in two cases for 202 and 414 days after a single block. Duration was inadequate in the other cases, but pain relief was maintained uniformly until death by second or third repetitions. In seven of the nine patients, duration of relief from the first block was under 10 days, suggesting that most patients will require repeated treatment, but this limitation was mitigated by ease of repetition. Motor and autonomic function were unaffected, and no other complications occurred. In a similar study on patients with bladder pain secondary to spasticity, Simon et al[64] obtained an average of 26.5 months of pain relief in respondants after sacral injections of 2 ml of 6% aqueous phenol. Most patients obtained relief with unilateral blockade of the third sacral nerve, although preliminary local anesthetic blocks identified some patients whose pain was mediated by S2 and S4. Several patients required repeat treatment, and no lasting complications were observed.

An isolated report of bladder atony after otherwise successful S3 and S4 alcohol block[65] emphasizes the need for careful observation of the results of preneurolytic prognostic blocks with local anesthetic. A recent well designed study[61] assessed the spread of a mixture of contrast medium and local anesthetic injected in 1- and 2-ml aliquots for sacral block. The authors demonstrated a wider spread of solution in the latter group, and concluded that 1 ml of anesthetic is sufficient to produce a selective sacral nerve root block, and moreover may be safer. They were able also to demonstrate that reflux into the sacral canal was much less likely when the needle tip was positioned at the anterior border of the sacrum rather than in the midportion of the sacral foramen. It is uncertain how these results apply to the spread of neurolytic solutions.

Successful treatment of penile pain and malignant priapism secondary to venous obstruction from bladder cancer has been reported anecdotally with injections of 5% aqueous phenol near the dorsal nerves of the penis close to the symphysis pubis.[66]

Feldman and Yeung[67] treated 26 patients for intractable claudication with paravertebral injections of lumbar somatic nerves with 5–10 ml of 7.5% phenol in myodil, and reported good long-term improvement without negative sequelae. Doyle[50,56] mentions performing two femoral nerve blocks with phenol in a patient with invasion of the femoral sheath area, but provides no other details. Our group performed an alcohol injection of the sciatic nerve in a patient with preexisting motor weakness from invasion of the nerve by pelvic tumor, with good short-term results.[17] We also have observed heightened distress and poor tolerance of resulting foot drop in other patients with less complete motor deficit who were exposed to trials of prognostic local anesthetic sciatic blockade. Rastogi and Kumar make a brief mention of "successful" alcohol block of the sciatic nerve in three patients with cancer.[14] Singler reported on a single case of successful sciatic and femoral neurolysis performed with 75% alcohol for intractable spasticity. A few reports have appeared documenting the injection of the lumbar somatic nerves with phenol within the psoas sheath for the relief of ischemic pain.[67,68] That 5–10 ml of 7.5% phenol[67] and 5 ml of 10% phenol[68] dissolved in contrast medium were injected without significant neurologic side effects is surprising, but suggests potential applications in patients with cancer.

OTHER PERIPHERAL NERVES: THE SPASTICITY EXPERIENCE

A review of the use of phenol in the treatment of spasticity is beyond the scope of this chapter, but several excellent papers are available on this subject.[69,70] It is of interest, however, that peripheral nerve blocks with phenol (in addition to subarachnoid and motor-point injections) have been advocated in spastic patients to improve balance, gait, self-care, and global rehabilitation. An important distinction between peripheral neurolytic blocks for pain versus spasticity is that, in the latter, motor or mixed nerves are targeted preferentially. Nevertheless, given the paucity of data on peripheral neurolytic blocks for the management of pain, it is worthwhile to try to extrapolate information obtained from work with spastic patients.

Moritz[69] reported on a series of 50 spastic patients who received a total of 90 peripheral nerve blocks (musculocutaneous, median, ulnar, tibial, obturator, femoral, and superior gluteal nerves) performed with either 2% phenol in saline or 3% aqueous phenol. A nerve stimulator was used for needle localization. Focal motor weakness lasted only about 1 week in 15% of patients, but the average duration of effect was 8 months. He noted a low incidence of transient dysesthesias (10%) that usually resolved in days or weeks, and no sensory disturbances; findings that are not surprising given the dilute solutions used. Reporting on 521 blocks of peripheral nerves performed with 6% aqueous phenol, Gibson[56] noted one serious complication, a 69-year-old hemiplegic patient, who, after five successful blocks, underwent a brachioradialis and musculocutaneous block, and subsequently developed an arterial occlusion in the upper limb that required a high amputation.

LOCAL INJECTION OF NEUROLYTICS

Local anesthetic and/or steroid injections of "trigger points" (see Chapter 19) is a well accepted means of managing chronic myofascial pain. The clinical effects of locally injected neurolytics are unknown, and local infiltration generally is avoided because of concerns about skin slough and worsening of pain due to local ischemia or necrosis. Cousins[2] refers to the practice of injecting persistent trigger points with 5%–6% aqueous phenol, but cautions that further research is needed to determine its safety and efficacy.

Ramamurthy et al[11] mention having performed three "myoneural" blocks with 6% aqueous phenol, but provide no further detail. In a study of patients with painful palpable peripheral neuromas, local injections of 0.1–0.5 ml of 5% phenol in glycerin were performed.[71] Fifteen neuromas were treated in 10 patients with a total of 20 blocks. Complete relief was obtained and maintained in all but one patient for the 8- to 22-month follow-up period, and no complications or neuritis were reported. In another series of patients with poststernotomy pain presumably due to scar neuroma,[72,73] 17 patients were treated with multiple, serial local neurolytic injections of 2–3 ml of 6% aqueous phenol or 1.5–2.0 ml of absolute alcohol. Complete relief was obtained in most patients, and no complications referable to neurolysis were observed. Finally, Defalque[74] obtained complete relief in 63 of 69 patients by performing repeated trigger-point injections near surgical scars with 1.0 ml of absolute alcohol, and noted no complications other than localized numbness. The implications for this treatment modality in patients with cancer pain are uncertain.

We have had two experiences with periosteal injections of dilute aqueous phenol (3%–5%) for persistent refractory bone pain, a technique mentioned by Swerdlow.[53] Both patients had experienced minimal relief after regional blockade, but good, transient relief with periosteal injections of local anesthetic and steroid ultimately achieved lasting relief after a series of two neurolytic injections.

The use of local subcutaneous infiltration with absolute alcohol for intractable anal and vulvar pruritus has been reported by several authors.[75–77] Although the relevance to patients with carcinomatous pain is uncertain, this technique deserves mention due to its apparent safety in patients with nonmalignant pain and itch. In one representative series,[76] over two-thirds of patients experienced complete symptomatic relief that persisted for 1–5 years. Complications were limited to local skin reactions that, although initially distressing, subsided over 2–3 weeks.

CONCLUSION

Peripheral neurolysis has specific but important indications in the management of intractable cancer pain. As with all invasive procedures with potential utility for improving intractable cancer pain, careful attention must be paid to the applicability of more conservative alternatives, patient selection, and technical aspects.

REFERENCES

1. Cousins MJ: Anesthetic approaches in cancer pain. In Foley KM, Bonica JJ, Ventafridda V (eds): Advances in Pain Research and Therapy, vol 16, p 249. New York, Raven Press, 1990.
2. Cousins MJ, Dwyer B, Gibb D: Chronic pain and neurolytic neural blockade. In Cousins MJ, Bridenbaugh PO (eds): Neural Blockade, 2nd ed, p 1053. Philadelphia, JB Lippincott, 1988.
3. Abrams S: Neurolytic blocks of peripheral nerves. In Racz GB (ed): Techniques of Neurolysis, p 185. Boston, Kluwer, 1989.
4. Murphy T: Treatment of chronic pain. In Miller RD (ed): Anesthesia, p 2097. New York, Churchill Livingstone, 1986.
5. Bonica JJ, Buckley FP, Moricca G et al: Neurolytic blockade and hypophysectomy. In Bonica JJ (ed): Management of Pain, 2nd ed, p 1980. Philadelphia, Lea and Febiger, 1990.
6. Swerdlow M: Role of chemical neurolysis and local anesthetic infiltration. In Swerdlow M, Ventafridda V (eds): Cancer Pain, p 105. Lancaster, England, MTP Press, 1986.
7. Moore DC: Regional Block, 4th ed, pp 148, 329. Springfield, IL, Charles C Thomas, 1965.
8. Pitkin GP: Blocking the trigeminal nerve. In Southworth JL, Hingson RA, Pitkin WM (eds): Conduction Anesthesia, 2nd ed, p 360. Philadelphia, JB Lippincott, 1953.
9. Pender JW, Pugh DG: Diagnostic and therapeutic nerve blocks: Necessity for roentgenograms. JAMA 1951;146:798.
10. Patt R: Neurosurgical interventions for chronic pain problems. Anesthesiology Clinics of North America 1987;5:609.
11. Ramamurthy S, Walsh NE, Schoenfeld LS et al: Evaluation of neurolytic blocks using phenol and cryogenic block in the management of chronic pain. Journal of Pain and Symptom Management 1989;4:72.
12. Raj PP, Rosenblatt R, Montgomery S: Uses of the nerve stimulator for peripheral blocks. Reg Anaesth 1980;5:14.
13. Raj PP, Montgomery SJ, Nettles D et al: The use of the nerve stimulator with standard unsheathed needles in nerve blockade. Anesth Analg 1973;53:827.
14. Rastogi V, Kumar R: Peripheral nerve stimulator as an aid for therapeutic alcohol blocks. Anesthesiology 1983;38:163.
15. Moore DC: Intercostal nerve block and celiac plexus block for pain therapy. In Benedetti C et al (eds): Adv Pain Res Ther 1984;7:309. New York, Raven Press, 1984.
16. Bonica JJ: Management of Pain, 1st ed. Philadelphia, Lea and Febiger, 1953.
17. Patt RB, Millard R: A role for peripheral neurolysis in the management of intractable cancer pain. Pain 1990; (Suppl 5):S358.
18. Szalados J, Patt R: Management of a patient with displaced orthopedic hardware. Journal of Pain and Symptom Management 1991 (in press).
19. Takagi Y, Koyama T, Yamamoto Y: Subarachnoid neurolytic block with 15% phenol glycerin in the treatment of cancer pain. Pain 1987; (Suppl 4):133.
20. Ischia S, Luzzani A, Pacini L et al: Lytic saddle block: Clinical comparison of the results, using phenol at 5, 10, and 15 percent. In Benedetti C et al (eds): Advances in Pain Research and Therapy, vol 7, p 339. New York, Raven Press, 1984.
21. Churcher M: Peripheral nerve blocks in the relief of intractable pain. In Swerdlow M, Charlton JE: Relief of Intractable Pain, 4th ed, p 195. Amsterdam, Elsevier, 1989.
22. Swerdlow M: Spinal and peripheral neurolysis for managing Pancoast syndrome. In Bonica JJ, Ventafridda V, Pagni C (eds): Advances in Pain Research and Therapy, vol 4, p 135. New York, Raven Press, 1982.
23. Roviaro GC, Varoli F, Fascianella A et al: Intrathoracic intercostal nerve block with phenol in open chest surgery. Chest 1986;90:64.
24. Mandl F: Paravertebral Block. New York, Grune and Stratton, 1947.
25. Katz J: Current role of neurolytic agents. Adv Neurol 1974;4:471.
26. Smith AE: Block Anesthesia and Allied Subjects. St. Louis, CV Mosby, 1920.
27. Madrid JL, Bonica JJ: Cranial nerve blocks. In Bonica JJ, Ventafridda V (eds): Advances in Pain Research and Therapy, vol 2, p 347. New York, Raven Press, 1979.
28. Hakanson S: Trigeminal neuralgia treated by the injection of glycerol into the trigeminal cistern. Neurosurgery 1981;9:638.
29. Shulman M: Treatment of cancer pain with epidural butyl-amino-benzoate suspension. Reg Anaesth 1987;12:1.
30. Shulman M: Intercostal nerve block with 10% butamben suspension for the treatment of chronic noncancer pain. Anesthesiology 1989;71:A737.

31. Shulman M, Joseph NJ, Haller CA: Local effects of epidural and subarachnoid injections of butylaminobenzoate suspension. Reg Anaesth 1987;12:23.
32. Sulman M: Epidural butamben for the treatment of metastatic cancer pain. Anesthesiology 1987;67:A245.
33. Evans PJD, Lloyd JW, Jack TM: Cryoanalgesia for intractable pain. J R Soc Med 1981;74:804.
34. Wilson PJEM: Neurosurgery and relief of pain associated with head and neck cancer. Ear Nose Throat J 1983;62:250.
35. Patt R, Jain S: Management of a patient with osteoradionecrosis of the mandible with nerve blocks. Journal of Pain and Symptom Management 1990;5:59.
36. Montgomery W, Cousins MJ: Aspects of the management of chronic pain illustrated by ninth cranial nerve block. Br J Anaesth 1972;44:383.
37. Labat G: Regional Anesthesia, p 114. Philadelphia, WB Saunders, 1922.
38. Twycross RG, Lack SA: Therapeutics in Terminal Care. Edinburgh, Churchill Livingstone, 1986.
39. Waldman SD, Feldstein GS, Allen ML et al: Cervical epidural implantable narcotic delivery systems in the management of upper body pain. Anesth Analg 1987;66:780.
40. Lobato RD, Madrid JL, Fatela LV et al: Intraventricular morphine for intractable cancer pain: Rationale, methods, clinical results. Acta Anaesthesiol Scand 1987;31:68.
41. Bonica JJ: The management of pain of malignant disease with nerve blocks. Anesthesiology 1954;15:280.
42. Grant FC: Surgical methods for relief of pain. Bull NY Acad Med 1943;19:373.
43. McEwen BW et al: The pain clinic: A clinic for the management of intractable pain. Med J Austr 1965;1:676.
44. Siegfried J, Broggi G: Percutaneous thermocoagulation of the gasserian ganglion in the treatment of pain in advanced cancer. In Bonica JJ, Ventafridda V (eds): Advances in Pain Research and Therapy, vol 2, p 463. New York, Raven Press, 1979.
45. Broggi G, Siegfried J: Percutaneous differential radiofrequency rhizotomy of glossopharyngeal nerve in facial pain due to cancer. In Bonica JJ, Ventafridda V (eds): Advances in Pain Research and Therapy, vol 2, p 469. New York, Raven Press, 1979.
46. Pagura JR, Schnapp M, Passarelli P: Percutaneous radiofrequency glossopharyngeal rhizotomy for cancer pain. Appl Neurophysiol 1983;46:154.
47. Kaplan R, Aurellano Z, Pfisterer W: Phenol brachial plexus block for upper extremity cancer pain. Regional Anesthesia 1988;13:58.
48. Neill RS: Ablation of the brachial plexus. Anaesthesia 1979;34:1024.
49. Mullin V: Brachial plexus block with phenol for painful arm associated with Pancoast's syndrome. Anesthesiology 1980;53:431.
50. Doyle D: Nerve blocks in advanced cancer. Practitioner 1982;226:539.
51. Moore D, Bridenbaugh DL: Intercostal nerve block in 4333 patients: Indications, techniques, complications. Anesth Analg 1962;41:1.
52. Vernon S: Paralgesia: Paravertebral block for pain relief. Am J Surg 1932;21:416.
53. Swerdlow M: Role of chemical neurolysis and local anesthetic infiltration. In Swerdlow M, Ventafridda V (eds): Cancer Pain, p 119. Lancaster, MTP Press, 1987.
54. Thompson GE, Moore DC: Celiac plexus, intercostal, and minor peripheral blockade. In Cousins MJ, Bridenbaugh PO (eds): Neural Blockade, 2nd ed, p 503. Philadelphia, JB Lippincott, 1988.
55. Conacher ID, Kokri M: Postoperative paravertebral blocks for thoracic surgery: A radiological appraisal. Br J Anaesth 1987;59:155.
56. Gibson IIJM: Phenol block in the treatment of spasticity. Gerontology 1987;33:327.
57. Atkinson GL, Shupack RC: Acute bronchospasm complicating intercostal nerve block with phenol. Anesth Analg 1989;68.
58. Mehta M, Ranger I: Persistent abdominal pain. Anaesthesia 1971;26:330.
59. Plancarte R, Amescua C, Patt R et al: Superior hypogastric plexus block for pelvic cancer pain. Anesthesiology 1990;73:236.
60. Plancarte R, Amescua C, Patt RB: Presacral blockade of the ganglion impar (ganglion of Walther). Anesthesiology 1990;73:A751.
61. Robertson DH: Transsacral neurolytic nerve block: An alternative approach to intractable perineal pain. Br J Anaesth 1983;55:873.
62. Clark AJ, Awad SA: Selective transsacral nerve root blocks. Reg Anaesth 1990;15:125.
63. Rockswold GL, Bradley WE, Chou SN: Effect of sacral nerve blocks on the function of the urinary bladder in humans. J Neurosurg 1974;40:83.
64. Simon DL, Carron H, Rowlingson JC: Treatment of bladder pain with transsacral nerve block. Anesth Analg 1982;61:46.
65. Goffen BS: Transsacral block. Anesth Analg 1982;61:623.
66. Wilson F: Neurolytic and other locally acting drugs in the management of pain. Pharmacol Ther 1981;53:431.
67. Feldman SA, Yeung ML: Treatment of intermittent claudication: Lumbar paravertebral somatic block with phenol. Anaesthesia 1975;30:174.

68. Jack ED: Regional anaesthesia for pain relief. Br J Anaesth 1975;47:278.
69. Moritz U: Phenol block of peripheral nerves. Scand J Rehabil Med 1973;5:160.
70. Papo I, Visca A: Intrathecal phenol in the treatment of pain and spasticity. Prog Neurol Surg 1976; 7:56.
71. Kirvel, Nieminen S: Treatment of painful neuromas with neurolytic blockade. Pain 1990;41:161.
72. Defalque RJ, Bromley JJ: Poststernotomy neuralgia: A new pain syndrome. Anesth Analg 1989; 69:81.
73. Todd DP: Poststernotomy neuralgia: A new pain syndrome. Anesth Analg 1989;69:691.
74. Defalque RJ: Painful trigger points in surgical scars. Anesth Analg 1982;61:518.
75. Stone HB: A treatment for pruritus ani. Bull Johns Hopkins Hosp 1916;27:242.
76. Woodruff JD, Babkinia A: Local alcohol injection of the vulva: Discussion of 35 cases. Obstet Gynecol 1979;54:512.
77. Woodruff JD, Thompson B: Local alcohol injection in the treatment of vulvar pruritus. Obstet Gynecol 1972;40:18.

Chapter 22

Neurolytic Blocks of the Sympathetic Axis

Ricardo Plancarte
Ruben Velazquez
Richard B. Patt

INTRODUCTION

The sympathetic nervous system has been implicated in the maintenance of numerous cancer pain syndromes (see Chapter 1).[1,2] Sympathetically mediated pain may be neuropathic in origin,[3] that is, associated with injury to nervous tissue *per se* (eg, Pancoast's syndrome, lumbosacral plexopathy, causalgia/reflex sympathetic dystrophy), or of visceral origin.[4,5] In visceral pain, there is damage to a sympathetically innervated end organ, and the intact sympathetic fibers are responsible for the transmission of noxious stimuli (eg, hepatic metastases, intestinal obstruction, and ischemia). In addition, occult microscopic deposits of perineural tumor invasion may contribute to pain in the latter group.[1] This premise is supported by autopsy findings of direct tumor invasion of peripancreatic nerves in 84% of a group of patients with pancreatic cancer.[6]

Historically, interruption of sympathetic pathways has been applied widely to relieve oncologic pain,[2,7,8] and modifications of classic techniques continue to be advocated enthusiastically in contemporary practice.[9-13] Surgical approaches, well described by Leriche, Cotte, Fontaine, Wertheimer, Putnam et al,[1] are used less frequently in preference to chemical interruption (neurolytic blocks), as the latter techniques have both been improved on and do not require the preterminal patient to be exposed to the rigors of surgery. In addition to the classic targets of sympatholysis (stellate or cervicothoracic ganglion, celiac plexus, and lumbar chain), new approaches to anesthetize the hypogastric plexus[13] and ganglion impar[14] have been reported recently, and are described here (Fig. 22–1).

FUNDAMENTAL CONSIDERATIONS

Essential to the consideration of instituting sympathetic blockade for a pain problem is an

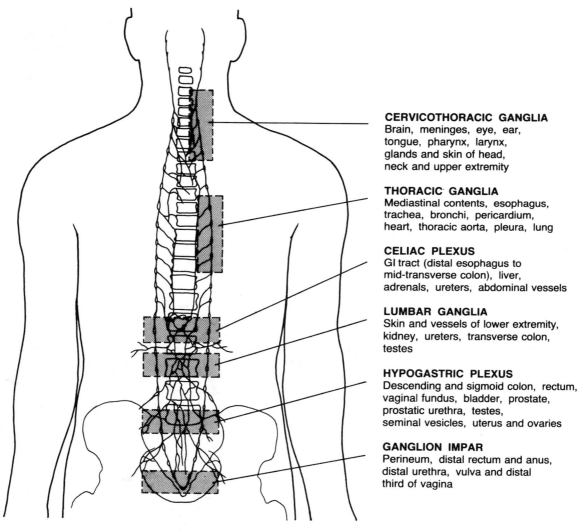

CERVICOTHORACIC GANGLIA
Brain, meninges, eye, ear, tongue, pharynx, larynx, glands and skin of head, neck and upper extremity

THORACIC GANGLIA
Mediastinal contents, esophagus, trachea, bronchi, pericardium, heart, thoracic aorta, pleura, lung

CELIAC PLEXUS
GI tract (distal esophagus to mid-transverse colon), liver, adrenals, ureters, abdominal vessels

LUMBAR GANGLIA
Skin and vessels of lower extremity, kidney, ureters, transverse colon, testes

HYPOGASTRIC PLEXUS
Descending and sigmoid colon, rectum, vaginal fundus, bladder, prostate, prostatic urethra, testes, seminal vesicles, uterus and ovaries

GANGLION IMPAR
Perineum, distal rectum and anus, distal urethra, vulva and distal third of vagina

Figure 22–1.   Schematic outline of the sites for anesthetic blockade of the sympathetic nervous system and affected structures. Note that the system is contiguous, and that there is considerable overlap and variation of innervation. Modified from Bonica JJ: The Management of Pain, Philadelphia, Lea and Febiger, 1953.

Table 22–1.
Tumor-induced Reflex Sympathetic Dystrophy
___

Quality of pain
  Neuralgic or dysesthetic
  • Constant, unbearable
  • Burning, numbing, tingling
  • Pressing, squeezing, itching
  • Occasionally sharp and stabbing
  • Superimposed lancinating (shooting) pain

Distribution of pain
  • Predominantly vascular

Altered sensory threshold (evoked pain)
  • Allodynia, hyperesthesia, hyperpathia

Vasomotor and sudomotor abnormalities
  • Intermittent cyanosis, rubor, or pallor
  • Edema, atrophy of muscle, skin, nails
  • Anhidrosis, hypohidrosis, hyperhidrosis
  • Abnormal sweat test
  • Increased or decreased skin temperature

Horner's sign

___

Subtle sympathetic dysfunction may be an early harbinger of tumor infiltration of the sympathetic chain, often preceding radiologic evidence of recurrence by months or even years.

___

understanding of its etiology. Assessment is primarily clinical, and is on the basis of the presence of historical, physical, and/or radiologic findings consistent with a sympathetic mechanism for pain. Characteristic cancer pain syndromes and diagnostic features of sympathetically mediated pain have been discussed in Chapter 1. The features of tumor-induced reflex sympathetic dystrophy are described immediately below, and are summarized in Table 22–1.

Pain often is multifactorial. When a mixed etiology is suspected, assessment should be geared further to determine the relative contributions of somatic and visceral mechanisms so that correct treatment can be selected. In this regard, diagnostic blocks with local anesthetics (see Chapters 19 and 21) help establish the predominant underlying pain mechanism.[15] In addition, the results of local anes-

thetic blockade have prognostic value for predicting the response to more definitive therapeutic neurolytic (destructive) interventions.[16]

Nerve blocks rarely are used as the sole means of pain relief in patients whose symptoms are due to cancer.[17] Before instituting invasive modalities, it is assumed that careful trials of pharmacotherapy and other conservative measures have failed to produce adequate pain relief.[17] Visceral pain tends to be less opioid-sensitive than somatic pain, and neuropathic pain least sensitive of all,[18,19] so standard opioid therapy may be ineffective in a proportion of patients. Treatment with co-analgesics such as antidepressants, anticonvulsants, vasodilators, and oral local anesthetics is sometimes effective, and should be considered (see Chapter 10). It should be borne in mind, however, that effective coanalgesic therapy is often difficult to institute, in that 1) dose response is unpredictable, within excess of 4 weeks often cited as the time necessary to evaluate the efficacy of each trial[20]; and 2) analgesic doses may be poorly tolerated in debilitated, polypharmacized patients.[21] Of the painful conditions associated with malignancy, neurolytic blockade is in some respects the most appropriate treatment for the sympathetically mediated syndromes (Table 22–2).

Table 22–2.
Advantages of Neurolytic Blockade for Sympathetically Mediated Cancer Pain
___

1. In contrast to somatically mediated pain, visceral and causalgic pain often is more effectively relieved by neural blockade than with pharmacologic management.
2. When performed properly, destruction of sympathetic nerves is not accompanied by alterations in muscle strength or tactile sensation (numbness).
3. Localized improvements in blood flow may be beneficial.
4. In contrast to the destruction of somatic nerves, neuritis and the development of deafferentiation pain are not significant risks.
___

TUMOR-INDUCED REFLEX SYMPATHETIC DYSTROPHY
(Causalgia)

The term **reflex sympathetic dystrophy** is used to describe a spectrum of incompletely understood syndromes (including causalgia) characterized by neuropathic pain (see Chapter 1) and vasomotor disturbances.[22,23,23a] Sympathetic dystrophy classically is a post-traumatic process, but variations induced by tumor invasion and/or antitumor therapy have been recognized.[24–26]

The quality of pain tends to be neuralgic and/or dysesthetic,[3] and when constant it is usually characterized as burning, numbing, tingling, pressing, squeezing, itching, and/or unbearable. Patients may complain of a sharp and stabbing or superimposed lancinating (shooting) component, as well.[24] Pain tends to be distributed along vascular channels, although there also may be elements of dermatomal pain, particularly when there is concomitant somatic nerve involvement. Evoked pain and alterations in resting sensory threshold (allodynia, hyperesthesia, and hyperpathia) are common (see Chapter 1).[27]

Associated findings may include a combination of vasomotor and sudomotor abnormalities, including intermittent cyanosis; rubor or pallor; edema; atrophy of muscle, skin, subcutaneous tissue, and nails; anhidrosis, hypohidrosis, or hyperhidrosis; and increased or decreased skin temperature. Classically, but not invariably, the limb is hyperperfused and sweaty in the early stages of disease, with atrophic changes being more prominent in advanced cases.[23] Horner's syndrome may be present when the upper limb is involved.

Reflex sympathetic dystrophy may be associated with invasion of the brachial plexus and cervicothoracic sympathetic chain by lung carcinoma or metastatic breast carcinoma (superior sulcus or Pancoast's syndrome),[28] and tumor infiltration of the lumbosacral plexus (see Chapter 1).[29] Radiation myelopathy and fibrosis of the major plexuses can contribute to this syndrome as well.[30,31] Some authorities believe that subtle sympathetic dysfunction may be an early harbinger of tumor infiltration of the sympathetic chain, often preceding radiologic evidence of recurrence by months or even years.[24]

Over a 2-year period, Warfield evaluated 15 patients with intractable pain secondary to carcinoma of the lung.[32] All of six patients who had pain referred primarily to the upper extremity were administered trials of local anesthetic stellate ganglion blocks. Of the six treated patients, three experienced profound and lasting relief of pain after a single stellate block, essentially confirming the diagnosis of tumor-induced reflex sympathetic dystrophy. Neither the quality of pain nor the presence of vasomotor changes correlated well with this group of patients' response to treatment, emphasizing the diagnostic utility of local anesthetic blockade. Independent of its etiology, reflex sympathetic dystrophy is sufficiently variable in its presentation that the diagnosing clinician should maintain a high index of suspicion. A trial of local anesthetic blockade of the sympathetic system should be considered early even in ambiguous cases, since, in experienced hands, the effects of treatment are relatively innocuous, and, when performed in a timely fashion, they may affect resolution of otherwise intractable symptoms.

PATIENT PREPARATION

DIAGNOSTIC VERSUS THERAPEUTIC BLOCKADE

As noted in Chapter 19, lytic blocks generally are preceded by diagnostic/prognostic local anesthetic blocks separated by an interval sufficient to permit adequate evaluation of efficacy and side effects by both patient and physician. This time-honored principle is of added importance when pain is suspected to be causalgic in nature. In causalgia or reflex sympathetic dystrophy, a single local anesthetic block sometimes will produce relief that persists in excess of the expected local anesthetic action (sometimes days to weeks), and a series of local anesthetic blocks may result in complete resolution of symptoms, obviating the need for neurolysis.[22-32] If extended relief is observed after a single local anesthetic block, treatment with a series of six to eight injections administered every 1–2 days has been observed to relieve symptoms for 4–6 months.[24]

It is common, however, to perform both the local anesthetic and neurolytic block on the same occasion, separated by only a brief interval, when 1) the diagnosis is relatively straightforward, 2) the recommended procedure is stressful and/or requires radiologic guidance (eg, celiac plexus block), and 3) it is performed in a debilitated patient who might withstand the stress of repeated procedures poorly.

INFORMED CONSENT

It is essential that informed consent be obtained, preferably from both the patient and a family member. This process serves multiple purposes (see Chapter 2). So-called "medico-legal" reasons have been cited, although experience shows that even an exhaustive consent process is no protection against a lawsuit,[33] and is certainly no substitute for the establishment of a close physician–patient relationship. Our experience is that even in the case of poor outcome, cancer patients tend to be nonlitigious, particularly when compassion and good intent on the part of the treatment team are well established. The consent process ideally serves as part of the educational process, and in this regard should be presented in a manner that is reassuring rather than threatening. By allaying anxiety and instilling confidence, cooperation and participation of the patient is enhanced. The informed consent should include a thorough explanation of the potential advantages, disadvantages, alternatives, and risks associated with the procedure, as well as a discussion of realistic expectations regarding its outcome.

PRETREATMENT

A careful physical examination with special attention to the neurologic system is per-formed before the procedure to verify physical findings and document preexisting deficits. When a major or bilateral sympathetic block is planned (celiac or hypogastric plexuses, lumbar sympathetic chain), hypotension may occur secondary to venous pooling, particularly in the presence of chronic dehydration or ongoing drainage from a surgical wound. In patients at risk for hypotensive sequelae, oral fluid intake is increased for several days before the procedure if there is no medical contraindication. Patients are advised to limit their diet to clear fluids for the period immediately preceding the block. Venous access is established, and if hypotension is anticipated 500–1,000 ml of balanced salt solution is infused.

SEDATION AND ANALGESIA

Intravenous sedatives and analgesics should not be administered routinely, but may be used on an individualized basis to facilitate positioning and patient comfort. Pharmacosedation is no substitute for personal attention and reassurance by health care providers. When required, short-acting agents should be used, and are administered cautiously on an incremental basis so as to avoid disorientation that might impair patient cooperation or interfere with the interpretation of the results of diagnostic/prognostic blockade. Patients should be accompanied by a responsible individual who can assure safe transportation home after a suitable period of observation has elapsed.

ANATOMY OF THE SYMPATHETIC NERVOUS SYSTEM

The peripheral portion of the sympathetic nervous system consists of a pair of ganglionated paravertebral chains that extend from the base of the skull to the coccyx, several major prevertebral plexuses (cardiac, celiac, and hypogastric), and numerous, small intermediate and terminal ganglia. The ganglia of the sympathetic chain lie on the anterolateral aspect of the vertebral column: they are positioned anterior to the transverse processes in the cervical region, anterior to the heads of the ribs in the thoracic region, along the sides of the vertebral bodies in the abdomen, and in front of the sacrum in the pelvis. The ganglia are inconstant in number due to fusion of adjacent components and anatomic variability among individuals, but the usual arrangement consists of 3 paired cervical ganglia, 12 paired thoracic ganglia, 4 paired lumbar ganglia, 4 paired sacral ganglia, and a single unpaired ganglion impar located near the sacrococcygeal junction.

Preganglionic sympathetic fibers originate from cells located within the anterolateral horn of the thoracolumbar spinal cord (T1–L2), are myelinated, exit the spinal cord with the anterior somatic motor roots, and then separate to become white rami communicantes, which enter the paravertebral chain of ganglia. Some white fibers synapse in the ganglion that corresponds segmentally to their site of origin, others travel up or down the chain to synapse in adjacent ganglia, and still others pass through the chain uninterrupted. Fibers in the latter group contribute to the formation of the splanchnic nerves (see "Celiac Plexus Block: Anatomic Considerations," below), and terminate by synapsing in more distant prevertebral ganglia (mesenteric, celiac, aorticorenal, renal, etc.) that subserve the abdominal viscera.

Some postganglionic fibers whose cell bodies are located within the paravertebral chain of ganglia form the nonmyelinated gray rami communicantes that rejoin and travel with the spinal nerves to be distributed segmentally as vasomotor, secretory, and pilomotor fibers to the blood vessels, sweat glands, and smooth muscle of the hair follicles.[34] Other postganglionic neurons originating in the paravertebral chain of ganglia supply the thoracic, abdominal, and pelvic viscera after first contributing to the formation of the major prevertebral, periaortic plexuses (cardiac, celiac, hypogastric). These major perivascular plexuses are aggregations of nerves and ganglia. Their fibers terminate either directly in neighboring viscera, or in more distant visceral after contributing to the formation of secondary plexuses, usually named for the branching arteries with which they are associated.[35] For example, branches of the celiac plexus contribute to the formation of the phrenic, splenic, hepatic, gastric, renal, testicular/ovarian, and mesenteric plexuses.

The complexity of the above system is apparent, and is amplified further by the existence of anomalous pathways and interindividual anatomic variation.[36] The regional anatomy of the sympathetic chain and its major peripheral or prevertebral plexuses is of greater clinical relevance, is depicted schematically in Figure 22–1, and is described in subsequent sections.

CERVICOTHORACIC (STELLATE GANGLION) SYMPATHETIC BLOCK

CLINICAL ANATOMY

The stellate or cervicothoracic ganglion usually is formed by the fusion of the inferior cervical and first thoracic paravertebral sympathetic ganglia. It is located characteristically at the base of the neck, anterior to the junction of the first rib and transverse process of the first thoracic vertebra, often extending cephalad to the level of the seventh cervical transverse process (Figs. 22–2 to 22–4). Its anatomic boundaries include the vertebral column and its fascial covering (longus colli muscle) posteriorly and medially, the subclavian artery and origin of the vertebral artery anteriorly, the scalenus muscles laterally, and the dome of the pleura inferiorly.

In practice, the stellate ganglion usually is accessed by an injection at the level of the C6 or C7 transverse process (Fig. 2–4), somewhat cephalic to its precise location. This technique is traditionally preferred because the risks of pneumothorax and arterial puncture are reduced, while efficacy is in most cases preserved. Its success depends on the ganglion's location within the same fascial plane as the remainder of the cervicothoracic sympathetic chain, and on diffusion of the injected solution caudally. If the correct fascial plane has

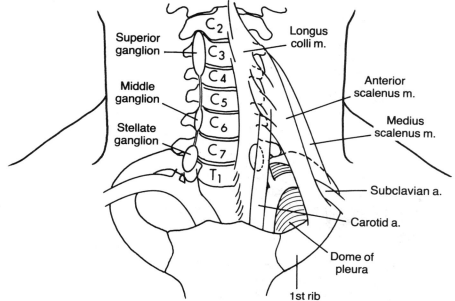

Figure 22–2. Anteroposterior schematic depicting regional anatomy pertinent to stellate ganglion block. Note ganglion's location at the C7–T1 level overlying the longus colli muscle level. Note proximity of the dome of the pleura, vascular structures, and epidural and subarachnoid space (via somatic nerve root sleeves).

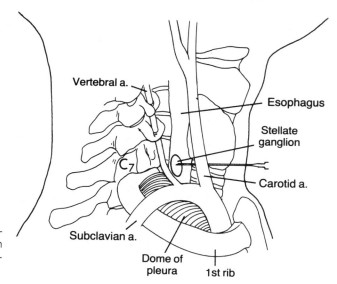

Figure 22–3. Oblique schematic view of the regional anatomy pertinent to stellate ganglion block, demonstrating features described for Figure 22–2.

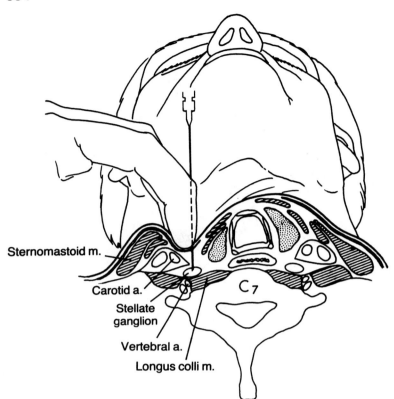

Sternomastoid m.

Carotid a.

Stellate ganglion

C7

Vertebral a.

Longus colli m.

Figure 22–4. Cross-sectional schematic demonstrating technique of stellate ganglion block at the C7 level. Technique is similar when block is performed at C6 level (see text). Note that the pressure exerted by the nondominant hand both retracts the carotid artery laterally and minimizes the distance between the skin and transverse process.

been located, injected material spreads freely along its craniocaudal axis (Fig. 22–5). Bonica has observed the following correlation between volume and spread of contrast medium: 5 ml—C6–T2; 10–12 ml—C5–T4; 20 ml—C3–T5.[36]

TECHNIQUE

At least 12 techniques for anesthetizing the stellate ganglion have been described, including anterior, lateral, anterolateral, and superior approaches. The anterior paratracheal approach, introduced by LeRiche in 1934,[37] is applied almost universally because of its simplicity and relative safety.

The patient lies supine with the neck neutral or slightly extended, and a wide field is cleansed aseptically to allow palpation of regional landmarks. Mild cervical extension thins out the intervening prevertebral tissue, and may pull the esophagus away from the transverse process on the left. Overextension is avoided to abrogate undesirable tension of the strap muscles; the patient is instructed to open his or her mouth slightly to relax the strap muscles further. The C6 transverse process is located either by tracing a horizontal line from the level of the cricoid cartilage or by palpating Chassaignac's tubercle. The index and middle fingers of the nondominant hand are inserted gently but firmly between the trachea and the anterior belly of the sternocleidomastoid muscle and are directed downward and laterally. The downward motion compresses the soft tissue of the neck against the vertebral column, minimizing the distance to be traversed by the needle. Lateral traction "hooks" the sternocleidomastoid muscle and

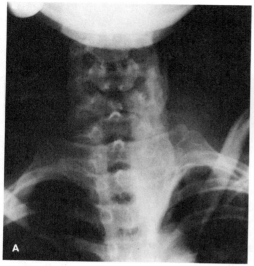
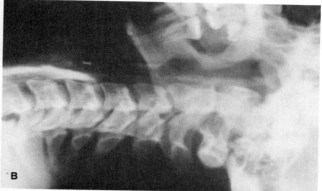

Figure 22–5. Characteristic spread of contrast medium after stellate ganglion block with 10 ml radiopaque solution injected at C7 (needle removed). **(A)** Note homologous column of widely spread dye, the caudal aspect of which is rounded and outlines the pleural apex. **(B)** Contrast is layered over vertebral bodies and longus colli muscle.

carotid artery away from the needle path. Carotid artery puncture is avoided by assuring that the carotid pulse is felt against the pads of the index and middle finger. A slight separation between the middle and index fingers marks the point of needle insertion, and corresponds to the transverse process of C6. A skin wheal may be raised here, but is usually unnecessary because, when performed properly, the procedure is quick and minimally painful. Patients are cautioned not to move, swallow, or phonate during the procedure, and may benefit from instructions to clear their throat and swallow before commencing.

When assistance is available, it is preferable to work with a needle attached to a syringe by means of sterile extension tubing,[38] so that the operator can stabilize the needle better during injection, while his or her assistant aspirates gently and continuously during insertion. A 1.5-inch (3.8-cm) 22-gauge needle is introduced perpendicular to the skin in all planes, and is steadily advanced until bone is contacted, usually at a depth of about 0.5–1 inch (1–4 cm). Before injecting, the needle is withdrawn about 2 mm to free its tip from the substance of the longus colli muscle. Most authorities recommend rotating the needle in several planes while continuing aspiration to detect blood or cerebrospinal fluid. A test dose of 1 ml is then injected to exclude aberrant placement and to dislodge any tissue from the lumen of one needle. Resistance to injection may indicate periosteal or intramuscular placement, and should prompt repeating contact with the bone to verify the needle's depth. If aspiration is negative and the test dose is injected without sequelae, then the remainder of the solution is injected relatively rapidly. A total of 10 ml usually is sufficient to produce desired results when injection is at the level of C6,[39] although Löfström recommends 15–20 ml,[40] and Carron only 5 ml.[41] If treatment is directed toward relieving upper limb pain, most authorities recommend that once the injection is complete, the patient assume a semisitting position in order to facilitate caudad diffusion.[42] Factors suggesting successful blockade of the cervicothoracic chain include ipsilateral Horner's sign (ptosis, enophthalmos, miosis, anhidrosis, facial flushing), chemosis of the ocular conjunctiva, nasal stuffiness, and elevated temperature and vasodilation of the ipsilateral upper extremity. Other sequelae sometime include shoulder pain, hoarseness (superior laryngeal nerve block), and dysphagia.

Aspirated blood usually indicates that the needle has passed between the transverse processes and that the vertebral artery has been punctured deep to the chain. The injection of even small amounts of anesthetic here should be avoided scrupulously because of the likelihood of the onset of immediate seizure and loss of consciousness. Resuscitation equipment should be immediately available. If local anesthetics are being used, the needle is withdrawn, and repositioned slightly more cephalad or caudad. If bone is contacted, the injection usually can be performed safely after careful aspiration and observation of the patient's response to several small test doses. Intra-arterial injection of a neurolytic agent may precipitate a stroke. If arterial puncture has occurred during attempted neurolysis, it is prudent to interrupt the procedure for a short period of time to reduce further the risk of intra-arterial injection.

MODIFICATIONS

Block at the Level of C7

The above approach may be modified slightly for needle placement at the level of the C7 transverse process to increase the likelihood of a more complete block of the brachial sympathetic outflow.[42,43] A smaller volume of solution (5–8 ml) can be used, and hoarseness due to superior laryngeal block is less likely to occur. The patient is placed in a semi-Fowler's position (supine with the back raised 15°), and a firm pad is placed beneath the shoulders to improve access to the base of the neck. The site of injection lies one to two fingerbreadths lower than in the latter description, or 3 cm above the sternoclavicular junction. The apex of the lung is closely related to the sympathetic chain, especially in tall, thin people, and

this technique is associated with an increased risk of pneumothorax. As a further safety precaution, the patient may be instructed to expire deeply before needle insertion.

Stellate Ganglion Neurolysis

The advisability of stellate ganglion neurolysis is considered controversial by almost all authors.[40,42] Repeated local anesthetic blocks have been favored as an alternative because of the hazards posed by the proximity of other important structures. Inaccurate needle placement or excessive spread of the neurolytic solution may result in long-lasting injury to neurologic structures (brachial plexus, superior laryngeal nerve, phrenic nerve, epidural and subarachnoid space) and non-neurologic structures (vertebral and carotid arteries, larynx, esophagus). However, if local anesthetic injections have been documented to provide consistent but temporary relief of pain, surgical extirpation of the ganglia may be considered, or neurolysis may be performed cautiously using radiologic guidance and small volumes of injectate.

Racz et al[12] reported successful stellate gangliolysis in over 100 patients without any serious complications, and they recently described their modifications to the classic technique in detail (summarized here). The site for needle entry is at the C7 level, as noted immediately above. To decrease the risk of injury to pleura, adjacent nerve roots, a dural cuff, or the vertebral artery, the ventrolateral aspect of the C7 vertebral body is targeted instead of its transverse process (Fig. 22–6). This is accomplished by orienting the needle 15°–30° toward the midline and observing its passage under fluoroscopy. Once bony contact occurs (just medial rather than anterior to the insertion of the longus colli muscle), the needle is withdrawn 1–2 mm to free its tip from the substance of the anterior longitudinal ligament. The needle is stabilized with a hemostat, and 1 ml of nonionic contrast medium is injected. Racz et al recommend the injection of 5 ml of phenol, saline, local anesthetic, and steroid mixed to achieve an ultimate concentration of 3% phenol (2.5 ml 6%

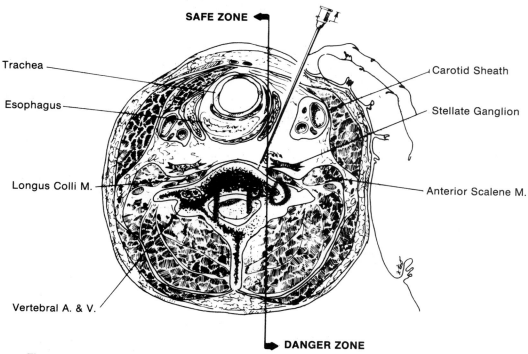

Figure 22–6. Schematic demonstrating Racz's technique for neurolytic stellate ganglion block. Note that the standard anterior approach has been modified by the introduction of a mesiad inclination to the needle, which is placed at the C7 level. The needle tip is intended to reach the vertebral body medial to the indention of the longus colli muscle. An imaginary line separates the "safe zone" from the "danger zone," where complications related to injection near the vertebral artery, exiting spinal nerve root, and epidural space may be less likely to occur. Reproduced with permission from Racz BG, Holubec JT: Stellate ganglion phenol neurolysis. In Racz GB (ed): Techniques of Neurolysis p 137. Boston, Kluwer, 1989.

phenol in saline, 2.5 ml 0.5% bupivacaine, 80 mg methylprednisone). This displaces the previously injected contrast medium, the margins of which then correspond roughly to the extent that the phenol solution has spread. After injections, patients are maintained in the supine position with the head slightly elevated for 30 minutes. In a series of over 100 patients, pain relief and alteration in vasomotor changes accrued rapidly and were relatively long-lasting, although repeated injections (1–4, mean of 1.6) frequently were needed, probably because the phenol solution used was relatively dilute. The only negative sequelae in patients treated in this fashion were transient chest wall pain in one patient, transient dysphagia in another, and Horner's syndrome of moderate duration (6–8 months) in a third.

Serial Transcatheter Blockade

A method of continuous or serial stellate ganglion blockade has been described that involves anterior paratracheal placement of a catheter under radiologic control.[44] Displacement of the catheter tip secondary to patient movement is possible, and caution is recommended if this approach is used. It is likely that continuous stellate ganglion blockade will be relied on more in the near future as a result of the development of more specialized catheter technology (see Appendix F).

Pediatrics

Therapeutic local anesthetic block of the stellate ganglion in a 2-week-old premature infant with arterial insufficiency[45] has been reported, suggesting that the above techniques could be adapted for pediatric patients.

THORACIC SYMPATHETIC NERVE BLOCK

FUNDAMENTAL CONSIDERATIONS

The thoracic sympathetic ganglia are selected infrequently as targets for neural blockade relative to other sites within the sympathetic nervous system.[40,42] This is in part because of hazards posed by the chain's regional anatomy (see below), and the relative simplicity and efficacy of alternative techniques such as intrathecal, epidural, and paravertebral somatic blocks. A posterior, paravertebral approach to the thoracic sympathetic chain first was suggested by Kappis[46] in 1912, and subsequently was modified and further described by Labat,[47] Adriani,[48] and Bonica.[36]

The thoracic sympathetic chain lies posterolateral to the vertebral bodies and anterior to the neck of the ribs (Figs. 22–7 and 22–8). Unlike the sympathetic chain in the cervical and lumbar regions, which is separated from the roots of the segmental somatic nerves by the longus colli and psoas muscles, respectively, no effective anatomic barrier exists between the sympathetic and somatic nerves in the thoracic region.[40] As a result, extremely precise needle localization and careful limitation of injected volume are essential to avoid spillage on to somatic roots and consequent risks of segmental numbness, motor weakness, and dysesthesia. Further, the thoracic sympathetic chain is related laterally to the pleura and medially to the intravertebral foramina, introducing risks of pneumothorax or accidental subarachnoid or epidural anesthesia from aberrant needle placement.

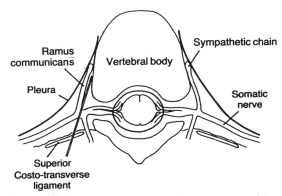

Figure 22–7. Cross-sectional schematic view of thoracic sympathetic block with needle in proper position. Note proximity of pleura, somatic nerve root, and epidural and intrathecal compartments.

INDICATIONS

Upper Limb

Oncologic conditions affecting the upper limb that are amenable to treatment with sympathetic blockade have been discussed (see above). Anesthesia of the second and third thoracic sympathetic ganglia usually results in complete interruption of the sympathetic fibers subserving the upper limb. Treatment can be provided either with cervicothoracic (stellate) block by the anterior paratracheal approach (see above), or by blockade of the upper thoracic ganglia by the posterior approach, each of which have distinct advantages and disadvantages. To obtain full sympathetic denervation with stellate block, the volume of drug required imposes risks of permanent Horner's syndrome and spread to the neighboring brachial plexus, superior laryngeal nerve, and even phrenic nerve.[49] The technique, however, is familiar, and may be warranted if diagnostic blocks with local anesthetic have yielded good results. Racz et al[12] have proposed several modifications intended to promote safe neurolysis (see "Stellate Ganglion Neurolysis," above). The presence of fascial barriers has been cited as a factor that may further impede the spread of

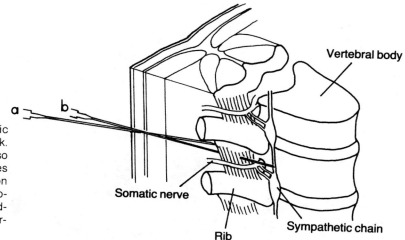

Figure 22–8. Lateral schematic view of thoracic sympathetic block. Needle initially is introduced so that its tip intentionally impinges on the superior rib near its junction with corresponding transverse process (a), then is withdrawn, readjusted, and advanced into the paravertebral space (b).

injected solutions to an appropriately caudal level when the cervicothoracic approach is used.[36] The posterior approach to the upper thoracic ganglia is less familiar, and is associated with the potential for pneumothorax and neuraxial spread. The advantages of the posterior approach are that when it is performed with careful attention to detail, it allows for more precise blockade with smaller volumes of drug, obviating the risks of the anterior approach. Radiologic guidance is essential.[40]

Thorax

The main indication for thoracic sympathetic blockade in the midthoracic region is visceral pain from esophageal neoplasm or pleuritic pain secondary to underlying lung cancer.[36] Performing multiple injections of the thoracic chain is technically challenging, and may be poorly tolerated in a debilitated patient, so consideration should be given to alternative techniques such as subarachnoid or epidural neurolysis (see Chapters 20 and 23).

Abdomen

The midthoracic and lower thoracic ganglia contribute to the formation of the splanchnic nerves, which ultimately provide sympathetic innervation to the abdominal viscera. Because

of the above considerations and the relative ease and efficacy of celiac plexus and splanchnic nerve block (see below), these latter techniques are preferred for pain due to abdominal neoplasm.

TECHNIQUE

The prone position is preferred when permitted by the patient's overall condition, but alternatively the lateral decubitus position with the painful side positioned upward may be used. Radiologic guidance is strongly recommended, particularly when a neurolytic block is proposed, and a scout film or fluoroscopy is used to locate the vertebral level that corresponds to the patient's pain. A skin wheal is raised 3 cm lateral to the cephalad aspect of the spinous process of the targeted segment. A 22-gauge, 8–10-cm needle initially is inserted perpendicular to the skin in all planes until rib or transverse process is contacted, usually at a depth of 2.5–3.5 cm (Fig. 22–8). Some craniocaudad adjustment from the perpendicular may be required, and is aided by fluoroscopy. The needle is withdrawn so that its tip lies just beneath the skin, and it is redirected slightly cephalad. A saline-filled syringe is attached to the needle hub, and gentle

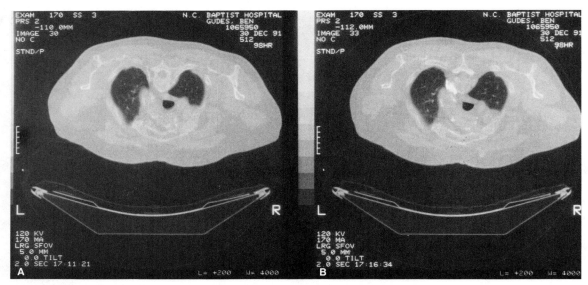

Figure 22–9. Computed tomography scan demonstrating correct needle placement for paravertebral thoracic sympathetic nerve block. **(A)** Depicts needle placement before the injection of contrast medium. **(B)** Postinjection of contrast medium. Courtesy of Richard Rauck, MD, Pain Control Center, North Carolina Baptist Hospital.

unremitting or intermittent pressure is exerted on its barrel as the needle is reintroduced until its tip impinges on the superior border of the rib. As the needle is slowly advanced beyond the depth at which osseous contact was previously noted, the operator may first appreciate increased resistance to its passage and to attempted injection, which corresponds to the superior costotransverse ligament, then decreased resistance, indicating that the paravertebral space containing the sympathetic chain has been entered. Passage through the ligament may be heralded by a transmitted palpable "click," better appreciated as experience accrues and amplified by the use of a blunt-tipped or larger-gauge needle. The position of the needle tip should lie anterior and inferior to the exiting somatic nerve root. Confirmation of accurate placement is assured further by the observation of the spread of injected contrast medium (Fig. 22–9), which should be confined to the paramedian and should spread freely in the craniocaudad axis. After careful aspiration, a test dose of 1–3 ml of local anesthetic is performed

to further exclude subarachnoid, epidural, and somatic nerve root involvement. Finally, 2–3 ml of neurolytic solution (6%–7% aqueous phenol) is injected, and the needle is cleared with air before its removal to prevent spillage along the needle track.

LUMBAR SYMPATHETIC BLOCK

Mandl first described a technique for blockade of the lumbar sympathetic chain in 1926[50] that subsequently has been modified by Bryce-Smith,[51] Reid,[52] Boas,[53] Raj,[42] and others. Despite these variations, the basic technique is similar to Kappis' approach to the celiac plexus (see below), but is carried out at a lower level.

INDICATIONS

The greatest utility for neurolytic lumbar sympathetic block is in the management of nononcologic sympathetically maintained pain due either to intractable sympathetic dystrophy or nonoperable ischemic pain.[40] Neoplastic causes of lower extremity pain usually are somatically mediated, and must be differentiated from pain associated with involvement of the sympathetic nervous system. Lumbar plexopathy due either to tumor invasion or radiation fibrosis may present with dysesthetic pain resembling reflex sympathetic dystrophy,[54] which may be amenable to treatment with neural blockade of the lumbar sympathetic chain. Several cases of painful hot foot due to tumor involvement of the lumbar sympathetic chain have been well described in patients with cervical and rectal carcinoma.[55,56] Painful lymphedema of the lower extremity likewise is treatable by lumbar sympatholysis.

Before the recent introduction of superior hypogastric plexus block,[13] lumbar sympathetic block had been used with some frequency to treat lower abdominal, pelvic, and some perineal pain problems,[57] and probably still has significance (see below). Visceral pelvic pain of lower urogenital and rectal origin may be amenable to treatment with lumbar sympathetic blockade, although time may prove blockade of the superior hypogastric plexus to be more specific and effective. Pain of renal origin, due either to invasion of surrounding structures or stretching of the perinephric capsule, is an indication for a trial of lumbar sympatholysis, as is the dysesthetic pain that sometimes follows nephrectomy (so-called "phantom kidney").[58] In these cases, blockade may need to be extended to include the T12 ganglia in order to be most effective. Lumbar sympatholysis performed with 5–12 ml of 6% phenol in water injected bilaterally produced long-term relief of rectal tenesmus in 10 of 12 patients with pelvic cancer.[59] Isolated case reports documenting relief of nononcologic abdominal[60] and prostatic pain[61] treated with phenol lumbar sympatholysis suggest applicability for patients with cancer as well. The testes are multiply innervated due in part to their *in utero* descent from the abdominal wall, and pain here may be amenable to lumbar sympathetic block. Lower abdominal complaints are often multifactorial,

and are usually sufficiently vague that diagnostic blockade with local anesthetics should be considered a prerequisite to neurolysis.

In contrast to subarachnoid injection, risks of bowel, bladder, and motor dysfunction are virtually nil, particularly when radiologic guidance is used.

REGIONAL ANATOMY

The anatomic arrangement of the lumbar sympathetic chain is said to be the most variable of the entire sympathetic system.[36] In addition to variation among individuals, its disposition often is asymmetric within the same person. Most commonly, there is fusion of the T12 and L1 ganglia and a total of four ganglia on each side, although the number of ganglia frequently varies between three and five. The location of the chain and its ganglia also is inconstant: the chain may be closely related to the vertebral bodies or situated anterior to the aponeurotic arcades of the psoas muscle; ganglia may be segmentally distributed or closely grouped and concentrated over a particular segment. Most commonly, ganglia are grouped between the cephalad portion of the L2 body and the caudad aspect of the L4 body. Umeda et al[62] analyzed the morphology of the lumbar sympathetic system in 19 cadavers. They reported that the ganglia most frequently are located at the level of the intravertebral disc at L2 and L3, usually extending cephalocaudad to relate to the neighboring margins of the vertebral bodies above and below. Ganglia range in size from 3–5 mm in width and 10–15 mm in length.

The lumbar part of the sympathetic chain lies within a fascial plane close to the anterolateral aspect of the vertebral bodies, separated from the somatic chain by the psoas muscle and psoas fascia (Figs. 22–10 and 22–11). Injection of a large volume of solution (*eg*, 25 ml) at any single level generally will fill the entire space, and bathe all of the ganglia. This approach commonly is used at L2 or L3 to achieve local anesthetic blockade, but when a neurolytic block is planned, most authorities recommend injecting smaller volumes

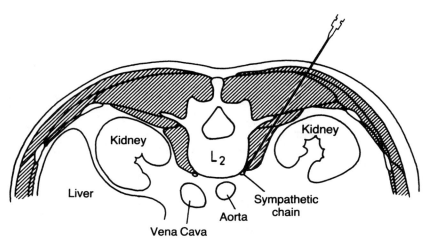

Figure 22–10. Cross-sectional schematic view of lumbar sympathetic block demonstrating passage of paravertebral needle through anterior psoas fascia.

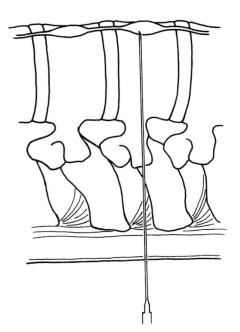

Figure 22–11. Lateral schematic view of lumbar sympathetic block depicting needle's ultimate destination in proximity to sympathetic chain.

through two to three needles placed at different levels. The latter approach is intended to promote cephalocaudad spread while limiting lateral extension at any single level. This at least theoretically promotes more complete blockade, and reduces the likelihood of complications from passage of solution across the psoas muscle to the genitofemoral nerve, through a fibrous tunnel to the somatic chain, or into the dural cuff region. Based on extensive experience with chemical sympathectomy performed with two needles versus one needle, Boas et al recently have recommended the use of a single needle placed at L2 or L3 as being equally safe and efficacious as the use of multiple needles, although the latter practice still is common.[63]

TECHNIQUE

The patient is positioned prone on a radiolucent table with a firm bolster placed beneath the pelvis to extend the lumbar spine. Surface landmarks and fluoroscopy are used to help identify the spinous processes of L2–L4 at a distance of 8–10 cm (four fingerbreadths) from the midline. This distance should correspond to the lateral border of the erector spinae muscle group, which is readily palpable in most individuals. The L1 spinous process generally corresponds to the junction of the lateral border of this muscle mass and the 12th rib, and the inferior portion of the L4 spinous process to a line joining the iliac crests.

Since the procedure is potentially uncomfortable, especially when performed at multiple levels or bilaterally, intravenous premedication and/or generous local infiltration should be considered. When the three-needle technique is used, skin wheals are raised at the levels of the L2, L3, and L4 spinous processes. A 3.5-inch (9 cm), 25-gauge needle is introduced through each wheal, and the muscle mass between the point of insertion and the corresponding vertebral body is infiltrated freely with local anesthetic, roughly along a 45° angle.

Needle length varies from 5–7 inches (12–18 cm), depending on the patient's body habitus. Twenty- or 22-gauge needles may be used. The former are less likely to bend, and are sometimes favored because they more readily transmit differences in tissue compliance and an absence of resistance to injection. Nevertheless, the use of 22-gauge needles is less painful and traumatic and generally is preferred, especially when fluoroscopy can be depended on to compensate for perceived differences. Needles are introduced at about a 45° angle with the midline and are advanced until the vertebral body is contacted, usually at a depth of about 4 inches (10 cm). Premature bony contact, usually about 5 cm deep to the skin, indicates that the transverse process has been contacted. The transverse process is distinguished further from the vertebral body with the aid of fluoroscopy and by the former's marble-like hardness, noticeably distinct from the gritty, yielding sensation that is transmitted when the body is contacted. If transverse process has been contacted, the needle is withdrawn and redirected slightly cephalad. The depth at which the body has been contacted is noted, and the needle is withdrawn to the level of the skin and redirected so that its tip slides just past the lateral margin of the corresponding vertebral body to a depth of about 1 cm beyond the prior

insertion (Fig. 22–12A,B). A palpable "click" is sometimes appreciated as the psoas fascia is breached. Some authors advocate attaching a glass syringe and using a loss-of-resistance technique to assist further in identifying the correct fascial plane.[64]

Once preliminary needle placement and aspiration tests are complete, 1–3 ml of non-ionic contrast medium is injected through each needle, and the spread of dye is observed (Fig. 22–13). The characteristic appearance on lateral views is of a thin column of dye anterior to the vertebral bodies, with a smooth posterior contour corresponding to the anterior border of the psoas fascia. Anterior views should demonstrate contrast medium confined to the paramedian region with no tracking along the psoas muscle. Most commonly, a total of 5 ml of 6%–7% aqueous phenol is injected subsequently on each side that is to be treated. Alternatively, computed tomography (CT) guidance may be used (Fig. 22–14).

CELIAC PLEXUS BLOCK

Celiac plexus block remains one of the most effective and commonly used nerve blocks performed to provide prolonged relief of cancer pain. Blockade of the celiac plexus has potential utility to relieve pain stemming from a variety of conditions, including, most prominently, cancer involving the upper and mid-abdomen,[65-68] but also acute visceral disease,[69,70] other chronic visceral disorders,[71-73] and discomfort associated with hepatic embolization for the treatment of carcinoma.[74] The most common indication for celiac axis block is in the management of upper abdominal and referred back pain secondary to pancreatic cancer, which, contrary to traditional teaching, frequently is associated with painful rather than painless jaundice.[65] Despite its location deep within the body (Figs. 22–15 to 22–17), the proximity of major organs (aorta, vena cava, kidneys, pleura, etc), and requirements for a large volume of neurolytic (up to 50 ml of 50% alcohol), complication rates are uniformly low.[65] Success has even been reported recently in a 4-year-old child,[75] albeit

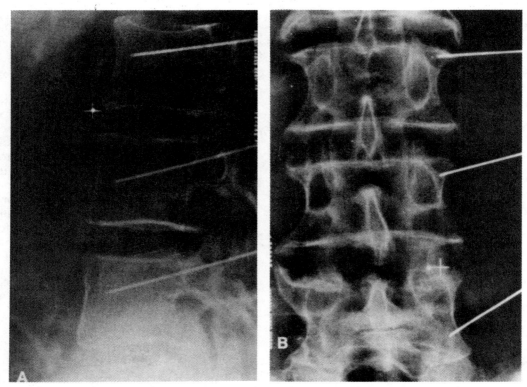

Figure 22–12. Lateral **(A)** and posteroanterior **(B)** radiographs demonstrating correct needle placement (before instillation of contrast medium) for lumbar sympathetic block. Classic three-needle technique (L2, L3, L4) is depicted, although procedure alternatively may be performed with a single needle (see text). Reproduced with permission from Lofstrom JB, Lloyd JW, Cousins MJ: Sympathetic neural blockade of upper and lower extremity. In Cousins MJ, Bridenbaugh PO (eds): Neural Blockade, 1st ed, p 375. Philadelphia, JB Lippincott, 1980.

under general anesthesia. The introduction and widespread acceptance of radiologic control and modifications of classic techniques have contributed to this technique's favorable risk-to-benefit ratio.

The celiac plexus contributes to the innervation of all of the intra-abdominal structures derived from embryonic foregut, including much of the gastrointestinal tract (distal esophagus, stomach, duodenum, small bowel, ascending and proximal transverse colon), pancreas, adrenal glands, spleen, and liver and biliary system. Although most experience is derived from the treatment of pancreatic cancer pain,[66] celiac block has

been demonstrated to be effective for a variety of painful conditions emanating from other intra-abdominal malignant neoplasms as well.[67,68]

DEVELOPMENT OF THE TECHNIQUE

Kappis[76] was the first investigator to introduce anesthesia of the splanchnic nerves in a preliminary report presented in 1914 to the Congress of Surgery in Berlin, which was documented further in a published report of a series of 200 cases in 1918.[77] His technique, which used two needles introduced posteri-

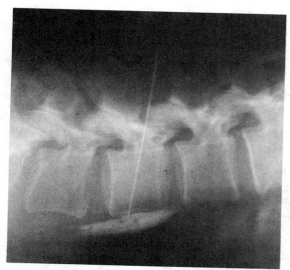

Figure 22–13. Lateral radiograph of lumbar sympathetic block performed at the L4 level with a single needle. Note smooth contours of contrast medium injected anterior to the psoas muscle, and absence of vascular run-off.

orly, has undergone numerous subsequent modifications, but still serves as the basis for techniques used in contemporary practice. At around the same time, Wendling[78] suggested an anterior approach to the splanchnic nerves that involved the introduction of a long needle through the intact anterior abdominal wall a little below and to the left of the ensiform cartilage. Passage through the left lobe of the liver and lesser omentum was required to reach the retroperitoneal nerves and ganglia. This method was demonstrated to be inaccurate and dangerous, and was quickly abandoned. Interestingly, 70 years later, a modified percutaneous anterior approach using CT guidance was introduced again, and has gained enthusiastic acceptance.[10] Braun, in 1919,[79] introduced direct anesthesia of the splanchnic nerves and the solar plexus at the time of laparotomy. Labat, in 1920,[80] also described a technique of anesthetizing the splanchnic nerves by a posterior route, similar to that of Kappis, but modifying the inclination of the needles from an angle of 30° to one of 45° (see Fig. 22–16).

Roussiel, in 1923, also used a posterior approach, naming this method paravertebral anesthesia, a term that has remained in continuous use.[81] In the same year, Lewen[82] demonstrated that by infiltrating procaine hydrochloride around the lower thoracic and upper lumbar white rami, the sensory fibers transmitting painful sensations from the upper ab-

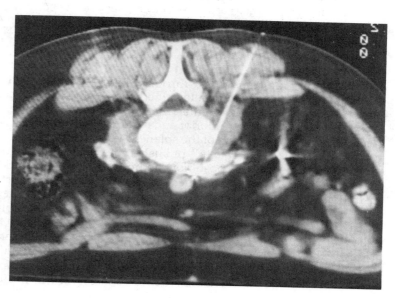

Figure 22–14. Cross-sectional CT of bilateral lumbar sympathetic nerve block with needle tips and contrast medium visualized anterior to psoas muscles. Left side easier to visualize than right. Courtesy Dr. Steven Waldman, Kansas City Pain Consortium.

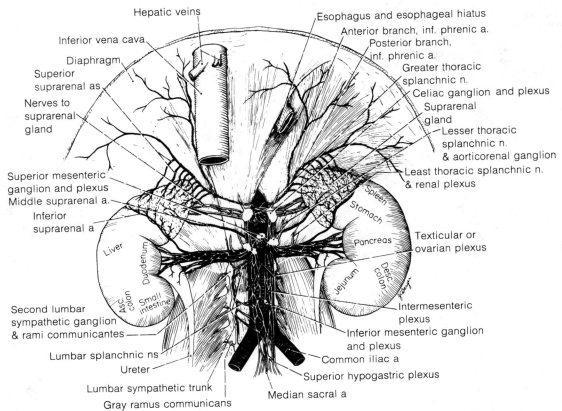

Figure 22–15. Anterior view of regional anatomy pertaining to celiac plexus block, with intraperitoneal organs and other structures removed for better visualization. Reproduced with permission from Woodburne RT, Burkel WE: Essentials of Human Anatomy, p 495. New York, Oxford University Press, 1988.

dominal viscera are transmitted through the splanchnic nerves, and also determined the levels at which these fibers enter the cord. Labat, in 1924, detailed the anterior and posterior approaches to the region of the splanchnic nerves.[83,84] In 1927, De Takats[85] published a study of the anterior and posterior methods of anesthetizing the splanchnic nerves, demonstrating both experimentally and clinically that bilateral splanchnic block produces anesthesia of the upper abdominal organs. In 1947, Gage and Floyd[86] described the posterior approach with the patient in either the prone or lateral position. In 1949, Esnaurizzar[87] recommended splanchnic block for the relief of ab-

dominal pain. Blockade of the splanchnic nerves was postulated to relieve acute pain by alleviating vasospasm, emptying blocked secretions by relaxing the sphincter of Oddi, and reducing sympathetic stimulation of pancreatic secretions. Popper[88] reported on both the therapeutic and diagnostic efficacy of left-sided paravertebral block of T8–T10 in four cases of acute pancreatitis. Mallet-Guy and associates[89] produced acute pancreatitis in dogs by electrical stimulation of the left splanchnic nerves, and later reported the efficacy of a limited splanchnicectomy in relief of the pain of chronic pancreatitis.[90]

It was in 1959 that Jones[91] first described a

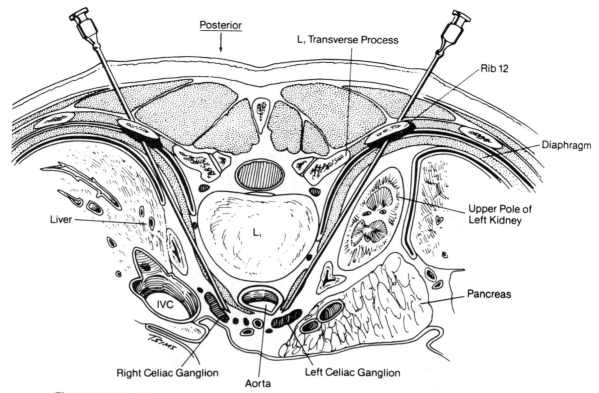

Figure 22–16. Cross-sectional schematic view of the celiac plexus and its regional anatomy. Figure depicts classic retrocrural technique of Kappis. Reproduced with permission from Raj PP: Chronic pain. In Raj PP (ed): Clinical Practice of Regional Anesthesia, p 496. New York, Churchill Livingstone, 1991.

technique for injecting the splanchnic nerves with alcohol to produce more enduring pain relief. Bridenbaugh et al reported the first 41 cases documented for the management of upper abdominal cancer.[92] Moore, in 1965, refined the technique of Kappis.[43]

Pancreatic cancer pain, and, secondarily, pain from other intra-abdominal neoplasms, have evolved as the most frequent applications for celiac block. Significant relief of pain, although often inadequately characterized[92a], generally is reported to result in between 70%–94% of patients,[65,93] with most studies reporting successful results in the higher ranges. Duration of relief varies considerably between weeks and a year or more, although the majority of treated patients experience rel-

atively pain-free deaths.[65] In one study of 136 patients with pancreatic cancer, celiac plexus block resulted in good pain relief in 85% of cases, 75% of whom died relatively free of pain.[66] In a study of patients with pain secondary to other intra-abdominal neoplasms performed by one of the same authors, 73% of 66 patients had good initial relief, of whom 59% died relatively free of pain.[68] The efficacy and duration of the pain relief are presumed to be related to the completeness of celiac ablation and the relative presence of concomitant pain of somatic origin, which requires other therapeutic measures.

In 1978, Boas[53] differentiated between the retrocrural and transcrural approach (see below), a distinction that was refined further by

Anatomy and Two Approaches to Celiac and Splanchnic Nerve Block

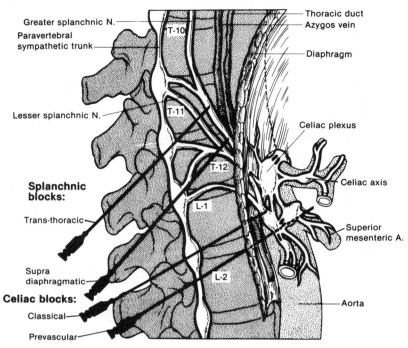

Figure 22–17. Lateral schematic view of alternate approaches to the splanchnic nerves and celiac plexus. The uppermost needle depicts a new approach advocated by Boas that uses a standard 22 g spinal needle introduced through the eleventh intercostal space (see reference). The adjacent needle represents the classic approach to splanchnic nerve block with ultimate placement at the T12 level above and behind the diaphragm. The lowest two insertions depict celiac plexus block performed at the L1 level using a transcrural and transaortic approach, from top-to-bottom respectively. Reproduced with permission from Abram SE, Boas RA: Sympathetic and visceral nerve blocks. In Benumof JL: Clinical Procedures in Anesthesia and Intensive Care. Philadelphia, JB Lippincott, 1992, p 798.

Singler's[9] CT-guided approach (see below). In 1982, Ischia described a transaortic method of celiac block (see below),[11] and 6 years later a CT-guided anterior approach was introduced.[10]

ANATOMIC CONSIDERATIONS

Different references have used terms such as celiac plexus, splanchnic plexus, solar plexus, semilunar ganglia, celiac ganglia, and abdominal brain of Bichat to refer to part or all of this great sympathetic nerve center. The etiology of these terms relates variously to the proximity of the adjacent artery (celiac), contributing nerves (splanchnic), or the general shape and body location (solar, semilunar).

The celiac plexus is the largest of the three great sympathetic nervous system plexuses: the cardiac plexus innervates thoracic structures, the celiac plexus innervates abdominal organs, and the hypogastric plexus supplies pelvic viscera.[94] All three contain visceral afferent and visceral efferent sympathetic fibers as well as parasympathetic fibers.

The regional anatomy of the celiac plexus is clinically important, and must be understood thoroughly to optimize results and minimize complications. The general location of the plexus is within the epigastrium, usually at the level of the upper portion of the L1 vertebral body, although in one study of cadavers the height of the ganglia ranged between the L2 vertebral body and T12–L1 intravertebral disc.[95] It lies within the retroperitoneal space behind the stomach and omental bursa, and in front of the crura of the diaphragm and vertebral column. The plexus can be conceived of as a diffuse network of interconnected neural fibers distributed around the aorta, embedded in loose, fatty areolar tissue. Its location and configuration are subject to considerable variation, but the plexus tends to be most consolidated around the roots of the celiac and superior mesenteric arteries, although it may extend as far caudad as the renal plexus. Although periaortic in location, fibers tend to be concentrated ventral to the aorta. In addition to other ganglionated structures, the plexus usually contains two large, relatively discrete semilunar ganglia, the mean measurements of which in one study were 2.79 × 1.43 cm on the right and 2.39 × 1.83 cm on the left.[95] The relatively lower position of the left versus the right celiac ganglion contrasts with the general tendency of paired abdominal organs (kidneys, adrenal glands). On the right, the ganglion lies behind and medial to the inferior vena cava, as well as behind the upper part of the head of the pancreas, part of the duodenum, and the lower end of the portal vein. The left ganglion is covered by the splenic vessels as well as the pancreas, and is more intimately related to the aorta. The phrenic arteries are superior and the renal vessels are inferior to the plexus, whereas the suprarenal vessels often pass through interstices within its substance. The entire plexus occupies an area about 3 cm in length and 4 cm wide that, in the transverse plane, occupies the region between the adrenal glands and upper poles of the kidneys on each side, and extends beyond the lateral

borders of the aorta on both sides. In the longitudinal plane, it occupies the area delineated by the celiac artery above and the renal arteries below. It is thus situated in front of the entire L1 vertebra, and often the upper portion of L2 and the lower portion of T12. The pleura and base of the lungs form another important cephalic relation (see Figs. 22–15 to 22–17).

Numerous structures converge to comprise the plexus. These include the greater, lesser, and least splanchnic nerves (composed of preganglionic branches from the thoracic ganglia 5–9, 10–11, and 12, respectively), white rami from the neighboring sympathetic trunk, and fibers of both vagus nerves. In addition to the celiac ganglia *per se*, the plexus also is made up of the superior mesenteric, aorticorenal, and inferior mesenteric ganglia.

The celiac plexus gives off secondary plexuses to the diaphragm, liver, spleen, stomach, adrenal glands, pancreas, ovary and fundus of the uterus, spermatic cord, abdominal aorta, mesentery, small intestine, and colon. Although sympathetic and parasympathetic motor fibers themselves probably do not transmit pain, afferent (sensory) nerve fibers that course with them transmit nociceptive impulses from the viscera.[2,5,96]

TECHNIQUE

Classic Retrocrural Technique

The most straightforward and frequently applied approach to blocking the celiac plexus is the retrocrural technique described in 1919 by Kappis[77] and subsequently refined by Moore.[43]

As with other techniques, preparation includes insertion of an intravenous catheter and consideration of prehydration (see above, "Patient Preparation: Diagnostic Versus Therapeutic Blockade"). The patient is positioned prone, and, if tolerated, either the table is flexed or a pillow is placed under the abdomen to reverse the normal lordosis, thus increasing the interval between the inferior margin of the rib cage and the iliac crests. The patient's head is turned to the side, flat to the table, and the arms are permitted to dangle freely off each side of the table. The field is widely prepped in a standard aseptic fashion, after which it may be elected to delineate the pertinent landmarks with a sterile marker. These include the iliac crests, 12th ribs, dorsal midline, vertebral bodies (T12–L2), and the lateral borders of the paraspinal (sacrospinalis) muscles. Moore[43] recommends that the intersection of the 12th rib and the lateral border of the paraspinal muscles on each side (which corresponds to L2) be connected with lines to each other and the cephalic portion of the L1 spine, forming an isosceles triangle, the sides of which serve as an additional guide to the correct needle trajectory.

Skin wheals are raised at the points of entry, just beneath the 12th ribs, about four fingerbreadths or about 7.5 cm lateral to the midline, and the underlying musculature is generously infiltrated with local anesthetic. Twenty- or 22-gauge needles (12–15 cm or 5–7 inches in length) are inserted bilaterally, as shown in Figure 22–11. The needles initially are oriented 45° toward the midline and about 15° cephalad, so as to contact the L1 vertebral body. Once this has been verified with anteroposterior fluoroscopy, the depth at which bony contact occurred is noted, and the needles are withdrawn to the level of the skin and redirected slightly less mesiad (about 60° from the midline), so as to "walk off" the surface of the L1 vertebral body (see Figs. 22–16 and 22–17). Once the needles have been replaced to their previous depth and contact with bone is found to be absent, the left sided needle is first gradually advanced 1.5 to 2 cm,[97] or until the pulsation emanating from the aorta and transmitted to the advancing needle is noted.[65] The right-sided needle is then advanced slightly further (ie, 3–4 cm past contact with the bone), with the ultimate result aimed at placement of the tips of the needles just posterior to the aorta on the left and at its anterolateral aspect on the right (see Figs. 22–16 and 22–17).[97] A small amount of contrast material is injected through each needle, and its spread is observed radiographically. Ideally, on the anteroposterior view, contrast is confined to the midline and concentrated

near L1, and on the lateral view a smooth posterior contour can be observed that corresponds to the psoas fascia (Figs. 22–18 and 22–19). Alternatively, CT can be used either throughout the procedure or at its conclusion to verify needle position (see below).[98]

Transcrural Technique

The diaphragm separates the thorax from the abdominal cavity while still permitting the passage of the thoracoabdominal structures, including the aorta and splanchnic nerves. The diaphragmatic crura are bilateral structures that arise from the anterolateral surfaces of the upper two or three lumbar vertebrae and discs and transmit the splanchnic nerves, effectively separating them from the celiac ganglia and plexus, below. The classic, modified Kappis approach to celiac plexus block described above is retrocrural, that is, the needles and injected solution are placed posterior and cephalad to the diaphragm. Recent modification to celiac block involves transcrural needle placement (ie, the needles and injectate are placed anterior and caudad to the diaphragm [see Fig. 22–12]). Transcrural celiac block maximizes the spread of injected solutions anterior to the aorta where the celiac plexus is most concentrated. Based on CT[9,97] and cadaver studies,[97] it has been suggested recently that the classic method of retrocrural block is more likely to produce splanchnic nerve block, and does not result in the deposition of injected material around the aorta and directly on to the celiac plexus at the level of L1, as previously thought. Rather, the injectate appears to 1) concentrate posterior to the aorta, in front of and along the sides of the L1 vertebral body, where it may anesthetize retroaortic celiac fibers; 2) diffuse cephalad to anesthetize the splanchnic nerves at a site rostral to the origin of the plexus; and 3) only finally encircle the aorta at the site of the celiac plexus when a sufficient volume of drug is injected to transgress the diaphragm by diffusing caudad through the aortic hiatus.

Singler[9] and Boas[53] recommend a transcrural approach using CT and fluoroscopic guidance, respectively, as an important option to

Distribution of Local Anesthetic Solution Following Splanchnic and Celiac Block

Composite posteroanterior projection

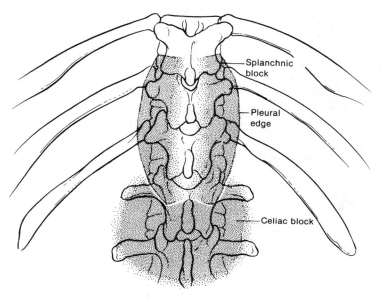

Splanchnic block

Pleural edge

Celiac block

Lateral projection

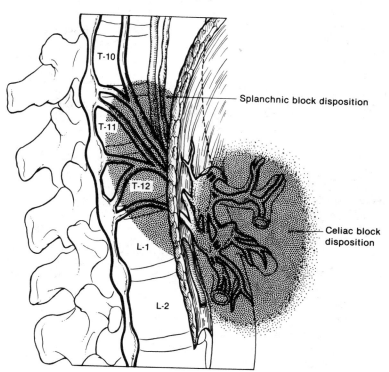

T-10

T-11

T-12

L-1

L-2

Splanchnic block disposition

Celiac block disposition

Figure 22–18. Schematic demonstrating proper spread of contrast medium (stippled area) after celiac and splanchnic block on posteroanterior and lateral radiographic projections. Reproduced with permission from Abram SE, Boas RA: Sympathetic and visceral nerve blocks. In Benumof JL (ed): Clinical Procedures in Anesthesia and Intensive Care, Philadelphia, JB Lippincott, 1992, p 787.

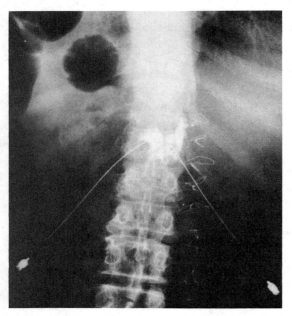

Figure 22–19. Anteroposterior radiograph of patient undergoing therapeutic celiac plexus block. Note needles impinging on first lumbar vertebral body and spread of contrast medium confined to the region surrounding the midline. Courtesy Dr. Subhash Jain, Memorial Sloan Kettering Cancer Center.

the traditional retrocrural technique. Brown et al[99] recommend an initial trial of retrocrural block that, if unsuccessful, is followed by a combined left-sided retrocrural and right-sided transcrural block. Transcrural block is carried out in a manner that is essentially the same as retrocrural block, except that needles are advanced further and the risk of vascular puncture is increased, especially on the left. Singler recommends the use of CT scan for transcrural block.[9] Ischia's transaortic technique (see below), which can be achieved with fluoroscopy, is an alternative means of accomplishing transcrural placement on the left.

Transaortic Technique

In 1983, Ischia and colleagues[11] introduced the concept of deliberately transgressing the abdominal aorta with a single, posteriorly placed needle in order to assure spread of the in-

jected solution in the preaortic region. Obviously, this technique results in a transcrural block. This method is in some respects analogous to the transaxillary approach to brachial plexus block, and the likelihood of its safety is suggested by previous experience with both axillary block and translumbar aortograms. Translumbar aortography, although no longer in common use, is associated with low incidences of clinically significant hemorrhage (0.1%–0.5%), despite the use of large-caliber (14–18-gauge) needles.[100,101] Despite concerns about the potential for aortic tears and subsequent occult retroperitoneal hemorrhage with this technique,[102] its proven safety thus far has been demonstrated in this and other larger series,[103,104] perhaps in part due to the use of fine needles and because the aorta is relatively well supported in this region by the diaphragmatic crura and prevertebral fascia.[102]

The authors suggest that their technique is 1) safe, 2) relatively simple, 3) effective, and 4) avoids the risks of neurologic complications related to posterior spread. Their approach uses the usual landmarks and technique for posterior placement of a left-sided 20-gauge needle to the points at which the depth of the L1 vertebral body has been exceeded. The needle is then gradually advanced continuously until its tip rests in the preaortic fat. Serially, 1) penetration of the posterior aortic wall is heralded by transmitted pulsations to the needle and increased resistance both to needle passage and injection of saline; 2) presence of the needle within the aortic lumen is evidenced by easy aspiration of arterial blood; and finally 3) transgression of the anterior wall is indicated by increased resistance that gives way to a new loss of resistance, indicating the needle tip's probable location within the preaortic fatty connective tissue and the substance of the celiac plexus. The authors recommend obtaining confirmatory fluoroscopic views of injected contrast medium (Fig. 22–20). On anteroposterior views, the contrast medium should be confined to the midline, with a tendency toward greater concentration around the lateral margins of the aorta (Fig. 22–21). Lateral views should demon-

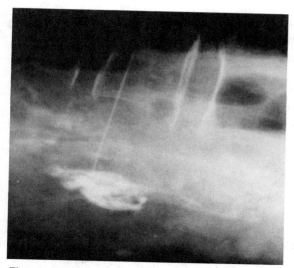

Figure 22–20. Lateral radiograph of patient undergoing transaortic celiac plexus block. Note single needle advanced well beyond the anterior margin of the vertebral column, and spread of contrast medium anterior to the aorta.

strate a predominantly preaortic orientation extending from around T12–L2, sometimes accompanied by pulsations. Incomplete penetration of the anterior wall is indicated by a narrow longitudinal "line image." A failure of the contrast medium to consolidate may occur with extensive infiltration of the preaortic region by tumor. Twelve of the 28 patients studied by Ischia's group underwent intraprocedural CT scanning to confirm the details of placement, and 6 patients underwent postprocedural scanning to insure an absence of retroperitoneal hematoma. Using 20 ml of 2% mepivacaine with epinephrine, and, 30 minutes later, 30 ml of 75% alcohol, all patients experienced immediate complete relief of pain. Pain recurred in nine patients over a period ranging from 2 days to 3 weeks, and the remainder of patients either died painlessly (mean, 40 days) or were pain-free on last follow-up (mean, 2 months). In two patients with an early return of pain, splanchnic alcohol neurolysis was carried out with excellent lasting results, suggesting that preaortic tumor may have prevented complete neurolysis.

Lieberman and Waldman[103] recommend CT guidance in all cases (Fig. 22–22), and go on to suggest that the transaortic approach should be deferred if screening reveals significant aortic aneurysm, mural thrombus, or calcifications. Once intraluminal placement is verified, their group recommends a slight modification of Ischia et al's technique that involves instituting a loss of resistance to the continuous instillation of saline maneuver as the needle is advanced, to ascertain further that its tip has traversed the anterior wall of the aorta. Computed tomography verification of a characteristic spread of contrast medium was followed by the injection of 15 ml of absolute alcohol. Their group reported marked immediate relief of pain in 91% of 124 patients studied that persisted in a large proportion of patients. At 6 weeks, 39% of surviving patients were pain-free and did not require opioid analgesics. An additional 50% of patients reported great improvement, but required adjunctive treatment with opioids. No unusual complications or side effects were encountered in this large series of patients.

Anterior Approaches

Percutaneous Gangliolysis. In 1988, Matamala and colleagues[10] described an anterior approach to blocking the celiac plexus that has since been adopted by others.[105,106] Of the five patients studied in their initial report, four reported complete relief of pain at 2 weeks post-block, and, at 6 months, of the four surviving patients, two reported complete and one moderate relief from pain. No complications were observed in this series and others using similar approaches.

A percutaneous anterior approach to the plexus was advocated early in this century,[78] only to be abandoned later.[83] The advent of fine needles, improvements in radiologic techniques, and the maturation of interventional radiology have since revitalized this option for ablating the celiac plexus. Widespread experience with transabdominal fine-needle aspiration biopsy has confirmed the relative safety of this approach, and provides a rationale and the methodology for the modi-

Transvascular Celiac Block and Distribution of Local Anesthetic Solution

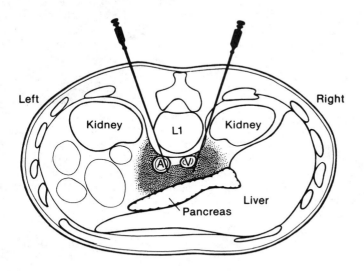

Figure 22–21. Schematic demonstrating proper spread of contrast medium (stippled area) after transaortic celiac plexus block on posteroanterior radiographic projection. Reproduced with permission from Abram SE, Boas RA: Sympathetic and visceral nerve blocks. In Benumof JL (ed): Clinical Procedures in Anesthesia and Intensive Care, Philadelphia, JB Lippincott, 1992, p 787.

fication of these well accepted radiologic techniques. These techniques necessarily involve the passage of fine needles through liver, stomach, small and large bowel, vessels, and the pancreas, but are associated with very low rates of complications.[107–109]

The cardinal advantages of using an anterior approach include relative ease, speed, and reduced periprocedural discomfort. Patients are spared the need to remain prone for prolonged periods, only one needle is used, and since needles do not impinge on either periosteum or nerve roots, sedation and adjunctive analgesia are less strongly indicated. Finally, there is less risk of accidental neurologic injury related to retrocrural spread of drug to somatic nerve roots and the epidural and subarachnoid space. One important disadvantage of the anterior approach is the need for CT guidance (Figs. 22–23 and 22–24), which is costly and in some settings inconvenient or unavailable. Potential disadvantages include risks of infection, abscess, hemorrhage, and fistula formation. Although preliminary findings indicate that the risks of these complications are low, further experi-

ence is needed to make a definitive conclusion. By the same token, although preliminary data suggest efficacy, further experience is needed to permit adequate comparisons to more well established techniques.

Anterior techniques involve targeting either the L1 vertebral body[105] or root of the celiac artery[10] with CT scout films, and then plotting coordinates to determine the proper point of insertion, needle trajectory, and depth. This necessarily involves the close cooperation of an experienced radiologist. The abdominal wall is infiltrated with local anesthetic, and a 22-gauge, 7-inch needle is introduced to the predetermined depth, usually in a roughly perpendicular direction. Ten milliliters of contrast medium is injected, and should be observed to remain within the confines of the preaortic space. For neurolytic block, a preliminary injection of local anesthetic (which can be combined with the contrast medium) is recommended to verify placement further. Matamala's group recommends the administration of 35 ml of 50% alcohol.[10] An alternative technique uses fluoroscopy to guide the passage of a single needle

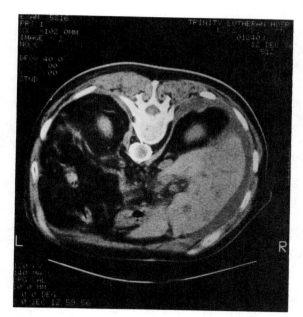

Figure 22–22. Cross-sectional CT of transaortic celiac plexus block. Note markers (L and R) for orientation. Left-sided needle transgresses aorta in its entirety, although image of distal needle is obscured by signals from aortic wall and injected contrast medium (which encircles the aorta, indicating satisfactory placement). Reproduced courtesy of Dr. Stephen Waldman, Kansas City Pain Consortium.

just to the right of the center of the L1 vertebral body, after which it is withdrawn 1–3 cm.[105] Important precautions include the administration of intravenous antibiotics and the use of no larger than a 22-gauge needle to minimize the risks of infection and trauma.

Intraoperative Gangliolysis. Intraoperative periceliac injection of neurolytic drugs is a further option for the management of intractable abdominal pain of malignant origin. With the availability of effective percutaneous methods of achieving celiac block, this method cannot be recommended except when laparotomy is already planned for exploration or bypass of the gastrointestinal or biliary tract.[110] Even in these settings its use is controversial, especially given many surgeons' unfamiliarity with the technique. A valuable alternative in

such a case is the placement of surgical clips in the vicinity of the celiac axis to facilitate postoperative neural blockade.[111] A recent report documenting a single case involving the intraoperative placement of a percutaneously tunneled epidural catheter that was used after surgery to produce neurolysis suggests another intriguing option.[112]

An intraoperative anterior approach first was advocated by Braun[79] as a means to provide intraoperative visceral anesthesia in combination with field block of the abdominal wall. This approach involved gentle retraction of the stomach and placement of a digit between the aorta and vena cava to serve as a guide to the injection of an anesthetic over the ventral surface of the first lumbar vertebral body.

Kraft and colleagues[110,113] described their technique and its results in 41 patients, and in addition reported on its histopathologic correlates in canines. Their method is similar to Braun's, and targets the area between the splanchnic nerves and the plexus, slightly lateral, posterior, and cephalad to the origin of the celiac artery. A 20-gauge spinal needle is advanced over the exploring finger, and 15–20 ml of 6% phenol is injected. Of patients with severe preoperative pain, 88% experienced significant relief that persisted for a mean of 4.3 months, and of patients with pain relief, 84% of patients experienced no return of pain before death (mean survival of 84%). There was a 15% perioperative mortality, but in no case was celiac block implicated. Canine studies revealed an absence of gross abnormalities, microscopic evidence of severe degeneration involving the nerves and ganglia, and only a mild subacute inflammatory response involving the adventitia of major blood vessel walls and surrounding adipose and muscular tissue.

The main advantage of intraoperative celiac block is the elimination of the need for a further procedure. In addition, it provides an opportunity to administer prophylactically to patients with only mild pain or an absence of pain. In addition to potential problems related to the average surgeon's unfamiliarity with the regional anatomy or injection technique,

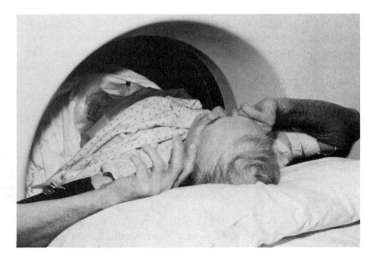

Figure 22–23. Patient with needle in place for celiac plexus block by anterior route, entering scanner.

safe access to the specified injection site may be prohibited by bulky intra-abdominal disease and phlegmon. Also, the risk of neurologic injury may be increased both because intraoperative dissection may result in the injected solution's leaking out of the intended injection site, and concurrent general anesthesia will prevent the use of a test dose of anesthetic.

Catheter Techniques

Isolated reports have appeared documenting the efficacy and safety of placement of a temporary catheter to facilitate repeat periceliac

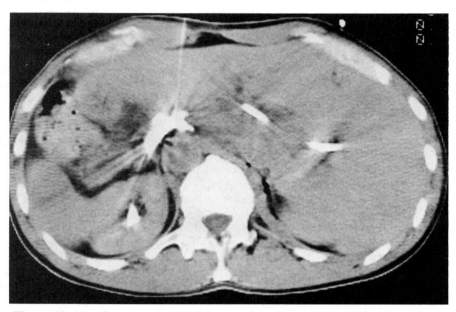

Figure 22–24. Cross-sectional CT image of needle placement for celiac plexus block by anterior route. Note needle's passage through enlarged left lobe of liver, and periaortic distribution of contrast medium.

injections.[114–116] One report used a percutaneous Teflon catheter for 14 days in a patient with pancreatitis, during which time serial injections of local anesthetic were administered before performing a definitive neurolytic block.[116] Fluoroscopy and CT scan performed 13 days after placement revealed an absence of catheter migration, and no perivascular erosion or pleural reaction. Our experience with a catheter placed for a similar indication was succeeded by persistent hematuria and CT evidence of transrenal catheter placement, suggesting that CT should be considered strongly as an adjunct to the application of catheter techniques in this region. Although indications for periceliac catheterization are not well defined and ultimately may prove more persuasive in patients with chronic nonmalignant conditions, the availability of improved catheters (see Appendix F) and imaging technology is likely to result in increased use and refinement of this technique.

Splanchnic Nerve Block

The supracrural anatomy of the splanchnic nerves[53] already has been considered (see above). The technique for splanchnic nerve block differs little from the classic retrocrural approach to the celiac plexus, except that the needles are aimed more cephalad at a site that corresponds to the anterolateral margin of the T12 vertebral body (Figs. 22–19 and 22–25). Thompson et al[94] recommend that both needles closely hug the vertebral body to reduce the the incidence of pneumothorax, a risk that, together with thoracic duct injury, is probably greater when the splanchnics are targeted. Generally, lesser volumes are needed to produce complete blockade at this level. Six to 15 ml of 10% phenol has been recommended.[53,94] Splanchnic nerve block may be particularly useful when the retroperitoneum is widely infiltrated by tumor or after failed celiac block.

Preliminary studies in cadavers and experience with 13 blocks in 6 patients formed the basis for a recent report on a new approach to splanchnic nerve block.[117] This approach uses 3.5-inch needles placed just 3–4 cm lateral to the midline at the T12 or T12–L1 level. Needles are placed just below the 12th ribs and are angled slightly mesiad so that their tips come to rest at the anterolateral margin of the T12 body. Good results were obtained in all cases, and no complications occurred.

Boas recommends an additional new technique for its ease of performance. This paravertebral transthoracic method is achieved with standard 22 gauge spinal needles introduced bilaterally 6 cm from the midline through the 11th intercostal space. Contact with the anterolateral aspect of the T11 vertebral body is readily attained and 10 ml of 12% phenol is injected bilaterally. While a risk, pneumothorax has not occurred in ten patients treated in this fashion. Precautions include attendance to a medial entry point and observation of the lower limits of the lung which, during quiet breathing, are generally observed to lie one segment higher in the costophrenic angle, allowing the needles to traverse the transpleural spaces safely at this point.[117a]

Choice of Agent, Volume, Needle, Technique, and Radiographic Guidance

Various authorities have recommended different combinations of volume, agent, and concentration of agent. Diagnostic blockade typically is achieved with a total of 20–30 ml of 0.25% bupivacaine or a similar agent (0.5%–1% lidocaine, 2% 2-chloroprocaine, 1% etidocaine) injected through one or two needles.[53] Although 50 ml is also advocated,[65] local anesthetic spreads more readily in tissue than do the commonly used neurolytic solutions, and smaller volumes of local anesthetic therefore can be used. For therapeutic blockade, classically, 25 ml of 50% ethanol and 0.125% bupivacaine or saline is administered through each needle.[43,65] Moore's overall voluminous clinical experience[126] and analysis of drug spread within patients and cadavers has led him to advocate strongly the use of a 50-ml volume administered through two needles,[97] at least for retrocrural block. Phenol and other strengths of alcohol (25%–100%)

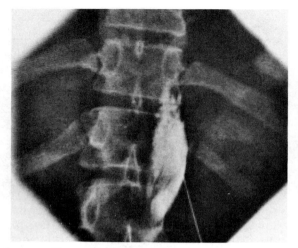 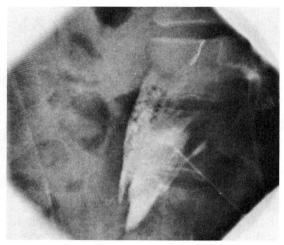

Figure 22–25. Radiographs demonstrating needle placement and spread of contrast medium following splanchnic nerve block performed at the T12 vertebral level. Courtesy Michael Stanton-Hicks, MD, Cleveland Clinic Foundation.

have been used in volumes ranging from 20–80 ml without apparent differences in efficacy or side effects.[72,67]

Alcohol (see Chapters 20, 21, and 23) has the disadvantage of producing severe, though transient pain on injection, and is not miscible with contrast medium.[53] Although, except in the case of accidental intravascular injection, actual intoxication from alcohol injection should not occur,[65,118,119] patients occasionally may be subject to acetaldehyde syndrome (see "Complications," below), a relatively innocuous sequela.[118] Several authors have recommended the use of 6%–10% phenol (see Chapters 20, 21, and 23).[53,110,113] An important advantage is that phenol and contrast medium can be combined to provide documentation of the distribution of injectate during therapeutic blockade, instead of relying on verification of needle placement before the actual block. Boas et al[63,120] have reported on their experience with mixtures of 10% phenol and iodinated contrast medium (Conray 420 [Mallinckrodt Medical, St. Louis, MO] or Renograffin 76 [Squibb Diagnostics, Princeton, NJ]), and have determined in the laboratory that both compounds remain stable for periods of up to 3 months. The use of nonionic

contrast is desirable in many patients. That phenol is not commercially available and must be prepared by a pharmacist (see Appendix C) is a practical disadvantage, whereas the apparent greater affinity of phenol for vascular rather than neurologic tissue is a theoretical disadvantage.[121] Again, controlled comparisons between alcohol and phenol for this application have not been conducted, and their use appears to be equally safe and efficacious.

Both 20- and 22-gauge needles have been advocated.[94] Thompson and Moore[94] correctly point out that the resistance to injection provided by a long 22-gauge needle interferes with the appreciation of differences in tissue compliance that can provide much useful information. In addition, it is more difficult to maintain a straight trajectory when 22-gauge needles are used. It is our practice to use 22-gauge needles to minimize pain and tissue trauma, and to rely on radiologic guidance to offset their disadvantages. The use of a 22-gauge needle is preferred for anterior or transaortic approaches.

The advisability of radiologic guidance, once highly controversial, is less so in contemporary practice. Provided precautions are observed, local anesthetic blockade can be accomplished safely in experienced hands with reliance on topographic guidance alone,[65] although radiologic control is preferred. In the opinion of the authors and others[53,98] radiologic guidance is virtually mandatory when neurolytic block is planned. Interestingly, when large series of cases are compared, it is not clear that the use of fluoroscopy actually results in a reduced incidence of complications,[122] although its use still must be encouraged on practical, empirical, and medico-legal grounds. Our review and another have disclosed few reports of serious complications when CT scanning has been used.[122] It is clear that (even sophisticated) radiologic guidance in and of itself does not insure an absence of complications. The routine application of simple measures (careful serial aspiration and the use of a local anesthetic test dose) is essential to minimize the likelihood of an adverse outcome. Computed tomography scanning permits the visualization of not just bony structures, but vascular and soft tissue elements (including tumor spread) as well. It is particularly useful when anterior and transcrural approaches are planned. The disadvantages of CT scanning include its restricted availability and restrictive cost, the need for specialized personnel, and the potential for claustrophobia in some patients.

As has been reviewed, numerous approaches have been advocated to achieve celiac plexus block. The bulk of experience is with the classic retrocrural technique, and as a result it can be regarded as being extremely reliable. It is anticipated that the newer techniques will gain greater acceptance as experience accrues, since they appear safe and efficacious and offer certain practical and theoretical advantages. The transaortic approach is attractive because it requires only a single needle, the position of which is verified readily, and anterior deposition of the drug is reliable. The anterior approach, although it requires CT scanning, is quick and relatively painless, and is an excellent option for patients who cannot assume the prone position. The transcrural approach, with or without CT scanning, is theoretically desirable, again be-

Table 22–3.
Some Possible Side Effects and Complications of Celiac Axis Blockade

Pain during and after procedure
Failure to relieve pain
Hypotension
Diarrhea
Paresthesia of lumbar somatic nerve
Deficit of lumbar somatic nerve
Subarachnoid or epidural injection
Intrapsoas muscle injection
Intravascular injection (venous or arterial)
Vascular thrombosis or embolism
Retroperitoneal hematoma
Pneumothorax
Chylothorax
Renal injury
Abscess
Peritonitis
Perforation of cysts or tumor
Paraplegia
Lower chest pain
Failure of ejaculation
Sensation of warmth or fullness in lower extremity
Urinary abnormalities

cause injections spread reliably around the aorta.

Ultimately, the choice of technique should be individualized to the available facilities, the patient's physical status, the extent of tumor spread, and the clinician's experience and preparedness.

Complications

In the hands of the skilled clinician, serious complications should be extremely rare events. However, multiple side effects and complications may occur (Table 22–3), particularly due to the close proximity of other vital structures and the use of large volumes of neurolytic drug.

Hypotension, Altered Gastrointestinal Motility, and Pain. Hypotension[123] and diarrhea are sufficiently common that they should be anticipated with either prophylaxis or a well conceived management plan. Hypotension, especially orthostatic hypotension, occurs as a result of regional vasodilation and pooling of blood within the splanchnic vessels, and is more likely in patients who are elderly, debilitated, and chronically or acutely dehydrated. Our only serious encounter with hypotension occurred in a patient who, in addition to chronic dehydration, continually lost fluid from a drain left at a biopsy site. Without prophylaxis, clinically significant hypotension can be expected in 30%–60% of patients,[126] but may be prevented to a large extent by administering 500–1,000 ml of balanced salt solution intravenously before commencing the procedure. Preadministration of oral ephedrine (50 mg), and postprocedural use of support hose and abdominal binders are often mentioned in the older literature,[126] but rarely are used in contemporary practice. Small increments of intravenous ephedrine occasionally are required. Monitoring of blood pressure during the procedure and recovery is mandatory.

Gastrointestinal hypermotility may occur as a result of unopposed parasympathetic activity. This occasionally manifests itself as a patient voiding spontaneously on conclusion of the procedure, usually a sign of an effective block, but more often, since patients tend to be chronically constipated from high doses of opioids, the result is simply improved bowel habit. Self-limited diarrhea lasting 36–48 hours has been reported in up to 60% of patients undergoing alcohol celiac block,[11] is occasionally severe and persistent,[124] and if unrecognized may even be life-threatening.[125]

Although not a complication *per se*, our practice is to include "pain during and after the procedure" and "failure to relieve pain" in our standard consent form. Time to maximal pain relief is variable. In the majority of patients, relief will be immediate and complete, in others it will accrue over a few days.[67] It is not uncommon for patients to experience new (generally self-limited) pain, either in the form of dull backache or pleuritic pain.[94]

Neurologic and Vascular Complications. Out of 3,000 cases, Moore[126] reported 18 episodes of dural puncture (0.006%), which in all but one case was manifested by the appearance of clear fluid. In the majority of these cases radiographic guidance was not used, and the results of more recent series suggest that this complication as well as epidural puncture can be avoided by the consistent use of radiographic guidance. One case of unilateral paraplegia has been reported in a patient who, because of obesity and ascites, was positioned laterally.[65] No form of radiologic guidance was used in this case, and it is probable that this complication occurred as a result of intrapsoas injection and accidental neurolysis of lumbar somatic nerve roots. Even when correct needle placement has been confirmed, the drug conceivably may track backward, resulting in deposition near somatic nerves and consequent neurologic injury (*ie*, numbness over the anterior thigh and lower abdominal wall and quadricep weakness).[71] This outcome may be more likely when retrocrural techniques are used.[9]

A further potential mechanism of neurologic injury is disruption of or accidental injection into small nutrient vessels of the spinal cord (*ie*, the artery of Adamkiewicz). This mechanism was postulated to be responsible for the rapid development of persistent paraplegia after celiac plexus block with 6 ml of 6% aqueous phenol in a patient with carcinoma of the pancreas.[127] Neither test doses of local anesthetic nor radiologic guidance were used in this case. The use of a preneurolytic test dose of local anesthetic and fluoroscopy to detect "vascular run-off" are useful adjuncts to avert this very serious occurrence. It is not uncommon that larger vessels are entered either by accident or intention.[11,103] Intermittent aspiration, an obvious and essential precaution, is not entirely reliable at detecting intravascular placement (see Fig. 24–5), however, and the above methods therefore should be used as well. Clinically significant bleeding or hematoma formation have not been reported in the literature, even after transaortic blocks. It is essential, however, that each patient's coagulation status be investigated and, if necessary, optimized before the procedure.

Visceral Injury. Perforation of adjacent viscera, especially the kidney, probably occurs more frequently than is appreciated clinically. Renal puncture is characteristically a self-limited complication, suggested by the appearance of transient hematuria, but accidental injection of an appreciable volume of neurolytic drug may produce injury and infarction. Moore[126] believes that renal puncture is more likely when 1) needles are inserted in excess of 7.5 cm from the midline[97]; 2) the needle tip comes to rest excessively lateral to the vertebral body; and 3) when a higher vertebral body (T11) is targeted. Although with careful attention to technique, perforation of the viscera should not occur, an obvious advantage of intraprocedural CT scanning is the ability to visualize visceral structures, particularly in patients in whom normal anatomy is distorted by the presence of bulky tumor.

Pneumothorax is a known complication that may occur even with the benefit of radiologic guidance. Thoracostomy may not be required.[66] Pleural effusion has been reported.[128] The proposed mechanism in these two cases was that of diaphragmatic irritation, resulting from overflow of alcohol into the left subdiaphragmatic space. Other potential mechanisms include acute pancreatitis and hemorrhage. Chylothorax, an occasional complication of translumbar aortography,[129] has been reported on one occasion after phenol celiac plexus block.[130] Ejaculatory failure has been reported,[93] although this complication is unlikely to be of serious concern in individuals with advanced symptomatic cancer. Intraperitoneal injection has not, to our knowledge, been reported.

Metabolic. Although accidental intravascular injection of alcohol conceivably can produce intoxication, several investigators have measured serum ethanol levels after celiac block and have determined that circulating levels are insufficient to produce systemic effects.[65,119,131] After 50 ml of 50% alcohol, peak serum ethanol levels ranged between 21–39 mg/dl, well below the legal levels of intoxication. Accumulation of high levels of acetaldehyde in individuals with an atypical phenotype for the enzyme aldehyde dehydrogenase has been observed, and has been suggested to

be responsible for facial flushing, palpitations, and hypotension in susceptible individuals.[118] These patients all provided a history of facial flushing after the ingestion of small amounts of alcoholic beverages, potentially useful historical data.

Unchanged levels of preprocedural and postprocedural amylase in 20 patients suggests that pancreatic injury does not typically occur.[131] In the same series, alterations in creatine phosphokinase (CPK) levels were minimal in most patients, suggesting an absence of significant skeletal muscle injury. Interestingly, the only two patients with significantly elevated CPK levels (4,242 and 1,640 IU/L) also experienced side effects consistent with damage to nearby muscular tissue (bilateral L1 neuritis and back pain).

A single case of a generalized seizure and transient loss of consciousness has been reported after an apparent accidental intravascular injection of phenol.[132]

SUPERIOR HYPOGASTRIC PLEXUS BLOCK

THERAPEUTIC OPTIONS FOR PELVIC PAIN

The pelvis contains diverse, multiple, and intricately innervated structures that are potential sources of pain, particularly when the etiologic process is gynecologic cancer, which tends to spread locally either by direct invasion or metastases to regional lymph nodes. Pelvic pain is particularly difficult to manage because it is often vague and poorly localized, and tends to be bilateral or to cross the midline.

Because of the properties of pelvic pain noted above, neurosurgical interventions generally are not applicable. Of the various neurosurgical operations developed to control cancer pain, only percutaneous cordotomy (see Chapter 26) is still in common use.[133,134] Cordotomy produces analgesia that is strictly unilateral, and therefore represents a poor choice for the treatment of most pelvic pain.

Bilateral cordotomy rarely is elected because of the high associated risks of fatal sleep apnea and bladder dysfunction. The proximity of the nerves that govern bladder, bowel, and lower extremity function and those that subserve pelvic sensation make subarachnoid and epidural neurolytic injections hazardous in this region (see Chapter 23). Except in patients with preexisting colostomy and urinary diversions, neuraxial blocks should be considered only as last resorts, and even then great care must be taken to avoid limb paresis. Of note is one study that combined unilateral cordotomy with contralateral subarachnoid neurolysis with relatively good results.[135]

Intraspinal opioid therapy is one important option for selected patients with pelvic pain that is refractory to conventional pharmacologic management.[136] The utility of chronic intraspinal opioid therapy is potentially limited, however, by factors that include uneven availability of the technology required for its institution and maintenance, high cost, the development of tolerance, and ineffectiveness in a proportion of patients.

Although no published studies exist, bilateral lumbar sympathetic block has been reported anecdotally to be an effective management tool for some patients with pelvic pain.[36,57] The lumbar sympathetic chain does not innervate pelvic structures directly, but due to its continuity with the superior hypogastric plexus, large volumes of injected solutions probably diffuse caudally, resulting in relief of pelvic pain. As noted, however, lumbar sympathetic block has yet to be studied systematically for this indication, and may be subject to a high rate of failure in patients with large masses or retroperitoneal invasion that restrict the caudal flow of neurolytic solution.

Surgical interruption of the hypogastric plexus (presacral neurectomy) is a time-honored procedure that has been demonstrated to relieve a variety of painful pelvic conditions, predominantly of nononcologic origin (ie, dysmenorrhea).[137,138] Superior hypogastric plexus block, a percutaneous procedure that is analogous to presacral neurectomy, has emerged recently as an important option in the management of intractable pelvic pain of neoplastic origin.[139,140]

SUPERIOR HYPOGASTRIC PLEXUS BLOCK

Interruption of the sympathetic nervous system at the ganglionic level has long been employed to treat sympathetically mediated chronic pain of diverse etiologies. Classically, the stellate ganglion (C6–T1), celiac plexus (T12–L1), and lumbar sympathetic chain (L2–L3) have been targeted to treat head, neck, and upper limb pain; upper abdominal and back pain; and lower extremity pain, respectively (see previous sections). Until recently, little attention has been focused on the interruption of the sympathetic nervous system at alternate sites.

The superior hypogastric plexus is a retroperitoneal structure located bilaterally at the level of the lower third of the fifth lumbar vertebral body and upper third of the first sacral vertebral body at the sacral promontory, and in proximity to the bifurcation of the common iliac vessels.[141–143] This plexus is in continuity with the celiac plexus and lumbar sympathetic chains above, and innervates the pelvic viscera via the hypogastric nerves. Investigators have reported on the successful surgical interruption of the hypogastric plexus (presacral neurotomy) for the relief of a variety of painful pelvic conditions.[137,138] In one series, presacral neurectomy for chronic pelvic pain showed success rates of 73% in relieving dysmenorrhea, 77% in relieving dyspareunia, and 63% in relieving other pelvic pains.[137] The frequency of visceral pelvic pain in association with oncologic disease[135,144] and the limited options for management served as a motivation for our group to devise a reliable percutaneous approach to blocking the nerves in this region.

In the first published study on hypogastric block,[139] 28 patients with neoplastic involvement of pelvic viscera secondary to cervical (20), prostate (4), and testicular cancer (1) or radiation injury (3) were treated with neurolytic superior hypogastric plexus block. Pain was significantly reduced or eliminated in all cases, and no serious complications occurred. Using visual and oral analogue scales, a mean reduction in pain of 70% was observed, and residual pain seemed generally to be of somatic origin. Injections of epidural steroids, serial injections of 2%–3% epidural phenol, and/or the oral administration of non-narcotic analgesics were used to control the remaining somatic component of pain, resulting in a global reduction in pain scores of 90%. In all but two patients with pain due to neoplasm, there was no return of sympathetically mediated symptoms until their demise (3–12 months). In a variable percentage of patients there was recurrence or extension of somatically mediated pain that required further treatment, as noted above. In two patients with pain of neoplastic origin, sympathetically mediated symptoms recurred 2 weeks post-block. Significant retroperitoneal spread of tumor was present in both of these patients, and presumably interfered with the free spread of the neurolytic agent. In both cases, superior hypogastric plexus block was repeated under CT guidance, resulting in relief of sympathetically mediated pain until their deaths 2 and 4 months later. In the three patients with pain related to complications of radiotherapy, symptoms had not recurred at 2-year follow-up. Since publication of the initial report, our group has accumulated experience with a total of 128 patients. Our more limited experience in patients with nononcologic pain has produced similarly promising results, with the distinction that, when successful, residual pain is less common and other complementary interventions have not been required.

Recently, Kent et al[144a] reported their results using the above technique in 26 patients with pelvic pain due to cancer. Eighteen (69%) of patients achieved satisfactory lasting pain relief after one or two procedures (VAS reduced from 10 to below 3), and the remaining 8 patients achieved partial relief (VAS reduced from 10 to 4-7). No complications were encountered.

In a modification of the technique described above, using a single needle and CT routine scanning, Waldman et al[140] have observed bilateral spread of contrast medium. They recommend initial placement paravertebrally at the L4-5 interspace, and, once the needle tip's location has been verified within the retroperitoneum, injection of 10 ml of either 1% lidocaine or absolute alcohol. Our group's experience does not support bilateral spread, particularly in the presence of tumor invasion.

Superior hypogastric plexus block is an effective, minimally hazardous means of providing palliation for visceral pelvic cancer pain emanating from one or more of the following pelvic organs: descending colon and rectum, vaginal fundus and bladder, prostate and prostatic urethra, testes, seminal vesicles, uterus, and ovary. In addition, it is often effective for burning tenesmus after rectal anastomosis and radiation injury to the pelvic viscera. Our group's impressions that superior hypogastric plexus block is a useful, safe, relatively easy, and specific intervention for managing pelvic pain are shared by other investigators who have accumulated considerable experience with this procedure.[145,146]

AUTONOMIC NERVES AND GANGLIA IN PELVIS

Because of the complex nature of pelvic neurophysiology, in addition to that of the anatomy that pertains specifically to the superior hypogastric plexus, the entire autonomic innervation of the pelvic cavity is described here.[96]

The superior hypogastric plexus, sometimes referred to as the presacral nerve, is formed by the confluence of the lumbar sympathetic chains and branches of the aortic plexus that contains fibers that have traversed the celiac and inferior mesenteric plexuses. In addition, it usually contains parasympathetic fibers that originate in the ventral roots of S2–S4 and travel as slender nervi erigentes (pelvic splanchnic nerves) through the inferior hypogastric plexus to the superior hypogastric plexus.

As noted, the plexus is located in the retroperitoneum within loose connective tissue, anterior to the body of the lower portion of the fifth lumbar vertebra, sacral promontory, and upper portion of the first sacral vertebra. Its anterior relations include the bifurcation of the aorta, both common iliac arteries, the left common iliac vein, and the median sacral vessels.

The superior hypogastric plexus divides into the right and left hypogastric nerves, which descend lateral to the sigmoid colon and rectosigmoid junction, to reach the two inferior hypogastric plexuses. The superior plexus gives off branches to the ureteric and testicular (or ovarian) plexuses, the sigmoid colon, and to the plexus that surrounds the common and internal iliac arteries.

In addition to pathways that traverse the superior hypogastric plexus, sympathetic fibers also reach the pelvis through perivascular pathways that include the inferior mesenteric plexus (sigmoid colon and rectum), and renal plexus (ureteric and ovarian or testicular plexuses). The lumbar and sacral parts of the sympathetic trunks are directly contiguous at the level of the pelvic brim. The sacral sympathetic trunks lie in the parietal pelvic fascia behind the parietal peritoneum and rectum, and on the ventral surface of the sacrum, just medial to its anterior foramina and the exiting sacral nerves. Below, they converge and unite to form a solitary, small "ganglion impar," located anterior to the sacrococcygeal junction (see next section).

Generally, four or sometimes three sacral ganglia exist bilaterally. No white rami communicantes are present in this region, but each ganglion supplies one or more gray rami communicantes containing postganglionic sympathetic fibers that are distributed to the nearby sacral and coccygeal plexuses, vessels, sweat glands, piloerector muscles, striated muscle, bone, and joints. As noted, the pelvic sympathetic trunk ganglia also supply slender rami, the nervi erigentes or pelvic splanchnic nerves, that join the inferior hypogastric plexuses. The inferior hypogastric plexus is a bilateral structure situated on each side of the rectum, lower part of the bladder, and (in the man) prostate and seminal vesicles or (in the woman) cervix of the uterus and vaginal fornices. In contrast to the superior hypogastric plexus, which is situated in a predominantly longitudinal plane, the configuration of the inferior hypogastric plexus is oriented more transversely, extending posteroanteriorly parallel to the pelvic floor. The inferior hypogastric plexuses supply branches to the pelvic viscera and genitalia, and form subsidiary plexuses (eg, the superior and middle rectal, vesical, prostatic, and uterovaginal plexuses). Its branches contain visceral, glandular, vascular, and afferent fibers, often combined in the nerve fascicles supplying the various structures concerned.

TECHNIQUE

Superior hypogastric block may be preceded by a single-shot L4–5 epidural injection of 8–10 ml 1% lidocaine to enhance patient cooperation by reducing reflex muscle spasm, ameliorating the discomfort associated with contact of needles with periosteum, and reducing movement. Alternatively, these goals can be achieved with local infiltration of the intervening muscle planes.

The patient assumes the prone position with padding placed beneath the pelvis to flatten the lumbar lordosis. The lumbosacral region is cleansed aseptically. The location of the L4–5 interspace is approximated by palpation of the iliac crests and spinous processes, and then is verified by fluoroscopy. Skin wheals are raised 5–7 cm bilateral to the midline at the level of the L4–5 interspace (Fig. 22–26). A 7-inch, 22-gauge, short-beveled needle with a depth marker placed 5–7 cm along the shaft is inserted through one of the skin wheals, with the needle bevel directed toward the midline. From a position perpendicular in all planes to the skin, the needle is oriented about 30° caudad and 45° mesiad so that its tip is directed toward the anterolateral aspect of the bottom of the L5 vertebral body (Figs. 22–27 to 22–29). The iliac crest and the transverse process of L5, which sometimes is enlarged, are potential barriers to needle passage, and necessitate the use of

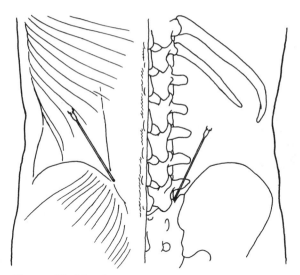

Figure 22–26. Posterior view illustrating approximate placement of skin wheals, needle trajectory, and relationships among needle path, iliac crests, and fifth lumbar transverse process.

the cephalolateral entrance site and oblique trajectory described. If the transverse process of L5 is encountered during advancement of the needle, the needle is withdrawn to the subcutaneous tissue and redirected slightly caudad or cephalad. The needle is readvanced until the body of the L5 vertebra is encountered or until its tip is observed fluoroscopically to lie at its anterolateral aspect. If the

vertebral body is encountered, gentle effort may be made to advance the needle further. If this is unsuccessful, the needle is withdrawn, and, without altering its cephalocaudal orientation, is redirected in a slightly less mesiad plane so that its tip is "walked off" the vertebral body. The needle tip is advanced about 1 cm past the depth at which contact with the body occurred, at which point a loss of resistance or "pop" may be felt, indicating that the needle tip has traversed the anterior fascial boundary of the ipsilateral psoas muscle and lies in the retroperitoneal space (see Figs. 22–27 to 22–29). At this point the depth marker should, depending on the patient's body habitus, lie close to the level of the skin. The contralateral needle is inserted in a similar manner, using the trajectory and the depth of the first needle as a rough guide.

Biplanar fluoroscopy is used during needle passage and to verify needle placement. Anteroposterior views should demonstrate the needle tips' locations at the level of the

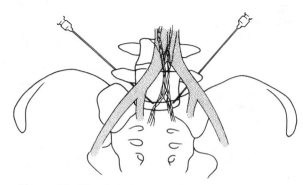

Figure 22–27. Anterior view of pelvis illustrating location of hypogastric plexus and correct bilateral needle placement.

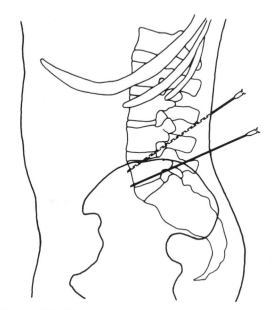

Figure 22–28. Lateral schematic view of bilateral hypogastric plexus block with paravertebral needles positioned with their tips just anterior to the sacral promontory.

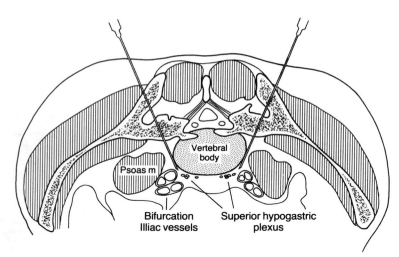

Figure 22–29. Cross-sectional schematic view illustrating bilateral hypogastric plexus block and needles' relationship to fifth lumbar vertebra, psoas muscle, and iliac vessels.

junction of the L5 and S1 vertebral bodies, and lateral views confirm placement of the needle tip just beyond the vertebral body's anterolateral margin. The injection of 3–4 ml of water-soluble contrast medium through each needle is recommended to further verify accuracy of placement. In the anteroposterior view, the spread of the contrast media should be confined to the paramedian region (Fig. 22–30). In the lateral view, a smooth posterior contour corresponding to the anterior psoas fascia indicates that needle depth is appropriate (Fig. 22–31). Alternatively, computerized axial tomography may be used, permitting visualization of vascular structures (Fig. 22–32).

Additional precautions include careful aspiration before injection and the use of "test" doses of local anesthetic. Vascular puncture with a risk of subsequent hemorrhage and hematoma formation are possible due to the close proximity of the bifurcation of the common iliac vessels. Intramuscular or intraperitoneal injection may result from an improper estimate of needle depth. These and less likely complications (subarachnoid and epidural injection, somatic nerve injury, renal or ureteral puncture) usually can be avoided by careful observation of technique.

Hypogastric plexus blockade can be used for diagnostic/prognostic and therapeutic pur-

poses. In the former case, a volume of 6–8 ml of 0.25% bupivacaine through each needle is recommended. For therapeutic (neurolytic) blocks, our group favors the use of a total of

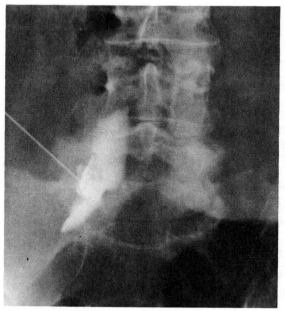

Figure 22–30. Posteroanterior radiograph demonstrating correct needle placement for unilateral hypogastric plexus block. Note contrast medium confined toward the midline over the sacral promontory.

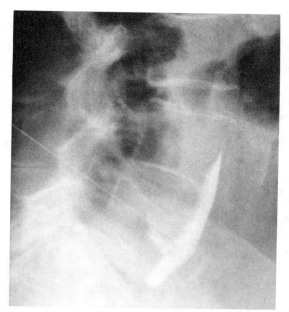

Figure 22–31. Lateral radiograph demonstrating correct needle placement for unilateral hypogastric plexus block. Note smooth margins of opacity formed by contrast medium, suggesting retroperitoneal placement anterior to the psoas muscle.

6–8 ml of 10% aqueous phenol through each needle. During manufacture, a small amount of glycerin is added to keep the phenol in solution.

GANGLION IMPAR
(GANGLION OF WALTHER)

Pain arising from disorders of the viscera and somatic structures within the pelvis and perineum is a frequent cause of discomfort and disability, especially among women. The perineum refers to the anatomic area immediately below the pelvis, and is comprised of diverse anatomic structures with mixed sympathetic and somatic innervation. Although various interventions have been proposed for the management of intractable perineal pain, their efficacy and applications are limited by the same factors that complicate the management of pelvic pain (see above). In addition, the target of nerve blocks in this region historically has focused on somatic rather than sympathetic components. Recently, blockade of the ganglion impar (ganglion of Walther) has

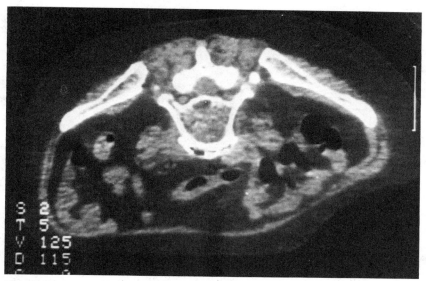

Figure 22–32. Computed tomography after the injection of air and contrast medium bilaterally at the level of the hypogastric plexus. Note retroperitoneal location of contrast medium.

been introduced as an alternative means of managing intractable neoplastic perineal pain of sympathetic origin.[147]

Characteristically, sympathetic pain in the perineal region has distinct qualities—it tends to be vague and poorly localized, and frequently is accompanied by sensations of burning and urgency. Although the anatomic interconnections of the ganglion impar rarely are described in any detail in even the anatomic literature, it is probable that the sympathetic component of these pain syndromes derives, at least in part, from this structure. The ganglion impar is a solitary retroperitoneal structure located at the level of the sacrococcygeal junction that marks the termination of the paired paravertebral sympathetic chains.

The first report of interruption of the ganglion impar for relief of perineal pain appeared in 1990.[147] Sixteen patients were studied (13 women, 3 men), ranging in age between 24 and 87 years (median = 48 years). All patients had advanced cancer (cervix, 9;

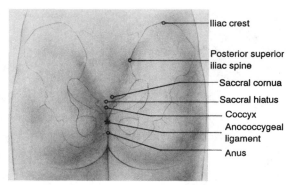

Figure 22–34. Surface anatomy pertinent to injection of the ganglion impar (see text).

colon, 2; bladder, 2; rectum, 1; endometrium, 2), and pain had persisted in all cases despite surgery and/or chemotherapy and radiation, analgesics, and psychological support. Localized perineal pain was present in all cases, and was characterized as burning and urgent in eight patients and of a mixed character in eight patients. Pain was referred to the rectum (7), perineum (6), or vagina (3). After preliminary local anesthetic blockade and subsequent neurolytic block, eight patients experienced complete (100%) relief of pain, and the remainder experienced significant reductions in pain (90% for one, 80% for two, 70% for one, and 60% for four) as determined with visual analogue scale. Blocks were repeated in two patients with further improvement. Follow-up depended on survival, and was carried out for 14–120 days. In patients with incomplete relief of pain, residual somatic symptoms were treated with either epidural injections of steroid or sacral nerve blocks.

TECHNIQUE

The patient is positioned in the lateral decubitus position and a skin wheal is raised in the midline at the superior aspect of the intergluteal crease, over the anococcygeal ligament and just above the anus (Figs. 22–33 to 22–36).

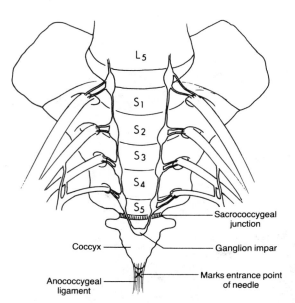

Figure 22–33. Anterior schematic view through pelvis demonstrating location of ganglion impar and pertinent regional anatomy.

4–6 ml 10% phenol is injected for therapeutic neurolytic blockade.

Under most circumstances, needle placement is relatively straightforward. Local tumor invasion, particularly from rectal cancer, may prohibit the spread of injected solutions. Observation that the spread of contrast material is restricted to the retroperitoneum is essential, as we have had experience with one case where epidural spread within the caudal canal was evident (Fig. 22–40). Also, unless care is taken to confirm the needle's posteroanterior orientation, perforation of the rectum or periosteal injection are possible. In

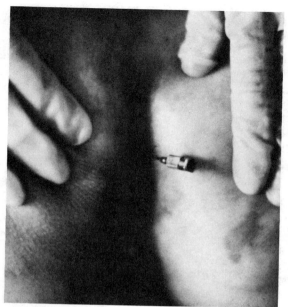

Figure 22–35. Photograph demonstrating needle placement for neural blockade of the ganglion impar.

The stylet is removed from a standard 22-gauge 3.5-inch spinal needle, which is then manually bent about 1 inch from its hub to form a 25°–30° angle (Fig. 22–37). This maneuver facilitates positioning of the needle tip anterior to the concavity of the sacrum and coccyx. The needle is inserted through the skin wheal with its concavity oriented posteriorly, and, under fluoroscopic guidance, is directed anterior to the coccyx, closely approximating the anterior surface of the bone, until its tip is observed to have reached the sacrococcygeal junction (see Figs. 22–36 and 22–37). Retroperitoneal location of the needle is verified by observation of the spread of 2 ml of water-soluble contrast medium (Figs. 22–38 and 22–39), which typically assumes a smooth-margined configuration resembling an apostrophe. Four milliliters of 1% lidocaine or 0.25% bupivacaine is injected for diagnostic and prognostic purposes, or, alternatively,

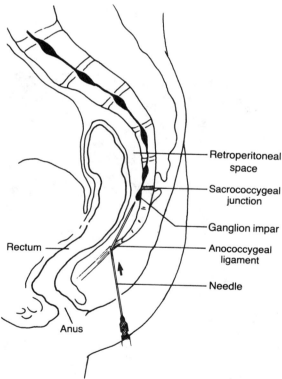

Figure 22–36. Lateral schematic view demonstrating correct needle placement for blockade of ganglion impar, and anatomic relations.

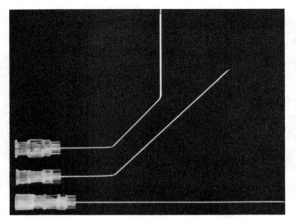

Figure 22–37. Note contrast among needles used for blockade of ganglion impar (upper two) with standard 20-gauge, 3.5-inch spinal needle (lowest needle). Middle needle is bent manually to permit access to anterior surface of sacrum. Upper needle is doubly bent to permit access in patients with an exaggerated sacral concavity.

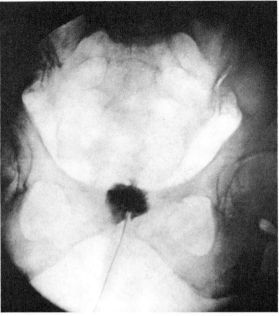

Figure 22–39. Posteroanterior radiograph after injection of contrast medium in the vicinity of ganglion impar. Note that contrast medium is confined to midline.

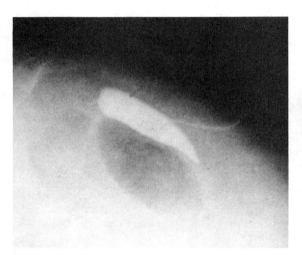

Figure 22–38. Lateral radiograph demonstrating correct placement of bent 22-gauge needle for block of the ganglion impar. Note smooth contours of contrast medium in retroperitoneum between sacrococcygeal region and rectal bubble.

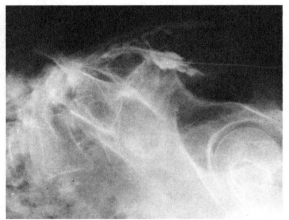

Figure 22–40. Similar to Figure 22–38 *except* for extension of contrast medium into the caudal epidural space. Needle needs to be repositioned before definitive injection is undertaken.

addition, anatomic abnormalities of the sacro-coccygeal vertebral column (*ie*, exaggerated anterior curvature) may inhibit access, in which case the needle may be modified further with an additional bend (see Fig. 22–37).

REFERENCES

1. Dargent M: Role of sympathetic nerve in cancerous pain. Br Med J 1948;1:440.
2. Bonica JJ: Autonomic innervation of the viscera in relation to nerve block. Anesthesiology 1968;29:793.
3. Tasker RR, Dostrovsky JO: Deafferentation and central pain. In Wall PD, Melzack R (eds): Textbook of Pain, 2nd ed. Edinburgh, Churchill Livingstone, 1989.
4. Cervero F: Mechanisms of visceral pain. In Liptons, Miles J (eds): Persistent Pain, vol 4, p 1. New York, Grune and Stratton, 1983.
5. Haugen FP: The autonomic nervous system and pain. Anesthesiology 1968;29:785.
6. Drapiewski JR: Carcinoma of the pancreas: A study of neoplastic invasion of nerves and its possible clinical significance. Am J Clin Pathol 1944;15:549.
7. DeBacker LJ, Kienzle WK, Keasling HH: A study of stellate ganglion block for pain relief. Anesthesiology 1959;20:618.
8. Pereira AD: Blocking of the splanchnic nerves and the first lumbar sympathetic ganglion: Technique, accidents and clinical indications. Arch Surg 1941; 53:32.
9. Singler RC: An improved technique for alcohol neurolysis of the celiac plexus. Anesthesiology 1982; 56:137.
10. Matamala AM, Lopez FV, Martinez LI: Percutaneous approach to the celiac plexus using CT guidance. Pain 1988;34:285.
11. Ischia S, Luzzani A, Ischia A et al: A new approach to the neurolytic block of the celiac plexus: The transaortic technique. Pain 1983;16:333.
12. Racz GB, Holubec JT: Stellate ganglion phenol neurolysis. In Racz GB (ed): Techniques of Neurolysis, p 133. Boston, Kluwer Academic, 1989.
13. Plancarte R, Amescua C, Patt R et al: Superior hypogastric plexus block for pelvic cancer pain. Anesthesiology 1990;73:236.
14. Plancarte R, Amescua C, Patt RB: Presacral blockade of the ganglion impar (ganglion of Walther). Anesthesiology 1990;73:A751.
15. Boas RA, Cousins MJ: Diagnostic neural blockade. In Cousins MJ, Bridenbaugh PO (eds): Neural Blockade in Clinical Anesthesia and Management of Pain, 2nd ed, p 885. Philadelphia, JB Lippincott, 1990.
16. Raj PP: Prognostic and therapeutic local anesthetic blockade. In Cousins MJ, Bridenbaugh PO (eds): Neural Blockade in Clinical Anesthesia and Management of Pain, 2nd ed, p 899. Philadelphia, JB Lippincott, 1990.
17. Ventafridda V: Continuing care: A major issue in cancer pain management. Pain 1989;36:137.
18. Arner S, Arner B: Differential effects of epidural morphine in the treatment of cancer related pain. Acta Anaesthesiol Scand 1985;29:32.
19. Coombs DW: Intraspinal Narcotics. In Abrams SE (ed): Cancer Pain, p 77. Boston, Kluwer Academic, 1989.
20. Kishore-Kumar R, Max MB, Schafer SC et al: Desipramine relieves postherpetic neuralgia. Clin Pharmacol Ther 1990;47:305.
21. Max MB, Culnane M, Schafer SC et al: Amitriptyline relieves diabetic neuropathy pain in patients with normal or depressed mood. Neurology 1987;37:589.
22. Payne R: Neuropathic pain syndromes, with special reference to causalgia and reflex sympathetic dystrophy. Clinical Journal of Pain 1986;2:59.
23. Rowlingson JC: The sympathetic dystrophies. Int Anesthesiol Clin 1983;21:117.
23a. Patt RB, Balter K: Posttraumatic reflex sympathetic dystrophy: Mechanisms and medical management. J Occupational Rehab 1991;1:57.
24. Gerbershagen HU: Blocks with local anesthetics in the treatment of cancer pain. In Bonica JJ, Ventafridda V (eds): Advances in Pain Research and Therapy, vol 2, p 311. New York, Raven Press, 1979.
25. Hitchcock CR: Practical neurosurgical techniques. In Swerdlow M, Ventafridda V (eds): Cancer Pain, p 129. Lancaster, England, MTP Press, 1987.
26. Abram SE: Role of nonneurolytic nerve blocks in the management of cancer pain. In Abram SE (ed): Cancer Pain, p 67. Boston, Kluwer Academic, 1989.
27. Merskey H (ed): Classification of pain. International Association for the Study of Pain. Subcommittee on Taxonomy. Pain 1986;(Suppl 3):S-217.
28. Swerdlow M: Spinal and peripheral neurolysis for managing Pancoast syndrome. In Bonica JJ, Ventafridda V, Pagni CA (eds): Advances in Pain Research and Therapy, vol 4, p 135. New York, Raven Press, 1982.
29. Jaekle KA, Young DF, Foley KM: The natural history of lumbosacral plexopathy in cancer. Neurology 1985;35:8.
30. Thomas JE, Cascino TL, Earl JD et al: Differential diagnosis between radiation and tumor plexopathy of the pelvis. Neurology 1985;35:1.
31. Foley KM: Brachial plexopathy in patients with

breast cancer. In Harris JR, Hellman S, Henderson IC et al (eds): Breast Diseases, p 103. Philadelphia, JB Lippincott, 1987.

32. Warfield CA, Crews DA: Use of stellate ganglion blocks in the treatment of intractable limb pain in lung cancer. Clinical Journal of Pain 1987;3:13.

33. Quimby CW: Medicolegal hazards of destructive nerve blocks. In Abram SE (ed): Cancer Pain, p 137. Boston, Kluwer Academic, 1989.

34. Ranson SW, Clark SL: Anatomy of the Nervous System: Its Development and Function, 10th ed, p 150. Philadelphia, WB Saunders, 1959.

35. Warwick R, Williams PL (eds): Gray's Anatomy: 35th British Edition. Philadelphia, WB Saunders, 1973.

36. Bonica JJ, Loeser DJ, Chapman RC et al (eds): The Management of Pain, 2nd ed. Philadelphia, Lea and Febiger, 1990.

37. LeRiche R, Fontain R: L'anesthesie isolee du ganglion etoile: Sa technique ses indications ses resultas. Presse Med 1934;42:849.

38. Winnie AP: An immobile needle for nerve blocks. Anesthesiology 1969;31:577.

39. Katz J: Atlas of Regional Anesthesia. Norwalk, CT, Appleton Century Crofts, 1985.

40. Lofstrom JB, Cousins MJ: Sympathetic blockade of upper and lower extremity. In Cousins MJ, Bridenbaugh PO (eds): Neural Blockade in Clinical Anesthesia and Management of Pain, 2nd ed, p 461. Philadelphia, JB Lippincott, 1988.

41. Carron H, Korbon GA, Rowlingson JC: Regional Anesthesia, Techniques and Clinical Applications. Orlando, FL, Grune and Stratton, 1984.

42. Stanton-Hicks M, Abram SE, Nolte H: Sympathetic blocks. In Raj PP (ed): Practical Management of Pain, p 661. Chicago, Yearbook, 1986.

43. Moore DC: Regional Block, A Handbook of Use in the Clinical Practice of Medicine and Surgery, 4th ed. Springfield, IL, Charles C Thomas, 1965.

44. Linson MA, Leffert R, Todd DP: The treatment of upper extremity reflex sympathetic dystrophy with prolonged continuous stellate ganglion blockade. J Hand Surg 1983;8:153.

45. Parns WCV, Reddy BC, White HW, McGrath DM: Stellate ganglion blocks in pediatric patients. Anesth Analg 1991;72:552.

46. Kappis M: Sensibilitt und local ansthesie in chirurgischen gebiet der bauchhohle mit besonderen bercksichtigung der Splanchnichus-ansthesie. Bruns Beitr Klin Cher 1919;15:161.

47. Labat G: Paravertebral and dorsal block: Blocking of the dorsal or thoracic nerves. In Labat G (eds): Regional Anesthesia: Its Technique and Clinical Application, 1st ed, p 255. Philadelphia, WB Saunders, 1924.

48. Adriani J: Thoracic sympathetic block. In Adriani J (ed): Nerve Blocks: A Manual of Regional Anesthesia for Practitioners of Medicine, 1st ed, p 47. Springfield, IL, Charles C Thomas, 1954.

49. Moore DC: Complications of Regional Anesthesia: Etiology, Signs and Symptoms, Treatment. Springfield, IL, Charles C Thomas, 1955.

50. Mandl F: Die Paravertebral Injection. Vienna, Springer Verlag, 1926.

51. Bryce-Smith R: Injection of the lumbar sympathetic chain. Anaesthesia 1951;6:150.

52. Reid W, Watt JK, Gray TG: Phenol injection of the sympathetic chain. Br J Surg 1970;57:45.

53. Boas RA: Sympathetic blocks in clinical practice. Int Anesthesiol Clin 1978;16:149.

54. Evans RJ, Watson CPN: Lumbosacral plexopathy in cancer patients. Neurology 35;1985:1392.

55. Dalmau J, Graus F, Marco M: "Hot and dry foot" as initial manifestation of neoplastic lumbosacral plexopathy. Neurology 1989;39:871.

56. Gilchrist JM, Moore M: Lumbosacral plexopathy in cancer patients. Neurology 1985;35:1392.

57. Cousins MJ: Anesthetic approaches in cancer pain. In Foley KM, Bonica JJ, Ventafridda V (eds): Advances in Pain Research and Therapy, vol 16, p 249. New York, Raven Press, 1990.

58. Stambaugh J: personal communication.

59. Bristow A, Foster JMG: Lumbar sympathectomy in the management of rectal tenesmoid pain. Ann R Coll Surg Engl 1988;70:38.

60. Duthie AM, Ingham V: Persistent abdominal pain: Treatment with lumbar sympathetic lysis. Anaesthesia 1981;36:289.

61. Johansson H: Chemical sympathectomy with phenol for chronic prostatic pain. Eur Urol 1976;2:98.

62. Umeda S, Arai T, Hatano Y et al: Cadaver anatomic analysis of the best site for chemical lumbar sympathectomy. Anesth Analg 1987;66:643.

63. Boas RA: The sympathetic nervous system and pain relief. In Swerdlow M, Charlton JE (eds): Relief of Intractable Pain, p 259. Amsterdam, Elsevier, 1989.

64. Arias LM, Woo R: Loss of resistance technique for lumbar sympathetic block. Reg Anaesth 1988;13 (Suppl):25.

65. Thompson GE, Moore DC, Bridenbaugh PO et al: Abdominal pain and celiac plexus nerve block. Anesth Analg 1977;56:1.

66. Brown BL, Bulley CK, Quiel EC: Neurolytic celiac plexus block for pancreatic cancer pain. Anesth Analg 1987;66:869.

67. Jones J, Gough D: Coeliac plexus block with alcohol for relief of upper abdominal pain due to cancer. Ann R Coll Surg Engl 1977;59:46.

68. Brown DL: A retrospective analysis of neurolytic

celiac plexus block for nonpancreatic intra-abdominal cancer pain. Reg Anaesth 1989;14:63.

69. Dale AW: Splanchnic block in the treatment of acute pancreatitis. Surgery 1952;32:605.

70. Kune GA, Cole R, Bell S: Observations on the relief of pancreatic pain. Med J Austr 1975;2:789.

71. Bell SN, Cole R, Roberts-Thomson IC: Coeliac plexus block for control of pain in chronic pancreatitis. Br Med J 1980;281:1604.

72. Hegedus V: Relief of pancreatic pain by radiography-guided block. AJR 1979;133:1101.

73. Leung JWC, Bowen-Wright W, Aveling PJ et al: Celiac plexus block for cancer and chronic pancreatitis. Br J Surg 1983;70:730.

74. Loper KA, Coldwell DM, Lecky J et al: Celiac plexus block for hepatic arterial embolization: A comparison with intravenous morphine. Anesth Analg 1989;69:398.

75. Tanelian D, Cousins MJ: Celiac plexus block following high dose opiates in a four-year-old-child. Journal of Pain and Symptom Management 1989;4:82.

76. Kappis M: Erfahrungen mit lokalansthesie bei bauchoperationen. Verhandlung der Deutschen Gesellschaft fur Cir 1914;43:87.

77. Kappis M: Die ansthesierung des nervus splanchnicus. Zentalbl 1918;45:709.

78. Wendling H: Ausschaltung der nervi splanchnici durch leitungsansthesie bei magenoperationen und anderen eingriffen in der oberen bauchhhle. Beitr z Klin Chur 1918;110;517.

79. Braun H: Ein Hilfsinstrument zur ausfuhrung der splanchnicusansthesie Zentralbl Chir 1921;48:1544.

80. Labat G: L'anesthesie splanchnique dans les interventions chirurgicales et dans les affections douloureuses de la cavite abdominale. Gaz d'Hop 1920;93:662.

81. Roussiel M: Anesthesie des nerfs splanchniques et des plexus mesenteriques spurior et inferieurs en chirurgie abdominal. Presse Med 1923:31;4.

82. Lewen A: Weitere ehrfahrungen uber paravertebrale schmerzaufhebung zur differentialdiagnose von erkrankungen der gallenblase, des magens, der niere, und des wurmfortsatzes. Zentralbl Chir 1923;50:461.

83. Labat G: Splanchnic Analgesia. In: Labat G (ed): Regional Anesthesia: Its Technique and Clinical Application, 2nd ed, p 398. Philadelphia, WB Saunders, 1928.

84. Pauchet V, Sourdat P, Labat G et al: Anesthsie des splanchiques. In: Pauchet V, Sourdat P, Labat G et al (eds). L'Anesthesie Regionale, 4nd ed, p 223. Paris, Gaston Dion et Cie, 1927.

85. De Takats G: Splanchnic anesthesia: A critical review of the theory and practice of this method. Surg Gynecol Obstet 1927;44:501.

86. Gage M, Floyd JB: The treatment of acute pancreatitis: With discussion of mechanism of production, clinical manifestations and diagnosis and report of four cases. Tr South SA 1947;59:415.

87. Esnaurrizar M: The surgical relief of abdominal pain by splanchnic block. Ann R Coll Surg Engl 1949;4:192.

88. Popper HL: Acute pancreatitis: An evaluation of the classification, symptomatology, diagnosis and therapy. Am J Digest Dis 1948;15:1.

89. Mallet-Guy P, Feroldi J, Reboul E: Experimental investigation of the pathogenesis of acute pancreatitis: Its provocation by stimulation of the left splanchnic nerve. Lyon Chir 1949;44:281.

90. Mallet-Guy P, Jaubert de Beaujeau M: Treatment of chronic pancreatitis by unilateral splanchnicectomy. Arch Surg 1950;60:233.

91. Jones RR: A technique of injection of the splanchnic nerves with alcohol. Anesth Analg 1957;36:75.

92. Bridenbaugh LD, Moore DC, Campbell DD: Management of upper abdominal cancer pain: Treatment with celiac plexus block with alcohol. JAMA 1964;190:877.

92a. Shartman WH, Walsh TD: Has the analgesic efficacy of neurolytic celiac plexus block been demonstrated in pancreatic cancer pain? Pain 1990;41:267.

93. Black A, Dwyer B: Coeliac plexus block. Anaesth Intensive Care 1973;1:315.

94. Thompson GE, Moore DC: Celiac plexus, intercostal and minor peripheral blockade. In Cousins MJ, Bridenbaugh PO (eds): Neural Blockade, 2nd ed, p 503. Philadelphia, JB Lippincott, 1988.

95. Ward EM, Rorie DK, Nauss LA et al: The celiac ganglion in man: Normal and anatomic variations. Anesth Analg 1979;58:461.

96. Woodburne RT, Burkel WE: Essentials of Human Anatomy, p 552. New York, Oxford Press, 1988.

97. Moore DC, Bush WH, Burnett LL: Celiac plexus block: A roentgenographic, anatomic study of technique and spread of solution in patients and corpses. Anesth Analg 1981;60:369.

98. Jain S: The role of celiac plexus block in intractable upper abdominal pain. In Racz GB (ed): Techniques of Neurolysis, p 161. Boston, Kluwer Academic, 1989.

99. Brown D, Moore DC. The use of neurolytic celiac plexus block for pancreatic cancer: Anatomy and technique. Journal of Pain and Symptom Management 1988;3:206

100. McAfee JG: A survey of complications of abdominal aortography. Radiology 1957;68:825.

101. Hessel SJ, Adams DF, Abrams HL: Complications of angiography. Radiology 1981;138:273.

102. Ostheimer GW: Pain and its treatment. In Miller RD,

Kirby RR, Ostheimer GW et al (eds): Year Book of Anesthesia, p 364. Chicago, Yearbook Medical Publishers, 1984.

103. Lieberman RP, Waldman SD: Celiac plexus neurolysis with the modified transaortic approach. Radiology 1990;175:274.

104. Feldstein GS, Waldman SD: Loss of resistance technique for transaortic celiac plexus block. Anesth Analg 1986;65:1089.

105. Lieberman RP, Nance PN, Cuka DJ: Anterior approach to the celiac plexus during interventional biliary procedures. Radiology 1988;167:562.

106. Mueller PR, vanSonnenberg E, Casola G: Radiographically guided alcohol block of the celiac ganglion. Semin Intervent Radiol 1987;4:195.

107. Lieberman RP, Crummy AB, Matallana RH: Invasive procedures in pancreatic disease. Semin Ultrasound CT MR 1980;1:192.

108. Wajsman Z, Gamarra M, Park JJ et al: Transabdominal fine needle aspiration of retroperitoneal lymph nodes in staging of genitourinary tract cancer. J Urol 1982;128:1238.

109. Kidd R, Crane RD, Dail DH: Lymphangiography and fine needle aspiration biopsy: Ineffectiveness for staging early prostate cancer. AJR 1984;141:1007.

110. Flanigan DP, Kraft RO: Continuing experience with palliative chemical splanchnicectomy. Arch Surg 1978;113:509.

111. Charlton JE: Relief of the pain of unresectable carcinoma of the pancreas by chemical splanchnicectomy during laparotomy. Ann R Coll Surg Engl 1985:67;136.

112. Illuminati M, Kizelshteyn G, Ackert M et al: Neurolytic celiac plexus block: Intraoperative catheter technique. Reg Anaesth 1989;14 (Suppl):90.

113. Copping J, Willix R, Kraft RO: Palliative chemical splanchnicectomy. Arch Surg 1969;98:418.

114. Corbitz C, Leavens M: Alcohol block of the celiac plexus for control of upper abdominal pain caused by cancer and pancreatitis. J Neurosurg 1971;34:575.

115. Balamoutsos NG: Infiltration block of the coeliac plexus using plastic catheter. Reg Anaesth 1982;5:64.

116. Humbles FH, Mahaffey JE: Teflon epidural catheter placement for intermittent celiac plexus blockade and celiac plexus neurolytic blockade. Reg Anaesth 1990;15:103.

117. Parkinson SK, Mueller JB, Little WL: A new and simple technique for splanchnic nerve block using a paramedian approach and 3 1/2 inch needles. Reg Anaesth 1989;14 (Suppl):41.

117a. Abram SE, Boas RA: Sympathetic and visceral nerve blocks. In Benumof JL (ed): Clinical Procedures in Anesthesia and Intensive Care. Philadelphia, JB Lippincott, 1992, p 787.

118. Noda J, Umeda S, Mori K et al: Acetaldehyde syndrome after celiac plexus block. Anesth Analg 1986;65:1300.

119. Jain S, Hirsh R, Shah N et al: Blood ethanol levels following celiac plexus block with 50% ethanol. Anesth Analg 1989;68 (Suppl):S135.

120. Boas RA, Hatangdi VS, Richards EG: Lumbar sympathectomy: A percutaneous chemical technique. In Bonica JJ, Albe-Fessard D (eds): Advances in Pain Research and Therapy, vol 1, p 685. New York, Raven Press, 1976.

121. Nour-Eldin F: Preliminary report: Uptake of phenol by vascular and brain tissue. Microvasc Res 1970;2:224.

122. Lieberman RP, Lieberman SL, Cuka DJ et al: Celiac plexus block and splanchnic nerve block: A review. Semin Intervent Radiol 1988;5:213.

123. Myhre J, Hilsted J, Tronier B et al: Monitoring of celiac plexus block in chronic pancreatitis. Pain 1989;38:269.

124. Teeple E, Ghia JN: Problems with neurolytic blocks for cancer pain in patients receiving narcotics and psychoactive drugs. Reg Anaesth 1981;6:152.

125. Matson JA, Ghia JN, Levy JH: A case report of a potentially fatal complication associated with Ischia's transaortic method of celiac plexus block. Reg Anaesth 1985;10:193.

126. Moore DC: Celiac (splanchnic) plexus block with alcohol for cancer pain of the upper intra-abdominal viscera. In Bonica JJ, Ventafridda V (eds): Advances in Pain Research and Therapy, vol 2, p 357. New York, Raven Press, 1979.

127. Galizia EJ, Lahiri SK: Paraplegia following coeliac plexus block with phenol. Br J Anaesth 1974;46:539.

128. Fujita Y, Takaori M: Pleural effusion after CT-guided alcohol celiac plexus block. Anesth Analg 1987;66:911.

129. Cook FE, Flaherty RA, Willmarth CL et al: Chylothorax: A complication of translumbar aortography. Radiology 1960;75:251.

130. Fine PG, Bubela C: Chylothorax following celiac plexus block. Anesthesiology 1985;63:454.

131. Lubenow TR, Ivankovich AD: Serum alcohol, CPK and amylase levels following celiac plexus block with alcohol. Reg Anaesth 1988;13 (Suppl):64.

132. Benzon HT: Convulsions secondary to intravascular phenol: A hazard of celiac plexus block. Anesth Analg 1979;58:150.

133. Patt RB: Neurosurgical interventions for chronic pain problems. Anesthesiology Clinics of North America 1987;5:609.

134. Patt R: Pain Therapy. In Frost EAM (ed): Clinical Anesthesia in Neurosurgery, 2nd ed, p 347. Boston, Butterworth, 1990.

135. Ischia S, Luzzani A: Subarachnoid neurolytic block (L5–S1) and unilateral percutaneous cervical cordotomy in the treatment of pain secondary to pelvic malignant disease. Pain 1984;20:139.
136. Wang JK: Intrathecal morphine for intractable pain secondary to pelvic cancer of pelvic organs. Pain 1985;21:99.
137. Lee RB, Stone K, Magelssen et al: Presacral neurotomy for chronic pelvic pain. Obstet Gynecol 1986; 68:517.
138. Frier A: Pelvic neurectomy in gynecology. Obstet Gynecol 1965;25:48.
139. Plancarte R, Amescua C, Patt R et al: Superior hypogastric plexus block for pelvic cancer pain. Anesthesiology, 1990;73:236.
140. Waldman SD, Wilson WL, Kreps RD: Superior hypogastric plexus block using a single needle and computed tomography guidance: Description of a modified technique. Regional Anesthesia 1991;16:286.
141. Pitkin G: In Southworth JL, Hingson RA, Pitkin WM (eds): Conduction Anesthesia, 2nd ed. Philadelphia, JB Lippincott, 1953.
142. Snell RS, Katz J: Clinical Anatomy for Anesthesiologists, p 271. Norwalk, CT, Appleton and Lange, 1988.
143. Brass A: Anatomy and physiology: Autonomic nerves and ganglia in pelvis. In Netter FH (ed): The Ciba Collection of Medical Illustrations, vol 1: Nervous System, p 85. USA, Ciba Pharmaceutical Co., 1983.
144. Wang JK: Intrathecal morphine for intractable pain secondary to pelvic cancer of pelvic organs. Pain 1985;21:99.
144a. Kent E, deLeon-Cassasota OA, Lema M: Neurolytic superior hypogastric plexus block for cancer-related pelvic pain. Regional Anesthesia 1992;17 (Suppl):19.
145. Jain S: personal communication.
146. Racz GB: personal communication.
147. Plancarte R, Amescua C, Patt RB et al: Presacral blockade of the ganglion of Walther (ganglion impar). Anesthesiology 1990;73:A751.

Chapter 23

Neurolytic Blocks of the Neuraxis

Mark Swerdlow

INTRODUCTION

The accessibility of the spinal cord makes it a relatively easy and logical site to accomplish blockade of the spinal nerve roots for diagnostic, prognostic, and therapeutic purposes. This chapter considers the various methods used for producing neurolysis of the spinal nerve roots (rhizolysis), with emphasis on their clinical utility and the potential problems associated with their use. In practice, the nerve roots may be approached via either the subarachnoid or the epidural routes, and the relative value of both of these methods is discussed.

INTRATHECAL INJECTION

Corning,[1] in 1885, was the first to attempt subarachnoid injection (with cocaine). More than 30 years then elapsed before the first intrathecal chemical neurolysis was reported by Dogliotti,[2] whose landmark paper recently has been translated and reprinted.[3] The history of the development of spinal neurolysis has been described in detail elsewhere.[4]

Neurolysis of spinal nerve roots is a valuable means of relieving severe, well localized cancer pain. It is applicable in patients who are elderly and debilitated, and occasionally even is performed at the bedside. Although effects are generally impermanent, when beneficial results of insufficient duration have been obtained, the procedure can be repeated readily. Minimal or no hospitalization and limited equipment or technical facilities are required. The short-term results are often good, even seductively good. The long-term results, however, frequently are inadequate, which, together with significant risks of unacceptable side effects, emphasize the need for careful patient selection. In particular, the application of a neurolytic agent near the outflow to the brachial or lumbar plexus may result in inadequate relief of pain, and is associated with a risk of limb paresis and/or bowel and bladder dysfunction. The balance of potential advantage versus disadvantage must be considered carefully for each case, and discussed with the patient and family in a clear and honest way before these techniques are applied. However, when used properly, spinal neurolysis is a relatively simple, effective, and economical therapeutic method with little risk of serious morbidity.

INDICATIONS AND CONTRAINDICATIONS

As has been emphasized throughout the text, effective pain management requires that treatment be selected on a carefully individualized basis. Most indications and contraindications are relative, but serve as important clinical guidelines.

Indications

1. Pain of oncologic origin that is expected to persist.
2. Life expectancy, ideally, of 6–12 months.*
3. Pain that is intractable despite adequate trials of analgesic drugs, either because pain has persisted or therapy is limited by unacceptable side effects (see Chapters 8–12).
4. Pain that is severe and is localized to two to three dermatomes.*

---

* Cordotomy (see Chapter 26) is the preferred method of treatment for pain that is more widespread or when life expectancy is longer. However, if surgery is unavailable or if the patient is unfit for, or refuses it, then it is worthwhile trying to produce adequate relief by chemical neurolysis.

5. Pain that is predominantly somatic in origin, without prominent visceral or neuropathic characteristics.
6. Evidence of a favorable response to prognostic local anesthetic block (see Chapter 19).

Contraindications

1. Pain that is primarily neuropathic in character (deafferentation pain). Spinal neurolysis is a relatively ineffective intervention for pain of neuropathic origin. In fact,[5] neurolytic block, especially in the periphery, may produce denervation sufficient to cause neuropathic pain (see Chapters 1–3, 10, and 21).
2. Pain that is largely of sympathetic origin (see Chapters 1, 2, and 22).
3. Extensive, mainly nonlocalized pain (see Chapter 18).
4. The presence of impaired mobility or sphincter incompetence should be taken into account carefully. There is a significant risk that neurolysis may increase preexisting disability, and this scenario must be acceptable to the patient and family.
5. The presence of incident pain (see Chapters 1 and 9), particularly when characterized by pain on movement due to pathologic fracture of a long bone or collapsed vertebra. The treatment here, when feasible, is fixation or immobilization of the affected part.
6. Inability to assume and maintain the position required to accomplish the procedure safely.
7. Pain that is secondary to brachial or lumbosacral plexopathy (see Chapters 1 and 3). Effective neurolytic blockade in this setting is likely to be associated with muscle paresis.
8. Inadequate relief of pain after prognostic local anesthetic nerve block (see Chapter 19).
9. Presence of tumor within the cord or spinal column at the level of the proposed injection (see Chapter 20). Tumor infiltration may reduce efficacy by limiting contact between the targeted roots and the neurolytic drug. Of greater concern is the

risk that bleeding or pressure from the injection can compress the spinal cord and produce neurologic compromise. If local tumor growth is suspected, it is advisable to perform myelography before undertaking either subarachnoid or epidural neurolysis.

10. The presence of complete obstruction of the subarachnoid space by tumor. Hollis et al[6] report that lumbar puncture and removal of cerebrospinal fluid (CSF) below the level of the obstruction may result in downward coning and herniation of the cord. If complete obstruction is suspected in a patient who is a candidate for neurolytic subarachnoid block myelography, computed tomography or magnetic resonance imaging are recommended to exclude this possibility.

GENERAL CONSIDERATIONS

Spinal blockade is only one aspect of the management of intractable pain. Regardless of the degree of success achieved by any given procedure, pharmacologic, psychological, and social support will also be needed.

Two different neurolytic agents are in common use (see Chapter 20): phenol (which is hyperbaric and is usually used 5%–7% concentration in glycerin solution), and absolute alcohol (which is hypobaric). In skilled hands, phenol and alcohol are equally effective. A less commonly used agent is chlorocresol (1 in 30 or 1 in 40 in glycerin), which is used in a similar manner to phenol. This and other more obscure agents are discussed thoroughly in Chapter 20. The use of glycerin prevents the neurolytic agent from mixing with the CSF on injection, and helps localize the neurolytic, which then is gradually released from the glycerin. In addition to its neurolytic properties, phenol has an initial local anesthetic effect, so it is not painful on injection, whereas ethyl alcohol can cause burning pain or marked paresthesia when it comes in contact with the spinal sensory roots. Spinal neurolysis, whether by the subarachnoid or the epidural route, should be carried out on an

operating table that allows the patient to be tilted readily in any direction.

Most nociceptive impulses from the periphery pass to the spinal cord via the posterior roots. By positioning the patient properly for the use of a hyperbaric or hypobaric neurolytic solution, the chemical can be brought into contact with, and will destroy the axons of the posterior rootlets, usually avoiding the anterior roots. However, because the cell bodies are not destroyed, axon regeneration is likely eventually to occur. By localizing the injection with the use of a small volume of solution, the concentration of neurolytic at the rootlets will be higher, there will be less spread of solution, and fewer complications. No attempt should be made to block more than two or three nerve roots at one injection. If there is pain in more than one area, treatment of the most severe pain should be undertaken first. If there is bilateral pain, the more painful side should be treated first, and if results are adequate, the other side can be injected a few days later. A technique has been described for producing bilateral block by a single injection, but this involves a larger volume of solution, and most workers believe that it is safer to treat each side separately. The doses and concentrations of neurolytic agents recommended here should not be exceeded. Ignoring this recommendation is likely to result in a greater increase in side effects than in analgesia. The aim should be accurate placement of the smallest volume and lowest concentration that will produce the desired result. When possible, it is better to omit premedication because the patient's cooperation is necessary to report the localization of the sensations produced when the neurolytic is injected. However, if the patient is very apprehensive, a minimal dose of sedative can be given.

The neurolytic agents produce demyelination and degeneration of the dorsal nerve root (see Chapter 20). The degree of block depends on the number rather than the nature of the fibers destroyed, and is related to the quantity and concentration of neurolytic injected.[7] At its origin, the posterior nerve root consists of 6 to 10 filaments called fila radicularia.[8] These present a large surface area to the neurolytic solution. Phenol in glycerin tends to deteriorate on storage, and should be used within 1 year of manufacture. Absolute alcohol can be used up to 2 years from the date of preparation.

SUBARACHNOID PHENOL INJECTION

TECHNIQUE

The patient is positioned laterally on the half of the table furthest from the operator, with the painful side dependent. The patient is then curled into a standard "lumbar puncture position," with the back flexed and at right angles to the surface of the table. The site of puncture should be determined carefully in advance. The nerve roots that innervate the center of the painful dermatomes (see Appendix D) are targeted. The vertebral interspace is selected based on inspection of a chart that indicates the level of the cord from which the targeted roots (fila radicularia) emerge (Fig. 23–1), usually somewhat cephalad to the corresponding bony interspace. The spinal puncture site is widely cleansed with an antiseptic preparation and is toweled dry, after which a skin wheal is raised over the chosen spinal interspace, and the space itself is infiltrated with local anesthetic. A 20–22-gauge spinal needle is inserted gradually into the interspace with its bevel directed downward toward the floor, until a free flow of spinal fluid indicates that the dura has been punctured. Lumbar puncture usually is not difficult, since the spinous processes in this region are roughly at right angles to the spinal axis and are separated by relatively wide interspaces. When dural puncture is attempted above the level of L2, great care must be taken to avoid puncturing the underlying spinal cord. The advancing needle should therefore be arrested as soon as the dura has been breached. A free flow of CSF should be present, however, before the neurolytic agent is injected.

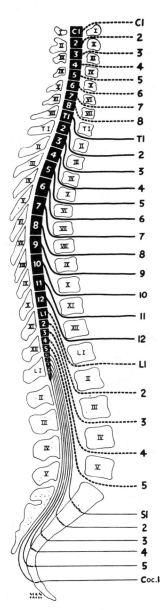

Figure 23–1. Diagram depicting the relationship between adult spinal cord and vertebral column intended to be used before neurolytic intrathecal blockade to localize the vertebral interspace that corresponds to the targeted nerve roots.

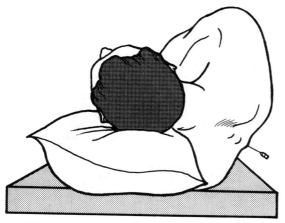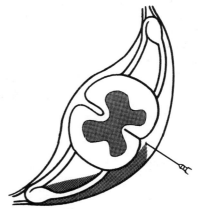

Figure 23–2. Proper positioning of the patient with left-sided pain for intrathecal injection of phenol in glycerine. Note 45° posterior tilt intended to bathe the posterior (sensory) nerve roots with hyperbaric phenol while sparing the anterior (motor) roots.

Once dural puncture has been achieved, the patient should be tilted posteriorly so that his or her back is at a 45° angle to the surface of the table (Fig. 23–2). After confirming a free flow of CSF, the syringe containing the neurolytic solution is attached carefully to the needle. Care must be exercised that the seal between the syringe and needle hub is firm, and that the needle is not moved in the process. Phenol in glycerin is very viscid, and ease of injection can be facilitated by immersing the ampule containing the neurolytic solution in hot water before it is drawn up, and using a 1-ml tuberculin type syringe. Then, 0.2 ml of solution is injected and the patient is asked to describe the nature of new sensations and their location. Intrathecal phenol injection characteristically produces relatively mild feelings of tingling, warmth, prickling, or pain in affected dermatomes. If the sensations reported are distant from the level of the pain that is being treated, the needle should be removed and reinserted at a more appropriate level, in preference to tilting the table to attempt moving the neurolytic solution toward the targeted roots. If, however, the reported

sensations are felt close to, but not quite at, the painful site, small adjustments in the angle of the table may be corrective.

Once proper needle placement is confirmed, the remainder of the dose is injected slowly, usually in increments of 0.1–0.2 ml/minute, interrupted by serial neurologic examinations. The total dose of phenol depends on a number of factors, including the number of nerve roots being treated, and the patient's response to treatment. The maximum doses recommended by this author for use in a single treatment are 0.5 ml in the lumbar region, 1.0 ml in the thoracic region, and 0.6 ml in the cervical region. Other reputable workers have recommended different limits. Stovner and Endressen used 5% phenol in volumes of up to 1.2 ml and 2.0 ml in the lumbosacral and thoracocervical regions, respectively.[9] This author recommends the use of 5%–7% phenol in glycerin. Although it should be noted that the use of concentrations of 10%[10,11] and even 15%[10] have been reported in the literature, they are not recommended by this author. Despite an absence of controlled comparisons, the volume and concentration of drug probably influence both efficacy and complication rates (see below), and should be selected carefully on an individualized basis, within the limits discussed. To assure that a track of neurolytic solution is not left behind, which may cause skin injury or sinus formation, the stylet either is replaced before the spinal needle is withdrawn, or the needle is cleared with a gentle injection of air. The injection position is maintained with the aid of helpers, pillows, and other support for 20 minutes to prevent redistribution of the injected drug.

CERVICAL SUBARACHNOID PHENOL INJECTION

The results of neurolytic injections into the cervical subarachnoid space often are not as good as for injections at lower levels of the cord.[12] This may be due to anatomic factors that reduce the contact between the neurolytic drug and the targeted nerve roots: 1) the cervical roots have a relatively short intrathecal course, and 2) the canal is narrower in the cervical region, and a current of CSF tends to dissipate the neurolytic relatively rapidly.

Intrathecal block at the level of the cervical roots may produce cranial nerve dysfunction or paralysis of the arm. In order to reduce the risk of the neurolytic spreading intracranially or to the anterior (motor) roots, the volume of solution should be minimized carefully. Other elements that will help avoid unwanted neurologic effects include selecting the proper position for the patient at the outset (Fig. 23–3), maintaining it during the procedure, and performing serial neurologic examinations as the drug is injected in increments. The needle should be advanced very gently and gradually to avoid injury to the spinal cord. Some workers advocate removal of the stylet before the needle enters the theca, attaching a syringe, and gently aspirating continuously so that the emergence of CSF might be observed, indicating that the needle need not be advanced further.[8]

Performing thecal puncture at the cervical level is not difficult. If the patient's neck is maximally flexed, the spinous processes ordinarily will not be much angulated, and the interspinous spaces will be reasonably wide. When using a hyperbaric solution, the foot of the table should be tilted slightly downward to prevent the neurolytic solution from diffusing cephalad toward or beyond the foramen magnum. Up to 0.6 ml of phenol solution can be injected. Results obtained using this method to treat pain localized to the upper chest and arm have been disappointing. Papo and Visca[13] report that only lower thoracic pain (below T6) was relieved permanently in a significant proportion of cases.

THORACIC SUBARACHNOID PHENOL INJECTION

The spinous processes of the midthoracic vertebrae are acutely angled, and as a result it may be difficult to introduce a needle into the subarachnoid space in this region. This difficulty sometimes is obviated by using a paramedian approach. If access still is prohibited, the needle may be introduced either more cephalad or more caudad, in a segment of the thoracic column where the spines are less imbricated. The second or third thoracic interspinous spaces are used when the T4, T5, or T6 segments are targeted and the 10th or 11th spaces are used for blockade at the T7, T8, or T9 levels. The table then is tilted so that the injected solution diffuses toward the desired nerve roots. Since the thoracic cord is relatively distant from both the outflow to the brachial and lumbar plexuses and the nerve supply to the bladder and bowel, there is little risk of complications from thoracic injections, except for when the uppermost nerves are targeted. As a result, a larger volume of solution (up to 1.0 ml phenol) may be used.

LUMBAR SUBARACHNOID PHENOL INJECTION

Caution is advised when blocks in this region are considered for the management of intractable lower extremity pain, because of the vul-

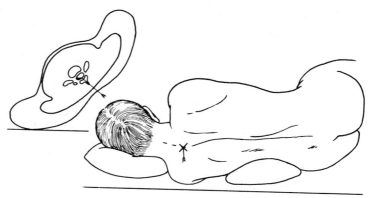

Figure 23–3. Patient positioned for cervical intrathecal phenol injection. Note that the vertebral column at the level of the injection site has been rendered most dependent by placement of padding (and/or table tilt), and that the patient simultaneously is tilted posteriorly: these maneuvers are intended to limit spread of hyperbaric phenol to the posterior (sensory) roots that correspond to the dermatomes affected by pain. See text for pertinent technical details.

nerability of motor fibers. Although careful positioning of the patient (Fig. 23–4) and limiting the volume injected predispose to a selective (sensory) block, limb paresis remains a distinct risk. Percutaneous cordotomy is a better option when pain is unilateral and motor function is normal.

LUMBOSACRAL SUBARACHNOID PHENOL INJECTION

Intrathecal neurolysis is a very useful technique for the relief of pelvic and for perineal pain. Although the lower sacral roots can be accessed easily, there is a risk that damage to the second and third sacral nerve roots may result in deficits in bowel and/or bladder function. When a colostomy and Foley catheter or nephrostomy tube are in place, as after pelvic exenteration for gynecologic cancer, these considerations are unimportant. The procedure is performed with the patient seated in a standard lumbar puncture position. The injection made at L4–5 or L5–S1, and the neurolytic solution is allowed to diffuse downward in the midline with the patient tilted backward 45° to spare the motor roots, as illustrated in Figure 23–5. If, however, bladder and bowel function are still intact, an attempt should be made to produce unilateral blockade by tilting the seated patient over toward the painful side, as demonstrated in Figure 23–6. Pelvic pain often is vague and difficult for patients

to characterize, and sometimes pain that was originally described as bilateral will be obviated with a unilateral block performed on the most painful side. If pain persists, the alternate side can be blocked after an interval of a few days.

When it is important to preserve urinary continence, an alternative means of relieving perineal pain is by transsacral blockade of the sacral roots (see Chapter 21). The innervation of the perineum is mainly by S4, and this nerve should be injected bilaterally via the sacral foramina with 2.5 ml of 6% phenol. A repeat injection may be needed 7–10 days later.[14,15] The use of a large volume or a high concentration of neurolytic increases the risk of complications. It is a wise precaution to do a prognostic block with 0.5% bupivacaine before deciding to apply the neurolytic technique.

SUBARACHNOID ALCOHOL INJECTION

TECHNIQUE

Absolute alcohol (specific gravity = 0.789–0.807) is considerably lighter than CSF (specific gravity 1.07–1.08), so in order to isolate maximally the injected alcohol to the posterior nerve roots, a position opposite to that described for phenol injection is adopted. For subarachnoid alcohol injection, the patient is

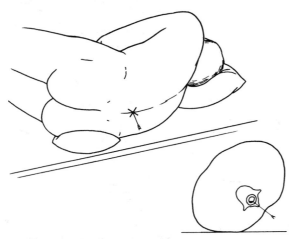

Figure 23–4. Patient positioned for lumbar intrathecal phenol injection. Note that the vertebral column at the level of the injection site has been rendered most dependent by placement of padding (and/or table tilt), and that the patient simultaneously is tilted posteriorly: these maneuvers are intended to limit spread of hyperbaric phenol to the posterior (sensory) roots that correspond to the dermatomes affected by pain. See text for pertinent technical details.

positioned laterally with the painful side uppermost, and before injection is tilted 45° forward with respect to the plane of the surface of the table, as illustrated in Figure 23–7. The table is then "broken" or flexed so that the targeted nerve roots lie at the apex of the curve of the spine, as shown in Figure 23–1. With the patient effectively in a semiprone position, CSF pressure may be inadequate for spontaneous flow through the needle, and aspiration may be necessary to confirm arachnoid puncture. Cousins has suggested[4] that this position may reduce the incidence of postdural puncture headache.

Once the patient is positioned, the spinal needle is introduced into the interspinous space with its bevel pointing upward at the level corresponding to the point at which the nerves subserving the center of the painful dermatomes exit the cord. Owing to the discrepancy between the length of the adult spinal cord and the surrounding vertebral column, the level that the roots originate from

the cord is somewhat cephalad to the vertebral level at which they exit the bony spinal column via the intervertebral foramen, as shown in Figure 23–1. Alcohol exerts its main effects on the fine rootlets (fila radicularia) that compose the origin of the root at the cord. Treatment commences with an initial injection of 0.2 ml alcohol, administered slowly and gently to limit CSF turbulence and avoid excessive spread. Contact between the alcohol and the sensory roots is heralded by transient burning pain and paresthesias occurring in a dermatomal pattern. In advance, the patient is informed that these disagreeable sensations will occur, cautioned that he or she must remain immobile, and instructed that he or she will be expected to describe their location. If these sensations are felt at the desired level, further increments of 0.2 ml of alcohol can be injected slowly at 1- or 2-minute intervals, interrupted by testing for sensory and motor function after

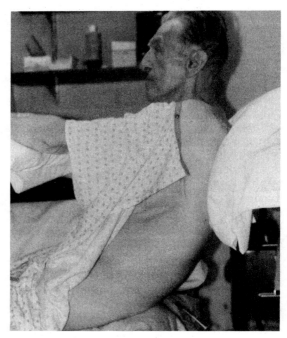

Figure 23–5. Patient positioned for neurolytic saddle block (bilateral lumbosacral intrathecal phenol block) with needle in place (L5–S1). Note 45° posterior tilt intended preferentially to bathe the posterior roots.

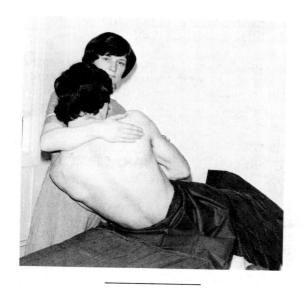

Figure 23–6. Patient positioned for unilateral lumbosacral intrathecal phenol injection. Note posterolateral tilt intended to limit spread of hyperbaric phenol to the posterior (sensory) roots that correspond to the dermatomes affected by pain. See text for pertinent technical details.

each dose. If motor weakness appears, the injection should be terminated. There is general consensus that 2.0 ml is the maximum dose of alcohol for intrathecal injection at any one session. If more than two nerve roots are being treated, some workers[8] prefer to introduce a spinal needle into the relevant two or three contiguous interspinous spaces, and to inject a small amount of alcohol through each. Occasionally, erythema of the affected dermatomes is noted postinjection.

CERVICAL SUBARACHNOID ALCOHOL INJECTION

Cerebrospinal fluid pressure is low in the cervical region, especially when the patient is in the semiprone position, and gentle aspiration may be required to confirm intrathecal placement. To avoid the passage of alcohol cephalad through the foramen magnum, the injection should take place in 0.1–0.2 ml increments, administered slowly and gently, with the cervical spine flexed so that the head is

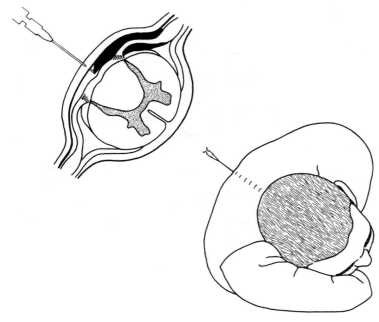

Figure 23–7. Proper positioning of the patient with left-sided pain for intrathecal injection of alcohol. Note 45° anterior tilt intended to bathe the posterior (sensory) nerve roots with hypobaric alcohol while sparing the anterior (motor) roots.

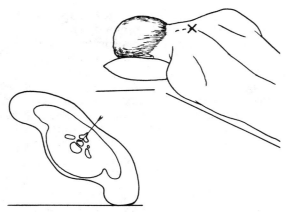

Figure 23–8. Patient positioned for cervical intrathecal alcohol injection. Note that the vertebral column at the level of the injection site has been rendered least dependent by placement of padding (and/or table tilt), and that the patient simultaneously is tilted anteriorly: these maneuvers are intended to limit spread of hypobaric alcohol to the posterior (sensory) roots that correspond to the dermatomes affected by pain. See text for pertinent technical details.

lower than the injection site (Fig. 23–8). The patient is monitored for the location of paresthesias, and the position is modified accordingly. Bonica[8] recommends the placement of multiple spinal needles into the two or three neighboring relevant interspaces, and injecting smaller increments of absolute alcohol through each needle.

THORACIC SUBARACHNOID ALCOHOL INJECTION

The considerations for thoracic subarachnoid injection of alcohol (Fig. 23–9) are similar to those described for the use of phenol except with respect to positioning of the patient, which is reversed (painful side up, wedge under the targeted segments, 45° anterior tilt). As was noted for phenol injection, needle placement may be difficult because of anatomic factors, but complications are unlikely because the outflow from the major plexuses to the limbs and sphincters are relatively distant.

LUMBAR SUBARACHNOID ALCOHOL INJECTION

The considerations for alcohol injection of the lumbar region for the relief of lower extremity pain are similar to those cited for phenol injection (see above), except that the patient's position is reversed (Fig. 23–10).

LUMBOSACRAL SUBARACHNOID ALCOHOL INJECTION

For lumbosacral block, the patient is placed in the prone, jackknife position with the sacral region as elevated as possible. Lumbar puncture is performed at the L5–S1 intervertebral space, and after aspiration of CSF, 1.0–1.5 ml of alcohol is injected slowly in small increments. Because of the risk of causing S2–3 deficits, this technique is reserved best for patients who already have a colostomy and indwelling catheter.

After completion of subarachnoid alcohol injection, the patient should be retained in the injection position for 20–30 minutes to avoid the spread of alcohol. The maximum therapeutic effect often takes several days to be-

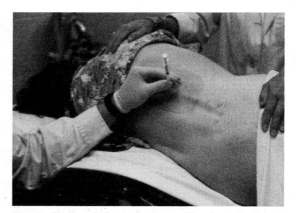

Figure 23–9. Patient positioned for thoracic injection of subarachnoid alcohol. Note the presence of padding beneath the thoracic column to render it the least dependent portion of the spinal axis which, together with a 45° anterior tilt to expose the targeted posterior roots preferentially to the hypobaric alcohol.

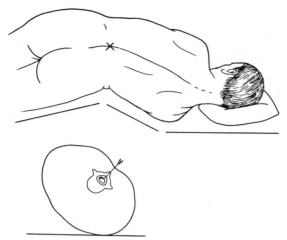

Figure 23–10. Patient positioned for lumbar intrathecal alcohol injection. Note that the vertebral column at the level of the injection site has been rendered least dependent by placement of padding (and/or table tilt), and that the patient simultaneously is tilted anteriorly: these maneuvers are intended to limit spread of hypobaric alcohol to the posterior (sensory) roots that correspond to the dermatomes affected by pain. See text for pertinent technical details.

come apparent. If results are inadequate or short-lived, the block can be repeated.

POSTNEUROLYTIC BLOCK MANAGEMENT

When possible, bed rest should be maintained for the remainder of the day to minimize the risk of postdural puncture headache. This also is beneficial because it is extremely common for patients to experience marked fatigue after completion of the procedure. A thorough neurologic examination should be performed, and results should be documented in the medical record. Motor and sensory deficits and bowel and bladder activity likewise should be documented. If motor weakness becomes evident, it is important to initiate corrective physical therapy as soon as possible. Failure or delay in treating complications of nerve block is one basis for litigation.[16]

The need for a repeat injection is suffi-

ciently common that patients should be advised in advance that it may be necessary. The need for a further injection can be judged after 2 days with phenol, but the maximum effect of alcohol is not seen for about 5 days. Gershagen[17] reports that after intrathecal neurolysis with alcohol, 20% of patients required a second injection. However, if the second injection also is unsuccessful, this author believes that a third injection should not be contemplated because it is unlikely to be effective, and the risk of complications is increased.

RESULTS

It is difficult to assess and compare the results reported by different investigators for a variety of reasons. Criteria for patient selection differ among series, as do standards for what constitutes a given degree and duration of relief. Older reports tend to group results in broad categories, and tend not to make use of analogue scales for pain assessment or statistical methodology. Unfortunately, reports usually do not specify changes in narcotic use after treatment, nor are changes in activity, mood, or other indirect measures of pain usually reported. That patients may have other painful foci in addition to the one being treated may not be adequately characterized, and, in addition, the development of new, often undocumented metastases further interferes with assessment.

Most workers report an average duration of relief of 2–4 months. Pain relief often is of a much shorter duration, and occasionally is much longer.

The cumulative results of subarachnoid phenol neurolysis in a total of 1,150 patients reported by four investigators are as follows: good relief, 51%; moderate relief, 23%; and poor relief, 26%. The composite results for subarachnoid alcohol injection reported by five different investigators in a total of 1,006 patients are as follows: good relief, 55%; moderate relief, 25%; and poor relief, 20%. Unfortunately, the duration of the relief obtained was not reported.

Gerbershagen[14] reviewed the results of

2,125 subarachnoid alcohol blocks, and reported that 12% had complications of muscular paresis, bowel or bladder dysfunction, or altered sensation after the block, but such complications were permanent in only 2% of patients. On the other hand, Porges and Zdrahal[18] reported on 47 patients given subarachnoid alcohol for pain of rectal carcinoma. At the time of the injection, 35 patients had no urinary problems, but after the block 11 required permanent bladder catheterization.

Failure may occur for a number of reasons. Pain may return shortly after the injection as a result of the spread of tumor outside the anesthetized area, or because of regeneration of partly destroyed fibers. Infiltration by intraspinal tumor may result in failure by sheltering the nerve roots from the neurolytic solution. If such infiltration is suspected, radiologic evaluation is recommended before the procedure is carried out. Prior radiotherapy to spinal roots or a previous neurolytic injection also can make good results more difficult to obtain. Sometimes failure occurs because there is a large sympathetic nervous component to the etiology of the pain.

There is no clear consensus on the relative merits of phenol and alcohol. Most often, the choice is made based on the clinical circumstances and the clinician's experience. For patients who are extremely uncomfortable lying on the painful side, the use of alcohol is advantageous so that the patient can be positioned on the asymptomatic side. If dyspnea prevents a head-down tilt, then phenol might be indicated. Some workers consider that alcohol may be more effective for block of cervical roots.[19]

COMPLICATIONS OF SUBARACHNOID NEUROLYTIC BLOCK

A number of complications can result from neurolytic subarachnoid block (see Chapter 24). Some, such as headache and backache, may follow any spinal injection, and are unrelated to the neurolytic agent. It might be expected that postdural puncture headache would be a relatively common event, especially after the injection of phenol, which necessitates the use of a relatively large-caliber needle to accommodate its viscosity, but nevertheless the incidence of headache is not great. Other complications are due to unintentional contact between the neurolytic agent and vulnerable tissues (such as autonomic nerves, motor nerves, or blood vessels) adjacent to the targeted nerves.

A number of factors affect the incidence of serious complications, particularly the volume and concentration of the neurolytic, the level of injection, positioning, and patient selection. Although their study included only a relatively small number of patients, results reported by Ischia et al[10] suggest that whereas greater efficacy is associated with the use of higher concentrations of phenol (10%–15%) in the lumbosacral area, there is a greater incidence of rectal and vesical problems than when lower concentrations (7.5%) are used. It is important that the presence of preexisting, even subtle neurologic deficits be recorded so that deficits observed after the block are not misconstrued. However, it must be realized that the block may intensify preexisting conditions such as paresis or incontinence.

Damage to the vascular supply of the spinal cord is a much more serious complication that can result in major spinal cord injury and permanent, severe disability.[20] Nour-Eldin[21] believes that phenol has a greater affinity for blood vessels than for nervous tissue. Although they are rare events, both posterior[22] and anterior[23] spinal artery thrombosis have been described as a result of the effect of a neurolytic agent on the blood supply of the cord. For a detailed account of the complications that can follow subarachnoid neurolysis, the reader is referred to Swerdlow.[4,24]

The complications that follow spinal neurolysis usually are temporary and of a minor nature, but some persist for some time and a few are permanent. In an analysis of the results of 2,125 subarachnoid alcohol blocks performed in 1,478 patients, Gerbershagen determined the incidence of transient complications to be 12%, and lasting complications as 2%. Reporting on 232 complications, he noted that 66 (28.5%) resolved within 3 days, 53 (23%) within 1 week, 50 (21.5%) within 1 month, 21 (9%) within 4 months, and that in 42 cases (18%), the problem persisted for greater than 4 months. Similar results have been reported after intrathecal phenol neurolysis.[9,25] In this author's analysis of a series of 300 cases performed personally, it was found that 177 patients experienced no complications at all. In general, headache, paresthesias, and intense numbness of the blocked area are not uncommon events. Urine retention should occur in only a small proportion of well selected patients, and then usually should be transient. In Gerbershagen's review, bladder dysfunction occurred in 6% of cases, and was permanent in only 0.66%. Anal incontinence occurs even less frequently. Muscular paresis most often affects the lower limb, and also usually is of short duration. In Gerbershagen's review, limb paresis or paralysis occurred transiently in 4.3% of cases, and was lasting in 0.85%. When this complication occurs, it is important to arrange for appropriate splinting, a walking aid, and physical therapy.

As noted above, for a more detailed account of the complications that can accompany subarachnoid neurolysis, the reader is referred to Swerdlow.[3,4,21,24]

EPIDURAL INJECTION

The first documented successful use of the epidural route for the relief of pain was by Sicard[26] in 1901, who administered cocaine into the caudal epidural space. That there have been relatively few reports of epidural neurolysis is somewhat surprising, particularly given that the epidural route is in such wide contemporary use by anesthesiologists.

ADVANTAGES

Theoretically, epidural neurolytic injection has potential advantages over subarachnoid block, particularly for pain with a more extensive anatomic distribution. The risk of spread to the cranial cavity and meningeal irritation is avoided, and the incidence of sphincter dysfunction, motor weakness, and headache should be less.

DISADVANTAGES

Although no controlled studies have been conducted comparing epidural and subarachnoid neurolysis, the above potential advantages are offset by impressions that inferior results historically have been obtained with epidural as compared to subarachnoid neurolysis. There has, however, been a resurgence of interest in epidural neurolysis related to improved results associated with modifications in technique (see below).

Independent of results *per se*, certain technical aspects deserve mention. When using subarachnoid techniques, return of CSF verifies correct needle placement, whereas localization of the epidural space must be inferred from the results of epidurograms or test doses of local anesthetic. One of the advantages of subarachnoid injection is that it is a relatively simple procedure, and usually can be performed on an outpatient basis. Recent recommendations that epidural neurolysis be accomplished by repeated administrations of phenol through an indwelling catheter (see below) are time consuming and mandate inpatient hospitalization. Also, although reports suggest that gravity and position can be relied on partially to control the effect of epidural block with hyperbaric phenol,[27] these factors can be used to exert more precise control in the case of subarachnoid injection.

RESULTS

A few workers have reported favorable results with epidural alcohol, and others have used phenol successfully.[28,29] Overall, though, the intensity of analgesia and duration of effect of epidural neurolytic techniques as used by early workers (using a single-injection technique) compared unfavorably with the results of subarachnoid injection. The modest results obtained may have been due to insufficient direct contact between the targeted nerve roots and the neurolytic drug. However, recent studies suggest that this shortcoming may be overcome by repeated administration over time through an indwelling epidural catheter. Korevaar[30] administered alcohol on 3 successive days to 30 patients via an indwelling catheter, and reported that 70% of the patients obtained appreciable relief for an average duration of 5–8 months. Racz[31,32] used a specially designed epidural catheter formulated from spiraled stainless steel coils coated with fluoropolymers, designed to facilitate radiologic localization, aspiration, and repositioning. The catheter was advanced through a specially designed, nonshearing needle under fluoroscopy until the desired spinal level was reached. Doses of 2.5–5.0 ml of 5.5% phenol in saline were then injected daily until complete or nearly complete relief was obtained for 24 hours. The procedure was halted if signs of motor involvement appeared at any stage. Jain and coworkers[33] employed epidural phenol to relieve extensive chest wall pain from cancer. They injected 5 ml of 5% aqueous phenol daily for 3 days via an epidural catheter, and of the seven patients treated in this preliminary report, three experienced complete relief, and four reported moderate relief.

Further trials of these new methods are necessary before it can be determined reliably that they are associated with real advantages over intrathecal neurolysis or single-dose epidural block. Meanwhile, it seems reasonable to use these methods in suitable cases of malignant pain arising from cervical or upper thoracic sites, particularly if other relevant therapies have been unsuccessful.

TECHNIQUE

The patient is positioned on the painful side in a 45° tilt, as for intrathecal phenol block. After antiseptic skin preparation and infiltration of the skin and the chosen interspace with local anesthetic, a spinal or Tuohy type needle is introduced into the epidural space at the level of the middle of the painful dermatomes, with its bevel oriented downward. Because the volume of solution used is relatively large, the greatest possible care should be taken to avoid accidental intrathecal injection. Whether a needle or a catheter is being used, a small amount of nonionic contrast medium ideally should be injected preceding or along with the neurolytic to confirm epidural placement. If radiologic facilities are unavailable, some workers recommend the use of a small volume of local anesthetic such as 2.0 ml 1% lidocaine for the test dose, in which case a period of 2 hours or more should be allowed for the affects of the local anesthetic to dissipate before giving the definitive dose of phenol. It is wise to administer a test dose of 0.2 ml phenol for each nerve root to be blocked. In the cervical region the dose should be 1.5 ml per dermatome. Recent research[34] suggests that epidurally injected phenol spreads further than is clinically appreciated. If a standard catheter is being used, difficulties will be encountered if a standard viscous glycerin–phenol preparation is used, even when warmed and administered through a tuberculin syringe. This problem is overcome by using either aqueous phenol or phenol dissolved in a combination of water and glycerin.

Because there is a large venous plexus in the epidural space, intravascular placement of the catheter tip should be excluded before injection of the neurolytic agent. If a unilateral block is desired, the patient should be kept on his or her side in the injection position for about 40 minutes after completion of the injection. It should be noted that, in contrast to subarachnoid injection, after epidural injection the patient usually cannot immediately verify the anatomic localization of the neurolytic solution relative to the affected nerve roots. Pain usually disappears about 10–15 minutes after each injection.

A special use of epidural neurolysis has been recommended by Doughty.[35] He administers 10% phenol in glycerin epidurally at the level of T12 to L1 to relieve attacks of tenesmus and burning pain in rectal cancer. On several occasions, the present author has found this method to be valuable.

COMPLICATIONS OF EPIDURAL NEUROLYSIS

Epidural neurolysis rarely is followed by complications other than backache, and, after the administration of alcohol, occasionally neuritis. However, both urinary incontinence[23] and muscular paresis[27] have been reported. It is advisable not to administer epidural injections to patients who are anticoagulated because of the risk of massive epidural hemorrhage if a vein is injured. Cousins[5] recommends that computed tomography or magnetic resonance imaging scan should be carried out before performing epidural block, to exclude local tumor invasion and the potential for hemorrhage, spinal cord compression, and neurologic injury. Furthermore, the distortion of the epidural space induced by tumor can cause the neurolytic solution to spread unpredictably.

SUBDURAL BLOCK

The subarachnoid and epidural routes are the normal means of accessing the posterior spinal nerve roots for neurolysis. Less frequently, the subdural route has been used. It is a potential space located between the dura and the arachnoid, and is most approachable in the cervical region. Several nerve roots can be blocked bilaterally, as they pass through the subdural space, with a small volume of solution. The subdural technique is technically difficult, and radiologic guidance is essential. So far, very few cases have been reported, and it is not yet clear whether this technique merits a permanent place in the armamentarium of pain specialists. Those seeking further information are directed to the references.[36,37]

REFERENCES

1. Corning JL: Pain, p 247. Philadelphia, JB Lippincott, 1894.
2. Dogliotti AM: Traitement des syndromes douloureux de la peripherie par l'alcoolisation subarachnoidienne. Presse Med 1931;67:11.
3. Dogliotti AM: A new therapeutic method for peripheral neuralgias: Injection of alcohol into the subarachnoid space. Pain Clinic 1987;3:197.
4. Swerdlow M: History of neurolytic block. In Racz GB (ed): Techniques of Neurolysis, p 1. Boston, Kluwer Academic, 1989.
5. Cousins, MJ: Chronic pain and neurolytic neural blockade. In Cousins MJ, Bridenbaugh PO (eds): Neural Blockade, p 1053. Philadelphia, JB Lippincott, 1988.
6. Hollis PH, Malis LI, Zapulla RA: Neurological deterioration after lumbar puncture below complete spinal subarachnoid block. J Neurosurg 1984;64:253.
7. Smith MC: Histological findings following intrathecal injections of phenol solutions for relief of pain. Br J Anaesth 1964;36:387.
8. Bonica JJ: Neurolytic blockade and hypophysectomy. In Bonica JJ (ed): The Management of Pain, 2nd ed, p 1980. Philadelphia, Lea and Febiger, 1990.
9. Stovner J, Endressen R: Intrathecal phenol for cancer pain. Acta Anaesthesiol Scand 1972:16;17.
10. Ischia S, Luzzani A, Ischia A et al: Subarachnoid neurolytic block (L5–S1) and unilateral percutaneous cervical cordotomy in the treatment of pain secondary to pelvic malignant disease. Pain 1984;20:139.
11. Lifshitz S, Debacker LJ, Buchsbaum HJ et al: Subarachnoid phenol block for pain relief in gynecologic malignancy. Obstet Gynecol 1976;48:316.
12. Swerdlow M: Spinal and peripheral neurolysis for managing Pancoast syndrome. In Bonica JJ, Ventafridda V, Pagni CA (eds): Advances in Pain Research and Therapy, vol 4, p 135. New York, Raven Press, 1982.
13. Papo I, Visca A: Phenol subarachnoid rhizotomy for the treatment of cancer pain. In Bonica JJ, Ventafridda V (eds): Advances in Pain Research and Therapy, vol 2, p 339. New York, Raven Press, 1979.
14. Robertson DH: Transsacral neurolytic nerve block. Br J Anaesth 1985;55:873.
15. Simon DI, Carron H, Rowlingson JC: Treatment of bladder pain with transsacral nerve block. Anesth Analg 1982;61:46.
16. Swerdlow M: Medicolegal aspects of complications following pain relieving blocks. Pain 1982;13:321.
17. Gerbershagen HU: Neurolysis: Subarachnoid neurolytic blockade. Acta Anaesthesiol Belg 1981;1:45.
18. Porges P, Zdrahal F: Die intrathekale Alkoholneurolyse der unterensakralen Wurzeinbeim inoperablen Rectumkarzinom. Anaesthesist 1985;34:627.
19. Swerdlow M: Intrathecal and extradural block in pain relief. In Swerdlow M, Charlton JE (eds): Relief of Intractable Pain, 4th ed, p 223–257. Amsterdam, Elsevier, 1989.

20. Superville-Sovak B, Rasminnsky M, Finlayson MH: Complications of phenol neurolysis. Arch Neurol 1975;32:226.
21. Nour-Eldin F: Preliminary report: Uptake of phenol by vascular and brain tissue. Microvasc Res 1970;2:224.
22. Hughes JT: Thrombosis of the posterior spinal arteries. Neurology 1970;20:659.
23. Totoki T, Kato T, Nomoto Y et al: Anterior spinal artery syndrome: A complication of cervical intrathecal phenol injection. Pain 1979;6:99.
24. Swerdlow M: Complications of neurolytic neural blockade. In Cousins MJ, Bridenbaugh PO (eds): Neural Blockade, 2nd ed, p 719. Philadelphia, JB Lippincott 1988.
25. Swerdlow M: Intrathecal neurolysis. Anaesthesia 1978;33:733.
26. Sicard MA: Les injections medicamenteuses extradurales par voie sacro-coccygienne. Comptes Rendus Sociète Biologie (Paris) 1901;63:396.
27. Ferrer-Brechner T: Epidural and intrathecal phenol neurolysis for cancer pain. Anesthesiology Review 1981;8:14.
28. Grunwald I: Neurlise com fenol: Uso da via peridural no tratemonto da dor de cancer. Revue Brasil de Anestesia 1976;26:628.
29. Colpitts MR, Levy DA, Lawrence M: Treatment of cancer-related pain with phenol epidural block. Presented at the 2nd World Congress on Pain, 1978, Montreal, Canada.
30. Korevaar WC, Kline MT, Donelly CVC: Thoracic epidural neurolysis using alcohol. In Dubner R, Gebhart GF, Bond MR: Pain Research and Clinical Management, vol 3. Amsterdam, Elsevier: Proceedings 5th World Congress on Pain, p S133, 1987.
31. Racz GB, Heavner J, Haynsworth R: Repeat epidural phenol injections in chronic pain and spasticity. In Lipton S, Miles J (eds): Persistent Pain, vol 5, p 157. Orlando, FL, Grune and Stratton, 1985.
32. Racz GB, Sabonghy M, Gintautus J: Intractable pain therapy using a new epidural catheter. JAMA 1982;248:646–647.
33. Jain S, Foley K, Thomas J et al: Factors influencing efficacy of epidural neurolysis therapy for intractable cancer pain. In Dubner R, Gebhart GF, Bond MR: Pain Research and Clinical Management, vol 3. Amsterdam, Elsevier: Suppl 4, Proceedings 5th World Congress I.A.S.P., 1987.
34. Salmon JB, Lovegrove FTA, Finch PM: Mapping the spread of epidural phenol in cancer pain patients by radionuclide admixture and epidural scintigraphy. In Bond MR, Charlton JE, Woolf CJ: Pain Research and Clinical Management, vol 4. Proceedings 6th World Congress on Pain, p S94. Elsevier, Amsterdam, 1990.
35. Wise RP: Treatment of pain. In Wiley WD, Churchill Davidson H (eds): A Practice of Anaesthesia, 4th ed, p 1085. Philadelphia, WB Saunders, 1979.
36. Charlton JE: Current views on the use of nerve blocking in chronic pain. In Swerdlow M (ed): The Therapy of Pain, 2nd ed, p 133–164. Lancaster, England, Kluwer Academic, 1986.
37. Ischia S, Maffezzoli GF, Luzzani A et al: Subdural extra-arachnoid neurolytic blocking cervical pain. Pain 1982;314:347.

Chapter 24

Complications of Invasive Procedures

Subhash Jain
Richard B. Patt

Complications specific to each given procedure are discussed elsewhere within the text (see Chapters 18–23), as is the influence of the risk of complications on decision-making (see Chapters 6 and 17). Complications are discussed here in a general way, together with strategies intended to reduce their occurrence and consequences. For a more detailed description of specific complications, the reader is referred to the excellent work of Moore,[1] Bridenbaugh,[2] and Swerdlow.[3]

INTRODUCTION

The clinical practice of neural blockade involves diagnostic, prognostic, and therapeutic nerve blocks, as well as careful decision-making as regards their application. The use of neurolytic substances to provide relief of pain has been practiced since these techniques were popularized by Dogliotti,[4] Mandl,[5] and others. Initially, neurolytic techniques were associated with problems stemming from lack of clear indications, faulty aseptic technique, lack of experience, and difficulty in localizing injections and therefore limiting the effect of treatment to the nerve responsible for transmitting the pain without compromising the integrity of other adjacent structures. As a result of these past deficiencies and other factors, the utility of such procedures has long been underrecognized. Contemporary treatment is safer as a result of improved understanding of cancer pain, accumulated experience, and modifications of various techniques (see Chapters 18–23), the availability of alternative therapies, and the integration of neural blockade into the comprehensive management of patients with symptomatic cancer. Nevertheless, neurolytic blockade still is associated with risks of morbidity and mortality that must be taken into account when procedures are considered, explained, and performed. The introduction of intraspinal opioid therapy as a means to control chronic cancer pain has had far-reaching influences on decision-making, and has improved the outcome of invasive procedures, but has also introduced new risks, mostly relating to the maintenance of implanted drug delivery systems.

COMPLICATIONS VERSUS COROLLARY EFFECTS AND SIDE EFFECTS

Bridenbaugh,[2] in an excellent discussion of the complications of local anesthetic blockade, has emphasized the distinction between side effects and complications, to which might be added the category of corollary effects. According to *Webster's Dictionary*, a **corollary effect** is one that ". . . follows as a normal result," and a **side effect** is a "secondary and usually adverse effect." By implication, the occurrence of corollary and side effects can be anticipated in a high frequency of cases. In contrast, whereas the risk of a complication may be known, its occurrence is unanticipated: according to *Webster's*, a "difficult factor or issue, often appearing unexpectedly . . ." This distinction between anticipated and unanticipated events (corollary and side effects versus complications) must be appreciated if outcome is to be characterized accurately, and must be explained to patients, their families, and referring physicians. The term **complication** implies an adverse outcome, which may or may not be the case for a corollary or side effect.

Swerdlow[3] has pointed out that, notwithstanding the smaller quantities of drug that usually are injected, the risk of adverse outcome is, in general, more serious for neurolytic than local anesthetic blockade. The substances that are injected are (by design) irritating, sclerosing, and destructive to tissue, and hence an adverse effect is likely to endure for a prolonged period of time, and may even be permanent. This factor makes both the avoidance of complications and the distinction between anticipated and unanticipated events all the more critical.

COROLLARY EFFECTS

The purpose of most nerve blocks is to relieve pain, and as a result all other effects reasonably can be considered as undesirable (ie, as corollary effects, side effects, or complications). Corollary effects are those that are associated predictably with a given procedure. Since they are anticipated, they should be carefully explained before undertaking any procedure. If the patient is made to understand that certain sequelae are inevitable or highly likely, then he or she is apt to be more accepting when these events occur. For example, numbness after blockade of somatic sensory nerves, weakness after blockade of motor nerves, and increased local warmth after sympathetic blockade are anticipated corollary events, and should be presented as such. Part of the reason for the upsurge in the popularity of intraspinal opioid therapy is its relative selectivity: the main consequence of treatment is analgesia, and unsought effects are usually minimal, especially in the opioid-tolerant patient.

SIDE EFFECTS

Other intercurrent effects occur with less frequency, but sufficiently often that patients ought to be informed of their relative likelihood. For example, diarrhea and orthostatic hypotension after celiac plexus block, keratitis and symptomatic masseter palsy after trigeminal block, and Horner's syndrome after stellate block are not inevitable but can be predicted to occur in a proportion of cases. In addition, although they are not side effects *per se*, it is advisable to forewarn patients of the potential for pain during a procedure and the potential for failure of the procedure to relieve pain.

COMPLICATIONS

The term "complication" implies an unanticipated adverse outcome. Although complications are by definition iatrogenic (caused by treatment), the occurrence of a complication or of adverse outcome does not in and of itself imply negligence. **Negligence** refers to an injury caused by a breach of duty, that is, a preventable error associated with poor outcome.[6] Neurolytic blockade involves a number of factors that predispose to injury, independent of the role of physician competence. These include 1) passage of a sharp needle through tissue; 2) the potential for movement of the needle or of the patient; 3) dependence on some degree of inference to determine actual needle placement (even with the benefit of radiologic guidance, procedures are performed without the benefit of direct vision, relatively blindly); 4) normal anatomic variation as well as distortion of normal tissues by tumor mass; 5) the injection of substances that are indiscriminately destructive to biologic tissue; 6) relative unpredictability of spread of the neurolytic agent; and 7) proximity of other vital structures. Due to the above factors, and independent of any contribution from physician error, if a sufficient number of procedures are undertaken, some incidence of complications is inevitable.

Regrettably, in addition to the above factors, physician error contributes to many occasions of adverse outcome, although the actual incidence and degree is unknown. Given the serious nature of potential complications, every conceivable effort obviously should be made to eliminate preventable errors. In addition, it is essential that once a complication has occurred, it be recognized promptly so treatment or rehabilitation can be instituted.

PREVENTION AND MANAGEMENT

To achieve the most successful outcome, a fundamental knowledge of the pertinent anat-

omy and physiology, and the pharmacologic effects of the various neurolytic agents is essential. A thorough understanding of the possible complications of a given procedure and of strategies aimed at their prevention also is essential. Access to monitoring and resuscitation equipment and knowledge in their use is expected.

Unfortunately, standardization in training for pain specialists is lacking. Some level of experience with the given procedure or a related one is assumed. Individuals with limited or accruing experience would do well to consult with a more expert authority. Even with ample experience, a review of reference material before a procedure is prudent.

SAFEGUARDS

Much of the potential for adverse outcome relates to the accuracy with which needles are placed. Knowledge of regional anatomy and the identification and use of anatomic landmarks is fundamental to success. In addition, the role of adjunctive measures intended to assure accurate needle localization cannot be overemphasized, particularly for neurolysis. These adjuncts include eliciting paresthesias, careful serial aspiration, and the use of a nerve stimulator, test doses, and radiologic guidance. The role of each of these techniques is specific to each procedure that is to be undertaken, and is discussed in Chapters 18–23.

INFECTION

Infection after neurolytic block may occur,[7] but is uncommon, perhaps because phenol and alcohol have bacteriostatic/bactericidal properties. Nevertheless, neurolysis produces devitalized tissue, and the introduction of even a small number of organisms may result in swelling, cellulitis, subcutaneous or deep abscess, and bacteremia, particularly in elderly, debilitated patients or those who are immunocompromised by antitumor therapy. The administration of prophylactic antibiotics

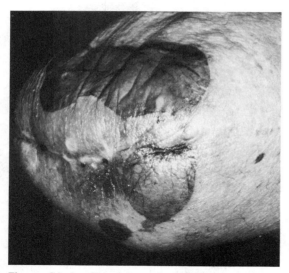

Figure 24–1. Skin injury after injection of phenol near a below-the-knee amputation stump neuroma. Injecting needle slipped out before it could be cleared with air or saline. Process resolved spontaneously.

is not recommended, but strict asepsis should be maintained, as well as vigilance after the procedure. Sloughing of the skin and subcutaneous tissue and sinus formation will predispose to infection and should be avoided (see below).

SLOUGH

Necrosis and slough of the skin and subcutaneous tissues (Fig. 24–1), and sinus formation have been reported on numerous occasions.[3] This complication may be due to leakage of the neurolytic solution along the needle tract, especially when superficial sites are targeted (intercostal nerve, stump or scar neuroma). The occurrence of this complication can be reduced by instituting the practice of flushing the needle with air, saline, or local anesthetic immediately before and during its removal. Small areas of superficial injury usually heal spontaneously.

More extensive slough of the skin, subcutaneous tissue, and mucosa has been reported after maxillary block with both alcohol and phenol, presumably due to vasospasm and/or injury to a nutrient end-artery.[3,8,9] In such cases, stellate ganglion blocks have been instituted in efforts to improve local circulation, but ultimately the need for plastic surgical intervention is likely. It has been suggested that maxillary block be conducted with no more than 1.0 ml of neurolytic. This type of injury, however, has occurred with alcohol administered in quantities as small as 0.28 ml.[3]

HEMATOMA

Hematoma can form after any nerve block procedure, but is particularly common in areas characterized by the presence of loose connective tissue, such as the face (Fig. 24–2). As with local anesthetic blockade, subarachnoid and epidural hematoma are of greatest concern because they may not be readily apparent, and may result in neurologic compromise (see Chapter 29). The injection of alcohol often is followed by the appearance of transient local erythema, or, in the case of subarachnoid block, erythema that is dermatomal in distribution.[10]

VASCULAR INFARCTION

Vascular infarction of nutrient vessels of the spinal cord has been advanced as an explanation for occasional reports of extensive, persistent neurologic injury after lytic injections near the spinal cord.[11–13] *In vitro* studies have demonstrated that phenol has a higher affinity for vascular than neurologic tissue.[14] As a result, some authorities have suggested that high concentrations of phenol should be avoided,[15] although others, including the present authors, have used high concentrations of phenol (10%–15%) without incidents of a vascular nature.[16,17]

INTRAVASCULAR INJECTION

This complication usually is avoidable by scrupulous attention to technique. Once the needle has been positioned, it must be immobi-

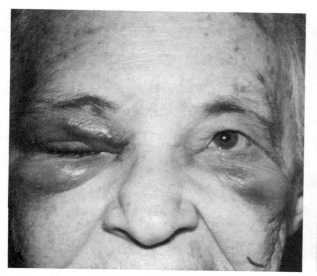
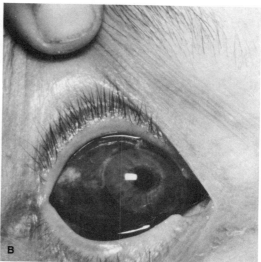

Figure 24–2. **(A)** Patient with bilateral periorbital hematomas after a unilateral (right-sided) alcohol injection of the supraorbital nerve for postherpetic neuralgia. Resolved spontaneously. **(B)** Subconjunctival hematoma in same patient after repeat procedure.

lized carefully to render the results of tests for intravascular injection valid. Racz and colleagues[18] recommend the use of a clamp for this purpose, although most authorities rely on the maintenance of a firm grip (Fig. 24–3), combined with maximizing contact between the hand and the patient's body surface (Fig. 24–4) and/or the use of extension tubing[19] to limit the effects of actions of the injecting hand on the hand holding the needle. Serial aspira-

tion should be carried out frequently. Rotation of the needle by 180° has been recommended to assure that negative aspiration does not simply reflect impingement of the needle's bevel on the surface of the vessel wall (Fig.

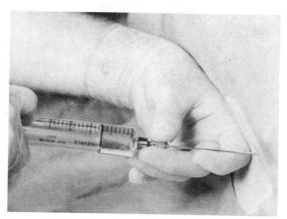

Figure 24–4. Note firm grip combined with maximal contact of hand and patient's body surface to stabilize needle, especially during removal or replacement of syringe.

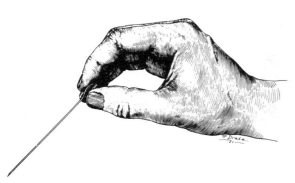

Figure 24–3. Schematic demonstrating firm, sure grip that should be adopted during needle placement.

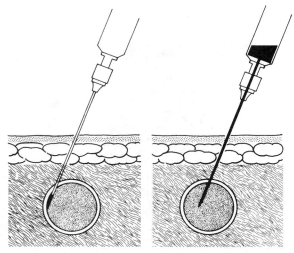

Figure 24–5. Schematic demonstrating how negative aspiration at least theoretically can occur despite intravascular placement due to unrecognized contact between vessel wall and needle bevel. This occurrence probably would be avoided by aspirating in multiple planes.

24–5). Aspiration always should be carried out as a two-step process, as recommended by Bonica[20]: initial negative aspiration is followed by the administration of a small volume of drug to clear the needle lumen of any tissue or blood clot, after which aspiration is repeated. Negative aspiration does not guarantee that intravascular or intrathecal placement has not occurred, especially when small-caliber catheters are used that may collapse or kink (Fig. 24–6). Avoiding the application of excessive negative pressure to the syringe will minimize the likelihood that the catheter will collapse on itself, and yield false-negative results.

In addition to aspiration, the use of a test dose of local anesthetic is recommended. The preferred content and volume of injectate is a subject of some debate.[21] The dosage and volume should be sufficient to produce signs of intrathecal anesthesia (lidocaine 60–100 mg, bupivacaine 10–15 mg) or systemic toxicity (5 ml). Increases in heart rate of ≥20 beats/minute after the injection of an epinephrine-

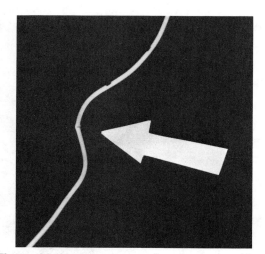

Figure 24–6. Appearance of a standard epidural catheter after withdrawal from patient who experienced symptoms consistent with intravascular injection. Arrow denotes kinked segment that presumably was responsible for falsely negative aspiration test. Courtesy Dr. Gabor Racz, Texas Tech University, Lubbock, TX.

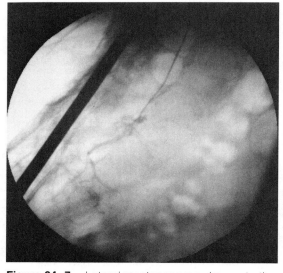

Figure 24–7. Lateral roentgenogram demonstrating the passage of a radiopaque epidural catheter in a patient with Harrington rods. Vertebral column is osteoporotic and difficult to visualize, but epidural catheter can be seen, together with a small amount of contrast in the epidural space and "venous run-off."

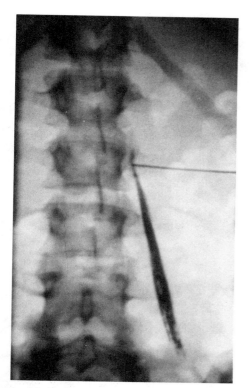

Figure 24–8. Anteroposterior radiographic view after attempted lumbar sympathetic block, demonstrating that needle has been advanced inadequately. Note column of contrast medium dispersing away from the midline, corresponding to an intrapsoas muscle injection (so-called "psoas streak").

well as distinguishing other aberrant placement (Figs. 24–8 to 24–10).

Systemic toxicity of local anesthetics has been well described elsewhere,[23] and is heralded by tinnitus, "tunnel-hearing," perioral numbness, and central nervous system (CNS) depression or excitation. Due to their sclerosant effects, intravascular injections of phenol and alcohol may result in thrombosis of the affected vessel with consequent end-organ injury. Small intravascular injections of phenol may produce severe tinnitus and flushing, usually followed by rapid and complete recovery.[24] The intravascular administration of larger amounts of phenol produces initial CNS stimulation accompanied by tremor and eventually loss of consciousness, hypotension, and convulsion.[25,26] Hepatic and renal injury may occur as well.[27] Intravenous alcohol produces the same effects as when alcohol

containing solution (15 μg) are suggestive of intravascular injection. Pain relief consequent to the administration of a test dose of anesthetic also helps confirm the likelihood of a good therapeutic response to the subsequent injection of neurolytic solutions, and reduces the pain of injection. Although the use of a test dose before neurolysis has detractors[22] who claim that its use may dilute the therapeutic injection, in most other quarters its use is heartily recommended.

Finally, in selected circumstances, the use of fluoroscopy will accurately detect intravascular placement by the observation of rapid disappearance of injected contrast medium (so-called "venous run-off") (Fig. 24–7), as

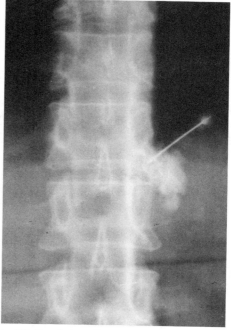

Figure 24–9. Anteroposterior radiograph after T12 paravertebral nerve block, demonstrating spread of contrast medium in epidural space. Courtesy Dr. Douglas Justins, St. Thomas' Pain Management Centre, London.

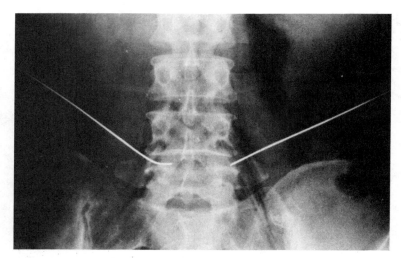

Figure 24–10. Anteroposterior radiograph during bilateral hypogastric plexus block, demonstrating two technical errors. Note psoas streaks on left produced by the instillation of air before positioning the needle more deeply. Note deviation of right-sided needle, indicating that its tip is embedded in the L4–5 intervertebral disc. Courtesy, Dr. Ricardo Plancarte, National Cancer Institute, Mexico City, Mexico.

is ingested socially: inebriation in small doses and respiratory depression and loss of consciousness in large doses.

SENSORY LOSS AND MOTOR WEAKNESS

It has been emphasized throughout this text that neurolytic substances must be deposited accurately on or near the targeted nerve to produce reliable pain relief. Neurolysis usually is associated with hypalgesia rather than complete anesthesia. Pain may persist in the presence of incomplete denervation, more proximal central injury, when an area is innervated by multiple afferent nerves the origin of which are widely separated, and in the case of highly invasive cutaneous lesions (Fig. 24–11). As is discussed in Chapter 21, hypalgesia may progress over time to dysesthesia, an annoying, often burning sense of discomfort in the denervated region, so-called "anesthesia dolorosa." The intensity of this phenomenon varies widely, and in some cases may exceed that of the original complaint. Clinically, this condition shares some characteristics of phantom limb pain and postherpetic neuralgia, and patients have likened it

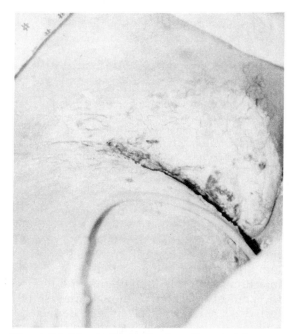

Figure 24–11. Patient with ulcerative, draining, cutaneous groin lesion due to recurrent vulvar carcinoma. White material is a combination of yogurt and metronidazole powder intended to control local infection and odor. Pain was blunted with two subarachnoid alcohol injections, but persisted at a sufficient level to require high doses of opioid analgesics.

to the sensation that accompanies the return of circulation after a limb has "fallen asleep." Postablative dysesthesias have been ascribed alternately to neuroma formation, perineural inflammation and adhesions, and deafferentation/plasticity. Treatment with centrally acting drugs (antidepressants, anticonvulsants, oral local anesthetics, opioids) is successful in a proportion of patients, as is repeat neurolysis, especially when performed at a more proximal site. In general, though, the results of treatment are sufficiently unsatisfactory that most authorities recommend that neurolytic blocks, particularly in the periphery, be reserved for patients with a limited expectancy of life who will be unlikely to outlive the analgesic effects of these procedures. The frequency of postablative dysesthesias is greatest after peripheral blocks, and is said to be increased with alcohol versus phenol, although controlled studies have not been performed. Radiofrequency-generated thermal lesions have the advantage of being associated with a reduced incidence of aberrant sensory phenomena.

The indiscriminate nature of nerve injury after the perineural injection of lytic substances[28,29] has been emphasized in Chapters 20-23. The risk of motor weakness corresponds to a number of factors, but primarily to the procedure that is selected. Consideration of a procedure that is associated with a significant risk of motor block should never be undertaken lightly, but it should be recognized that the risk-to-benefit ratio is unique to each case. Lower extremity or bladder paralysis that may be devastating to an ambulatory patient may be of minimal consequence to a patient who is bed-bound or requires bladder drainage for other reasons. It should be emphasized that desperation may drive patients to submit to practically any intervention, and that as a result the physician would be prudent to regard his or her role partially as that of a "gatekeeper." For example, a partially weak upper limb due to tumor invasion of the brachial plexus still serves to oppose its functional counterpart for simple tasks like getting dressed, and as a result, neurolytic

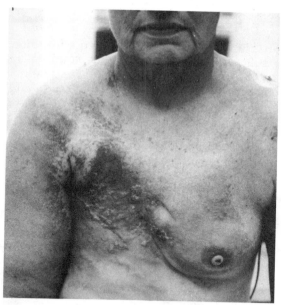

Figure 24-12. Patient with advanced locally and systemically invasive breast cancer with functionless limb due to infiltration of the brachial plexus, lymphedema, and disuse. In the absence of adequate relief with the application of more conservative measures, these clinical findings qualify the patient as a candidate for neurolytic brachial plexus block. Percutaneous cordotomy was not considered in this case because of concomitant pulmonary metastases and the risk of nocturnal respiratory failure.

brachial plexus block should be avoided if at all possible so as not to increase disability. Alternatively, in the case of a limb that is totally functionless (Fig. 24-12), brachial block not only may be considered favorably (see Chapter 21), but a relatively strong concentration of neurolytic may be used to maximize analgesia, since motor function is not, in such cases, a consideration.

Due to its initial local anesthetic effect,[30] early results obtained after the injection of phenol may diminish in intensity and shrink topographically over 24 hours, although this cannot be relied on. In contrast, the topographic limits of the neurologic sequelae of alcohol injection tend to persist, and the denervated area may even increase slightly over 24 hours.

DYSPNEA

Breathing difficulties after a procedure may result from multiple iatrogenic sources, including pneumothorax (Fig. 24–13), chylothorax and hemothorax, phrenic nerve palsy, and intercostal paralysis. Great care to avoid pneumothorax always should be taken when performing intercostal blocks, particularly in individuals with a bulky frame, and for contralateral procedures after pneumonectomy. It is now recognized that subclinical phrenic nerve paralysis occurs much more often after brachial plexus block than was previously thought, particularly when undertaken by the intrascalene route.[31] Patients undergoing intrathecal neurolysis usually can be positioned to avoid paralysis of the intercostal muscles, although, should such weakness occur, respiratory status still actually may improve due to decreased splinting. Finally, the systemic administration of opioids is well known to ease air hunger,[32] and for this reason it may be prudent to continue their administration in dyspneic patients.

NEW PAIN

Postablative dysesthesias already have been discussed (see above, and Chapter 21). For the first 24–48 hours after a procedure, patients may complain of burning over a denervated area or muscle soreness, particularly after celiac plexus block, phenomena that are usually self-limited and are presumably due to perineural inflammation. New complaints of pain in distant sites are not uncommon in individuals with multiple foci of tumor involvement. Presumably, a particularly intense pain problem may prevent the appreciation of pain in other sites, which later may be unmasked when nociceptive traffic is reduced by denervation. In such patients, a technique that provides more generalized, systemic relief of pain, such as intraspinal opioids or pituitary ablation, may be preferable.

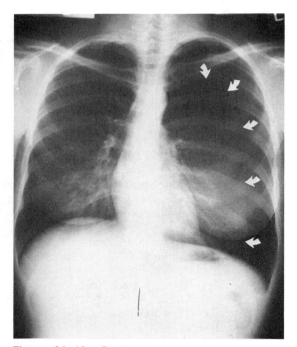

Figure 24–13. Radiograph demonstrating moderate-large pneumothorax associated with chest pain and dyspnea in a patient after thoracic trigger point injection performed with a 25 gauge needle. Arrows denote interface of collapsed lung margin and free air (6 cm from apex, 4 cm from lateral wall). A flexible cannula was inserted and placed on suction.

FATIGUE AND OVERSEDATION

It is extremely common that patients will experience extreme fatigue after a neurolytic block, although it is not clear whether this is due to systemic or metabolic effects, psychological stress, or prior sleep deprivation. Of greater concern is the potential for patients on high doses of opioids to become obtunded soon after a procedure is completed. Pain acts as an antagonist to the CNS-depressant effects of opioids, and reduced nociception consequent to a nerve block may result in a relative overdose if opioids are not gradually withdrawn.

COMPLICATIONS ASSOCIATED WITH SPECIFIC PROCEDURES

Complications related to peripheral nerve blocks, celiac and other sympathetic blocks, and axial blocks are discussed in greater detail in Chapters 21–23, respectively. As noted, for a more detailed description of specific complications, the reader is referred to the excellent work of Moore,[1] Bridenbaugh,[2] and Swerdlow.[3]

Problems related to intraspinal opioid therapy may be pharmacologic or technical in nature. The diagnosis and management of side effects and complications of intraspinal opioid therapy are described in Chapter 18. Selected technical problems are highlighted in Figures 24–14 to 24–26.

(text continues on p. 460)

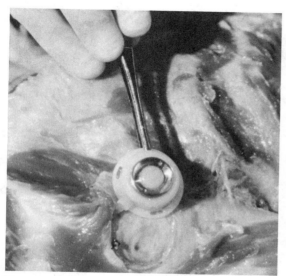

Figure 24–14. Normal appearance of subcutaneously implanted epidural portal at autopsy. Courtesy Dr. F.P. Boersma, The Netherlands.

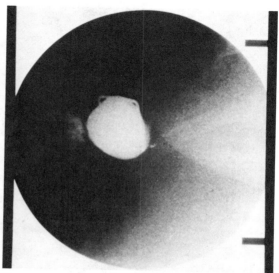

Figure 24–15. Radiographic study demonstrating dysfunction of a subcutaneously implanted intraspinal portal. Injected contrast medium can be seen filling port and extravasating at nine o'clock, due to perforation of the distal segment of the epidural catheter by the portal's outlet tube. Courtesy Dr. F.P. Boersma, The Netherlands.

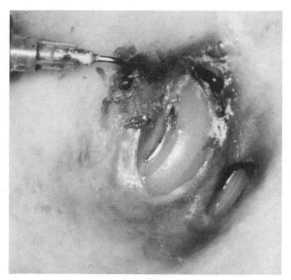

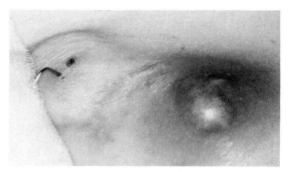

Figure 24–17. "Pseudoabscess" alongside functioning subcutaneously implanted portal, representing collection of bile around neighboring gall bladder drain. Area was drained and allowed to heal by secondary intention while epidural treatment continued uninterrupted. Courtesy Dr. F.P. Boersma, The Netherlands.

Figure 24–16. Necrosis of skin overlying subcutaneously implanted epidural portal subsequent to severe progressive weight loss (>30 kg). Courtesy Dr. F.P. Boersma, The Netherlands.

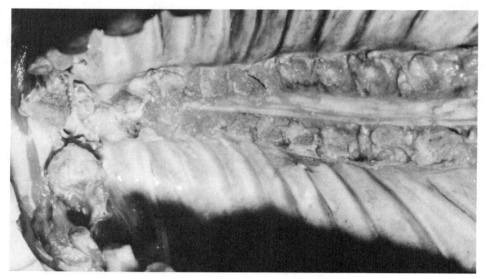

Figure 24–18. Appearance of spinal cord at autopsy. Cord is exposed in continuity by means of an anterior approach facilitated by the use of an oscillating saw. Courtesy Dr. F.P. Boersma, The Netherlands.

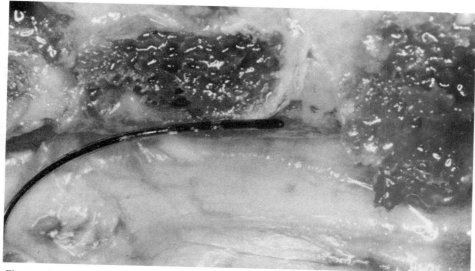

Figure 24–19. Normal appearance of correctly situated epidural catheter at autopsy. Courtesy Dr. F.P. Boersma, The Netherlands.

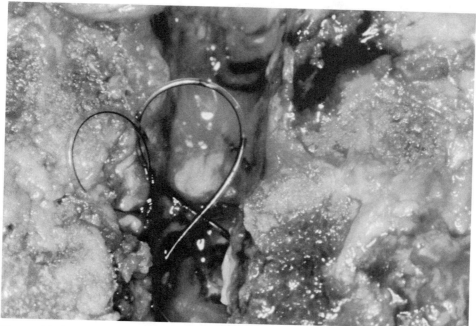

Figure 24–20. "Figure-of-eight" appearance of redundant epidural catheter at autopsy; catheter has been advanced excessively. Courtesy Dr. F.P. Boersma, The Netherlands.

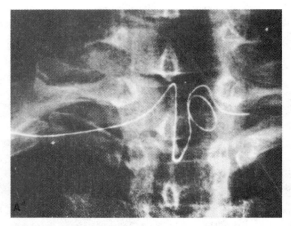

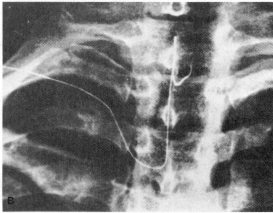

Figure 24–21. **(A)** Demonstrates radiographic appearance of epidural catheter after the injection of contrast medium. Catheter has been advanced excessively, has kinked, curled, and eventually its tip can be observed to be exiting through a neural foramen. **(B)** Demonstrates correct appearance of catheter after partial withdrawal.

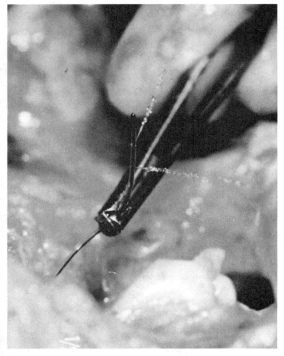

Figure 24–22. Appearance of standard epidural catheter at autopsy, demonstrating occlusion of distal orifice and patency of side holes. Courtesy Dr. F.P. Boersma, The Netherlands.

Figure 24–23. **(A)** Appearance of epidural catheter *in situ* at autopsy embedded in epidural ➤ fibrosis after 3 months of infusion. **(B)** Catheter has been removed along with adherent fibrotic tissue. **(C)** Microscopic view of epidural tissue, demonstrating mild inflammatory reaction and foreign body giant cells. **(D)** Microscopic view of epidural tissue, demonstrating the presence of calcium deposits. Courtesy Dr. F.P. Boersma, The Netherlands.

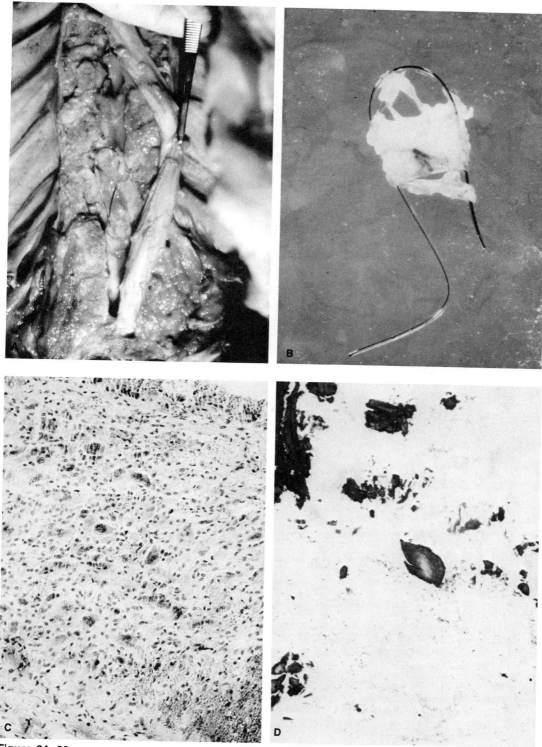

Figure 24-23.

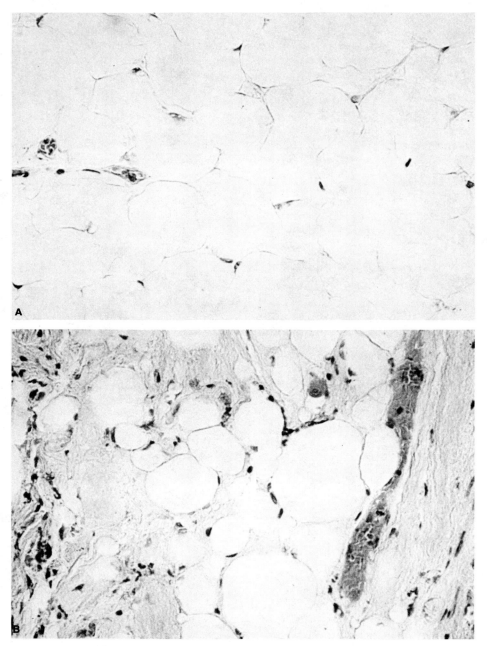

Figure 24–24.   **(A)** Microscopic view of epidural tissue, demonstrating normal appearance of epidural fat.**(B)** Microscopic view of epidural tissue in cachectic patient, demonstrating a paucity of normal fat cells and proliferation of vascular tissue. Relative absence of fatty tissue may predispose to abnormal pharmacokinetics and pharmacodynamics. Courtesy Dr. F.P. Boersma, The Netherlands.

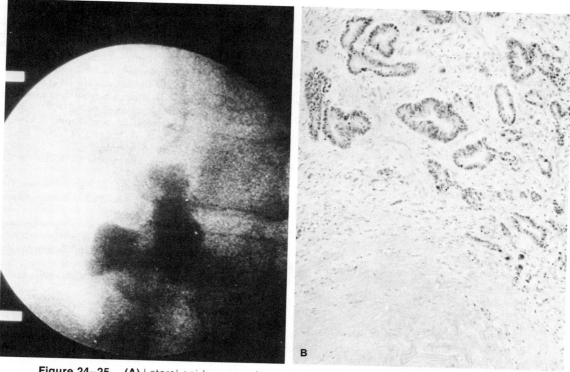

Figure 24–25. **(A)** Lateral epidurogram demonstrating "pseudopocket" formation with localized collection of contrast medium and failure of even epidural spread. Study was obtained subsequent to deterioration of quality of pain control. **(B)** Magnified section of spinal cord of above patient, demonstrating tumor infiltration by rectal carcinoma, presumably responsible for defect. Courtesy Dr. F.P. Boersma, The Netherlands.

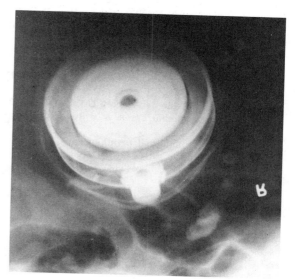

Figure 24–26. Radiograph of subcutaneously implanted drug delivery system (type V) obtained after a period of failed analgesia. Radiograph depicts coiling of radiopaque intraspinal catheter around base of drug pump, suggesting a failure of the stitches intended to immobilize the pump subcutaneously; the pump subsequently rotated with normal movement, withdrawing the catheter from its correct position. Courtesy Leonard Hirsch, MD, Chief of Neurosurgery, Crozer Chester Medical Center, Pennsylvania.

REFERENCES

1. Moore DC: Complications of Regional Anesthesia. Springfield, IL, Charles C Thomas, 1955.
2. Bridenbaugh PO: Complications of local anesthetic neural blockade. In Cousins MJ, Bridenbaugh PO (eds): Neural Blockade, 2nd ed, p 695. Philadelphia, JB Lippincott, 1988.
3. Swerdlow M: Complications of neurolytic neural blockade. In Cousins MJ, Bridenbaugh PO (eds): Neural Blockade, 2nd ed, p 719. Philadelphia, JB Lippincott, 1988.
4. Dogliotti AM: A new therapeutic method for peripheral neuralgias: Injection of alcohol into the subarachnoid space. Pain Clin 1987;1:197.
5. Mandl F: Aqueous solution of phenol as a substitute for alcohol in sympathetic block. J Int Coll Surg 1950;13:566.
6. Quimby CW: Medicolegal hazards of destructive nerve blocks. In Abram SE (ed): Cancer Pain, p 137. Boston, Kluwer Academic, 1989.
7. Beddard JRJ: Twenty years of clinical nerve blocking. Br J Anaesth 1958;30:367.
8. Churcher M: Peripheral nerve blocks. In Swerdlow M (ed): Relief of Intractable Pain, 3rd ed, p 133. Amsterdam, Elsevier, 1983.
9. Macomber DW: Necrosis of the nose and cheek, secondary to treatment of trigeminal neuralgia. Plast Reconstr Surg 1953;11:337.
10. Stern EL: Relief of intractable pain by the intraspinal (subarachnoid) injection of alcohol. Am J Surg 1934;25:217.
11. Hughes JT: Thrombosis of the posterior spinal arteries. Neurology 1970;20:659.
12. Totoki T, Kato T, Nomoto Y et al: Anterior spinal artery syndrome: A complication of cervical intrathecal phenol injection. Pain 1979;6:99.
13. Souperville-Sovak B, Rasminky M, Finlayson MH: Complications of phenol neurolysis. Arch Neurol 1975;32:226.
14. Nour-Eldin F: Preliminary report: Uptake of phenol by vascular and brain tissue. Microvasc Res 1970;2:224.
15. Swerdlow M: Spinal and peripheral neurolysis for managing Pancoast syndrome. In Bonica JJ, Ventafridda V, Pagni C (eds): Advances in Pain Research

and Therapy, vol 4, p 135. New York, Raven Press, 1982.
16. Ischia S, Luzzani A, Ischia A et al: Subarachnoid neurolytic block (L5–S1) and unilateral percutaneous cervical cordotomy in the treatment of pain secondary to pelvic malignant disease. Pain 1984;20:139.
17. Lifshitz S, Debacker LJ, Buchsbaum HJ et al: Subarachnoid phenol block for pain relief in gynecologic malignancy. Obstet Gynecol 1976;48:316.
18. Racz GB, Holubec JT: Stellate ganglion phenol neurolysis. In Racz GB (ed): Techniques of Neurolysis, p 133. Boston, Kluwer Academic, 1989.
19. Winnie AP: An immobile needle for nerve blocks. Anesthesiology 1969;31:577.
20. Bonica JJ, Loeser DJ, Chapman RC et al (eds): The Management of Pain, 2nd ed. Philadelphia, Lea and Febiger, 1990.
21. Blomberg RG, Lofstrom JB: The test dose in regional anesthesia. Acta Anaesthesiol Scand 1991;35:465.
22. Moore DC: Regional Block, 4th ed, p 330. Springfield, IL, Charles C Thomas, 1965.
23. Covino BG: Recent advances in local anaesthesia. Can Anaesth Soc J 1986;33;S5.
24. Reid W, Watt JK, Gray TG: Phenol injection of sympathetic chain. Br J Surg 1970;47:45.
25. Benzon HT: Convulsions secondary to intravascular phenol: A hazard of celiac plexus block. Anesth Analg 1979;58:150.
26. Felsenthal G: Pharmacology of phenol in peripheral nerve blocks: A review. Arch Phys Med Rehabil 1974;55:1.
27. Goodman LS, Gilman A: A Pharmacologic Basis of Therapeutics, 4th ed. London, MacMillan, 1970.
28. Smith MC: Histological findings following intrathecal injections of phenol solutions for relief of pain. Br J Anaesth 1964;36:387.
29. Labat G: The action of alcohol on the living nerve: Experimental and clinical considerations. Anesth Analg 1933;12:190.
30. Nathan PW, Sears TA: Effects of phenol on nervous conduction. J Physiol 1960;150:565.
31. Urmey WF, Talts KH, Schraft S et al: Ipsilateral hemidiaphragm paresis associated with intrascalene brachial plexus anesthesia. Anesthesiology 1989;71:A728.
32. Regnard C. Dyspnea in advanced cancer: A flow diagram. Palliative Medicine 1990;4:311.

Chapter 25

Orthopedic Management of Cancer Pain

Randy N. Rosier

Musculoskeletal manifestations of cancer include both the occurrence of primary cancers of the bone and soft tissues, or sarcomas, as well as metastatic carcinomas that involve the skeletal system. Pain may be the presenting complaint with any cancer involving the musculoskeletal system, and lesions involving bone are particularly likely to cause pain. For sarcoma involving bone or soft tissues, surgical removal of the tumor is generally the principal treatment, often accompanied by adjuvant chemotherapy or radiation. In such cases, pain generally resolves with removal of the tumor, and is rarely a subsequent problem for the patient. However, sarcomas are extremely rare in comparison to carcinomas that metastasize to bone, and the latter comprise the great majority of orthopedic cancer pain management problems. Although almost any type of cancer can metastasize to bone, the five carcinomas with the greatest predisposition for bony metastases are breast, prostate, lung, kidney, and thyroid cancers (Table 25–1).[1] The other common cancer that causes skeletal pain is multiple myeloma, which is a primary marrow cell tumor involving bone. Most of these disorders affect individuals in older age groups (ie, fifth to sixth decade and above).

A number of clinical problems can be caused by cancers involving the skeletal system. Bone pain can result from metastatic deposits in bone, even in the absence of gross bone destruction.[2] The mechanisms for production of pain by tumor deposits is unclear, but a variety of cytokines are released from tumor cells that mediate bone resorption, changes in bone blood flow, and inflammatory reactions. Elevated bone marrow pressure may result from these events, and in some way may be transduced to the richly innervated periosteum, causing the pain

Table 25–1.
Incidence of Cancers With Bone Involvement

Cancer	Incidence	Percent Bone Involvement
Lung	17.8%	23%–44%
Breast	16.5%	48%–84%
Prostate	11%	47%–84%
Kidney	2.5%	33%
Thyroid	1.1%	27%–50%
Myeloma	1.1%	100%
Bone sarcoma	0.3%	100%
Soft-tissue sarcoma	0.8%	—

This table shows the incidence in the United States of the cancers most commonly involving bone. This is based on data from the National Cancer Data Base,[1] and the percentage multiplied by 1,000,000 (estimated total new cases in U.S. per year) gives the number of cases. The figures for bone involvement give the ranges reported in various autopsy studies. The incidences of bone and soft tissue sarcoma are shown for comparison.

signal. There are no nerve endings within bone except for unmyelinated sympathetic nerves that are thought to modulate bone blood flow.[3] However, pain is known to occur in association with elevated hydrostatic pressure within the marrow in bone infarctions, and in these cases is relieved by surgical decompression of the marrow.

Pain also may result from bone destruction with pathologic fracture or impending pathologic fracture. This is a very common situation with multiple myeloma or metastatic carcinoma, and often requires orthopedic intervention. Pain due to an impending pathologic fracture generally is aggravated by physical activity involving the extremity or by weight-bearing on the extremity, and characteristically is somewhat relieved by rest. This is in contrast to the situation discussed above where there is no gross bone destruction, in which case pain more commonly is constant, unrelated to activity, and often worse at night.

A pattern of pain on weight-bearing in the presence of a lytic bony lesion actually is a very reliable clinical indicator of an impending pathologic fracture.

Metastatic carcinomas show a predilection for involvement of the axial skeleton, with the thoracic and lumbar spine representing the most common focus. Therefore, impingement on neural structures such as the spinal cord or nerve roots is another common cause of musculoskeletal cancer pain. Similarly, any peripheral nerve can be impinged on or invaded by a skeletal or soft tissue metastasis, causing both pain and neurologic symptoms. Examples include axillary nodal metastases, which can cause brachial plexus symptoms, or pelvic masses impinging on the lumbosacral plexus, leading to sciatica. Pain induced by such neural compression can be particularly severe and difficult to treat, and there is the compounding problem of loss of function due to neurologic deficit. Postradiation neuritis can occur after cancer treatment, causing pain, neurologic symptoms, or both. Additionally, cancer patients may develop painful causalgias or reflex sympathetic dystrophy after injury or surgical interventions to an extremity, although the incidence is probably no higher than in the general population.

Orthopedic problems other than pain that result from musculoskeletal manifestations of cancer include muscle weakness, impaired ambulation, joint stiffness or contractures, spinal deformities, osteopenia from inactivity, thromboembolic phenomena, and hypercalcemia. Most of these problems can be improved by interventions directed toward maintenance of a maximal functional activity level. Therefore, a relatively aggressive approach generally is adopted by orthopedic oncologists with regard to surgical fixation of impending or completed pathologic fractures, maintenance of ambulatory status, and rehabilitative programs such as physical therapy and occupational therapy.

The different types of cancer that can involve the skeletal system exhibit varying patterns of bony involvement and associated clinical problems. Some tumors characteristically demonstrate a purely lytic radiographic appearance, such as multiple myeloma, lung carcinoma, and renal cell carcinoma. This implies minimal reaction of the bone to the presence of the tumor, and purely lytic lesions are much more prone to pathologic fractures. Other tumors such as prostatic carcinoma have a blastic radiographic appearance, indicating that they secrete factors that induce host osteoblasts in the area of the tumor to form excess bone. Acid phosphatase may be one of these factors, and acts via the insulin-like growth factor II receptor to directly stimulate osteoblasts adjacent to the tumor cells.[4] The resulting sclerotic metastases are less apt to fracture than are lytic lesions because of the locally increased bone mass. Many tumors, such as metastatic breast carcinoma, typically exhibit a mixed picture of both lytic and blastic areas, with fractures usually occurring through the lytic areas. Again, locally secreted cytokines are thought to mediate the bone resorption as well as the local bony reaction to the lesion, although these factors have not yet been fully defined. Tumor-produced factors thought to mediate local bone resorption include prostaglandins, interleukin-1, tumor necrosis factor, and transforming growth factor.[5] Factors that may stimulate bone formation or inhibit its resorption include insulin-like growth factors, transforming growth factor beta, calcitonin, and calcitonin generated peptide.[6] In addition to local growth factors, some tumors can mediate a systemic resorption of bone resembling that which occurs with hyperparathyroidism. This is due to secretion of parathyroid hormone-related peptide (PTHrP), a protein with homology to parathyroid hormone, and with similar actions. This is most commonly seen with lung cancers, and occasionally with breast or renal carcinoma, and is the cause of the so-called humoral hypercalcemia of malignancy.[7] However, secretion of PTHrP accounts for only a small percentage of cases of hypercalcemia in malignancy, with the majority of cases resulting from local osteolysis by multiple metastases. Table 25–2 summarizes the role of cytokines in skeletal lesions.

The course of skeletal involvement also varies greatly with the type of tumor, and the capability of treatment to control the disease. Patients with metastatic lung cancer tend to have rapid progression of disease in both skeletal and extraskeletal sites, and lytic bone lesions frequently progress to fracture. Patients with metastatic breast or prostatic carcinoma, however, may have a much more indolent and protracted course, particularly in the case of hormonally responsive tumors. The degree of histologic differentiation of a given tumor also may correlate somewhat with the expected rate of progression of disease. Of patients with skeletal metastases, only about 10% have involvement of the long bones, and there is a predilection for the proximal appendicular skeleton over the more distal extremities. One exception to this is lung carcinoma, which occasionally metastasizes to the small bones of the hands or feet. Eighty percent of skeletal metastases involve the axial skeleton, and an additional 10% the calvarium. In the axial skeleton, the thoracic spine is involved most frequently, followed by the lumbar spine, ribs, pelvis, clavicle, and sternum. The most frequent significant orthopedic problems result from involvement of the femur, humerus, and spine.

The major goals of orthopedic treatment are control of musculoskeletal pain while maintaining a maximal level of functional activity. Control of pain may be as simple as providing appropriate opioid or anti-inflammatory pain medication. Anti-inflammatory medication may have an additional beneficial effect of decreasing prostaglandin synthesis by tumor cells in bone, and thereby slowing local osteolysis (see Chaps. 7 and 10). However, careful evaluation of the cause of pain is extremely important in formulating treatment decisions. A fundamental concept in understanding the course of skeletal metastases is that tumor cells initially tend to take the path of least resistance within bone. Consequently, the marrow elements are displaced initially by metastatic tumor cells, and only later does erosion of the trabecular bone begin, either through stimulation of host osteoclasts by cytokines, or by direct enzymatic destruction of bone matrix by tumor cells. Figure 25–1 shows a histologic example of breast carcinoma infil-

Table 25–2.
Cytokines Involved in Regulation of Bone Formation and Resorption[3–5]

Mediators of Resorption	Inhibitors of Resorption	Stimulators of Formation
Prostaglandin E_2	Calcitonin	Insulin-like growth factor I
Interleukin-1	Calcitonin gene-related peptide	Insulin-like growth factor II
Tumor necrosis factor α		Transforming growth factor betas
Transforming growth factor α		? Acid phosphatase

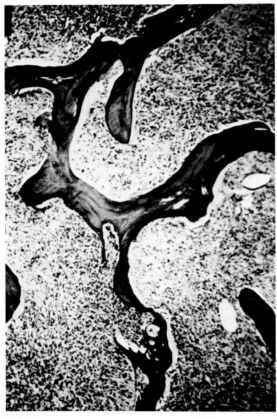

Figure 25–1. This histologic specimen is from a bony metastasis in a patient with breast carcinoma. Note the complete replacement of the marrow elements with tumor before erosion of the trabecular bone, which remains fairly well preserved. Several areas of beginning lysis of the trabecular bone are evident.

tration into bone, with complete replacement of bone marrow by the lesion, yet preservation of the architecture of most of the bone. The clinical significance of this phenomenon is that a patient may present with persistent pain due to a bony lesion, and yet the radiographs of the involved bone can appear normal. In fact, nearly 50% of trabecular bone must be destroyed before a lytic lesion becomes evident on a plain radiograph. A much more sensitive indicator of bone involvement is the bone scan, which usually will demonstrate subtle bony reaction to an occult lesion long before the lesion is evident on plain films. Thus, involved areas can be assessed and followed to allow local treatment to a problematic area before progression to fracture. The one exception to this is multiple myeloma, in which the tumor has the ability to suppress local bony reaction through unknown mechanisms. This accounts for the "punched-out" radiographic appearance of myelomatous lesions, and leads in many cases to negative bone scans. An additional important diagnostic modality in evaluation of pain in patients with possible metastatic skeletal disease is magnetic resonance imaging. Magnetic resonance imaging can demonstrate the abnormal signal present in areas of marrow involvement. This modality is even more sensitive than the bone scan, but generally is not necessary as a screening tool. Magnetic resonance imaging also can be useful in assessing neural impingement by tumor in the spine.

Bone pain due to skeletal lesions without significant associated bone destruction (*ie*, lesions not likely to cause fractures) usually can be treated effectively with the administration of local radiotherapy. In fact, radiotherapy is really the mainstay of pain control in patients with metastatic carcinoma or myeloma. Radiation generally is administered to levels of 3,000 to 4,000 cGy to the affected area in divided doses over 10 to 14 daily fractions. Potential complications of radiation include bone necrosis, skin reaction, and delayed healing of wounds, but generally these moderate doses are well tolerated.

Pain caused by impending or actual fractures is rarely aided by bracing or casting of the involved extremity, presumably due to the continued presence of the tumor and progressive bone destruction. Protected weight-bearing with a walker or crutches may provide temporary or partial pain relief in the situation of an impending fracture, but is poorly tolerated as a long-term solution. Consequently, conservative treatment for fractures or symptomatic impending fractures of the extremities rarely is successful. However, in patients who are medically too ill to tolerate surgical intervention, orthoses may offer some benefit. Radiation to a fracture often will improve the pain by reducing the bulk of local tumor, but it also obliterates the callus response, and therefore usually leads to nonunion of the fracture. The cartilaginous component of the fracture callus is its more radiosensitive element, and osteoblastic bone formation is relatively radioresistant. If a fractured bone is rigidly fixed with a metal plate or rod, the bone heals primarily by osteoblastic bone formation, without a significant cartilaginous callus. Therefore, surgical stabilization of a long bone fracture, followed by radiotherapy, will achieve pain control through destruction of the local tumor, provide immediate stabilization of the fracture, and will allow healing of the fracture. This is the most common approach to pathologic fractures of the long bones, and has a high rate of success in eliminating pain and allowing a rapid return to function. Figure 25–2 demonstrates this approach.

In the axial skeleton, conservative treatment of painful pathologic fractures is suc-

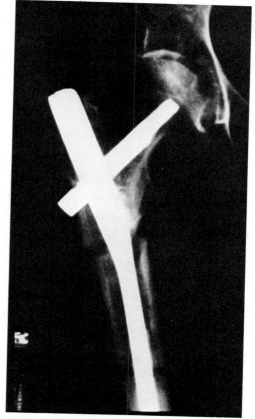

Figure 25–2. This patient with metastatic carcinoma to the femur developed a pathologic subtrochanteric fracture that was stabilized with an intramedullary device. Subsequently, the patient received local radiotherapy and the fracture healed uneventfully, enabling the patient to remain ambulatory.

cessful more often. Bones such as the vertebrae, clavicle, ribs, sternum, and pelvis have a much better blood supply, and therefore inherently heal more readily after fracture than the long bones. Consequently, fractures treated conservatively often will heal even after radiotherapy has been administered for tumor treatment. Tumors located in the bony spine tend to cause back pain before the development of significant bone destruction, thus facilitating earlier detection and intervention. Bracing may be quite effective, in combination with radiotherapy, for the control of pain from spinal lesions. These measures are aided in part by the stability afforded the thoracic spine by the rib cage. Pathologic vertebral compression fractures often will heal uneventfully when treated in this manner, relieving pain and preventing neurologic deficits.

There are a number of situations, however, in which surgical management of spinal lesions is necessary. Indications for surgery include the presence of a neurologic deficit that does not resolve rapidly with radiation therapy, recurrence or progression of a deficit after radiation, or bone destruction causing spinal instability. Decompression of the spinal cord or nerve roots is preferentially carried out through an anterior approach to the spine, as laminectomies may contribute to the instability. Stabilization of the spine can be anterior, posterior, or both, and usually involves the use of metal rods, methylmethacrylate bone cement, and wires. In addition, it is important also to obtain bony fusion of the spine, or the metal and cement constructs eventually will fail mechanically. Bony fusion may be facilitated by the use of allograft bone from a bone bank if the patient's own bone is diffusely involved with cancer. The same principles apply to lesions of the cervical spine, although metastases to this area are less common than in the thoracic and lumbar regions.

When a pathologic fracture occurs adjacent to a major joint, such as the hip, knee, or shoulder, replacement of the joint by prosthetic arthroplasty may have significant advantages over fixation of the fracture. For instance, displaced pathologic fractures of the femoral neck are characterized by a high rate of nonunion and avascular necrosis of the femoral head. Prosthetic replacement avoids these problems, and renders the patient fully ambulatory in a short time. Figure 25–3 shows a clinical example of this approach. If large areas of major bones are destroyed by tumor, stabilization may be mechanically difficult. Custom computer-designed implants may allow reconstruction of such bones. Allografts, or bone transplants, offer another alternative. In less severe cases of bone loss, stability may be provided by use of metal plates or intramedullary rods in conjunction with

methylmethacrylate bone cement. However, in such cases, as previously discussed for spinal lesions, supplementation of the hardware with bone grafts to allow eventual restoration of biologic continuity of the bone is essential to prevent late mechanical failures. This is most important in tumors that characteristically are associated with prolonged survival, such as hormonally responsive breast and prostatic cancers.

Occasionally, a painful metastatic lesion may warrant resection and limb reconstruction, similar to the usual approach for sarcoma (*eg*, radioresistant lesions such as renal cell carcinoma). In extreme situations of refractory tumor, palliative amputation of an extremity may be appropriate, and sometimes can provide marked improvement in pain control. This is particularly true with bulky, fungating, radioresistant tumors exhibiting extensive soft tissue and bone involvement.

With the many technical advances now available for surgical stabilization of the spine and extremities, the orthopedic approach to the cancer patient with skeletal involvement has become increasingly aggressive in recent years. Maintaining patients in an ambulatory, functional state dramatically improves the quality of life, and decreases the pain and suffering of these patients. Furthermore, such aggressive management prevents the many complications associated with patients becoming bedridden, thereby potentially improving longevity as well. Finally, this approach enables many patients to be cared for in the home setting rather than relying on institutional care. Obviously, the potential benefits of surgical intervention have to be tempered with careful medical assessment of the patient's ability to survive the surgical procedure, and, to this end, a coordinated team effort between the orthopedic surgeon, medical oncologist, and radiation oncologist is essential. With this important principle of maintaining function in mind, there has been an increasing trend toward prophylactic fixation of high-risk bony lesions. Patients who undergo prophylactic fixation recover from surgery more quickly, often require lesser surgical procedures, and are usually in better

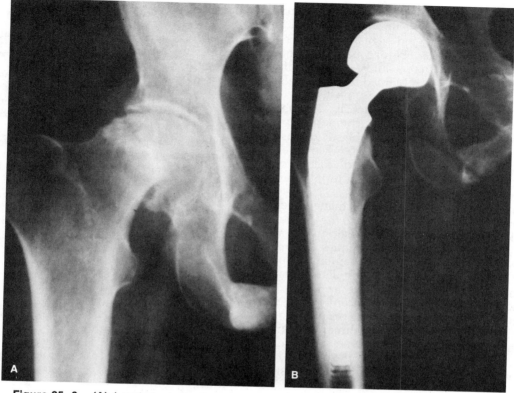

Figure 25–3. **(A)** A pathologic fracture of the femoral neck is demonstrated in a patient with metastatic breast carcinoma. Because of the high incidence of avascular necrosis of the hip with this type of fracture, replacement of the joint was undertaken, as shown in **(B)**.

overall health at the time of surgery than if intervention is delayed until fracture occurs. Zickel and Mouradian, Harrington, and others have proposed guidelines for prophylactic fixation.[8,9] Table 25–3 summarizes these surgical indications. In general, lesions in a weight-bearing bone that are larger than 2 to 3 cm, demonstrate more than 30%–50% cortical involvement circumferentially, or are associated with pain on weight-bearing, warrant fixation. This author has found pain on weight-bearing or use of the involved extremity to be an extremely reliable predictor of impending fracture. Presumably, such pain emanates from microfractures of the bony cortex causing disturbance of the richly innervated periosteum. For some locations, surgi-

Table 25–3.
Surgical Indications for Prophylactic Fixation[7,8]

Indications for Prophylactic Fixation	Additional Influencing Factors
Lesion >50% diameter of bone with cortical involvement	Degree of differentiation of lesion
Lesion >2–3 cm diameter	Radiosensitivity of lesion
Lesion involving >50% of cortex	Lytic vs. blastic disease
Lesion associated with avulsion fracture of the lesser trochanter of the femur	Medical condition of patient
	Estimated survival of patient
Pain on weight-bearing	

cal criteria must be modified, as in the femoral neck, where even a smaller lesion should be prophylactically pinned. This substitutes a minor surgical procedure for a major one (total hip replacement) that would be needed if a fracture were to occur. Many other factors also must be considered, such as the likelihood that the tumor will progress rapidly, its probable response to radiation or chemotherapy, predominance of lytic versus blastic disease, and the patient's activity level. All of these factors influence the likelihood of fracture occurrence, and thus the decision to intervene surgically.

In summary, the orthopedic management of cancer pain primarily relates to the problem of skeletal metastases and associated fractures. Improved surgical techniques and recognition of the importance of maintaining patients in a functional and ambulatory state have led to a more aggressive approach to orthopedic intervention in recent years. In conjunction with the widening array of non-surgical pain management techniques, rehabilitation and physical medicine, and more effective new tumor therapies, the outlook for orthopedic cancer patients is improving significantly.

REFERENCES

1. Menck HR, Garfinkel L, Dodd GD: Preliminary report of the national cancer data base. CA 1991; 41:7.
2. Edeiken J, Karasick D: Imaging in cancer. CA 1987; 37:239.
3. Cooper RR, Milgram JW, Robinson RA: Morphology of the osteon. J Bone Joint Surg 1966;48A: 1239.
4. Ishibe M, Rosier RN, Puzas JE: Human prostatic acid phosphatase directly stimulates isolated bone cells. Journal of Bone and Mineral Research 1990;5 (Suppl):307.
5. Galasko CSB: Skeletal Metastases, p 22. London, Butterworth, 1986.
6. Noda M, Camilliere JJ: In vivo stimulation of bone formation by transforming growth factor-beta. Endocrinology 1989;124:2991.
7. Broadus AE, Stewart AF: Humoral mechanisms of hypercalcemia. Journal of Bone and Mineral Research 1984;3:311.
8. Harrington KD: Orthopaedic Management of Metastatic Bone Disease, p 297. St. Louis, CV Mosby, 1988.
9. Zickel RF, Mouradian WH: Intramedullary fixation of pathological fractures and lesions of the subtrochanteric region of the femur. J Bone Joint Surg 1976;58A: 1061.

Section 4

Special Problem Areas

Chapter *26*

Neurosurgical and Neuroaugmentative Intervention

Ronald R. Tasker

GENERAL CONSIDERATIONS

Neurosurgery is at a crossroads regarding its role in the management of cancer pain. On the one hand, referrals are diminishing as oncologists and pain treatment facilities are adopting more aggressive approaches to the use of opioids administered by oral, subcutaneous, and intravenous routes (see Chapters 6–12). On the other hand, whereas the future appears to lead increasingly toward the direct delivery of specific neuroactive substances to discrete central nervous sites,[1] current treatment options remain relatively limited. The contemporary neurosurgeon therefore must choose between reliance on time-honored operations that interrupt nociception, and modulatory techniques that involve either the delivery of opioids to the central nervous system (see Chapter 18) or the localized application of electrical stimulation.

Notwithstanding the individualized considerations that form an essential part of the decision-making process on each occasion a patient is assessed, generic characteristics of each of these categories of options are identifiable. Destructive procedures performed in properly selected patients by competent surgeons using state-of-the-art equipment are associated with a very low but definite risk of (often irreversible) complications. In their favor, however, destructive procedures can be characterized as "once-only" events that do not require ongoing attendance at a health care facility. The direct delivery of opioids to the central nervous system minimizes the unwanted effects of the opioids by using the smallest possible doses. The risks of destructive procedures are avoided, but new risks are introduced (eg, infection, catheter malfunction). Chronic therapy requires implantation of a catheter–reservoir system (see Chapter 18) that must be either 1) accessed regularly for bolus injections through the same skin site (portal system); 2) serviced by one of a variety of external pumps, automated devices that are effective but costly and must be maintained (externalized catheter system); or 3) outfitted with one of the fully implantable automated pumps, sophisticated nonreusable devices that require less frequent filling, but, more often than not, are prohibitively expensive. Regardless of the means of administration, spinal opioid therapy requires continued attendance at a health care facility for supervision and drug replenishment. Systemically administered opioid analgesia depends on relatively higher doses of drugs that are biodistributed more widely, and entails other risks, predominantly of inadequate analgesia and drug toxicity (side effects). Although significant surgical procedures and expensive nonreusable equipment are avoided, the patient's dependence on the health care system is increased. This chapter reviews neurosurgical procedures that have been used widely to control cancer pain, other than implanted drug delivery systems (see Chapter 18).

HISTORICAL PERSPECTIVE: THE DEVELOPMENT OF NEUROSURGICAL TECHNIQUES FOR THE CONTROL OF CANCER PAIN

The early development of neurosurgical operations for the management of cancer pain was based on the Cartesian concept of pain, which postulated a direct circuit between the site of tissue injury and the brain. Early procedures were devised with the intention of physically isolating the peripheral nociceptors being stimulated by intractable cancer from conscious perception at the central level. The most obvious and frequently used approach

was that of surgical division of the relevant peripheral nerves or dorsal roots. The older literature is replete with accounts of open dorsal rhizotomy, performed predominantly for pain originating in the limbs and trunk, and multiple cranial nerve sections and high cervical rhizotomy for rostral pain due to head and neck cancer.

Despite moderate success characterized by limited but often adequate duration, such open procedures imposed major risks and significant requirements for convalescence on patients already debilitated and terminally ill. Even after the virtual replacement of open procedures by percutaneous surgery (see below), the results of neurectomy and rhizotomy often were suboptimal for multiple reasons, including:

1. The receptive fields of neighboring nerves tend to overlap, and if fibers of an adjacent, uninterrupted peripheral nerve or root contribute to the innervation of the painful area, relief will be incomplete.
2. Cancer is a dynamic, progressive process, and with the passage of time malignant invasion seldom remains localized to the domains of individual nerves or roots. Despite initially promising results, uncontrolled progression of tumor beyond the anatomic limits of surgical denervation may render surgery ultimately ineffective.
3. The nonselective nature of these procedures, with loss of all modalities of sensation after rhizotomy and additional loss of motor function after section of mixed nerves, often results in unacceptable outcomes.
4. Peripheral nerves regenerate and can form neuromas, the pain from which may rival or exceed the severity of the original complaint. Deafferentation also can lead to relentless neuropathic pain.

Nevertheless, in special situations these procedures still are valuable (see below). Whenever possible they should be performed by percutaneous means.

Even at an early date the merits of percutaneous versus open surgery were advanced, as with the introduction of trigeminal nerve cauterization by Hartel[2] and Kirschner.[3] These procedures were associated with a relatively high incidence of serious complications until Sweet and Wepsic[4] introduced the safer technique of radiofrequency coagulation, which since has become the standard neurosurgical means for producing a percutaneous neural lesion.

Although there is controversy as to whether percutaneous destructive surgery should be performed best with radiofrequency current or by chemical means (injection of alcohol and phenol), the radiofrequency technique usually is preferred because it is so easily coupled with various physiologic means of corroborating the intended site of the lesion (recording, stimulation, and impedance recording). In addition, the extent of the resulting lesion is controlled readily in response to information obtained by monitoring the current applied and/or the temperature achieved. In contrast to the more predictable nature of the radiofrequency lesion, the spread of injected solutions within biologic tissue is more likely to be indiscriminate and uneven, diminishing the reliability, effectiveness, and persistence of results.[5-11]

The focus of destructive neurosurgery for pain initially dictated by Cartesian concepts changed with the introduction of spinothalamic (anterolateral) cordotomy. In 1905, Spiller first demonstrated discrete transmission of pain and temperature sensation through the anterolateral spinothalamic tract,[12] and 7 years later Spiller and Martin reported the first case of relief of intractable pain by open surgical section of the anterolateral quadrant.[13] Although the subject of their first case did not suffer from cancer pain, cordotomy became the main choice in the neurosurgical armamentarium for the treatment of cancer pain.

Open cordotomy involves general anesthesia, cervical or thoracic laminectomy, and near complete section of the anterolateral quadrant. Thus, the extent of surgery imposes excessive risk and major requirements for convalescence in the medically unfit cancer patient. These drawbacks and others were overcome by the introduction of the percutaneous

method by Mullan et al in 1963.[14] Percutaneous cordotomy is performed under local anesthesia, and produces a stereotactically guided lesion in the spinothalamic tract within the cord's anterolateral quadrant. Mullan et al's original technique used ionizing radiation to produce a lesion at the C1–2 level by means of a strontium-tipped probe, but later was supplanted by Rosomoff's radiofrequency technique (1965).[15] The procedure has since been improved further with the introduction of myelography,[16] impedance monitoring,[17] and physiologic guidance.[18-22] As a result, percutaneous cordotomy is safer and more efficacious than the open technique,[23] has extended the relevance of tractotomy to more critically ill patients, and is easily repeatable if the need arises on the same or contralateral side.

In an attempt to improve on cordotomy, Armour, in 1927, introduced open midline commissurotomy (myelotomy).[24] Classic commissurotomy is intended to divide the spinothalamic fibers in the process of decussation in the midline, to secure a higher level of analgesia relative to the level of the surgical incision in the cord. This procedure, too, virtually has been replaced by a cervical percutaneous technique pioneered by Hitchcock.[25-27] Contrary to Armour's original thinking, commissurotomy appears to affect pain in some novel way, as the level of incision or coagulation in the cord bears no relationship to the somatotopographic distribution of pain relief, or to the (usually transient) analgesia that results.

Further developments in surgery for pain relief exploited the concept of cordotomy, but at the level of the brain-stem, with the introduction of trigeminal and spinothalamic tractotomy at the medullary level and mesencephalic tractotomy.[28-31] These procedures, however, were associated with extensive morbidity and mortality, so that the acceptance of this general approach likely would not have persisted had it not been for the introduction of the human stereotactic technique by Spiegel and Wycis,[32] which permitted percutaneous access to essentially any site within the brain. Initial efforts to achieve pain relief by stereotactic means were directed toward the mesencephalic spinothalamic tract, a procedure that proved safer, more effective, and, interestingly, less prone to inducing dysesthesias than the open procedure, and which often was coupled with dorsomedian thalamotomy with the intention of alleviating suffering.[33-36] It was only natural, also, that the possibility of thalamotomy in the ventrobasal complex be explored,[37-39] because this region was thought to represent the termination of the lateral somatotopographically organized spinothalamic tract. Lesions also were made in the medial thalamus, the presumed destination of the medial nonsomatotopographic portion of the spinothalamic tract. A series of studies by Mark and colleagues[40-45] suggested that the medial thalamus was a more suitable target than the lateral, and that targeting this area would avoid the generalized sensory loss and accompanying complications produced by ventrocaudal thalamotomy, as well as the risk of dysesthesia, exchanging them instead for usually transient cognitive dysfunction. Moreover, pain relief was said to be more complete, and the operation induced no sensory loss. An alternative that does not appear to have been explored adequately is stereotactic interruption of the thalamic relay for the somatotopographically organized part of the spinothalamic tract in Hassler's parvicellular ventrocaudal nucleus in the inferoposterior ventrobasal complex.[46-48]

Over the years, considerable experience with both stereotactic medial thalamotomy and mesencephalic tractotomy has accumulated for the treatment of pain, particularly for pain affecting the head, neck, and other sites not amenable to cordotomy. An interesting comparison of the two procedures by Frank et al[49] suggests that pain relief is less assured with medial thalamotomy (51.9% initial relief with 41% recurrence) than it is with mesencephalic tractotomy (83.5% persistent relief), but that the risks of the former procedure are less (ie, medial thalamotomy: no mortality, 1.9% aphasia, and 70% transient confusion; compared with 1.8% mortality and 10.1% oculomotor and dysesthetic complications with mesencephalic tractotomy).

The publication of the Gate Control Theory of Pain in 1965[50] had a major impact on thinking about pain, and, subsequently, clinical practice. Particularly, it focused attention not only on pain transmission but also on its modulation. The notion that pain transmission could be modulated initially was explored by Wall and Sweet[51] under the assumption that stimulation of large peripheral nerve fibers would suppress activity in small, presumably nociceptive fibers. As clinical experience with chronic stimulation at various sites in the nervous system accumulated, however, it became clear that the artificial production of paresthesias in the patient's area of pain was more effective for the treatment of central and deafferentation pain than for the nociceptive pain that typically characterizes cancer pain.[52] A particularly interesting development occurred with studies of chronic stimulation in the brain begun by Pool and Heath and their colleagues.[53-55] Whereas Mazars and his associates pioneered stimulation of the ventrobasal complex so as to produce regional paresthesias localized to the patient's area of pain,[56] Richardson and Akil[57,58] and Richardson,[59] exploiting the work of Reynolds,[60] demonstrated that chronic stimulation of the periventricular–aqueductal gray in humans also could reduce pain. In contrast to thalamic stimulation, the pain relief associated with stimulation of the periaqueductal–periventricular gray was of a more generalized topographic nature, thus potentially effective for bilateral and midline pain. Pain relief was postulated to occur as a result of activation of the brain's endogenous opioid receptors, activating descending circuits that modulated entry of nociceptive impulses into the spinothalamic tract at the level of the spinal cord. This technique, then, offered a nondestructive, reversible means of interrupting nociception, instead of cordotomy or tractotomy, though the cost of the necessary equipment has restricted its application in terminally ill cancer patients.

Finally, manipulation of the hypophyseal axis has been used in patients with cancer pain. It had long been observed that open hypophysectomy had a beneficial effect on the progress and pain of hormonally dependent cancers such as those of prostate and breast.[61-63] Morricca,[64] in an effort to simplify open hypophysectomy, advocated percutaneous alcohol injection into the pituitary, and subsequently made the surprising observation that the pain of nonendocrinologically dependent cancers also was relieved. The mechanism of pain relief is not reversed by naloxone administration and remains obscure, having been shown to be unrelated to pituitary function, hypothalamic involvement, or blood or cerebrospinal fluid (CSF) levels of substances such as the endorphins.[65-67] Initially used enthusiastically, the role for this procedure remains as yet incompletely defined because of numerous, usually transient complications, and a tendency for pain recurrence in 3–4 months. It remains, however, a simple, efficacious procedure in sick cancer patients.

Thus, a variety of interrupting and modulatory procedures have become available to the neurosurgeon for the treatment of cancer pain outside the realm of management with opioids. These will be reviewed in more detail after some comments on patient selection.

SELECTION OF PATIENTS FOR CANCER PAIN SURGERY

Appropriate patient selection, one of the keys to optimizing outcome, essentially involves two issues, the pathophysiologic nature of the pain, and general indications relative to the patient himself.

PATHOPHYSIOLOGY OF CANCER PAIN

Until recently, the classification of chronic pain of organic origin as being either "benign" or "malignant" was advocated. Fortunately, that era has lapsed, and there now is wide acceptance for the existence of two very different kinds of organic pain syndromes with distinct mechanisms—nociceptive pain and

neural injury pain (see Chapters 1, 8, and 10).[68-70] Nociceptive pain results from chronic stimulation of nociceptors with continual transmission along nociceptive pathways, essentially the medial and lateral spinothalamic systems.[71] Neural injury pain (neuropathic pain) consists of deafferentation and central types, depending on whether the lesion is located in the peripheral or central nervous system, respectively. Neuropathic pain follows neural injury, but in an idiosyncratic and unpredictable fashion, and then generally in the distribution of the sensory change produced by the lesion. Although deafferentation pain may be precipitated by a wide range of different neural lesions, the causes of central pain are fewer; pain of spinal cord origin is usually secondary to trauma, whereas pain from brain injury usually is the result of a stroke.

The differing pathophysiologies of nociceptive versus neural injury pain dictate different strategies of treatment. Whereas it is reasonable to expect that interruption or modulation of transmission in the spinoreticulothalamic tract will offer a reasonable chance of alleviating nociceptive pain, such is not the case with the constant, steady, usually causalgic and/or dysesthetic elements of neural injury pain. Such pain depends on mechanisms that are poorly understood, but that do not involve transmission along the classic pain pathways. It is too frequently overlooked that cancer pain, although usually nociceptive in character, and therefore potentially amenable to interruption or suppression of impulse transmission in the spinothalamic tract, also may contain an element of deafferentation pain.[72] This is not surprising, since compression of neural elements, particularly the lumbosacral and brachial plexuses, is one of the chief mechanisms by which cancer produces intractable pain, and this process ultimately leads to neural destruction as the disease progresses. Thus, earlier in the course of disease, cancer pain may be predominantly of the nociceptive-compressive type, and therefore will display a high degree of responsiveness to the administration of opioids and other measures such as interruption of nerves, roots, or the spinothalamic tract, and even to periventricular gray stimulation. Later, as the progressive compression of neural elements leads to irreversible injury, a dysesthetic causalgic discomfort often is superimposed on the original pain, usually within the distribution of the denervated area. This type of pain characteristically does not respond to the measures that typically are effective for the management of nociceptive pain—about which this chapter is chiefly concerned—any more than does post-traumatic deafferentation pain. Rather, this pain characteristically responds to the strategies usually applied for the treatment of deafferentation pain caused by nonmalignant lesions, such as with chronic stimulation of dorsal aspect of the spinal cord or of the medial lemniscal system.

GENERAL INDICATIONS FOR SURGERY

Before considering a neurosurgical procedure for the relief of cancer pain, a number of issues must be addressed. The pain for which surgery is proposed must be truly intractable to more conservative measures, and not amenable to therapy directed at the tumor *per se*. It should be clear that it is the pain and not some other symptom that is the chief cause of the patient's distress. The proposed procedure must be appropriate for relief of the type of pain from which the patient suffers. Finally, the delicate balance between the likelihood of success and of complications must be favorable and cost-effective in light of the patient's degree of suffering and probable life expectancy.

CHOICE OF NEUROSURGICAL PROCEDURES

Having decided that surgical treatment is appropriate for a particular patient with cancer pain, the surgeon then must decide which of the many procedures available is the most appropriate. Obviously, the simplest and safest technique that has a reasonable chance of success, whether modulatory or destructive, should be considered. In the infrequent cases of pain that is localized to the distribution of single or a few peripheral nerves, percutaneous radiofrequency neurectomy is an option, such as multiple intercostal neurectomy for cancer pain involving the chest wall, and trigeminal neurectomy in the case of pain confined to trigeminal distribution. For nociceptive pain in the lower extremity caused by neoplastic involvement of the lumbosacral plexus, percutaneous cordotomy is the treatment of choice. For pain in the head or neck, or for upper extremity pain that is not amenable to cordotomy, an intraventricular infusion of morphine is a simpler and safer option than is stereotactic mesencephalotomy. Although less effective than mesencephalotomy, medial thalamotomy is a further option associated with less risk. Overall, for bilateral truncal pain, epidural or intrathecal morphine infusion is preferable to bilateral percutaneous cordotomy, which is associated with significant risks of impairment of urinary function and failure of unconscious respiration. Percutaneous cervical commissurotomy also may be considered. Although the cost of the more elegant implantable automatic pump for opioid infusion may prohibit its realistic use in patients with only a few months to live, the patient or his or her relatives can be taught to inject an indwelling reservoir to provide serial bolus injections into the epidural or even the intrathecal space, or an external pump can be used with home care supervision. In cases for which intraspinal opioids are an alternative, decision-making is facilitated by the interpretation of the results of trials of test doses or short-term infusions through temporary catheters. Other options for the management of diffuse pain include pituitary ablation and chronic stimulation of the periventricular gray matter. In the latter case, the cost of an implanted or radiofrequency-coupled stimulating system may be avoided by the use of a chronically externalized electrode.

The following section examines regularly used destructive procedures and the role of periventricular gray stimulation.

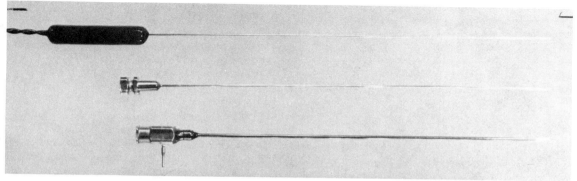

Figure 26–1. Electrode with thermistor (above) for radiofrequency coagulation of trigeminal nerve (provided by Diros Technology).

DESTRUCTIVE PROCEDURES

Attempts to interrupt pain transmission may target the peripheral nerves, roots, spinal cord, or brain. Peripheral procedures applicable to cancer pain will be considered first.

PERIPHERAL NEURECTOMY

The Trigeminal Nerve

Although radiofrequency percutaneous trigeminal neurectomy was originally developed for the treatment of tic douloureux, the procedure is equally applicable to those rare patients with cancer pain confined to the distribution of the trigeminal nerve in whom the cancer has not obliterated all of the landmarks necessary for the procedure (see Chapters 20 and 21). Using image intensification and brief general anesthesia,[73] an insulated 18- or 19-gauge lumbar puncture needle with a 3- to 4-mm exposed tip (Fig. 26–1) is introduced into Meckel's cave through the foramen ovale (Fig. 26–2) from a site a fingerbreadth lateral to the angle of the ipsilateral corner of the mouth. This is accomplished using surface landmarks, directing the needle tip toward the middle of the ipsilateral zygoma in the horizontal plane, and toward the pupil in its neutral position in the longitudinal plane. A free flow of CSF indicates a likelihood that the needle is located in the vicinity of the preganglionic rootlets, where the total denervation desirable for cancer pain is most likely to be achieved. The image intensifier guards against too deep an introduction, above the apex of the petrous pyramid. The procedure is completed with the electronic back-up provided by the OWL (Diros Technology, Inc., Toronto, Ontario, Canada; Fig. 26–3) or Radionics (Radionics Corp., Burlington, MA) systems. With the needle properly positioned, 2-Hz stimulation should cause 2-Hz contractions in the ipsilateral masticatory muscles at under 3 volts. The application of 100-Hz stimulation should produce paresthesias in trigeminal territory harboring the pain, preferably at less than 0.8 volt. Once physiologic corroboration of a suitable location is achieved, a graded radiofrequency lesion is made using the high-output mode of the OWL machine. Under brief general anesthesia, gradually increasing current flow is applied until current decline indicates the formation of a maximal lesion. Lesion temperature also is monitored, beginning at about 80°C. It is important that the current is not driven too high too fast, to avoid a premature decline in temperature that may result in an accompanying bubble of gas that will insulate the electrode tip, preventing the formation of a lesion of adequate size. Adequacy of sensory loss (and for cancer this preferably should be anesthesia in the entire trigeminal territory—see Chapter 21) is confirmed, and the procedure is terminated. During the introduction of the

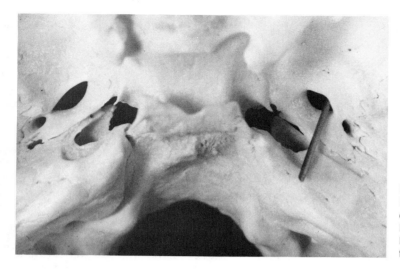

Figure 26–2. Electrode entering Meckel's cave through foramen ovale in a dried skull. Provided by Dr. H. Barr, Dept of Neurosurgery, Royal Victoria Hospital, London, Ontario, University of Western Ontario.

electrode it is important to hold a finger inside the patient's mouth to avoid its entrance into the buccal cavity and the subsequent risk of the development of meningitis and abscess formation. It is also important to monitor for and prevent severe rises in blood pressure during electrode placement in order to limit the risk of intracranial hemorrhage. Using this technique in 20 patients with cancer pain, Siegfried and Broggi[74] achieved enduring pain relief in all subjects. Complications are similar to those observed when this procedure is performed in patients with tic douloureux: tran-

sient masticatory weakness in about 25% of patients, dysesthesia in 14%–27%, transient diplopia in 2%, and keratitis from corneal anesthesia in 4%, even though corneal anesthesia may occur in up to 30%.[73,75]

Lower Cranial Nerves

A similar approach can be used to treat cancer pain in the distribution of the lower cranial nerves (see Chapter 21) by introducing the electrode into the jugular foramen (Fig. 26–4).[73,76–82] Complications include alterations of

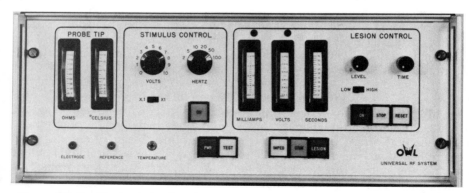

Figure 26–3. Electrode backup for percutaneous surgery provided by Diros Technology. Reproduced with kind permission of Grune and Stratton from Operative Neurosurgical Techniques, Indications, Methods, and Results 1st ed, vol 2, p 1143, 1982, edited by HH Schmidek and WH Sweet.

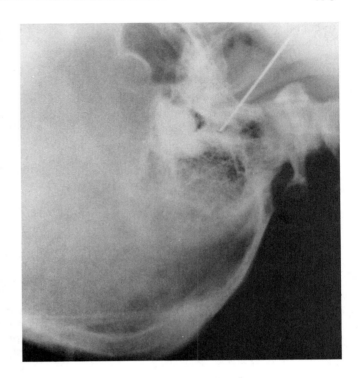

Figure 26–4. Electrode placed in jugular foramen for coagulation of lower cranial nerves. Reproduced from JB Lippincott Co. from Neural Blockade In Clinical Anesthesia and Management of Pain 2nd ed, 1988, p 1090, edited by MJ Cousins and PO Bridenbaugh.

vagal function such as dysrhythmia, blood pressure dysregulation, and dysarthria. Most published reports document results in patients with nonmalignant facial neuralgias. In the small series reporting on patients treated for cancer pain, pain relief ranged from 40%–89%.

Intercostal Nerves

In cases of neoplastic invasion of sternum, ribs, or chest wall (see Chapter 21), relief often can be achieved by multiple-level percutaneous radiofrequency neurectomy of the appropriate intercostal nerves. The principles are the same as for percutaneous trigeminal neurectomy, except that the preferred needle electrode possesses a curved tip (Fig. 26–5). The procedure can be carried out under general anesthesia, sliding the electrode in turn under the trailing edge of each rib at an appropriate distance along its course. Continuous 2-Hz stimulation at 10 volts is applied, and the tip is manipulated until intercostal muscle contractions are obtained at the lowest possible threshold, ideally 1–3 volts. A graded radiofrequency lesion then is created, and current flow is increased steadily until decline occurs. This should double the threshold required to produce stimulation of the corresponding in-

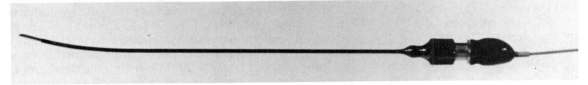

Figure 26–5. Electrode used for percutaneous radiofrequency intercostal neurectomy provided by Diros Technology.

tercostal muscles. To maximize the likelihood of a successful result, it is useful to create two separate lesions on each nerve. Although the procedure is mentioned by Uematsu,[83] there appears to be no reported experience in the literature. As mentioned, although this procedure is suitable for treatment of pain caused by cancerous invasion of the sternum or chest wall, it offers little more than a 25% chance of relieving the pain of post-thoracotomy syndrome. The only potential complication is that of pneumothorax, which we observed in 3 out of 52 procedures, 2 of which resolved spontaneously.

Splanchnicectomy

Another potential application for peripheral neurectomy in the treatment of cancer pain, particularly that arising in the pancreas, is splanchnicectomy. The procedure depends on the fact that abdominal visceral nociceptive fibers reach the spinal cord via the splanchnic nerves and the sympathetic trunks. Although similar effects may be accomplished with percutaneous alcohol injections of the celiac ganglion (see Chapters 22 and 24), splanchnicectomy is useful when there is an absence of experienced personnel to carry out a celiac block, or when the latter fails. The procedure is accomplished through bilateral incisions four fingerbreadths from the midline centered on the 11th rib, which is excised in its proximal course, allowing the pleura to be teased away from the undersurfaces of the 11th and adjacent ribs and from the vertebral column. The 2-mm diameter greater and the smaller lesser splanchnic nerves run longitudinally in parallel to the sympathetic trunk. All these structures, including as many ganglia as are accessible, are exposed over as great a length as possible and are excised. Pain relief has been reported as 36%–70% complete and 34%–40% partial in patients with cancer of the pancreas, though pain may recur in up to 25% of patients. Potential complications include empyema, pneumothorax, and even paraplegia, presumably from interference with vital segmental arteries.[84,85]

PERCUTANEOUS DORSAL RHIZOTOMY

Occasionally, the distribution of cancer pain is such that it lies within the distribution of expendable dorsal roots, allowing consideration of multiple dorsal rhizotomy as a means of control. Providing that the site of nociception is sufficiently distal along the course of the root that a lesion placed in or near the intervertebral foramen is proximal to the site of injury, the percutaneous radiofrequency technique, in principle identical to that described for neurectomy, can be used,[83,86] thus sparing the medically unfit patient the greater risk of the open procedure, but with about the same chances of success.[87–91] Thus, 50%–60% of properly selected patients should expect short-term, and 28%–50%, long-term relief of pain. Regardless of approach, dorsal rhizotomy is considered best in selected cases when pain involves a limited number of spinal dermatomes, and ideally when further local tumor growth is unlikely or predicted to be indolent. Except in the case of a functionless extremity, its practicality is limited to cases in which the pertinent spinal roots do not form a major part of the outflow to a limb plexus. A particularly valuable world literature review by Sindou et al[91] of 585 case reports of rhizotomy applied for the management of cancer pain suggested a 59% early and 47% enduring incidence of pain relief, but at the expense, with the open procedure, of a mortality of up to 20%. Smith[92] and Osgood[93] advocated open ganglionectomy to derive greater success with pain relief by interrupting any aberrant ventral root afferents.[94,95]

The percutaneous procedure consists of placing a needle electrode, similar to that used for radiofrequency trigeminal neurectomy, into the dorsal aspect of the appropriate intervertebral foramen under the guidance of image intensification. Stimulation at 2 Hz should ensure an absence of motor effects and stimulation at 100 Hz, ideally at or below 0.5 volt, should ensure location within the dorsal root, and in particular that portion of it involved with pain by induction of appropriate paresthesias. Uematsu reported a 53% success rate with various pain syndromes using this technique.[83,86] Pagura[96] observed relief of cancer pain in 76% of patients treated in this manner. It may be imprudent to carry out percutaneous radiofrequency coagulation at the T1–T4 and T11–L1 areas because of concern about damage to vital segmental end arteries, and possible infarction of the spinal cord. If sacral rhizotomy is proposed, the risks of bladder and sexual dysfunction must be considered.

DESTRUCTIVE PROCEDURES DIRECTED AT THE SPINAL CORD

Peripheral procedures are not appropriate for the control of cancer pain in most patients for the reasons stated above, and as a result the application of cord lesions needs to be explored. Of the two relevant procedures, commissurotomy and cordotomy, the latter is the only one with which this author has had clinical experience.

Commissurotomy

The advantage of commissurotomy lies with the fact that it is capable of producing bilateral, often extensive, pain relief. Unfortunately, analgesia is usually transient and not necessarily topographically related to the location of the spinal cord lesion. Various authors have reportedly achieved 65%–88% short-term, and 47%–55% long-term relief of various types of pain, mostly caused by cancer, using open commissurotomy. However, the reported mortality of the open procedure is 3%–21%, and serious morbidity is common: in representative studies 8%–26% of patients developed postoperative paresis, 71% temporary paresthesias, 4%–8% permanent paresthesias, up to 50% loss of position sense, and 12% bladder dysfunction.[87,97–102]

The risks of the open operation were reduced with Hitchcock's introduction of the percutaneous cervical radiofrequency technique.[25] With the patient seated, an electrode similar to that used for cordotomy (described below) is advanced into the space between the occiput and C1 to a midsagittal point 5 mm anterior to the dorsal cord margin, as outlined with contrast medium. Initial stimulation with the electrode located superficially in the dorsal columns is said to produce bilateral foot paresthesias. As the electrode is advanced toward the central canal, a sequence of paresthesias in face, opposite limbs, and both upper limbs is obtained. Lesions similar to those described below for cordotomy then are made anterior to or just at the level of lower limb responses. Hitchcock described 10 excellent and 2 good results in 14 patients with various types of pain. In the hands of others,[103–105] although initial pain relief was obtained in 78%–100% of patients, recurrence was frequent, and transient postoperative dysmetria and gait ataxia were common.

Trigeminal Tractotomy

Other procedures performed infrequently on the cord for the relief of cancer pain include percutaneous radiofrequency coagulation of the caudal nucleus and the descending tract of the fifth nerve, and dorsal root entry zone lesions.

The former can be performed in the medullary or upper cervical region.[26,106–113] If the medullary approach is selected, the patient is positioned prone, and the floor of the fourth ventricle, obex, and dorsum of the brain-stem are outlined with contrast medium in a manner similar to that used in percutaneous cordotomy. The electrode is advanced while impedance monitoring is carried out to the expected site in the medulla, where 50-Hz stimulation should produce facial paresthesia. A graded radiofrequency lesion then is made, interrupted by serial assessment of the patient's neurologic status. Fox[108,109] described transient pyrexia and ipsilateral ataxia in most of his patients, and contralateral body analgesia with sensory loss in the face in three of eight patients.

The cervical technique is performed in a manner similar to percutaneous cervical commissurotomy, with the patient seated. After the anteroposterior aspects of the cord and cisterna magna are outlined with contrast medium, a cordotomy-like electrode is advanced under impedance control, and, with the aid of serial stimulation, the expected location of the descending tract is identified by the appearance of facial paresthesias. A graded radiofrequency lesion is then made, again with careful serial monitoring of neurologic effects. Schvarcz[26,112] reported 84% relief of cancer pain. Complications included contralateral hypalgesia below the face and ipsilateral ataxia.

Dorsal Root Entry Zone Lesions

Hyndman[114] originally performed open Lissauer tract lesions as an adjunct to open cordotomy to raise the level of analgesia and pain relief one to two segments, and thus to make up for the two dermatomes' worth of spinothalamic input that, in the process of decussation, usually escapes section by standard cordotomy lesions. In 1972, Sindou[115–118] resurrected this procedure, making a 2-mm, 45° angle cut with a razor blade just lateral to the dorsal rootlets in an attempt to treat, in particular, Pancoast's syndrome. In the latter condition, percutaneous cordotomy often fails to achieve a high enough level of analgesia, and if extended for this purpose, exposes the patient to increased risks of postoperative respiratory failure (see below). Even so, Sindou cautions against making dorsal root entry zone lesions at the C4 level to avoid interference with diaphragmatic innervation. He reported 65% relief of patients with cancer pain, but at the expense of a 5% mortality rate with leg hypotonia in 15%. The dorsal root entry zone operation, performed with multiple, small radiofrequency lesions as introduced by Nashold and colleagues, has become much more accepted for the relief of the pain from brachial plexus avulsion and other related conditions than for neoplastic disorders.

Percutaneous Cordotomy

Percutaneous cordotomy, usually by the high lateral cervical approach, has become one of the most useful and frequently employed operations to treat cancer pain.[14–23,119–122] Although the open procedure still is advocated,[123,124] it involves greater surgical tres-

pass, and, in this author's opinion, is less elegant, effective, and safe.

Supposed obstacles to percutaneous cordotomy, such as local pathology and anomalies of the spine or cord, very rarely materialize as barriers in practice. Although it is usually stated that open cordotomy must be resorted to in uncooperative patients, the percutaneous procedure can be performed under general anesthesia, even bilaterally, in children and for other patients unwilling or unable to cooperate under local anesthesia.[23,122] The most valuable guide to lesion-making admittedly is lost under general anesthesia (ie, the induction of contralateral stimulation-induced sensory effects), but other important information derived from myelography, impedance monitoring, and motor stimulation is still present. Bilateral percutaneous cordotomy nearly always is quite feasible, apart from the as yet unavoidable 20% risk of bladder dysfunction, and the need to tailor the procedure to avoid respiratory difficulties.

Three techniques have been advocated for percutaneous cordotomy: the lateral high cervical,[14,15] the dorsal high cervical,[125,126] and the anterior low cervical approach.[127] This author prefers the first, since it does not require a stereotactic frame, is more convenient to carry out with the patient positioned supine, and a higher level of analgesia is achieved more readily. The supposed benefit for the latter option, mainly avoidance of respiratory complications (since the lesion is made below the level of the reticulospinal outflow to diaphragm), is mitigated by the substantially lower level of analgesia achieved, and the difficulty of making small incremental adjustments of electrode position, because the probe becomes anchored in the intervertebral disc, which must be traversed before the spinal cord is entered. Moreover, as will be mentioned below, it is possible to tailor a lesion made at the high cervical level to avoid excessively high levels of denervation that may endanger the reticulospinal phrenic outflow. This is accomplished by avoiding locations where 100-Hz stimulation causes contralateral sensory responses referred to the hand, in preference for evoking sensory responses in the trunk or lower extremity.

Percutaneous Cordotomy by the Lateral High Cervical Approach.

This procedure is the author's preference in cancer patients whose pain is not amenable to percutaneous radiofrequency neurectomy or rhizotomy. It is, however, unsuitable in the treatment of pain above the level of the C5 dermatome, since lasting analgesia usually cannot be achieved without excessive risk. Stereotactic procedures and intraventricular opioids remain alternatives for pain of more rostral origin. In patients with truncal, especially perineal, pain that does not extend into the legs also, cordotomy probably is not the preferred procedure. Pain of this type (*ie*, bilateral or midline) requires a bilateral procedure that introduces an approximately 20% risk of worsening bladder function, with the likelihood of poor pain relief.[6] Commissurotomy, periventricular gray stimulation, or intraspinal morphine infusion remain alternatives.

The chief contraindication to percutaneous cordotomy at the lateral high cervical level is, however, the risk that postoperative failure of unconscious respiration (Ondine's curse) might develop. The reticulospinal pathway that governs this function, in contrast to corticospinally controlled voluntary breathing (as, for example, when a patient is asked to take a deep breath), lies sandwiched between the cervical part of the spinothalamic homunculus and the ventral horn, and is distributed strictly ipsilaterally.[128,129] Whereas the patient with pain caused by Pancoast's syndrome extending high up the arm into shoulder and neck, and who is dependent on the solitary effective lung on the side of the cordotomy, may achieve an adequate level of analgesia from cordotomy, he will almost certainly die of failure of unconscious respiration, because the spinothalamic lesion in the high cervical dermatomes will spill over into the reticulospinal pathway. A "safe" lesion made by the low anterior cervical approach will not produce adequately high analgesia. Bilateral cordotomy, preferably performed in stages separated by at least 1 week in patients with two

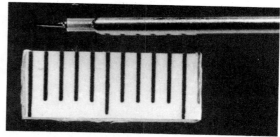

Figure 26–6. Cordotomy electrode provided by Diros Technology.

normally functioning lungs, is safe as long as excessively high levels of analgesia are not achieved on both sides. Levels of analgesia can be tailored by paying particular attention to the location of contralateral sensory effects achieved by 100-Hz stimulation. Some authors prefer to combine unilateral high percutaneous cordotomy with a lower, percutaneous rhizotomy induced either by radiofrequency coagulation or the injection of phenol. Patients are quite capable of functioning with unconscious respiration in only one lung as long as it is reasonably free of pathology.

The technique consists of introducing through a thin-walled, 18-gauge lumbar puncture needle a fine, sharpened Teflon-insulated electrode with a 2-mm exposed tip (Fig. 26–6) into the cord, under neuroleptanalgesia or brief general anesthesia. The needle is introduced near the mastoid process and is passed between the C1 and C2 vertebrae under image intensification. Small amounts of air and contrast material are injected intrathecally to outline the cord and dentate ligament, and the location of the needle tip just anterior to the ligament is verified (Fig. 26–7). The electrode locks into the hub of the lumbar puncture needle so that the Teflon insulation in turn projects 2 mm beyond the tip of the needle: a 2-mm extent of cord penetration seems about right for optimal interruption of the spinothalamic tract. Adequate penetration of the cord up to the point where the electrode is arrested by the shoulders of the Teflon insulation is monitored by recording electrical impedance, which usually is about 400 ohms in spinal fluid, and rises to 800–1,000 ohms or more as the cord is penetrated (Fig. 26–8). Location of the electrode in the spinothalamic tract is confirmed with electrical stimulation using the electronic support of equipment such as that provided by Diros Technology or Radionics Corporation. With 2-Hz stimulation, ipsilateral neck and sometimes upper limb motor responses should occur at 1–3 volts, whereas at 100 Hz no motor responses should be seen, but, rather, warm or cool paresthesias should be elicited in the contralateral body. Tetanization of the ipsilateral neck suggests electrode position in the anterior horn, elsewhere in the corticospinal tract. Contralateral sensory responses referred to the lower limb suggest a distal position in the spinothalamic homunculus, whereas responses referred to the hand suggest a central position. Sensory responses in upper trunk or contralateral neck suggest too rostral a location in the spinothalamic tract, with the likelihood of inadequate suspended sensory loss when the lesion is made. When the electrode is optimally located, a graded radiofrequency lesion is made with serial neurologic testing of, in particular, ipsilateral lower limb power and of contralateral analgesia. The lesion usually is initiated at 25 mA for 60 seconds under brief general anesthesia, and is gradually increased to 35–45 mA to achieve the level and depth of analgesia desired while avoiding sparing of sacral segments. Once the lesion has been initiated under a general anesthetic, it can be enlarged without further general anesthesia. If repeated lesioning at high levels of current flow at the same site fails to achieve the desired level of analgesia, the electrode must be reintroduced at a new site and the entire procedure repeated. Equipment is available that permits monitoring of the temperature of the lesion during its execution, if this is desired.

Reported pain relief after open cordotomy[23,123,124] varies from 54%–90%, with a mean of 75% after 3 months, subsequently declining to 50% at 18 months. Mortality ranges from 3%–21%, and the incidence of paresis from 0%–11% for unilateral, and 24% for bilateral cordotomy. Bladder impairment

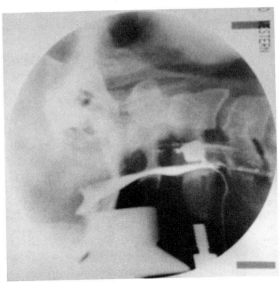

Figure 26–7. Lateral x-ray of C1C2 interspace with cordotomy electrode impinging on cord at site of spinothalamic tract near attachment of dentate ligament outlined with contrast medium.

is seen in 0%–8% of unilateral cordotomies, usually transiently. Postcordotomy dysesthesia occurs to some degree in 25%, and remains a serious problem in 6% of patients after 2–3 years.

Various series of unilateral percutaneous cordotomy[14–20,130–140] quote a 59%–96% incidence of pain relief at the expense of a 0%–6% mortality, 2.6%–4.2% respiratory complications, up to 80% initial paresis (with persistent paresis in 1%–20%), up to 19% transient and 0%–8.7% persistent bladder dysfunction, up to 20% incidence of postcordotomy dysesthesia, 0.5% gait ataxia, and up to 100% initial incidence of Horner's syndrome. In 4%, levels of analgesia fade after surgery. Ischia et al[139,140] noted a 48%–63% incidence of pain developing on the other side of the body, a 6.8%–14% incidence of pain persisting or developing below an apparently adequate level of analgesia (presumably deafferentation pain, which resists cordotomy, as has been discussed above), and a 4% incidence of new pain developing above the level of analgesia, associated with progression of the disease.

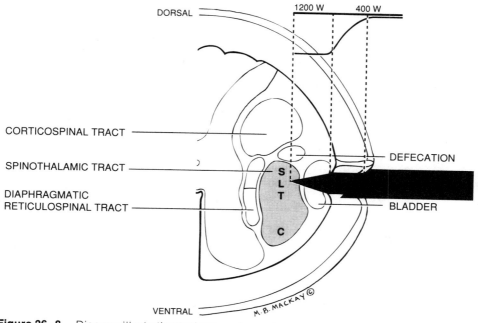

Figure 26–8. Diagram illustrating technique of percutaneous cordotomy by lateral high cervical technique. Impedance changes from CSF to cord impalation, the homuncular arrangement of the spinothalamic tract, and the locations of important pathways are shown.

After bilateral percutaneous cordotomy, the incidence of pain relief reported in the literature was 47%, of mortality up to 10%, respiratory difficulties up to 20%, initial paresis up to 36% (permanent in 1.8%), bladder dysfunction in 12%–100%, and of hypotension up to 36%.

Our own results with almost 400 cases, all carried out by the unilateral high cervical technique,[21–23,119,121,122] have been as follows: 99% of procedures were completed with location of the spinothalamic tract. In 2.6%, the level of analgesia receded within a few days, requiring repetition of the procedure. Analgesia apparently was adequate in 93% at postdischarge follow-up. At the time of discharge from hospital, 88% of patients had no pain in the area to which the cordotomy was directed, and 94% had no or only minor pain in this area. By the time of the latest follow-up, 72% had no pain and 84% had no significant pain

in the area to which the cordotomy was directed. Persisting pain after cordotomy fell into several categories; in addition to the small number with inadequate relief because of inadequate levels or depths of analgesia, 5% developed pain above their level of analgesia, presumably due to progress of the disease, 40.7% developed similar or worsening pain on the opposite side of the body, whereas about 34% continued to suffer or developed new pain below a level of apparently adequate analgesia, presumably because of the existence of deafferentation pain. In most cases these complaints were minor. Six percent of our cases developed postcordotomy dysesthesia, which was of significant severity in 3% of patients. Complications in our unilateral cases included a 0.3% mortality caused by failure of involuntary respiration, 0.5% transient failure of unconscious respiration, 16.8% transient and 0.5% persistent paresis, 6.6% minor or transient, 2.9% significant worsening of bladder function, and 33% (usually transient) Horner's syndrome.

For bilateral percutaneous cordotomy performed with the lateral high cervical approach, satisfactory pain relief occurred in 72%, roughly the square of the incidence for one side, as would be expected. The mortality was 1.6%. There was a 2.8% transient and 1.6% significant persisting incidence of paresis, 18.8% significant worsening of bladder function, and 9.4% minor additional bladder dysfunction.

DESTRUCTIVE PROCEDURES PERFORMED ON THE BRAIN

When procedures aimed at nerve roots or cord are inappropriate, and modulatory procedures are not options, the alternatives include stereotactic surgery. For cancer pain, stereotactic mesencephalic tractotomy and medial thalamotomy are the most frequently performed procedures.

Pontine Tractotomy

Although Hitchcock et al[141–143] introduced stereotactic pontine tractotomy as an alternative intervention for cancer pain when percutaneous cordotomy was contraindicated, it appears to have been used infrequently.[144] The operation is accomplished by stereotactically introducing an electrode into the pons, after definition of the aqueduct floor and fastigium of the fourth ventricle with contrast medium has been accomplished. Before executing a graded radiofrequency lesion, proper position of the electrode is confirmed by stimulation. Satisfactory relief of pain with acceptable risks appears to be achieved, suggesting that the operation should receive further evaluation.

Mesencephalic Tractotomy

Mesencephalic tractotomy, first by open, then stereotactic means, has been one of the main methods used to treat rostrally located cancer pain that is not amenable to cordotomy. For this procedure, the position of the spinoreticulothalamic tract at the level of the upper midbrain is approximated with respect to the anterior commissure–posterior commissure line, which is identified with computed tomography (CT) or a magnetic resonance imaging (MRI) scan and an appropriate stereotactic atlas. The spinothalamic tract is identified with macrostimulation by the induction of contralateral, somatotopographically referred sensations of warm or cold paresthesias at sites about 8–9 mm from the midline. These responses contrast sharply with the somatotopographically organized paresthesias induced a little more laterally in the medial lemniscus between 10 and 12 mm from the midline. Medial to the spinothalamic tract again, 2–8 mm from the midline, macrostimulation may produce diffuse, bilaterally referred, nonsomatotopographically oriented responses of varied and unusual quality, not always consistent from one patient to the next, similar or identical to those described below with stimulation of the periventricular gray.[145–149] In contrast to the dissociated sensory loss achieved by the lesions made in the spinothalamic tract, lesions medial to it are said to alleviate suffering, although they induce no sensory loss. Exploration of the mesencephalic tegmentum with microelectrodes also has been described.[150] Once the location of the spinothalamic tract vis-à-vis the medial lemniscus is physiologically confirmed, a graded radiofrequency lesion is made with serial testing, until adequate levels of contralateral analgesia are achieved, taking great care to spare the medial lemniscus but to include structures lying medially (Fig. 26–9). This analgesia usually is accompanied initially by contralateral loss of proprioception and pseudoparesis, undesirable findings that soon recede, leaving behind dissociated sensory loss that tends to be rostrally located, ideally corresponding to the area of the patient's pain.

Various authors have reported a 67%–100% (mean, 80%) incidence of initially satisfactory pain relief after stereotactic mesencephalic tractotomy for pain of various causes. Series consisting only of cancer pain patients

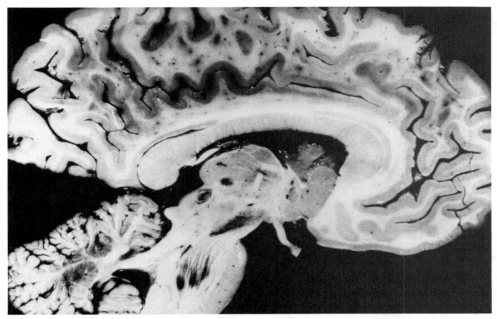

Figure 26–9. Sagittal section of autopsy specimen showing (dark ellipses) stereotactic mesencephalic tractotomy (upper midbrain) and parafascicular nucleus (caudal thalamus) lesions that abolished the patient's head and neck pain caused by gingival carcinoma.

are infrequent. Recurrence with time is observed frequently, occurring in up to 100% of cases according to some authors. Mortality varies from 6.5%–38%, whereas morbidity, which is usually transient, includes significant contralateral dysesthesia in 5%, paresis in 7%, oculomotor palsies in 13%–88% (with frank diplopia in 1%–5%), ataxia in 4%, and contralateral hearing loss in 50%.[33–36,49,145–147,150–167] Turnbull[165] recommends the combination of mesencephalic tractotomy with cingulumotomy to improve overall effectiveness.

Thalamotomy

As has been pointed out, from an early stage stereotactic lesions made in the thalamus to relieve pain have tended to be directed toward the medial thalamus rather than the ventrobasal complex. Although the specific relay for the spinothalamic tract in Hassler's parvicellular ventrocaudal nucleus is well recognized

(Fig. 26–10), few surgeons have made lesions here to relieve pain.

Other than the early experience with lesions made in the dorsomedian nucleus in efforts to relieve anxiety, common sites in the medial thalamus where lesions were made included the centrum medianum, parafascicular complex, internal thalamic lamina, and/or pulvinar.[33–36] Probably the parafascicular nucleus and internal thalamic lamina are the actual relays for the medial nonsomatotopographically organized portion of the spinothalamic tract, and are the sites at which medial thalamic lesions actually should be made (see Figs. 9, 10). The location of these structures must be extrapolated from the position of the anterior and posterior commissures as determined by imaging, for they cannot be recognized by stimulation.[148,149,168–170] Microelectrode recording techniques for their recognition have, however, been described.[171–174] Localization can be enhanced further by iden-

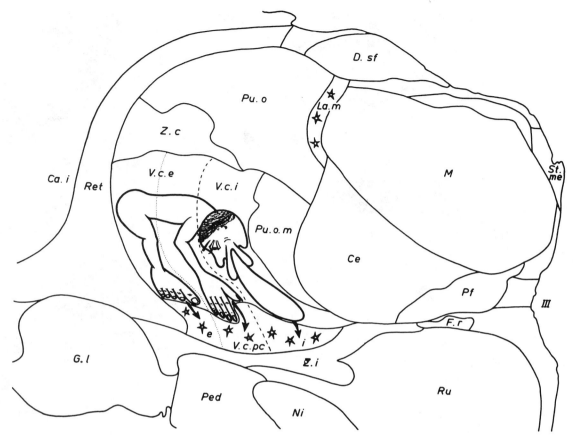

Figure 26–10. Diagram illustrating the medial non-somatotopographic and the lateral somatotopic relays (stars) of spinothalamic tract in medial thalamic lamina (La.m) and parvicellular ventrocaudal nucleus (v.c.pc) respectively. Ca.i = internal capsule; Ce = centrum medianum; D = dorsal nucleus; Fr = tegmental reticular formation; G.1 = lateral geniculate nucleus; M = dorsomedian nucleus; Pf = parafascicular nucleus; Ni. = substantia nigra; Ped = cerebral peduncle; Pu.e = pulvinar; Ret = reticular nucleus; Ru = red nucleus; St.me = stria medullaris of thalamus; V.c.e., V.c.i. = ventrocaudal nucleus; Z.c = central portion of caudal nucleus; Z.i = zona incerta; III = third ventricle. Reproduced with kind permission of Georg Thieme Publishers from Pain Basic Principles-Pharmacology-Therapy, 1972, p 106, edited by R Janzen, WD Keidel, A Herz, C Steichele.

tifying the medial margin of the ventrobasal complex with either macrostimulation or microelectrodes. Once the desired target is located and stimulation confirms that no untoward responses occur, a graded radiofrequency lesion similar to that made in the thalamus for Parkinson's disease is made, sufficient to interrupt the parafascicular complex and/or internal thalamic lamina about 6 mm from the midline. With the OWL machine (Diros Technology) and a thalamotomy electrode with a 3-mm exposed tip, this is achieved at the "low" output setting, with a current flow of 65–75 mA for 60 seconds.

Although experience with medial thalamotomy dates back 40 years and is extensive,[37–45,49,168,171–198] results for pain of varying etiologies are often pooled, so that it is difficult to discern the results for cancer pain *per se*. In a personal literature review,[151,168] 175 published protocols were identified that described results in patients suffering from nociceptive pain, nearly always caused by cancer, and were determined to be appropriate for separate review. Forty-six percent of patients experienced significant, and 11% fair relief of pain that was persistent. Ten percent to 20% of patients experienced nonfatal complications, usually consisting of transient confusion or other cognitive disorders.

CHEMICAL HYPOPHYSECTOMY

As has already been discussed, the classification of this procedure as destructive or modulating in effect is controversial. Percutaneous chemical hypophysectomy is accomplished under light general anesthesia. An 18-gauge needle is introduced through the nose, and gently hammered into the sella in the midline 2 mm inferior to its rim, with guidance provided by image intensification. When the appropriate position of the needle is confirmed, 1 ml of absolute alcohol is injected in 0.1-ml aliquots every 1 minute. Pain relief has been reported to occur initially in 41%–95% of treated patients with hormonally dependent cancer (breast, prostate), and in 69% of patients with nonhormonally dependent cancers. There is a tendency for the pain to recur in 3 to 4 months. Surprisingly, there is a rather high mortality of 2%–6.5%, a trend that seems to be reversing in more recently conducted studies. Significant but usually transient morbidity includes rhinorrhea in 3%–20%, meningitis in 0.3%–1%, visual and oculomotor disturbances in 2%–10%, and diabetes insipidus in 5%–60%. Hypothalamic disturbances and headaches are said to be common.[64–66,199–206]

PSYCHOSURGICAL PROCEDURES

One group of destructive procedures with which this author has had little experience are those that comprise psychosurgery. The strategy of psychosurgical procedures involves amelioration of suffering by modifying affect. One way of characterizing pain is as an event or experience that consists of two components: acute, reflex reactions to noxious stimuli (nociception), and emotional suffering induced by stimuli. Classically, neurosurgery for pain has focused on interrupting nociceptive pathways to eliminate the arrival of impulses at higher centers. Psychosurgery concentrates on destroying or stimulating integrative brain pathways involved in the assignment of meaning to peripheral stimuli. Pain continues, but emotional response and heightened reactivity are reduced, especially with respect to the anticipation and memory of pain.

In 1936 Freeman and Watts serendipitously observed decreased reports of pain in patients subjected to prefrontal leukotomy for the treatment of psychiatric illness.[207] The report on their first series of patients treated with lobotomy for persistent pain contains illustrative case histories, and is of considerable historical interest.[208] Frontal ablative procedures were performed with increasing frequency through the 1940s. By the mid-1950s, enthusiasm for psychosurgery as a remedy for mental illness waned due to ethical concerns, the recognition of a high incidence of postoperative seizures, and the development of more effective psychotropic drugs. In 1947, Spiegel and Wycis performed the first true stereotactic procedure performed in humans, a dorsomedian thalamotomy,[34] thus introducing human stereotactic surgery and paving the way for more precise and sophisticated psychosurgery. Destruction of the dorsomedian nucleus interrupted the thalamic relay for the frontal lobes, and in the early years of stereotactic surgery, that operation frequently was substituted for lobotomy.[168] Results were best when dorsomedian thalamotomy was carried out bilaterally, a procedure sometimes accompanied by recent memory loss. The notion that medial mesencephalic tractotomy reduced suffering has been mentioned. Anterior thalamotomy and destruction of the anterior thalamic radiations was also practiced.[168]

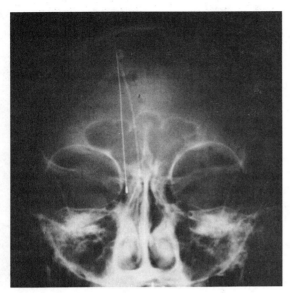

Figure 26–11. Anteroposterior skull x-ray showing chronic stimulating electrodes in periventricular grey (medial) and ventrocaudal nucleus (lateral).

Although psychosurgical procedures are not performed commonly, in more recent times bilateral cingulumotomy, ideally performed stereotactically either alone or in conjunction with lesions elsewhere, has been favored.[165] The procedure is considered most effective in patients with significant depression or anxiety, or when drug use is excessive. Bouckoms[207] has authored a current review of the subject, in which he reiterates the oft-stated impression that psychosurgery results in the patient not complaining of pain unless asked. He notes that nociceptive pain, such as that most commonly seen with cancer, and neural injury pain respond equally well, and that patients with anxiety or depression and those with pain fare equally well. He concluded that one-half to three-quarters of patients with pain derive short-term relief from cingulumotomy, but that long-term relief, particularly from cancer pain, was "equivocal." The mortality from the operation was 0.1%, physical morbidity was 0.3%, and psychological morbidity was 10%–30%.

Bouckoms believed that the other currently favored psychosurgical procedure,

inferoposteromedial frontal leukotomy (a fractional refinement of the classical leukotomy), also was useful for treating pain, but less clearly so, particularly in the long term, than cingulumotomy.

MODULATORY SURGERY

The second chief principle underlying the neurosurgical treatment of cancer pain is that of modulation. Central nervous system opioid therapy is discussed elsewhere in this book (see Chapter 18), but similar effects can be achieved with chronic stimulation of the periventricular–periaqueductal gray, a process that is thought to activate a descending pathway to inhibit the access of nociceptive impulses to the spinothalamic tract (Fig. 26–11). These techniques offer the great advantage of reversibility and therefore lowered risk, and it is unfortunate that the standard technique requires the purchase of costly radiofrequency-coupled or totally implantable stimulation devices. Meyerson et al,[209] however, have demonstrated that chronic periventricular stimulation can be used for prolonged periods in cancer patients by means of a transcutaneous lead, without infection.

Stimulation usually is carried out in the periventricular rather than the equally responsive periaqueductal gray, since stimulation at the latter site is reported to produce unpleasant effects and/or diplopia, although there is no general agreement on this point (Figs. 26–12 and 26–13).[57–59,149,210]

The usual target site is about 2–5 mm anterior to the posterior commissure along the intercommissural line, and 2 mm lateral to the wall of the third ventricle, a site whose coordinates can be obtained readily from a stereotactic CT or MRI scan. Macrostimulation then is carried out in 1–2-mm steps extending from 10 mm above to 5 mm below this site, and again possibly 2–3 millimeters rostral or caudal, seeking a site where a generalized feeling of satiety, well-being, pleasure, or a "glow" is achieved, together with pain relief (Fig. 26–12). Recognition of the site is also facilitated with microelectrode recording. As the

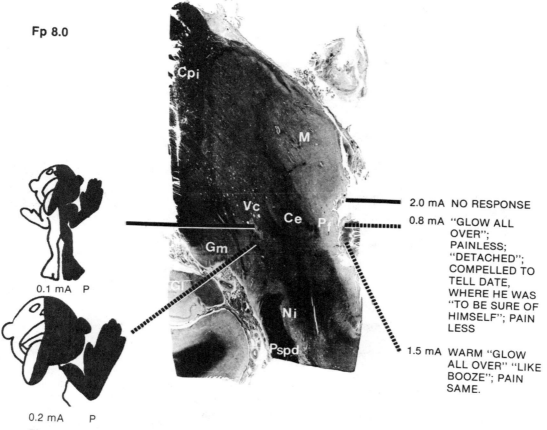

Fp 8.0

Cpi

M

Vc   Ce   Pf

Gm

Ni

Pspd

2.0 mA   NO RESPONSE

0.8 mA   "GLOW ALL
OVER";
PAINLESS;
"DETACHED";
COMPELLED TO
TELL DATE,
WHERE HE WAS
"TO BE SURE OF
HIMSELF"; PAIN
LESS

1.5 mA   WARM "GLOW
ALL OVER" "LIKE
BOOZE"; PAIN
SAME.

0.1 mA   P

0.2 mA   P

Figure 26–12. Reconstruction of stimulation sites in periventricular grey 8 mm caudal to mid-commissural point in a patient with central pain of cord origin. Reproduced by kind permission of Springer-Verlag from Samii M (ed): Surgery In and Around the Brainstem and the Third Ventricle, 1986, pp 164–165.

electrode is introduced, it usually traverses the dorsomedian nucleus where spontaneously bursting cells are common; a suitable target for stimulation occurs deep to the point where these cease, possibly in the parafascicular nucleus. In perhaps half of the patients, no sure clue to confirm electrode position is found on physiologic exploration, and a test stimulating electrode is placed on anatomic grounds alone. Although there is little published experience with treating cancer pain *per se* using periventricular gray stimulation, presumably the results are similar to those

obtained with other types of nociceptive pain, namely a 60%–80% chance of relieving pain, and low to moderate risks of neural trauma (up to 11%), infection (4%–5%), device failure (3%–9%), and lead migration (7%). Although it might be expected that the resulting pain relief would resemble that obtained from opioids, and thus would be characterized by tolerance, reversibility with naloxone, and efficacy for only nociceptive pain, there is considerable disagreement on these points.[57–59,209,211–224] Young and Chambi,[224] for example, found tolerance no

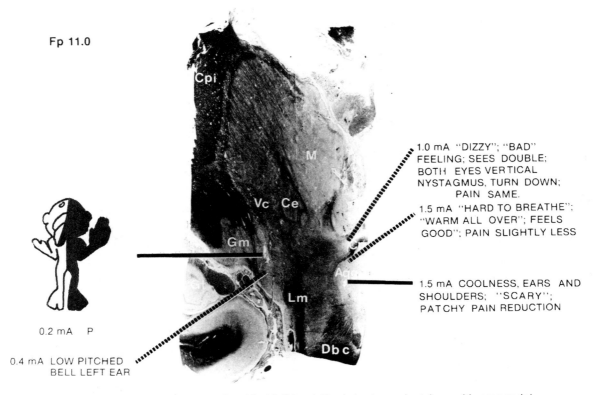

Fp 11.0

1.0 mA "DIZZY"; "BAD" FEELING; SEES DOUBLE; BOTH EYES VERTICAL NYSTAGMUS, TURN DOWN; PAIN SAME.

1.5 mA "HARD TO BREATHE"; "WARM ALL OVER"; "FEELS GOOD"; PAIN SLIGHTLY LESS

1.5 mA COOLNESS, EARS AND SHOULDERS; "SCARY"; PATCHY PAIN REDUCTION

0.2 mA   P

0.4 mA LOW PITCHED BELL LEFT EAR

Figure 26–13. Same patient as Fig. 26–12. Stimulation in periaqueductal grey 11 mm caudal to mid-commissural point. In Figs 12, 13 figurine charts show locations of paresthesiae elicited in ventrocaudal nucleus. Stimulation thresholds in mA. Agg = periaqueductal grey; Cpi = internal capsule; Dbc = decussation of brachium conjunctivum; Gm = medial geniculate nucleus; Lm = medial lamniscus; Pspd = cerebral peduncle. Abbreviations otherwise as in Fig. 26–10. Reproduced by kind permission of Springer Verlag from Samii M (ed): Surgery In and Around the Brainstem and the Third Ventricle, 1986, pp 164–165.

more frequent with periventricular or periaqueductal gray stimulation than with ventrobasal complex stimulation, and they could demonstrate no cross-tolerance between periventricular or periaqueductal gray stimulation and morphine administration. Young et al,[225] reviewing their experience with brain stimulation over 5 years, reported that they had placed electrodes in periventricular–periaqueductal gray with or without an additional electrode in other structures in 42 of 48 patients, only 7 of whom suffered from cancer. Three of the latter enjoyed excellent, and three partial relief of their pain.

CONCLUSION

Newer concepts of pain physiology, leading to the notion that clinical pain is the algebraic sum of nociceptive stimulation and inhibitory modulation, have altered our approach to treating cancer pain. One option open to the neurosurgeon remains the application of time-honored destructive procedures that isolate nociceptive input from consciousness. Refinement of technique, particularly of percutaneous radiofrequency techniques, has minimized the negative impact and maximized the efficacy of such procedures, of which percutaneous cordotomy is exemplary, in managing cancer pain. Although these are irreversible procedures, the risks are small, and they are "once-only" affairs not leading to long-term continued close supervision or the constant presence of expensive equipment.

Alternatively, modulatory techniques of two types now are available: those that rely on drug infusions, and on chronic stimulation for their effects. Although these are reversible procedures, they still carry definite risks of their own, require expensive equipment that may be difficult to provide for a cancer patient with a short life expectancy, and require ongoing medical supervision. There are preferred roles for both destructive and modulatory types of management; it is important not to neglect the one in the enthusiasm to use the other.

REFERENCES

1. Harbaugh RE, Saunders RL, Reeder RF: Use of implantable pumps for central nervous system drug infusions to treat neurological disease. Neurosurgery 1988;23:693.
2. Hartel F: Die Leitungsanasthesie und injectionsbehandlung des Ganglion Gasseri und der Trigeminustame. Archiv fur Klinische Chirurgie 1912;100:193.
3. Kirschner M: Elektrokoagulation des Ganglion Gasseri. Zentralblatt fur Chirurgie 1932;47:2841.
4. Sweet WH, Wepsic SG: Controlled thermocoagulation of trigeminal ganglion and results for differential destruction of pain fibers. J Neurosurg 1974;29:143.
5. Katz J: Current role of neurolytic agents. In Bonica JJ (ed): Advances in Neurology, vol 4, p 471. New York, Raven Press, 1974.
6. Meyerson BA, Arner S, Linderoth B: Pros and cons of different approaches to the management of pelvic cancer pain. Acta Neurochir 1984; (Suppl 33):407.
7. Moore DC: Role of nerve block with neurolytic solutions for pelvic visceral cancer pain. In Bonica JJ, Ventafridda V (eds): Advances in Pain Research and Therapy, vol 2, p 593. New York, Raven Press, 1979.
8. Ventafridda V, Martino G: Clinical evaluation of subarachnoid neurolytic blocks in intractable cancer pain. In Bonica JJ, Albe-Fessard D (eds): Advances in Pain Research and Therapy, vol 1, p 699. New York, Raven Press, 1975.
9. Papo I, Visca A: Phenol subarachnoid rhizotomy for the treatment of cancer pain: A personal account on 290 cases. In Bonica JJ, Ventafridda V (eds): Advances in Pain Research and Therapy, vol 2, p 339. New York, Raven Press, 1979.
10. Swerdlow M: Subarachnoid and extradural neurolytic blocks. In Bonica JJ, Ventafridda V (eds): Advances in Pain Research and Therapy, vol 2, p 325. New York, Raven Press, 1979.
11. Ventafridda V, Fochi C, Sganzerla EP et al: Neurolytic blocks in perineal pain. In Bonica JJ, Ventafridda V (eds): Advances in Pain Research and Therapy, vol 2, p 597. New York, Raven Press, 1979.
12. Spiller WG: The occasional resemblance between caries of the vertebra and lumbothoracic syringomyelia and the location within the spinal cord of the fibers of the sensation of pain and temperature. University of Pennsylvania Medical Bulletin 1905; 18:147.
13. Spiller WG, Martin E: The treatment of persistent pain of organic origin in the lower part of the body by division of the anterolateral column of the spinal cord. JAMA 1912;58:1489.
14. Mullan S, Harper PV, Hekmatpanah J et al: Percutaneous interruption of spinal pain tracts by means of a strontium 90 needle. J Neurosurg 1963;20:931.
15. Rosomoff HL, Carroll F, Brown J et al: Percutaneous radiofrequency cervical cordotomy: Technique. J Neurosurg 1965;23:639.
16. Onofrio BM: Cervical spinal cord and dentate delineation in percutaneous radiofrequency cordotomy at the level of the first to second cervical vertebrae. Surg Gynecol Obstet 1971;133:30.
17. Gildenberg PL, Zanes C, Flitter MA et al: Impedance monitoring device for detection of penetration of the spinal cord in anterior percutaneous cervical cordotomy: Technical note. J Neurosurg 1969;30:87.
18. Hitchcock ER, Tsukamoto Y: Distal and proximal sensory responses during stereotactic spinal tractotomy in man. Ann Clin Res 1973;5:68.
19. Taren JA: Physiologic corroboration in stereotactic high cervical cordotomy. Confinia Neurologica 1971;33:285.
20. Taren JA, Davis R, Crosby EC: Target physiologic corroboration in stereotactic cervical cordotomy. J Neurosurg 1969;30:569.
21. Tasker RR, Organ LW: Percutaneous cordotomy. Physiological identification of target site. Confinia Neurologica 1973;35:110.
22. Tasker RR, Organ LW, Smith KC: Physiological guidelines for the localization of lesions by percutaneous cordotomy. Acta Neurochir 1974;21 (Suppl):111.
23. Tasker RR: Open Cordotomy. In Krayenbuhl H,

Maspes PE, Sweet WH (eds): Progress in Neurological Surgery, pt II, vol 8: Pain, Its Neurosurgical Management, p 1. Basel, Karger, 1977.

24. Armour D: Surgery of the spinal cord and its membranes. Lancet 1927;ii:691.

25. Hitchcock ER: Stereotactic cervical myelotomy. J Neurol Neurosurg Psychiatry 1970;33:224.

26. Schvarcz JR: Spinal cord stereotactic techniques re trigeminal nucleotomy and extralemniscal myelotomy. Appl Neurophysiol 1978;41:99.

27. Cook AW, Nathan PW, Smith MC: Sensory consequences of commissural myelotomy: A challenge to traditional concepts. Brain 1984;107:547.

28. Sjoqvist O: Studies on pain conduction in the trigeminal nerve: A contribution to the surgical treatment of facial pain. Acta Psychiatr Scand 1938;(Suppl):171.

29. Schwartz HG, O'Leary JL: Section of the spinothalamic tract in the medulla with observations on the pathway for pain. Surgery 1941;9:183.

30. Walker AE: Relief of pain by mesencephalic tractotomy. Arch Neurol Psychiatry 1942;48:865.

31. Walker AE: Mesencephalic tractotomy: A method for the relief of unilateral intractable pain. Arch Surg 1942;44:953.

32. Spiegel EA, Wycis HT: Pallidothalamotomy in chorea. Presented at the Philadelphia Neurological Society, April 22, 1949, Philadelphia, PA.

33. Spiegel EA, Wycis HT: Mesencephalotomy in treatment of ''intractable'' facial pain. AMA Arch Neurol Psychiatry 1953;69:1.

34. Spiegel EA, Wycis HT: Mesencephalotomy for the relief of pain. Published in Anniversary Volume for Poetz O, Vienna, 1948, p 438. In Monographs in Biology and Medicine II Stereoencephalotomy Part II, p 206. Clinical and Physiological Applications. New York, Grune and Stratton, 1962.

35. Spiegel EA, Wycis HT: Stereoencephalotomy: II. Clinical and Physiological Applications. New York, Grune and Stratton, 1962.

36. Wycis HT, Spiegel EA: Long-range results in the treatment of intractable pain by stereotaxic midbrain surgery. J Neurosurg 1962;19:101.

37. Hecaen H, Talairach J, David M et al: Coagulations limitees du thalamus dans les algies du syndrome thalamique. Rev Neurol 1949;81:917.

38. Monnier M: Contributions techniques a l'exploration du thalamus chez le singe et chez l'homme. In IV Congres Neurol Internat, Paris, 1949, vol III, p 148. Masson, Paris, 1951.

39. Monnier M, Fischer R: Localisation, stimulation et coagulation du thalamus chez l'homme. J Physiol (Paris) 1951;43:818.

40. Ervin FR, Mark VH: Stereotactic thalamotomy in the human: II. Physiologic observations on the human thalamus. Arch Neurol 1960;3:368.

41. Mark VH, Ervin FR, Yakovlev PI: Correlation of pain relief, sensory loss, and anatomical lesion sites in pain patients treated by stereotactic thalamotomy. Transactions of the American Neurological Association 1961;86:86.

42. Mark VH, Ervin FR, Yakovlev PI: Stereotactic thalamotomy: III. The verification of anatomical lesion sites in the human thalamus. Arch Neurol 1963;8:78.

43. Mark VH, Ervin FR: Role of thalamotomy in treatment of chronic severe pain. Postgrad Med 1965;35:563.

44. Mark VH, Tsutsumi H: The suppression of pain by intra-thalamic lidocaine. In Bonica JJ (ed): Advances in Neurology, vol 4, p 715. New York, Raven Press, 1974.

45. Mark VH, Ervin FR, Hackett TP. Clinical aspects of stereotactic thalamotomy in the human: I. The treatment of chronic severe pain. Arch Neurol 1960;3:351.

46. Hassler R: The division of pain conduction into systems of pain sensation and pain awareness. In Janzen R, Keidel WD, Herz A et al (eds): Pain: Basic Principles—Pharmacology—Therapy, p 98. Stuttgart, George Thieme, 1972.

47. Halliday AM, Logue V: Painful sensations evoked by electrical stimulation in the thalamus. In Somjen GG (ed): Neurophysiology Studied in Man, p 221. Amsterdam, Excerpta Medica, 1972.

48. Hitchcock ER, Teixeira MJ: A comparison of results from center-median and basal thalamotomies for pain. Surg Neurol 1981;15:341.

49. Frank F, Fabrizi AP, Gaist G et al: Stereotactic lesions in the treatment of chronic cancer pain syndromes: Mesencephalotomy versus multiple thalamotomies in the treatment of chronic cancer pain syndromes. Appl Neurophysiol 1987;50:314.

50. Melzack R, Wall P: Pain mechanisms: A new theory. Science 1965;150:971.

51. Wall PD, Sweet WH: Temporary abolition of pain in man. Science 1967;155:108.

52. Tasker RR: Neurostimulation and percutaneous neural destructive techniques. In Cousins MJ, Bridenbaugh PO (eds): Neural Blockade in Clinical Anesthesia and Management of Pain, 2nd ed, p 1085. Philadelphia, JB Lippincott, 1988.

53. Pool JL: Psychosurgery in elderly people. J Am Geriatr Soc 1956;2:456.

54. Pool JL, Clark WK, Hudson P et al: In Fields WS, Guillemin R, Carton CA (eds): Laboratory and Clinical Assessment. Hypothalamic—Hypophyseal Interrelationships, p 114–124. Springfield, IL, Charles C Thomas, 1965.

55. Heath RG, Mickle WA: Evaluation of seven years' experience with depth electrode studies in human patients. In Ramey ER, O'Doherty DS (eds): Electrical Studies on the Unanesthetized Brain, p 214. New York, PB Hoeber, 1960.

56. Mazars GJ: Intermittent stimulation of nucleus ventralis posterolateralis for intractable pain. Surg Neurol 1975;4:93.

57. Richardson DE, Akil H: Pain reduction by electrical brain stimulation in man: Part I: Acute administration in periaqueductal and periventricular sites. J Neurosurg 1977;47:178.

58. Richardson DE, Akil H: Pain reduction by electrical brain stimulation in man: Part II. Chronic self-administration in periventricular gray matter. J Neurosurg 1977;47:184.

59. Richardson DE: Analgesia produced by stimulation of various sites in the human beta-endorphin system. Appl Neurophysiol 1982;45:116.

60. Reynolds DV: Surgery in the rat during electrical analgesia induced by frontal brain stimulation. Science 1969;164:444.

61. Luft R, Olivecroma H: Experiences with hypophysectomy in man. J Neurosurg 1953;10:301.

62. Perrault M, LeBeau J, Klotz B et al: L'hypophysectomie totale dans le traitement du cancer du sein; premier cas francais; avenir de la methode. Therapie 1952;7:290.

63. Tindall GT, Christy JH, Nixon DW et al: Trans-sphenoidal hypophysectomy for pain of disseminated carcinoma of the breast and prostate gland. In Lee JF (ed): Pain Management, p 172. Baltimore, Williams and Wilkins, 1977.

64. Morricca G: Chemical hypophysectomy for cancer pain. In Bonica JJ (ed): Advances in Neurology, vol 4, p 707. New York, Raven Press, 1974.

65. Takeda F, Fujii T, Uki J et al: Cancer pain relief and tumour regression by means of pituitary neuroadenolysis and surgical hypophysectomy. Neurol Med Chir (Tokyo) 1983;23:41.

66. Takeda F, Uki J, Fujii T et al: Pituitary neuroadenolysis to relieve cancer pain: Observations of spread of ethanol instilled into the sella turcica and subsequent changes of the hypothalamo-pituitary axis at autopsy. Neurol Med Chir (Tokyo) 1983;23:50.

67. Capper SJ, Conlon JM, Lahuerta J et al: Peptide concentration in the CSF following injection of alcohol into the pituitary gland. Pain 1984; (Suppl 2):S316.

68. Tasker RR, Organ LW, Hawrylyshyn P: Deafferentation and causalgia. In Bonica JJ (ed): Pain, p 264. New York, Raven Press, 1980.

69. Tasker RR: Pain resulting from central nervous system pathology (central pain). In Bonica JJ (ed): Management of Pain in Clinical Practice, p 262. Philadelphia, Lea and Febiger, 1988.

70. Tasker RR, Dostrovsky JO: Deafferentation and central pain. In Wall PD, Melzack R (eds): Textbook of Pain, 2nd ed, p 154. Edinburgh, Churchill Livingstone, 1988.

71. Willis WD: The origin and destination of pathways involved in pain transmission. In Wall PD, Melzack R (eds): Textbook of Pain, 2nd ed, p 88. Edinburgh, Churchill Livingstone, 1984.

72. Tasker RR: The problem of deafferentation pain in the management of the patient with cancer. Journal of Palliative Care 1987;2:8.

73. Tew JM Jr, Tobler WD: Percutaneous rhizotomy in the treatment of intractable facial pain (trigeminal, glossopharyngeal, and vagal nerves). In Schmidek HH, Sweet WH (eds): Operative Neurosurgical Techniques, Indications, Methods and Results, p 1083. New York, Grune and Stratton, 1982.

74. Siegfried J, Broggi G: Percutaneous thermocoagulation of the gasserian ganglion in the treatment of pain in advanced cancer. In Bonica JJ, Ventafridda V (eds): Advances in Pain Research and Therapy, vol 2, p 463. New York, Raven Press, 1979.

75. Tew JM Jr, Keller JT, Williams DS: Functional surgery of the trigeminal nerve. In Rasmussen T, Marino R (eds): Treatment of Trigeminal Neuralgia: Functional Neurosurgery, p 129. New York, Raven Press, 1979.

76. Broggi GC: Surgical treatment of glossopharyngeal neuralgia and pain from cancer of the nasopharynx. J Neurosurg 1984;61:952.

77. Broggi G, Siegfried J: Percutaneous differential radio-frequency rhizotomy of glossopharyngeal nerve in facial pain due to cancer. In Bonica JJ, Ventafridda V (eds): Advances in Pain Research and Therapy, vol 2, p 469. New York, Raven Press, 1979.

78. Isamat F, Ferran E, Acebes JJ: Selective percutaneous thermocoagulation rhizotomy in essential glossopharyngeal neuralgia. J Neurosurg 1981;55:575.

79. Lazorthes Y, Verdie JC: Radiofrequency coagulation of the petrous ganglion in glossopharyngeal neuralgia. Neurosurgery 1979;4:512.

80. Pagura JR, Schnapp M, Passerelli P: Percutaneous radiofrequency glossopharyngeal rhizolysis for cancer pain. Appl Neurophysiol 1983;46:154.

81. Salar G, Ori C, Baratto V et al: Selective percutaneous thermolesions of the ninth cranial nerve by lateral cervical approach: Report of eight cases. Surg Neurol 1983;20:276.

82. Giorgi C, Broggi G: Surgical treatment of glossopharyngeal neuralgia and pain from cancer of the nasopharynx: A 20 year experience. J Neurosurg 1984; 61:952.

83. Uematsu S: Percutaneous electrothermocoagulation of spinal nerve trunk, ganglion, and rootlets. In Schmidek HH, Sweet WH (eds): Operative Neurosurgical Techniques, Indications, Methods and Results, p 1177. New York, Grune and Stratton, 1982.

84. Ray BS, Console AD: The relief of pain in chronic (calcareous) pancreatitis by sympathectomy. Surg Gynecol Obstet 1949;89:1.

85. Sadar ES, Cooperman AM: Bilateral thoracic sympathectomy splanchnicectomy in the treatment of intractable pain due to pancreatic carcinoma. Cleveland Clinic Quarterly 1974;41:185.

86. Uematsu S, Udbarhelyi GB, Benson DW et al: Percutaneous radiofrequency rhizotomy. Surg Neurol 1974;2:319.

87. McLaurin RL: Neurosurgical approaches to pain in cancer. In Lee JF (ed): Pain Management, p 186. Baltimore, Williams and Wilkins, 1977.

88. Loeser JD: Dorsal rhizotomy: Indications and results. In Bonica JJ (ed): Advances in Neurology, vol 4, p 615. New York, Raven Press, 1974.

89. Onofrio BM: Rhizotomy: What is its place in the treatment of pain? In Bonica JJ (ed): Advances in Neurology, vol 4, p 621. New York, Raven Press, 1974.

90. Saris SC, Silver JM, Vieira JFS et al: Sacrococcygeal rhizotomy for perineal pain. Neurosurgery 1986; 19:789.

91. Sindou M, Fischer G, Mansuy L: Posterior spinal rhizotomy and selective posterior rhizidiotomy. Progress in Neurological Surgery 1976;7:201.

92. Smith FP: Trans-spinal ganglionectomy for relief of intercostal pain. J Neurosurg 1970;32:574.

93. Osgood CP, Dujovmy M, Faille R et al: Microsurgical lumbosacral ganglionectomy, anatomic rationale, and surgical results. Acta Neurochir 1976;35:197.

94. Coggeshall RE: Afferent fibers in the ventral root. Neurosurgery 1979;4:443.

95. Coggeshall RE, Applebaum ML, Fazen M et al: Unmyelinated axons in human ventral roots, a possible explanation for the failure of dorsal rhizotomy to relieve pain. Brain 1975;98:157.

96. Pagura JR: Percutaneous radiofrequency spinal rhizotomy. Appl Neurophysiol 1983;46:138.

97. Piscol K: Die "offenen" spinalen Schmerzoperationen (antero-laterale Chordotomie und kommissurale Myelotomie) in der modernen Schmerzbekampfung. Archiv fur Chirurgie 1976;91:342.

98. Wertheimer P, Lecuire J: La myelotomie commissurale posterieure. Acta Chir Belg 1953;52:568.

99. Payne NS: Dorsal longitudinal myelotomy for the control of perineal and lower body pain. Pain 1984; (Suppl 2):S320.

100. Adams JE, Lippert R, Hosobuchi Y: Commissural myelotomy. In Schmidek HH, Sweet WH (eds): Operative Neurosurgical Techniques, Indications, Methods and Results, p 1155. New York, Grune and Stratton, 1982.

101. Broager B: Commissural myelotomy. Surg Neurol 1974;2:71.

102. Sourek K: Mediolongitudinal myelotomy. In Krayenbuhl PE, Maspes PE, Sweet WH (eds): Progress in Neurological Surgery, vol 8, p 15. Basel, Karger, 1977.

103. Eivas J, Garcia J, Gomez J et al: First results with extralemniscal myelotomy. Acta Neurochir 1980; (Suppl 30):377.

104. Schvarcz JR: Stereotactic high cervical extralemniscal myelotomy for pelvic cancer pain. Acta Neurochir 1984; (Suppl 33):431.

105. Papo I: Spinal posterior rhizotomy and commissural myelotomy in the treatment of cancer pain. In Bonica JJ, Ventafridda V (eds): Advances in Pain Research and Therapy, vol 2, p 439. New York, Raven Press, 1979.

106. Crue BL Jr, Todd EM, Carregal EJA et al: Percutaneous trigeminal tractotomy: Case report utilizing stereotactic radiofrequency lesion. Bulletin of the Los Angeles Neurological Society 1967;32:86.

107. Crue BL, Todd EM, Carregal EJ: Percutaneous radiofrequency stereotactic trigeminal tractotomy. In Crue BL (ed): Pain and Suffering, p 69. Springfield, IL, Charles C Thomas, 1970.

108. Fox JL: Delineation of the obex by contrast radiography during percutaneous trigeminal tractotomy: Technical note. J Neurosurg 1972;36:107.

109. Fox JL: Percutaneous trigeminal tractotomy: Variations in delineation of the obex using emulsified pantopaque. Confinia Neurologica 1974;36:97.

110. Hitchcock ER: Stereotactic trigeminal tractotomy. Ann Clin Res 1970;2:131.

111. Hitchcock ER, Schvarcz JR: Stereotaxic trigeminal tractotomy for post-herpetic facial pain. J Neurosurg 1972;37:412.

112. Schvarcz JR: Stereotactic spinal trigeminal nucleotomy for dysesthetic facial pain. In Bonica JJ, Liebeskind JC, Albe-Fessard DG (eds): Pain Research and Therapy, vol 3, p 331. New York, Raven Press, 1979.

113. Todd EM, Crue BL, Carregal EJA: Posterior percutaneous tractotomy and cordotomy. Confinia Neurologica 1969;31:106.

114. Hyndman OR: Lissauer's tract section: A contribution to chordotomy for the relief of pain (preliminary report). Journal of International College of Surgery 1942;5:394.

115. Sindou M: Etude de la Jonction Radicellomedullaire Posterieure: La Radicellotomie Posterieure Selective dans la Chirurgie de la Douleur. Medical Thesis, Lyon, France, 1972.

116. Sindou M, Lapras C: Neurosurgical treatment of

pain in the Pancoast-Tobias syndrome: Selective posterior rhizotomy and open anterolateral C cordotomy. In Bonica JJ (ed): Advances in Pain Research and Therapy, vol 4, p 199. New York, Raven Press, 1982.

117. Sindou M, Fischer G, Goutelle A et al: La radicellotomie posterieure selective: Premiers resultats dans la chirurgie de la douleur. Neurochirurgie 1974;20:391.

118. Sindou M, Mifsud JJ, Boisson D et al: Selective posterior rhizotomy in the dorsal root entry zone for treatment of hyperspasticity and pain in the hemiplegic upper limb. Neurosurgery 1986;18:587.

119. Tasker RR: Percutaneous cordotomy: The lateral high cervical technique. In Schmidek HH, Sweet WH (eds): Operative Neurosurgical Techniques, Indications, Methods, and Results, p 1137. New York, Grune and Stratton, 1982.

120. Tasker RR: Surgical approaches to the primary afferent and the spinal cord. In Fields HL, Dubner R, Cervero F (eds): Advances in Pain Research and Therapy, vol 9, p 299. New York, Raven Press, 1985.

121. Tasker RR: Percutaneous cordotomy. Compr Ther 1975;1:51.

122. Tasker RR: Percutaneous cordotomy: The lateral high cervical technique. In Schmidek HH, Sweet WH (eds): Operative Neurosurgical Techniques, Indications, Methods, and Results, 2nd ed, p 1191. New York, Grune and Stratton, 1988.

123. Young FR: Cordotomy by open operative techniques. In Youmans JR (ed): Neurological Surgery, 3rd ed, vol 6, p 4059. Philadelphia, WB Saunders, 1990.

124. Poletti CE: Open cordotomy, medullary tractotomy. In Schmidek HH, Sweet WH (eds): Operative Neurosurgical Techniques, Indications, Methods, and Results, 2nd ed, p 1155. New York, Grune and Stratton, 1988.

125. Hitchcock ER: An apparatus for stereotactic spinal surgery: A preliminary report. J Neurosurg 1969; 31:386.

126. Crue BL, Todd EM, Carregal EJA: Posterior approach for high cervical percutaneous radiofrequency cordotomy. Confinia Neurologica 1968; 30:41.

127. Lin RM, Gildenberg PL, Polakoff PP: An anterior approach to percutaneous lower cervical cordotomy. J Neurosurg 1960;25:553.

128. Nathan PW: The descending respiratory pathway in man. J Neurol Neurosurg Psychiatry 1963;26:487.

129. Hitchcock E, Leece B: Somatotopic representation of the respiratory pathways in the cervical cord of man. J Neurosurg 1967;27:320.

130. Rosomoff HL: Percutaneous radiofrequency cervical cordotomy for intractable pain. In Sixth International Congress of Neurological Surgery: International Congress Series 148, p 110. Amsterdam, Excerpta Medica, 1977.

131. Lipton S: Percutaneous cordotomy. In Walls PD, Melzack R (eds): Textbook of Pain, p 632. Edinburgh, Churchill Livingstone, 1984.

132. Meglio M, Cioni B: The role of percutaneous cordotomy in the treatment of chronic cancer pain. Acta Neurochir 1981;59:111.

133. Lahuerta T, Lipton S, Wells JCD: Percutaneous cervical cordotomy: Results and complications in a recent series of 100 patients. Ann R Coll Surg Engl 1985;67:41.

134. Kuhner A: La cordotomie percutanee: Sa place actuelle dans la chirurgie de la douleur. Anesthesie, Analgesie, Reanimation (Paris) 1981;38:357.

135. Siegfried J, Kuhner A, Sturm V: Neurosurgical treatment of cancer pain: Recent results. Cancer Res 1984;89:148.

136. Lorenz R: Methods of percutaneous spinothalamic tract section. In Krayenbuhl H (ed): Advances and Technical Standards in Neurosurgery, Vol 3, p 123. Vienna, Springer-Verlag, 1976.

137. Ischia S, Luzzani A, Ischia A et al: Bilateral percutaneous cervical cordotomy: Immediate and long-term results in 36 patients with neoplastic disease. J Neurol Neurosurg Psychiatry 1984;20:129.

138. Ischia S, Luzzani A, Ischia A et al: Subarachnoid neurolytic block (L5–S1) and unilateral percutaneous cervical cordotomy in the treatment of pain secondary to pelvic malignant disease. Pain 1984; 20:139.

139. Ischia S, Luzzani A, Ischia A et al: Role of percutaneous cervical cordotomy in the treatment of neoplastic vertebral pain. Pain 1984;19:123.

140. Ischia S, Luzzani A, Ischia A et al: Results up to death in the treatment of persistent cervicothoracic (Pancoast) and thoracic malignant pain by unilateral percutaneous cervical cordotomy. Pain 1985;21: 339.

141. Hitchcock ER: Stereotaxic pontine spinothalamic tractotomy. J Neurosurg 1973;39:746.

142. Hitchcock E, Sotelo MG, Kim MC: Analgesic levels and technical method in stereotactic pontine spinothalamic tractotomy. Acta Neurochir 1985;77:29.

143. Hitchcock ER, Kim MC, Jotela M: Further experience in stereotactic pontine tractotomy. Appl Neurophysiol 1985;48:242.

144. Barbera J, Barcia-Salorio JL, Broseta M: Stereotaxic pontine spinothalamic tractotomy. Surg Neurol 1979;11:111.

145. Spiegel EA, Kletzkin M, Szekely EG et al: Pain reactions upon stimulation of the tectum mesencephali. J Neuropathol Exp Neurol 1954;13:212.

146. Nashold BS Jr, Wilson WP: Central pain: Observations in man with chronic implanted electrodes in

the midbrain tegmentum. Confinia Neurologica 1966;27:30.

147. Nashold BS Jr, Wilson WP, Slaughter DG: Sensations evoked by stimulation in the midbrain of man. J Neurosurg 1969;30:14.

148. Tasker RR, Organ LW, Hawrylyshyn P: In Wilkins RH (ed): The Thalamus and Midbrain of Man: A Physiological Atlas Using Electrical Stimulation, p 5–14. Springfield, IL, Charles C Thomas, 1982.

149. Tasker RR: Identification of pain processing systems by electrical stimulation of the brain. Human Neurobiology 1982;1:261.

150. Amano K, Tanikawa T, Iseki H et al: Single neuron analysis of the human midbrain tegmentum. Appl Neurophysiol 1978;41:66.

151. Tasker RR: Stereotaxic surgery. In Wall PD, Melzack R (eds): Textbook of Pain, p 639. Edinburgh, Churchill Livingstone, 1984.

152. Amano K, Iseki H, Notani M et al: Rostral mesencephalic reticulotomy for pain relief with reference to electrode trajectory and clinical results. Appl Neurophysiol 1979;42:316.

153. Amano K, Kawamura H, Tanikawa T et al: Long-term followup study rostral mesencephalic reticulotomy for pain relief: Report of 34 cases. Appl Neurophysiol 1986;49:105.

154. Frank F, Tognetti F, Gaist G et al: Stereotaxic rostral mesencephalotomy in treatment of malignant faciothoracobrachial pain syndromes. J Neurosurg 1982;56:807.

155. Gioia DF, Wallace PB, Fuste FJ et al: A stereotaxic method of surgery for the relief of intractable pain. Int Surg 1967;48:409.

156. Helfant MH, Leksell L, Strang RR: Experience with intractable pain treated by stereotaxic mesencephalotomy. Acta Chir Scand 1965;129:573.

157. de Montreuil CB, Lajat Y, Resche F et al: Apport de la neuro-chirurgie stereotaxique dans le traitement des algies des cancers cervico-faciaux. Ann Otolaryngol Chir Cervicofac 1983;100:181.

158. Mazars G, Pansini A, Chiarelli J: Coagulation du faisceau spino-thalamique et du faisceau quintothalamique par stereotaxie: Indications—resultats. Acta Neurochir 1960;8:324.

159. Mazars G, Roge R, Pansini A: Stereotactic coagulation of the spinothalamic tract for intractable trigeminal pain (abstract). J Neurol Neurosurg Psychiatry 1960;23:352.

160. Nashold BS, Wilson WP, Slaughter DG: Stereotaxic midbrain lesions for central dysesthesia and phantom pain. J Neurosurg 1969;30:116.

161. Nashold BS Jr, Wilson WP, Slaughter G: The midbrain and pain. In Bonica JJ (ed): Advances in Neurology, vol 4, p 191. New York, Raven Press, 1974.

162. Nashold BS, Slaughter DG, Wilson WP et al: Stereo-

tactic mesencephalotomy. In Krayenbuhl H, Maspes PE, Sweet WH (eds): Progress in Neurological Surgery, vol 8, p 35. Basel, Karger, 1977.

163. Nashold BS Jr: Brainstem stereotaxic procedures. In Schaltenbrand G, Walker AE (eds): Stereotaxy of the Human Brain: Anatomical, Physiological and Clinical Applications, p 475. Stuttgart, Georg Thieme, 1982.

164. Torvik A: Sensory motor and reflex changes in two cases of intractable pain after stereotactic mesencephalic tractotomy. J Neurol Neurosurg Psychiatry 1959;22:299.

165. Turnbull IM: Bilateral cingulumotomy combined with thalamotomy or mesencephalic tractotomy for pain. Surg Gynecol Obstet 1972;134:958.

166. Voris HC, Whisler WW: Results of stereotaxic surgery for intractable pain. Confinia Neurologica 1975;37:86.

167. Whisler WW, Voris HC: Mesencephalotomy for intractable pain due to malignant disease. Appl Neurophysiol 1978;47:52.

168. Tasker RR: Thalamic stereotaxic procedures. In Schaltenbrand G, Walker AE (eds): Stereotaxy of the Human Brain, p 484. Stuttgart, Georg Thieme, 1982.

169. Tasker RR: Effets sensitifs et moteurs de la stimulation thalamique chez l'homme: Applications cliniques. Rev Neurol (Paris) 1986;142:316.

170. Dostrovsky JO, Tasker RR, Yamashiro K et al: Sensations evoked by microstimulation in human ventral thalamus in neuronal receptive fields. Society for Neurosciences Abstracts 1986;12:329.

171. Sano K: Intralaminar thalamotomy (thalamolaminotomy) and posterior hypothalamotomy in the treatment of intractable pain. In Krayenbuhl J, Maspes PE, Sweet WH (eds): Progress in Neurological Surgery, vol 8, p 50. Basel, Karger, 1977.

172. Sano K: Stereotaxic thalamolaminotomy and posteromedial hypothalamotomy for the relief of intractable pain. In Bonica JJ, Ventafridda V (eds): Advances in Pain Research and Therapy, vol 2, p 475. New York, Raven Press, 1979.

173. Sano K, Yoshioka M, Ogashiwa M et al: Thalamolaminotomy: A new operation for relief of intractable pain. Confinia Neurologica 1966;27:63.

174. Sano K, Yoshioka M, Sekino H, et al: Functional organization of the internal medullary lamina in man. Confinia Neurologica 1970;32:374.

175. Pagni CA: Place of stereotactic technique in surgery for pain. In Bonica JJ (ed): Advances in Neurology, vol 4, p 669. New York, Raven Press, 1974.

176. Askenasy HM, Levinger M: Stereoencephalotomy for relief of pain. Harefuah 1968;74:85.

177. Bettag W, Yoshida T: Uber stereotaktische Schmerzoperationen. Acta Neurochir 1960;8:299.

178. Bulacio EN, Pozzetti A, Barros M: Dolor cronico

effedos de lesiones en nucleos centro-medianus y parafascicularis. Buenos Aires Medicine 1972;32: 363.

179. Cooper IS: Clinical and physiologic implications of thalamic surgery for disorders of sensory communication: Thalamic surgery for intractable pain. J Neurol Sci 1965;2:493.

180. Fairman D: Unilateral thalamic tractotomy for the relief of bilateral pain in malignant tumours. Confinia Neurologica 1967;29:146.

181. Fairman D: Hypothalamotomy as a new perspective for alleviation of intractable pain and regression of metastatic malignant tumours. In Fusek I, Kunc Z (eds): Present Limits of Neurosurgery, p 525. Prague, Avicenum, 1972.

182. Fairman D, Llavallol MA: Thalamic tractotomy for the alleviation of intractable pain in cancer. Cancer 1973;31:700.

183. Forster DMC, Leksell L, Meyerson BA et al: Gamma thalamotomy in intractable pain. In Janzen R, Keidel WD, Herz A et al (eds): Pain: Basic Principles—Pharmacology—Therapy, p 194. Stuttgart, Georg Thieme, 1972.

184. Hassler R, Riechert T: Klinische und anatomische Befunde bei stereotaktischen Schmerzoperationen im Thalamus. Archiv fur Psychiatrie und Nervenkrankheiten 1959;93:200.

185. Kudo T, Yoshi N, Shimizu S: Stereotaxic surgery for pain relief. J Exp Med 1968;96:219.

186. Leksell L, Meyerson BA, Forster DMC: Radiosurgical thalamotomy for intractable pain. Confinia Neurologica 1972;34:264.

187. Mundinger F: Stereotaktische Operationen gegen anderweitig unbehandelbar schwere Schmerz-zustande. Zeitschrift fur Allgemein Medizin 1974;50: 860.

188. Niizuma H, Kwak R, Saso S et al: Follow-up results of center median thalamotomy for central pain. Appl Neurophysiol 1980;43:336.

189. von Orthner H: Weitere klinische und anatomische Erfahrungen mit zerebralen Schmerzoperationen. Confinia Neurologica 1966;27:71.

190. von Orthner H, Roeder F: Further clinical and anatomical experience with stereotactic operations for relief of pain. Confinia Neurologica 1966;27:418.

191. Richardson DE: Recent advances in the neurosurgical control of pain. South Med J 1967;60:1082.

192. Richardson DE: Thalamotomy for control of chronic pain. Acta Neurochir 1974; (Suppl 21):77.

193. Steiner L, Forster D, Leksell L et al: Gamma thalamotomy in intractable pain. Acta Neurochir 1980; 52:173.

194. Sugita K, Musuga N, Takaoka Y et al: Results of stereotaxic thalamotomy for pain. Confinia Neurologica 1972;34:265.

195. Tsubokawa T, Moriyasu N: Follow-up results of centre median thalamotomy for relief of intractable pain. Confinia Neurologica 1975;37:280.

196. Uematsu S, Konigsmark B, Walker AE: Thalamotomy for alleviation of intractable pain. Confinia Neurologica 1974;36:88.

197. Urabe M, Tsubokawa T: Stereotaxic thalamotomy for the relief of intractable pain. Tohoku J Exp Med 1965;85:286.

198. Yoshimasu N, Ishijima B, Sano K: Pain and the internal medullary lamina. Appl Neurophysiol 1982; 45:498.

199. Lipton S: Percutaneous cervical cordotomy and the injection of the pituitary with alcohol. Anesthesia 1978;33:953.

200. Lipton S, Miles J, Williams N et al: Pituitary injection of alcohol for widespread cancer pain. Pain 1978; 5:73.

201. Madrid JL: Chemical hypophysectomy. In Bonica JJ, Ventafridda V (eds): Advances in Pain Research and Therapy, vol 2, p 381. New York, Raven Press, 1979.

202. Morricca G: Neuroadenolysis for diffuse intractable pain. In Bonica JJ, Albe-Fessard D (eds): Advances in Pain Research and Therapy, vol 1, p 863. New York, Raven Press, 1976.

203. Miles J: Chemical hypophysectomy. In Bonica JJ, Ventafridda V (eds): Advances in Pain Research and Therapy, vol 2, p 373. New York, Raven Press, 1979.

204. Miles J: Neurological advances in the relief of pain. Br J Hosp Med 1983;30:348.

205. Miles J: Pituitary destruction. In Wall PD, Melzack R (eds): Textbook of Pain, p 656. Edinburgh, Churchill Livingstone, 1984.

206. Yanagida H, Corssen G, Trouwborst A et al: Relief of cancer pain in man: Alcohol-induced neuroadenolysis vs electrical stimulation of the pituitary gland. Pain 1984;19:133.

207. Bouckoms AJ: Psychosurgery for pain. In Wall PD, Melzack R (eds): Textbook of Pain, 2nd ed, p 868. Edinburgh, Churchill Livingstone, 1988.

208. Freeman W, Watts JW: Pain of organic disease relieved by prefrontal lobotomy. Lancet 1946;i:953.

209. Meyerson BA, Boethius J, Carlsson AM: Percutaneous central gray stimulation for cancer pain. Appl Neurophysiol 1978:41:57.

210. Tasker RR, Yoshida M, Sima AAF et al: Stimulation mapping of the periventricular-periaqueductal gray (PVG-PAG) in man: An autopsy study. In Samii M (ed): Surgery in and Around the Brain Stem and the Third Ventricle, p 161. Berlin, Springer-Verlag, 1986.

211. Amano K, Tanikawa T, Kawarnura H et al: Endorphin and pain relief: Further observations on electrical stimulation of the periaqueductal gray matter during rostral mesencephalic reticulotomy for pain relief. Appl Neurophysiol 1982;45:123.

212. Boivie J, Meyerson BA: A correlative anatomic and clinical study of pain suppressed by deep brain stimulation. Pain 1982;13:113.

213. Gybels J: Electrical stimulation of the brain for pain control in humans. Verh Dtsch Ges Inn Med 1980; 86:1553.

214. Hosobuchi Y, Adams JE, Linchitz R: Pain relief by electrical stimulation of the central gray matter in humans and its reversal by naloxone. Science 1977; 179:181.

215. Hosobuchi Y: Analgesia induced by brain stimulation with chronically implanted electrodes. In Schmidek HH, Sweet WH (eds): Operative Neurosurgical Techniques, Indications, Methods and Results, 2nd ed, p 1089. New York, Grune and Stratton, 1988.

216. Levy RM, Lamb S, Adams JE: Treatment of chronic pain by deep brain stimulation: Long-term follow-up and review of the literature. Neurosurgery 1987; 21:885.

217. Meyerson BA: Aspects on the present state of intracerebral stimulation for pain. In Tsubokawa T (ed): Brain Stimulation and Neuronal Plasticity, p 33. Tokyo, Neuron, 1985.

218. Ray CD, Burton CV: Deep brain stimulation for severe chronic pain. Acta Neurochir 1980; (Suppl 30):289.

219. Richardson DE, Akil H: Long term results of periventricular gray self-stimulation. Neurosurgery 1977;1:200.

220. Richardson DE: Long-term follow-up of deep brain stimulation for relief of chronic pain in the human. In Brock M (ed): Modern Neurology, p 449. Berlin, Springer-Verlag, 1982.

221. Tsubokawa T, Katayama Y, Yamamoto T et al: Deafferentation pain and stimulation of the thalamic sensory relay nucleus: Clinical and experimental study. Appl Neurophysiol 1985;48:166.

222. Tsubokawa T, Hirayama T, Tamamoto T et al: Differential effects between thalamic sensory relay nucleus and peri-aqueductal gray stimulation on neural activity within the normal and deafferented trigeminal medullary dorsal horn. In Tsubokawa T (ed): Brain Stimulation and Neuronal Plasticity, p 65. Tokyo, Neuron, 1985.

223. Young RF, Brechner T: Electrical stimulation of the brain for relief of intractable pain due to cancer. Cancer 1986;57:1266.

224. Young RF, Chambi VI: Pain relief by electrical stimulation of the periaqueductal and periventricular gray matter. J Neurosurg 1987;66:364.

225. Young RF, Kroening R, Frelton W et al: Electrical stimulation of the brain in treatment of chronic pain: Experience over 5 years. J Neurosurg 1985;62:389.

Chapter *27*

Cancer Pain Management Problems in Developing Countries

Roberto D. Wenk

INTRODUCTION

Cancer, although comprising a heterogeneous group of disorders, is characteristically a multisymptomatic process, particularly in its advanced stages (see Chapter 13). Symptoms may be associated with tumor invasion or antitumor therapy (see Chapters 1 and 3), and have a variable but overall marked capacity to reduce patients' quality of life, as well as to affect negatively the well-being of members of the family and close community. Patients with advanced cancer often complain of weakness, anorexia, pain, dyspnea, constipation, cough, nausea and vomiting, dysphagia, and insomnia (see Chapters 10, 12, 13, and 30).[1-3] In most studies, significant pain is the most frequent symptom, observed in 60%–90% of patients in advanced stages of disease.[2,4,5]

The provision of adequate care for patients with established cancer is confounded by the following three conditions: 1) due to late detection, the aggressive nature of some neoplasms, and, frequently, an absence of efficacious antitumor therapy, a high proportion of cancer patients are beyond "cure,"[6] so that all that can be offered is symptom control and a management philosophy that aims to minimize suffering; 2) current knowledge of the pathophysiology of cancer pain syndromes and the pharmacology of the analgesics and adjuvant drugs applied under optimal circumstances allows adequate control of terminal symptoms[7]; and 3) notwithstanding 1) and 2), this group of patients continues to receive inadequate treatment in both industrialized and developing nations.[8,9] Various explanations have been cited as contributing to this global failure to provide adequate care despite the existence of adequate knowledge and technology.

Health care professionals often are unaware of accepted methods for the control of pain and other cancer-related symptoms,[7] and for the most part have not received proper instruction in principles of symptom control in either medical school, residency, or continuing professional education (see Chapter 8). As a result, many unscientific beliefs persist, such as the inevitability of cancer pain, the need to reserve the use of potent opioids for the preterminal stage of disease to preserve their efficacy, and the potential for respiratory depression and addiction to occur with chronic opioid use. A common factor among the barriers posed by the attitudes of health care professionals, patients, their families, and health care/government regulators is an excessive preoccupation regarding the potential for addiction to opioid analgesics. Prohibitions impeding access to appropriate opioid analgesics persist, and governments do not appear interested in changing this situation.

This regrettable gap between treatment that potentially could be provided and that which actually is provided refutes the only therapeutic alternative available to many cancer patients. This situation is amplified dramatically in developing nations. Developing nations are the source of more than half of the new cancer cases diagnosed annually, and by the time a diagnosis of cancer has been made in these settings, illness is most often incurable.[10] The World Health Organization (WHO) has proposed a pharmacologic ladder approach to the management of cancer pain (Fig. 27–1 and Chapters 6–10) that, when applied in the context of a global policy such as has been suggested recently by the WHO (Fig. 27–2), is pertinent to the cancer pain problem in developing nations.

THE SITUATION IN SOME DEVELOPING COUNTRIES

In 1989, a collaborative study designed to obtain information on the condition of cancer

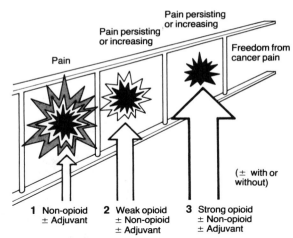

Figure 27–1. WHO-advocated pharmacologic ladder approach to the management of cancer pain. Depending on the severity of pain at initial presentation, the patient may access the ladder at any site. Note recommendations for combination and adjuvant therapy. See Chapters 6–10 for further details. Courtesy World Health Organization, Geneva, Switzerland.

patients at their first consultation for palliative care services was undertaken in three Argentine cities (Buenos Aires, Cordoba, and San Nicolas).[11] The authors observed that: 1) most of the 70 patients sampled had experienced

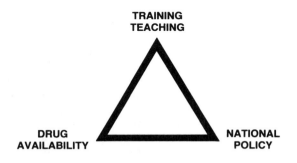

Keys to Resolving "Third World"
Cancer Pain Dilemma

Figure 27–2. Interdependent factors targeted by the WHO necessary for the development of an effective cancer pain program in developing nations. Courtesy World Health Organization, Geneva, Switzerland.

pain for greater than 1 month, and more than 60% of this group reported pain that was "strong" or "unbearable," although they were recipients of ongoing analgesic treatment; 2) 63% of patients described disturbances in sleep secondary to pain, resulting in less than 5 hours of sleep daily; and 3) intercurrent analgesic treatments shared the following common features that presumably contributed to their lack of effectiveness: prominent use of mild (nonopioid) analgesics, frequent use of agonist–antagonist and partial agonist opioids administered according to schedules inconsistent with their pharmacologic actions, frequent use of parenteral routes, and inadequate efforts to treat nausea, vomiting, and constipation.

The reasons typically cited for the undertreatment of cancer pain,[12,13] although perhaps contributory, are inadequate to explain entirely the situation described above, and like scenarios. For example, in Argentina: 1) publications in Spanish are available that describe appropriate pharmacologic measures for managing cancer pain[14]; 2) there are groups that actively spread information on cancer pain control in each of the three cities where this survey took place; 3) it is possible to obtain specially prepared preparations of codeine and morphine at public pharmacies in quantities sufficient to provide treatment for extended periods of time[15]; 4) sophisticated treatment methods are not required to relieve nausea, vomiting, and constipation; and 5) although handicapped by limited resources, private and public health care systems exist that can be adapted to promote the provision of palliative care.

The underuse of available resources and documentation of continued inadequate symptom control[10] serve to identify an additional etiologic factor, perhaps at the root of all others: a simple lack of motivation to provide assistance.

Various other published reports document the inadequate use of analgesics in cancer patients in Mexico, Vietnam, India, Brazil, China, and the Dominican Republic,[16–21] and unpublished data reveal that the situation in Chile and Colombia is similar.[22,23] Various opioid analgesics (Table 27–1), some of which are included on the list of basic drugs recommended by the WHO,[12] are available in Brazil, Chile, Colombia, the Dominican Republic, and Mexico. Many of these drugs can be used without serious restrictions, and although they perhaps are not as valuable as oral morphine, they can be used effectively.[24] Unarguably, it is preferable to provide treatment with available opioid analgesics than to defer treatment altogether, although this frequently does not occur. Information concerning analgesic approaches exists in the aforementioned countries. Initiatives to assist terminal patients either are recent or do not yet exist. The lack of motivation to reduce the human suffering advanced as a determinant of treatment inadequacies in Argentina can be argued to operate in these other nations as well.

The causes underlying deficits are uncertain and doubtlessly complex. A sociocultural phenomenon that tolerates the general acceptance of suffering and indifference has been proposed.[25] The ineffective use of educational techniques and the scarcity of attempts to modify the existing situation may play a part as well, or may be a result of this attitude. The consequences of such a system are that the affected population does not demand that it be improved, and effective initiatives are wanting, with resultant delays in acquiring and transmitting knowledge, legalizing the medical use of opioids, and developing terminal care programs that work. The sociocultural phenomenon of indifference referred to above generates attitudes that are difficult and slow to modify. Only effective education of health care personnel, representatives of the government, and the general population can alter this situation.

Experience has demonstrated that neither exhortation nor the simple dissemination of information are effective in altering entrenched practices of pain control,[26] and it has been suggested that new teaching strategies must be developed.[13] Our experience has shown that two elements are necessary to produce the desired change: 1) people must be motivated by the desire to help, and 2) access to a teaching program that includes relevant

Table 27–1.
Availability of Opioid Analgesics in South America

Opioid	Argentina	Brazil	Chile	Colombia	Dominican Republic	Mexico
Buprenorphine	P	O, P	—	O, P	—	O, P
Codeine	P	O	O	O	—	O
Fentanyl	P	—	P	P	P	P
Meperidine	P	P	P	O, P	P	P
Morphine	O, P	P	O, P	P	—	O, P
Nalbuphine	P	—	—	—	P	P
Oxycodone	—	—	—	O	O	—
Pentazocine	—	—	—	P	P	—
Propoxiphene	O, P	—	—	O	O	O

O = oral; P = parenteral
Data courtesy of M. T. Evangelista (Brazil), A. Felmer (Chile), L. Lima (Colombia), R. Paredes
(Dominican Republic), and J. R. Romo (Mexico).

information and an operative model is essential. The application of a model depending on foreign assistance models is of questionable value: although the influences on such a program will be multiple, the operative model must be developed *"in situ,"* and must be adapted to the area's distinctive socioeconomic situation. An understanding of local limitations on obtaining maximum yields of the available resources (equipment, personnel, and drugs) is critical. It is essential that the model establish assistance guidelines, but, more important, it must demonstrate the cause–effect relationship of the application of a certain therapeutic approach on a group of patients. The results obtained then can serve to attract the attention of the observers within the same country or in countries with similar problems, and generate in them the desire to reproduce or modify the assistance model.

The existence of an operative model designed to facilitate its replication in diverse regions within a country could potentially change customs. Terminal care programs cannot be demanded or organized if their benefits are unproven, and likewise regulations that control the availability of opioids cannot be modified if the benefits of appropriate opioid use have not been demonstrated. In countries

where no official plans exist to redress deficiencies in health care delivery, an effective sequence to produce change is the creation of an assistance model, demonstration of concrete results by its application, and, on this basis, influencing health authorities to make the changes necessary for its implementation on a large scale.

THE SAN NICOLAS PROGRAM: A PROPOSED MODEL FOR DEVELOPING COUNTRIES

The economic resources of Argentina are limited, and its health authorities and personnel historically have not shown an interest in providing assistance to the terminal patient. Opioid analgesics are available in public pharmacies. The community, when properly motivated, has collaborated in the past with aid programs. The operating model of the *Centro de Cuidados Paliativos de San Nicolas* (CCP) has adapted to these socioeconomic conditions in four specific areas: the palliative care team, the assistance activity, the therapeutic approach, and the relationship with the health care system.

Table 27–2.
Team Activity

Physicians 1 and 2	Thursdays—5:00–9:00 PM • Start and control outpatient treatments, in CCP office • Start treatments of patients who cannot reach the CCP (at home or in hospital)
Physician 1 (Director)	Mondays, Wednesdays—8:00–10:00 AM • Telephone advice to community physicians (by pager)
Physician 2 (Resident)	Monday–Friday—5:00–9:00 PM • Patient control at home or in hospital when requested by volunteers
Volunteers	Mondays, Saturdays—5:00–9:00 PM Assess patients at home or in hospital All Days 24-hour availability for family support by telephone Thursdays—5:00–9:00 PM (in CCP office) • Family support • Daily recording forms reception • Preparation of morphine solutions • Data collection • Computer data entry
Psychologist	Group work with CCP team

THE TEAM

Individuals willing to offer their time and efforts are welcomed. The ultimate requisite for participating in voluntary work in terminal care is a strong humanitarian concern. Over the course of 5 years of activity, two physicians and four lay persons abandoned the program, representing 50% and 40% of professional and nonprofessional volunteers, respectively. This spontaneous selection process has reflected an incapacity of individuals to function as part of a team, and/or a discrepancy between their expectations and the reality of the work.

Currently, the team is staffed by an anesthesiologist, a resident in anesthesiology, a psychologist, and six volunteers. All but the resident provide their efforts without reimbursement. The psychologist does not work with cancer patients, but instead works with the members of the team. The activities of the CCP are detailed in Table 27–2. The organization of the team establishes two lines of assistance/support that are activated in sequence: the lay volunteers and the physician volunteers. This system functions to reduce the demands on medical professionals, and consequently permits more effective attention at a lower "cost" to a greater number of patients.

The volunteers represent the first line of assistance. Their background is uniformly nonmedical, but over a 6-month period they receive theoretical information on cancer, and acquire knowledge of techniques in terminal care by working jointly with physicians and veteran volunteers. Table 27–3 lists the various topics included in their training. The principal activity of the volunteers is to monitor the condition of the patient and responses to treatment. The information thus obtained serves to complete the "information loop" during the time that elapses between weekly medical consultations. They form the first line of responsibility for the well-being of patients at home and in the hospital, as well as provid-

Table 27–3.
Training of Volunteers

Interpersonal communication skills
Quality control of analgesia
   Monitor/adjust doses
   Use combinations of analgesics
   Use of bedtime and rescue doses
Prophylaxis/treatment of constipation
Treatment of nausea and vomiting and of oral problems
Prevention of decubitus ulcers
Nonpharmacologic treatment of pruritus
Knowledge of nutritional support
Knowledge of subcutaneous infusion devices.

ing family support with telephone contact. They are able to make therapeutic decisions within certain preestablished limits that depend on their level of training and expertise. Their activities are supervised closely by the team physicians, who comprise the second line of responsibility/assistance, and are consulted when the clinical condition of the patient exceeds preestablished limits. Nonphysician volunteers are grouped into three pairs to perform home visits and to provide telephone assistance: two pairs work while the third rests during alternating 3-month periods. Discussion of active cases occurs during weekly team meetings. Twice monthly, the psychologist coordinates these meetings to discuss the emotions that arise from contact with terminal patients and their families.

The funds for the CCP activity (drugs, didactic material, printing, mail and telephone expenses, resident fees, etc.) are provided through public donations.

THE ASSISTANCE ACTIVITY

Patients are treated at home whenever possible. Treatment is the result of the combined actions of the family, the CCP, and the primary care physician.

The family is charged with the responsibility of administering analgesics as instructed,

providing adequate nutrition and general care, and endeavoring to cultivate a supportive means of interacting. The family also completes a daily report form that documents the patient's symptoms, and what medications were used in what doses. The supporting and teaching process is continuous, and is done during both the visits of the family to the CCP and the volunteers to the patients' homes; it is complemented with telephone assistance and illustrative fliers.

There is no charge for CCP intervention. Owing to its volunteer base, the CCP's activities are limited (see Table 27–2). Other restrictions include a maximum distance for home visits of 20 km, home visits by the resident physician only on the basis of a request by nonphysician volunteers, and an absence of coverage for emergencies. To reduce the impact of the latter deficit, the family is advised to make contact with a community emergency service that is informed of the patient's condition and instructed on specific palliative techniques. These restrictions are explained to the family, and a form stating their understanding of the conditions that guide the provision of care is signed at the time of the first consultation.

Another requirement is that the patient maintain a relationship with a primary care physician. If there is no primary care physician, patients are advised to engage one. The primary care physician is expected to follow the patient clinically and to be responsible for specific treatments, as well as administrative procedures, prescriptions, etc.

THE THERAPEUTIC APPROACH

The treatment approach is pharmacologically based and applied in accordance with WHO guidelines.[27] The CCP has no supporting structure to perform neurolytic blocks, and few patients have access to palliative radiotherapy. All patients receive analgesics by the oral route, except when it is precluded by their medical condition, in which case drugs are administered subcutaneously. A limited num-

Table 27–4.
Drugs Used by Volunteers Under Physician Supervision

Naproxen
Propoxyphene/dipyrone (commercial combination)
Oral morphine
Haloperidol
Danthron
Magnesium salts
Antacids
Benzynamide

ber of drugs are used (Table 27–4). When needed, the subcutaneous administration of morphine, hyoscine, and haloperidol is accomplished with the Edmonton Injector (see Chapter 11).[28] This reusable device is both economic and effective (Fig. 27–3), and allows intermittent subcutaneous infusion of preset doses of the selected medication in volumes of 0.5–3 ml. It is suitable for ambulatory or home use, and, with a minimum of training,

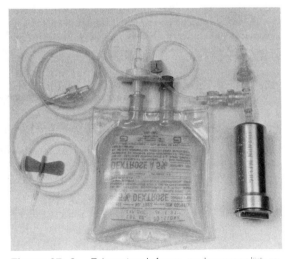

Figure 27–3. Edmonton Infusor, an inexpensive reusable device to provide intermittent subcutaneous infusions of opioids and other drugs at preset doses (limits 0.5–3.0 ml).

can be operated by the patient or family members.

Commercial preparations of morphine are not currently available in Argentina, and as a result, arrangements have been made for on-site preparation. Morphine hydrochloride is acquired in powder form, and is stored in a safe-deposit box located in a nearby bank that is opened weekly. Drug distribution to the patient and his or her family is accounted for carefully. The amount of drug, the date it was delivered, and the identity of the family member who received it are recorded in a data base.

For oral use, 6 g morphine is diluted in 1,000 ml of mineral water to a solution of 6 mg/ml, and is placed in a dark glass bottle that is kept refrigerated in a locked metal container. The key to maintaining a stable solution seems to lie in maintenance of sanitary materials. The solution is discarded if it has not been consumed within a period of 15 days.

For subcutaneous use, 1–2 g morphine hydrochloride is diluted in 50 ml saline (20–40 mg/ml) in a 50-ml graduated cylinder, and is sterilized at 120°C at 15 psi for 25–30 minutes. This solution often is combined with commercial preparations of hyoscine and/or haloperidol for combined parenteral use.

THE RELATIONSHIP WITH THE HEALTH CARE SYSTEM

Despite the CCP's unidisciplinary structure (anesthesiology), global independence, and nonprofit/charity status, multiple interactions with the health care system still take place. These include: 1) the referral of patients to primary care physicians in the community; 2) the provision of consultation for hospitalized patients who will continue to receive care by responsible medical and nursing staff; 3) the availability of telephone consultation with community physicians on issues related to symptom control; 4) the use of hospital beds for patients with intractable symptoms or for individuals without family support (hospital staff maintains overall responsibility for treatment); and 5) the provision of education for health care personnel.

CONCLUSION

Application of the assistance model described above has produced acceptable results.[29] It is a unique instrument, capable of facilitating the introduction and growth of palliative care in developing nations, and demonstrates that the presence of limited resources by no means represents an absolute barrier to program development.

Note: The author wishes to thank Ana and Jorge Laver and Dr. Patt for assistance in the English translation of this chapter.

REFERENCES

1. Baines M: Nausea and vomiting in the patient with advanced cancer. Journal of Pain and Symptom Management 1988;3:81.
2. Twycross RG, Lack SA: Therapeutics in Terminal Cancer. New York, Churchill Livingstone, 1986.
3. Twycross RG, Lack SA: Control of Alimentary Symptoms in Advanced Cancer. Edinburgh, Churchill Livingstone, 1986.
4. Walsh DT: Oral morphine in chronic cancer pain. Pain 1984;18:1.
5. Sutton PM, Khan SM, Khan M: Cancer pain can be relieved. World Health Forum 1990;11:210.
6. Silverberg E, Boring CC, Squires TS: Cancer statistics: 1990. CA 1990;40:9.
7. Foley KM: Treatment of cancer pain. N Engl J Med 1985;313:84.
8. International experts call for W.H.O. support of palliative care. Cancer Pain Release 1989;3(3):1.
9. Bonica JJ: Status of pain research and therapy. Seminars in Anesthesiology 1986;5:82.
10. Stjernsward J: All the world against cancer. World Health 1988:6.
11. Wenk R, DeSimone G, Pruvost MA: Los cuidados paliativos en la Argentina: La necesidad de centros de enseanza. Rev Arg Anest (in press).
12. Hill CS Jr: Relationship among cultural, educational and regulatory agency influences on optimum cancer pain treatment. Journal of Pain and Symptom Management 1990;5 (Suppl):S37.
13. Friedman DP: Perspectives on the medical use of drugs of abuse. Journal of Pain and Symptom Management 1990;5 (Suppl):S2.
14. World Health Organization: Alivio del Dolor en el Cancer. Geneva, WHO, 1987.
15. Wenk RD: Availability of analgesics in Argentina. Journal of Pain and Symptom Management 1987;2:191.
16. Romero Romo JI, Plancarte R, Amescua C et al: Mexico's W.H.O. cancer pain relief program. In Foley KM, Bonica JJ, Ventafridda V (eds): Advances in Pain Research and Therapy, vol 16, p 489. New York, Raven Press, 1990.
17. Vietnam: Making cancer pain relief a reality. Cancer Pain Relief 1988;2(1):1.
18. Vijayaram S et al: Experience with oral morphine for cancer pain relief. Journal of Pain and Symptom Management 1989;4:130.
19. Troccoli BT, Keller ML: Cancer pain relief in Paraiba, Brasil. Journal of Pain and Symptom Management 1989;4:110.
20. Merriman A: Better care for the terminally ill in Singapore. Journal of Pain and Symptom Management 1989;4:58.
21. Dominican Cancer Institute starts pain relief program in Santo Domingo. Cancer Pain Relief 1989;3(2):1.
22. Personal communication.
23. Personal communication.
24. Bruera E: Manejo farmacologico del dolor por cancer. In Pain Research Group (eds): Monografia Sobre Cuidados Paliativos, p 35. Madison, WI, University of Wisconsin–Madison, 1990.
25. Wenk, RD: Are we really ready to alleviate pain? Journal of Pain and Symptom Management 1989;4:1.
26. A report on the Wisconsin Cancer Pain Initiative. Journal of Pain and Symptom Management 1988;3 (Suppl):S2.
27. World Health Organization: Cancer Pain Relief. Geneva, World Health Organization, 1986.
28. Bruera E: Subcutaneous administration of opioids in the management of cancer pain. In Foley KM, Bonica JJ, Ventafridda V (eds): Advances in Pain Research and Therapy, vol 16, p 203. New York, Raven Press, 1990.
29. Wenk RD et al: Argentina's W.H.O. Cancer Pain Relief Program: A patient care model. Journal of Pain and Symptom Management (in press).

Chapter 28

The Management of Pain in Childhood Cancer

Neil L. Schechter

Steven J. Weisman

The management of pain traditionally has been a neglected aspect of the overall management of childhood cancer (see Chapter 4). Yet, for many children, it is the pain (often associated with procedures) or fear of that pain that dominates their experience while living with cancer.[1,2] The adequate management of pain, therefore, can significantly improve the quality of life for these children, and reduce some of the burden that these diseases place on them and their families.

Miser[3] and others[4] have summarized some of the differences between adult and childhood cancer. Children clearly have a different spectrum of malignancies. Carcinomas, the predominant cancer type in adults, are rare in children. Instead, leukemias and lymphomas predominate. These malignancies are associated with less disease-related pain than solid tumors. However, they are more likely to require painful diagnostic procedures such as lumbar punctures and bone marrow aspirations, which are particularly distressing for children. In addition, most children's malignancies are more responsive to initial therapies. Therefore, aggressive, multimodality therapy may alleviate disease-related pain very rapidly in children with cancer, whereas the response to treatment in adults may be more gradual. If children do not respond to chemotherapeutic regimens, their demise usually is rapid, leaving less time for chronic pain problems to emerge and predominate.

In addition, depending on their age, children respond psychologically in a different manner to the diagnosis of cancer and its treatment than do adults. Typically, for children, the word "cancer" does not have the same negative connotation that it does to adults; nor do children have the fear of death that often accompanies the diagnosis of cancer in an adult. Unlike adults, however, they are often so fearful of needles that preoccupation over procedures tends to dominate their relationships with health care providers.

CANCER PAIN SYNDROMES

Children's cancer pain syndromes can be conceptualized as follows:

1. *Procedure-related pain*: These are the pains associated with diagnostic and treatment procedures that are often a necessary part of cancer therapy. These include lumbar punctures, bone marrow aspirations, frequent venipunctures, placement of central venous lines, access to those lines, etc. For many children, procedures are the worst part of having their disease (see Chapter 4).[2]

2. *Disease-related pain*: Pain directly from cancer itself may result from a number of different etiologies. Leukemias, lymphomas, and neuroblastomas, the most common malignancies of childhood, commonly present as disseminated at diagnosis. Hence, children with these malignancies often present with bone and joint pain secondary to direct invasion by disease or by replacement of the bone marrow with malignant cells. When solid tumors arise in relatively closed anatomic locations, such as the head and neck or adjacent to the spine, bony destruction or nerve entrapment may occur. In addition, many brain tumors present with headache and vomiting from ventricular obstruction and associated intracranial pressure. Leukemic or lymphomatous meningeal disease usually will be associated with headache as well.

Many of the abdominal tumors of childhood present as painless masses. However, if acute hemorrhage into such a tumor occurs, pain is not uncommon. In addition, intra-abdominal lesions may result in obstruction of the urinary tract or the gastrointestinal tract, with subsequent colicky pain. Occasionally, an intra-abdominal tumor can result in intussusception or even volvulus. Neuropathic pain certainly can accompany any tumor that invades locally into neural tissue. This is not unusual in the soft-tissue sarcomas, especially those that arise paravertebrally. Pelvic rhabdomyosarcomas also may involve the lower lumbar or sacral roots and cause typical sciatic pain.

3. *Pain associated with treatment itself*: Pain also may result from a variety of treatment modalities (see Chapter 4). Chemotherapy may result in mucositis, particularly in association with bone marrow transplantation. This typically occurs in the pancytopenic patient, but also may be seen as a direct effect of drugs such as methotrexate. Neutropenia from chemotherapy predisposes patients to a variety of infections, in addition to those of the oral mucosa. Therefore, pain frequently will be seen in this situation. Perirectal infection should be suspected when perirectal pain or tenderness is noted. Local cellulitis or intra-abdominal processes related to infection also may present with pain in these patients.

Vincristine, a commonly used drug, causes a wide spectrum of symptoms by inducing peripheral neuropathy (see Chapter 3).[5,6] Such symptoms include constipation and even ileus. Jaw, hand, or foot pain with typical neuropathic dysesthesias, with burning, tingling, and motor changes also are frequent.

Radiation may cause dermatitis and mucositis. This is a particular problem in some of the soft-tissue sarcomas, like rhabdomyosarcoma, in sites such as the head and neck or pelvis. Since these tumors usually are treated with actinomycin D with or without an anthracycline, the additional problem of "radiation-recall" is seen.[7] In these children, even after radiation therapy is complete, administration of chemotherapy can cause recurrence of mucositis or dermatitis in the radiation field. In children receiving whole abdomen radiation, intestinal ulceration and ileus are possible. Some children with axial tumors that require a radiation field that includes the nerve roots or spinal cord, may have exacerbating vincristine neuropathy well after radiation treatments are complete.

Pain also may result from surgery for cancer or from amputations. Postamputation phantom limb pain in children has become increasingly recognized.[8]

The nature of the pain that the child experiences from any of these syndromes depends on the pathophysiology of the specific insult (see Chapter 1). Procedure pain stemming from stimulation of peripheral nociceptors is sharp and intense. Obstruction of a viscus usually yields colicky, crampy pain. Pain stemming from nerve injury characteristically is burning or shooting. The treatments for these entities vary, and therefore a clear understanding of the origin of the pain is essential for adequate treatment.

EPIDEMIOLOGY OF CANCER PAIN

The epidemiology of cancer pain in children has been examined in a number of studies (see Chapter 4). Cornaglia[9] reported that solid tumors in children have a much higher incidence of pain than the more common malignancies, such as leukemias and lymphomas. More methodically rigorous work in this area was done by Miser,[1] who sampled the prevalence of pain in children with cancer in inpatient and outpatient settings. Pain was present in 26% of the outpatients and 54% of the inpatients. The etiology of their pain was primarily treatment-related, such as mucositis, postoperative pain, and neuropathic pain. Tumor pain itself most often resulted from bony lesions. The group sampled, however, was not representative of children with cancer, as it included an extraordinarily high incidence of children with solid tumors. More recently, McGrath and colleagues[3] reported on the pain of 77 children from a pediatric oncology clinic. This group consisted primarily of children with leukemias and lymphomas, although some children with solid tumors also were included. This study suggests that almost three-quarters of children experience severe pain from bone marrow aspirations and procedures, 50% experience moderate to severe

pain from their treatment, and only about one-quarter of children have pain directly from their disease.

These studies all suggest that pain is a relatively common occurrence in childhood cancer. In particular, the management of pain associated with procedures, which often is not even considered in adults with cancer, is critical for the humane care of children.

ASSESSMENT

The assessment of pain is an essential element of the overall treatment of pain in children with cancer. This topic is well covered in Chapter 4. Developmentally appropriate pain assessment should be a routine part of the inpatient and outpatient care of children with malignancies. Virtually every child has a problem list developed as part of either the inpatient or outpatient medical record, and cancer pain should be an essential component of such problem lists. This list should incorporate the various types of pain the child may experience. In the inpatient setting, the bedside chart should include specific entry locations for pain assessment. In addition, there also should be ample space for the nursing staff to record side effects of therapy. This approach emphasizes the importance of routine pain assessment as an integral aspect of nursing care, and provides documentation for the use of pain management as a quality assurance indicator.

GENERAL TREATMENT PRINCIPLES

Some of the general principles of cancer pain management in children are summarized in Table 28–1. Effective treatment of cancer pain in children should be monitored in the various clinical settings through standard quality assurance methods.[10] Elevating pain management to this level of importance serves to educate a variety of health professionals involved in the care of children, as

Pain relief is a quality assurance issue for all children with cancer
The setting and staff should be child-oriented
Believe pain complaints of children with cancer
The staff should be skilled in pain assessment
Each child should have a pain problem list
Institute anticancer therapy as soon as possible
Use behavioral techniques early
Procedure pain should be treated aggressively
Use the pharmacologic ladder for analgesic choices
Parents must be involved in all phases of pain therapy

well as to reinforce the standards of care for cancer-related pain. Children with malignancies should be treated in a cancer treatment center that specializes in the care of children. This ultimately surrounds sick youngsters with an environment and health professionals committed to the developmental needs of children. Such bright, cheerful environments, filled with television, video games, books, and arts and crafts, serve to keep the ill child occupied and present certain behavioral tools that can be used to cope with the pain of cancer.

Each cancer treatment team should have access to nursing, physician, social work, or psychological health professionals who are skilled in the use of the various behavioral interventions for pain management. Such techniques should be introduced at the inception of the evaluation or treatment of a newly diagnosed malignancy. Parents must play a critical role in effecting a pain treatment plan for their child. In the face of an overwhelming medical diagnosis, even the parents may fail to overlook the comfort needs of their children. The parents and the child should receive preparation that includes information about the pain that might be expected from the disease or from the treatment. In addition, at every opportunity, parents should be encouraged to be present and assist their youngsters.

PHARMACOLOGIC MANAGEMENT

GENERAL PHARMACOLOGIC PRINCIPLES

The safest and simplest approach to analgesic use in children is recommended. The goal of therapy always should be adequate analgesia, as determined by the patient, family, and staff. Age and disease-related decisions must be used to determine the best route of delivery. Use of the analgesic ladder,[11] well described by others in this text (see Chapters 6–9), is the cornerstone of pharmacologic therapy. The clinician should be familiar with the side effects of the analgesics and their specific routes of administration so that prophylactic intervention can be planned. Although the oral route remains theoretically the preferred one in children, it is critical to remember that administration of any oral medicine in an uncooperative, traumatized child can be rather invasive.

The choice of an appropriate pharmacologic agent depends on the degree of pain that the child is experiencing. In general, three categories of drugs are useful: 1) peripherally acting analgesics, 2) opioids, and 3) adjuvants.

PERIPHERALLY ACTING AGENTS

These drugs, all of which effect prostaglandin synthesis, are useful for mild pain associated with childhood cancer (Table 28–2). Peripherally acting drugs all have ceiling effects (ie, unlike opioids, there is a dose beyond which further analgesic efficacy usually is not achieved). All of these drugs also have antipyretic effects that potentially might mask fever in an immunosuppressed child.

Acetaminophen is the most commonly used agent in this category. Typical doses are 10–15 mg/kg every 4 hours orally or 10–20 mg/kg every 4 hours rectally. The rectal route obviously should be used with caution in children with cancer because of the danger of perirectal irritation and infection. Acetaminophen appears to have no effect on platelet

Table 28–2.
Oral Analgesics for Mild Pain

Drug	Equianalgesic Dose (mg)	Pediatric Dose (mg/kg/dose)	Comments
Acetaminophen	650	10	Minimal anti-inflammatory properties
Aspirin	650	10	Gastritis; antiplatelet effect
Choline magnesium trisalicylate	650	10	Usually no antiplatelet effect; gastritis
Codeine	30–60	0.5–1.0	Weak opioid; dose-limiting nausea/vomiting
Nonsteroidal anti-inflammatory drugs	400	5–10	Gastritis; antiplatelet effect; hepatic or renal dysfunction

function, nor is it associated with gastritis. Unfortunately, it has minimal anti-inflammatory activity.

Choline magnesium salicylate (Trilisate; Purdue Frederick Co., Norwalk, CT) offers some of the anti-inflammatory activity of the salicylates, but appears to be associated with minimal inhibition of platelet function.[12]

Naproxen, ibuprofen, and tolmetin are nonsteroidal anti-inflammatory agents that are approved for use in children. They typically are administered three to four times daily. Unfortunately, they all are associated with gastritis and platelet dysfunction, but may have a role in the child with bony metastasis who has normal platelet counts. Ketorolac,[13] a recently approved nonsteroidal agent, is the only drug in this category that can be administered parenterally, and may have value in the child who is having problems tolerating opioids but is unable to take medication by mouth.

OPIOIDS

These agents are the mainstay of treatment for moderate and severe cancer pain (Table 28–3; see Chapters 6, 8, 9, and 11). They have no ceiling on their analgesic efficacy, and the correct dose is the dose that provides analgesia. The efficacy of some of these drugs may be limited by their side effects. These drugs have varying half-lives, oral–parenteral ratios, and side effect profiles.

Codeine. This agent and its analogues, oxycodone and hydrocodone, are the drugs of choice for pain of moderate intensity. They can be used in conjunction with a peripherally acting agent, and this combination provides more relief than either agent administered alone. A standard dosage of codeine is 0.5 to 1 mg/kg orally every 4 hours. If there is not significant relief from a two- to fourfold increase in dosage, then it is recommended that a more potent opioid be used.[14]

Morphine. Morphine remains the gold standard for management of moderate to severe cancer pain, and the agent against which most other drugs are measured. It may be administered via a number of routes, and is well tolerated and well studied in pediatrics. It can be administered orally, intravenously in a bolus or through continuous infusion, intramuscularly, or subcutaneously. It is the most common agent used in patient-controlled analgesia devices. Controlled-release morphine preparations are now available but have received only limited formal study in children.[15] They may allow a longer interval between administrations, and therefore permit the child sleep without interruption at night.

Hydromorphone. Hydromorphone has simi-

Table 28–3.
Analgesics for Moderate and Severe Pain

Drug	Equianalgesic Parenteral Dose	Equianalgesic Oral Dose (mg)	Suggested Pediatric Doses	
			Bolus	Infusion/Oral
Fentanyl	100 μg	None	1–2 μg/kg IV q1–2h	2–4 μg/kg/hr IV
Hydromorphone	1.5 mg	7.5 mg	0.02 mg/kg IV q3–4h	0.1 mg/kg PO q3–4h
Ketorolac	30 mg	None	1 mg/kg IV; load 0.5 mg/kg q6h	None
Meperidine	75 mg	300 mg	0.8–1.0 mg/kg IV q2–3h; 0.8–1.3 mg/kg SC q3–4h	3–4 mg/kg PO q3–4h
Methadone	10 mg	20 mg	0.1 mg/kg q4h load then q6–12h	0.1 mg/kg PO q4–12h
Morphine Sulfate	10 mg	30–60 mg	0.08–0.1 mg/kg IV q2h	0.03–0.06 mg/kg/h IV; 0.2–0.4 mg/kg PO q4h

Abbreviations: IV = intravenous; PO = by mouth; q...h = every ... hours; SC = subcutaneous

lar pharmacokinetic characteristics to morphine. It may be more palatable in oral elixir form than morphine elixir, which is somewhat bitter.[14]

Methadone. Methadone has a longer half-life and requires less frequent administration. Its oral–parenteral ratio is significantly better than that of morphine. Unfortunately, its prolonged half-life makes titration somewhat more difficult. It is therefore useful in stable pain, and not in the setting of rapidly escalating pain. Treatment requires careful monitoring, and accumulation of this drug has been reported in debilitated patients.[16,17]

Fentanyl. Fentanyl is a rapidly acting synthetic opioid that may have particular value in procedure pain. It also reportedly produces less pruritus than does morphine.[18]

Meperidine. Although meperidine traditionally has been an agent commonly used for pain relief, recent data suggest that normeperidine, a metabolite of meperidine with a long half-life, is associated with seizures and dysphoria.[19] Therefore, meperidine may be use-

ful in certain children with documented morphine allergies for a short period of time, but it should not be used for periods longer than 24 to 48 hours.

Routes

Depending on their characteristics, opioids can be administered via a variety of routes (see Chapter 11). Oral administration certainly is preferable, and methadone, morphine, and hydromorphone all can be administered via an elixir. If oral administration is not possible, than intravenous routes are preferred next. Intravenous boluses of morphine, fentanyl, and methadone all have been studied in children. Continuous intravenous infusion of morphine is appropriate for prolonged and predictable episodes of pain.[20] For children managed at home in whom intravenous access is a problem, continuous subcutaneous morphine seems appropriate.[21] Many children with cancer have surgically placed indwelling catheters that readily allow the administration of continuous infusions of opioids. A variation on intermittent bolus and continuous infusion is the use of patient-controlled analgesia. There is some literature on patient-controlled analgesia in children,[22,23] but an extremely limited literature on its usefulness in children with cancer. Clearly, there are significant developmental reasons why this is a good choice for children, particularly in the terminal phases of illness. It also has been used for treating the pain associated with mucositis.

In addition to these routes, transmucosal fentanyl citrate has been used for procedure pain in children with cancer,[24] and in adults for breakthrough pain.[25] Transdermal fentanyl patches also have been used in disease-related pain in children.[26] Sublingual routes, in particular with buprenorphine, have been explored.[27]

Rectal administration of opioids occasionally is necessary, but is to be avoided because of the possibility of perirectal abscess formation in immunocompromised children. Opioids also can be administered intrathecally, intraventricularly, and epidurally in a select group of children with cancer pain. Finally, intramuscular administration clearly should be discouraged. If at all possible, an alternative, less noxious route should be used.

Side Effects

Opioid side effects in children are similar to those found in adults (see Chapter 12).

Respiratory Depression. For the health care professional, respiratory depression clearly is the most anxiety-producing side effect of the opioids. Children on continuous doses of opioids rarely have respiratory arrests, but they can have respiratory depression manifested by oversedation, decreasing respiratory rate, and oxygen desaturation. If respiratory depression appears mild, then the patient should be stimulated, oxygen offered, and the dose subsequently reduced. Obviously, if respiratory depression is pronounced, careful reversal with naloxone and support of the airway should be provided.

Sedation. Somnolence is another potential side effect associated with these agents. There currently is a limited literature on the use of stimulants to decrease somnolence in adults[28] and in children[29] receiving opioids (see Chapter 10).

Constipation. Constipation is a common side effect that should be treated by prevention. Stimulant laxatives such as senna usually are necessary, and should be prescribed prophylactically.

Pruritus. Pruritus due in part to histamine release is another common side effect associated with opioid administration. Administration of an antihistamine usually is helpful. Occasionally, shifting to an opioid that is associated with less histamine release, such as fentanyl, may be necessary.

Nausea and Vomiting. Nausea and vomiting associated with opioids can be treated by administration of a neuroleptic, typically a phenothiazine. These agents also have the potential for causing respiratory depression and sedation, and therefore children receiving these agents in addition to opioids should be monitored carefully.

ADJUVANT MEDICATIONS

Other pharmacologic agents, although not primarily analgesic, may reduce pain and suffering in the child with cancer.

Tricyclic Antidepressants

The tricyclic antidepressants have been clearly demonstrated to provide pain relief in adults with cancer.[30] These agents appear to enhance nighttime sleep, provide some sedation, and may provide some analgesia on their own. There is no literature on the use of tricyclic antidepressants for children with cancer pain, but anecdotally, they have been used frequently for children, particularly when neuropathic pain is present. Classically, they are used in very small doses. For example, amitryptiline starting at about 0.1 mg/kg (usually around 10 mg) at bedtime is a typical starting dose. The initial dose can be increased gradually until the desired effect is achieved.

Stimulants

Stimulants such as dextroamphetamine and methylphenidate have been used in adults in whom a pain-relieving dose of opioids causes oversedation.[29] The administration of stimulants sometimes can decrease such sedation, and, in fact, often allows for a slight reduction in the dose of opioids.

COGNITIVE/BEHAVIORAL APPROACHES

Psychological techniques (see Chapters 4, 5, and 14) have a large role to play in the pain associated with childhood cancer. These approaches can help the child and family cope with the fear, anxiety, and depression that inevitably accompanies a diagnosis of cancer in a child. In addition, they offer techniques that allow the child directly to reduce disease-related and procedure-related pain.

A general review of these techniques is presented in this section. The applicability of these techniques to specific painful situations will be explored later on in this chapter.

PSYCHOLOGICAL SUPPORT/ EDUCATION

Few problems are as distressing to a family as the diagnosis of cancer in a child. This diagnosis affects not only the child, but the parents, siblings, extended family, and the neighborhood. Relationships suddenly change, and the family often becomes more dependent on the health care system and on family and friends. The unpredictable outcome associated with the cancer, the frequent hospitalizations and toxic treatments that often are necessary, and the financial burdens all enormously strain the coping abilities of any family. Thus, psychological support aimed at providing information and at opening lines of communication is always helpful. It is clear that different families have different styles of coping, but the availability of ongoing psychosocial support to discuss these important issues is essential to enhance coping, which in turn clearly reduces anxiety, depression, and pain.

PARENTAL INVOLVEMENT

Parents have a critical role in helping their children cope with medical illness. Parents should be kept informed of their child's progress and what to expect in terms of symptoms from therapeutic agents. They should have some role in decision-making. Such empowerment decreases their anxiety, which should have a positive impact on their child.

The nature of the parental role in helping children cope with painful procedures is far less clear. Some studies imply that parental presence during a procedure is a detriment to the child and the health care team, whereas other studies indicate parental presence is valuable.[31,32] If one asks the child what helps most during a procedure, however, parental presence is clearly paramount.

Current literature suggests that parents should have a specific role in helping their child cope with a painful procedure. Parents can be taught techniques that they can apply during painful procedures.[33] These techniques allow the parent to have a role in comforting and helping the child during times when he or she ordinarily might feel helpless. This benefits the parent, the child, and the health care team. Kuttner's videotape on the parental use of behavioral techniques is an excellent teaching aide in this regard.[34]

SELF-CONTROL

Many studies have demonstrated that increasing the patients' sense of control over their illness and its therapy has beneficial impact on their experience of the discomfort associated with that illness. Kavanaugh's work on children with burns[35,36] clearly has demonstrated that by increasing the predictability of the child's day, and by increasing his or her control over some of the surroundings, dramatic decreases in pain associated with burn dressing changes can be realized. This principle is one of the cornerstones of patient-controlled analgesia, which allows the patient direct control over his or her therapy (see Chapter 11). Although there is no published literature on the use of patient-controlled analgesia for children with cancer pain, anecdotally, most pediatric pain clinics have experience with the use of this modality for cancer pain in children over age 7 years.

DISTRACTION

By distracting the child away from his or her discomfort, we can often reduce the pain experienced. Distraction is helpful both for disease-related pain and for pain associated with painful procedures. Distraction may be accomplished by having children focus on their breathing, having them become involved in a book, having them blow bubbles, and, in general, drawing their attention away from their discomfort or from an upcoming procedure. A recent study by Manne and colleagues[37] reported the successful use of party blowers to distract children from the pain of intravenous cannulation. Other investigators have used cognitive distraction methods such as video games to alleviate distress from chemotherapy.[38]

VISUAL IMAGERY

Another technique that involves distracting a child away from his or her discomfort is the use of visual imagery. During this task, the child is encouraged to think of a more pleasant scene and recall its details[39] (ie, thinking about a family vacation). The child is asked to recall the sites, smells, and sounds of that vacation. To use this technique effectively, one must know some details of the child's life, which makes parents the ideal individuals to help the child with this technique.

HYPNOSIS/IMAGINARY INVOLVEMENT

This technique is distinguished from visual imagery because the child is involved more actively in a fantasy. The child is asked to focus his or her attention on imaginary activities, such as taking a magic carpet ride. Other variations of this technique involve focused attention and suggestion, such as the use of "pain switches" and "imaginary anesthetic gloves." These techniques are particularly helpful during painful procedures.[40-42]

MODELING

Another technique that has been used for children with cancer who are about to undergo painful procedures is the use of modeling. The child may be shown a film of another child undergoing this procedure, or talk with another child who has undergone a similar procedure. This approach gives the child very direct knowledge of what will happen, thus decreasing some of the anxiety about the limits of pain for a given procedure.

DESENSITIZATION/REHEARSAL

In this technique, the child rehearses what will happen during the procedure. If extremely anxious about a procedure, he or she gradually can be desensitized to what will happen. For example, if the child is fearful of an upcoming needle stick, he or she can be brought to the room where it will take place, can look at the needle, can play with the needle while leaving the cap on, etc. This way, in gradual steps, anxiety gradually can be decreased.

These, then, are some of the behavioral techniques that have been developed for children with cancer. Many are specifically relevant to procedure pain, whereas others can be used during more prolonged, painful periods. Most require minimal training to implement, although some of the hypnotic techniques may require more sophisticated skills that may be obtained from organizations such as The Society for Clinical and Experimental Hypnosis.

ANESTHETIC AND PHYSICAL APPROACHES

Anesthetic techniques have value in providing relief to a small subgroup of children with cancer. For children who have undergone significant cancer surgery, continuous epidural anesthesia may be the most effective way of providing pain relief without undue sedation. The use of cervical epidural anesthesia has been reported as the mainstay of pain relief in a young child with painful bony metastases in the terminal phase of her illness.[43]

In children with localized cancer pain and a limited survival potential, some of the neurodestructive techniques have demonstrated efficacy. Celiac plexus blocks and lumbar sympathetic blocks may offer temporary pain relief for some children. Other anesthetic techniques such as on-demand nitrous oxide and intrathecal morphine have been used to offer relief to children in the terminal phases of their disease.

The use of physical therapy techniques such as splinting and bracing have value for some children with cancer pain. In addition, the use of transcutaneous electrical nerve stimulation may be beneficial in localized pain or for children with phantom limb pain.

MANAGEMENT OF SPECIFIC PAIN PROBLEMS

PAIN ASSOCIATED WITH DIAGNOSTIC AND TREATMENT PROCEDURES

As previously mentioned, the pain associated with diagnostic and treatment procedures in children with cancer is probably the greatest source of distress associated with their disease.[44] These necessary procedures often set

in motion for the child a cycle of fear and dread of the next procedure that often generalizes to the child's caregivers. Despite the well known distress that these procedures cause in children, little has been done in a formalized way to address this problem. We[45] surveyed children's cancer programs around the United States in an attempt to identify how frequently routine premedication was used for bone marrow aspirations, and what types of medications were chosen when it was used. We found, in fact, that routine premedication was used only approximately 30% of the time. When it was used, a variety of different drugs and drug combinations were used. The most commonly used regimen was the DPT (demerol-phenergan-thorazine) cocktail, a 40-year-old concoction that makes limited pharmacologic sense, has a high incidence of reported side effects, and requires an intramuscular injection. Other reported regimens solely used sedative hypnotic agents that provide no analgesia, and are therefore inappropriate choices.

In an attempt to address this lack of uniformity in clinical practice and void in research, the Consensus Conference on the Management of Pain in Childhood Cancer[46] was held, and offered a series of recommendations regarding the conduct of such procedures. Many of these recommendations will be included in the following discussion.

Pain management related to diagnostic and medical procedures in children needs to be individualized based on the age of the child and on the degree of intrusiveness and distress that the given procedure will cause.

General Principles

A number of general principles can be gleaned from the available literature. It is clear that the child and parents should be prepared for the procedure. This preparation should be done in a developmentally appropriate manner so that the child can understand it. Preparation should have both a cognitive component (ie, What will be done?) and a sensory component (ie, How it will feel?). If at all possible, the parents should be involved during the procedure, and given a specific role as coach and comforter of the child. Another general principle that emerged from the Consensus Conference is the suggestion that if multiple procedures are anticipated for a child, the pain of the initial procedures should be addressed in an aggressive manner.[47] If these are painful and intrusive procedures, then pharmacologic intervention should be maximized. This may prevent the cycle of ongoing pain and fear in the child that was described previously.

All medical staff involved in performing procedures on children should have an adequate knowledge of both the behavioral and pharmacologic approaches that are available. They also should have adequate mechanical skills to perform these procedures. Children who will be subjected to multiple procedures should not be part of the learning curve of a house officer. If a physician or student requires training in how to perform a bone marrow aspiration, that training should take place when the child is anesthetized.

These procedures always should take place in a treatment room, and not in the patient's room. The treatment room should be as pleasant and attractive as possible. There should be appropriate monitoring and resuscitative equipment in the procedure room, as well as resuscitative drugs.

Finally, pain assessment should be an ongoing part of the procedure and its aftermath. If the child has done well with one type of intervention, it should be continued. If it has not been adequate, then alternative interventions should be brought into the treatment repertoire.

Nonpainful Procedures Requiring Sedation

For most children, procedures such as computed tomography and magnetic resonance imaging scans can be performed merely by using preparation and behavioral interventions. For young children, however, and older children who may be fearful, pharmacologic interventions may be necessary. Oral chloral hydrate or intravenous pentobarbital are the most appropriate choices for these procedures.

Minor Invasive Procedures

Although a finger stick, heel stick, or intravenous cannulation may not be minor to the child, these procedures clearly are less painful then bone marrow aspirations or other more intrusive procedures. As a general rule, blood drawing and intravenous cannulations all should be done at the same time so the same stick can be used for a variety of purposes, thus avoiding multiple sticks. Local anesthetics should be used if at all possible. A local anesthetic combination, EMLA (eutectic mixture of local anesthetics), will soon be available. This preparation, which is topically applied, provides adequate anesthesia to allow for almost pain-free needle sticks.[40] It should be used if at all possible before blood drawing or venous cannulation. Until this preparation is available, the use of buffered lidocaine, which burns less then lidocaine alone, is advised.

A number of nonpharmacologic strategies clearly are advantageous in helping with these procedures. Distraction, through the use either of bubble blowing, pop-up books, or party blowers, has been shown to be effective. Young infants appear to benefit from nonnutritive sucking and stroking. Older children might benefit from hypnotic strategies. Physical methods, such as ethylene chloride spray, also may be helpful.

Lumbar Punctures

Lumbar punctures are believed, in general, to be more intrusive than blood drawing procedures, but somewhat less painful than bone marrow aspirations. Local anesthetics should be used for lumbar punctures. When it becomes available, EMLA would appear to be quite helpful, and is in use for this purpose in England at this time.[48] Because there is a profound anxiety associated with lumbar punctures in some children, it may be beneficial to use a benzodiazepine in selected children. In addition, conscious sedation with an opioid and a benzodiazepine may be helpful for some children.

Behavioral approaches similar to those previously described may have efficacy for lumbar punctures. These include hypnosis and clusters of behavioral techniques that involve rehearsal, modeling, and a variety of distraction techniques.

Bone Marrow Aspirations

These appear to be among the most intrusive and painful procedures for children with cancer. Zeltzer,[49] in a survey of a group of children with cancer, reported that these procedures averaged 4.5 out of 5 in terms of pain score. Clearly, aggressive pharmacologic intervention, especially during initial procedures, is necessary. General anesthesia using either inhalational agents such as halothane and nitrous oxide, or intravenous agents such as propofol or ketamine, can be considered, depending on the preference of the anesthesiologist. An alternative is the use of conscious sedation combining an opioid and a benzodiazepine. A number of combinations have been developed (flunitrazepam and fentanyl,[50] fentanyl and midazolam,[47] etc.). Use of any of these combinations requires adequate monitoring, presence of an individual skilled at airway management, and availability of resuscitative equipment and drugs. Another alternative that soon may be available is the use of oral transmucosal fentanyl citrate,[51] which provides an alternative way of rapidly administering analgesia in children who do not have intravenous access. Nonpharmacologic approaches similar to those already described are available for use in this population as well.

Postoperative Pain

Even in the child who does not have a formal surgical tumor resection, it is common for surgery to take place around the time of the initial diagnosis of a malignancy. Most children with malignancies that require chemotherapy will have some type of indwelling venous access placed. This procedure and its attendant anesthesia should be taken advantage of by the cancer treatment team. This is an excellent opportunity to complete any diagnostic testing (ie, lumbar puncture for a new leukemic) or repeat tissue sampling (ie, repeat bone marrow aspiration for additional testing) without subjecting the child to pain from these procedures.

Traditional surgical postoperative pain encountered after deep tissue biopsy or resection of a mass should be managed aggressively and creatively in children with cancer. These children should be afforded all of the skills of the anesthetist, and regional analgesia should be part of the preoperative planning. As with other procedure-related pains, postoperative pain is treated on a continuum depending on the degree of tissue damage associated with a particular surgery. In general, children with abdominal or thoracic surgery require opioid analgesics for the first few days after surgery. These should be administered via a non-noxious route. Medication should be offered in a preventative manner (around the clock, by constant infusion, or by patient-controlled analgesia) rather than on an as-needed basis, and the goal should be to prevent the pain rather than to treat it once it occurs.

A number of routes are available, but for young children the continuous infusion of morphine has been well studied, and offers many advantages.[52,53] For children over 6 or 7 years, patient-controlled analgesia, if available, offers an attractive alternative.[22]

A number of anesthetic approaches can help with the management of postoperative pain. Intraoperatively, epidural opioids and/or local anesthetic and local anesthetic infiltrated into the wound or applied via a peripheral nerve block clearly have been demonstrated to be efficacious. Children who receive such intraoperative opioids require close monitoring in the early postoperative period. In addition, continuous epidural administration of local anesthetics and/or opioids is available, but requires sophisticated monitoring, and a team of experts who are familiar with the use of these drugs and their potential side effects to provide ongoing supervision.[54]

Like adults, children undergoing amputation can be expected to experience some phantom limb pain. Although complaints are not uncommon in the first few months after surgery, the long-term prognosis for this type of pain is excellent in children. Most amputation-related pain in children is related to direct trauma to the stump. The pain can become dysesthetic if postoperative neuromas occur. There is some literature in adults to suggest that the administration of epidural opioids 24 to 48 hours before the amputation significantly diminishes the incidence of postoperative phantom limb pain.[55] As yet, this work has not been reproduced in children.

DISEASE-RELATED PAIN

An overall approach to the treatment of disease-related pain can be found in Figure 28–1, which emerged from the Consensus Conference on the Management of Pain in Childhood Cancer. A number of basic principles for the treatment of disease related pain require further emphasis.

Anticancer therapy, in and of itself, often provides significant pain relief (see Chapters 15 and 16). Radiation or chemotherapy, which shrinks the tumor mass, can have a very direct and immediate impact on the pain associated with the child's cancer.

The use of the analgesic ladder,[11] as defined by the World Health Organization Cancer Unit, offers a general framework for how to approach these problems. It is critical, however, to remember that the appropriate dose is the one that works. Analgesic dosing should be escalated rapidly to provide relief as quickly as possible for the child. Many would suggest that it is perhaps advantageous to rapidly gain control of the pain, even at the risk of causing somnolence initially, and then to back off, rather than to titrate analgesics slowly, leaving the child to suffer for a longer period of time and perhaps lose confidence. The approach to any given child, however, should be tailored to the specific needs of that child and family.

Many families continue to have persistent concerns about addiction. These should be put to rest in the strongest possible terms. Some families may feel that they would prefer to hold morphine in reserve in case it is necessary in the terminal phases of the illness. The child and family should be informed that this philosophy is incorrect, and that there is no need for the child to suffer unnecessarily.

Tolerance usually is not a significant issue when using opioids in children with cancer, once an effective dose is established. Rapid escalation of pain usually represents progressive disease, not tolerance. Once escalating doses are required, an investigation for spread of disease should be undertaken.

Heiligenstein[56] has reported that some mental health symptoms in children with cancer, such as depression, sometimes represent undertreated pain. Therefore, ongoing pain assessment is a critical dimension in children with cancer, even when the disease-related pain appears to be stable.

A final consideration in the discussion of disease-related pain involves the importance of neuropathic pain. Neuropathic pain may result from nerve injury secondary to direct tumor invasion of neural tissue. Neuropathic pain classically is described as sharp and burning. Occasionally, a pattern of sympathetically maintained pain may emerge. Tricyclic antidepressants appear to be the treatment of choice for these problems.[57–59] Anesthetic approaches involving neural blockade may be of diagnostic and therapeutic benefit in selected cases.

TREATMENT-RELATED PAIN

Pain associated with treatment of cancer is a significant contributor to the discomfort the child experiences.

Mucositis

One of the most common treatment-related pains is mucositis, which occurs typically in patients who are pancytopenic, but also may stem from the direct effect of certain anticancer agents, such as methotrexate. Mucositis often initially is managed best with locally act-

Assess the patient. Consider:
1. Character of the pain, mechanism of the pain
2. Directly remediable causes (fractures, abscesses, etc)
3. Context:
   Course of the disease
   Anxiety and depression
   Family milieu

→

Treat remediable conditions
(eg, fractures, abscesses, etc)
Apply tumor therapy
(chemotherapy, radiotherapy, steroids)

Initiate nonpharmacologic modalities as indicated
1. Cognitive-behavioral measures: Relaxation, guided imagery, hypnosis, activities therapy, reassurance, art or music therapy, distraction
2. Where indicated by initial assessment, individual or family counseling, psychologic or psychiatric consultation as needed
3. Physical measured: transcutaneous electrical nerve stimulation, heat, cold, massage

Analgesic Management (Analgesic Ladder)
1. Mild pain
   a. Acetaminophen
   b. If not contraindicated, may use choline-magnesium salicylate or nonsteroidal anti-inflammatory agents
   c. If oral route is not accessible, may use reduced doses of "strong opioids," listed under "severe pain," by parenteral routes.
   d. Assess adequacy of pain relief. If adequate, continue; of inadequate, progress to "moderate pain" recommendations.
   e. Treat side effects of associated symptoms. ————
2. Moderate pain
   a. Continue nonopioid medications as per "mild pain."
   b. Begin codeine 0.5–1 mg/kg orally every 4 hours.
   c. If oral route is not accessible, may use reduced doses of "strong opioids," listed under "severe pain" recommendations.
   d. Assess adequacy of pain relief. If adequate, continue; if inadequate, progress to "severe pain," by parenteral routes.
   e. Treat side effects or associated symptoms. ————
3. Severe pain
   a. Continue nonopioid medications as per "mild pain" if tolerated and noncontraindicated
   b. Begin a strong opioid agonist; eg, morphine or methadone.
      Use oral route, if feasible
      Use parenteral route (intravenous, subcutaneous), if necessary.
   c. Assess adequacy of pain relief. If adequate, continue; if inadequate, increase dosing as limited by side effects, and consider addition of adjunctive medications. ————
   d. In the vast majority of cases, titration of opioids and use of adjunctive medications will produce adequate analgesia and acceptable side effects. If analgesia cannot be produced without unacceptable side effects, consider anesthetic or neurosurgical approaches.

Side Effect Management, Symptom Management, and Use of Adjunctive Medications
1. Nausea and vomiting
   Phenothiazines, butyrophenones, steroids
2. Constipation
   Cathartics, stool softeners
3. Pruritus
   Antihistamines
4. Sleep disturbance
   Increased opioid doses
   Tricyclics (low dose)
5. Somnolence
   Reduced opioid doses
   Stimulants
6. Neuropathic character to the pain
   Tricyclics (low to moderate dose)
   Anticonvulsants
7. Somatic signs of depression
   Tricyclics (antidepressant doses, with psychiatric consultation)
8. Urinary retention
   Encouragement, physical maneuvers, intermittent or short-term bladder catheterization, cholinergics
9. Respiratory depression (mild)
   Stimulation, encouragement, careful observation, reduced opioid doses
10. Respiratory depression (severe)
    Ventilatory support until opioid effects subside,
    Stop opioid administration,
    Intensive care observation
    Avoid naloxone whenever possible
    If naloxone is needed and time permits, titrate tiny doses,
    When opioid is restarted, use reduced opioid doses.

Figure 28–1. Algorithm for management of pediatric cancer pain. Reprinted with permission from Berde C, Ablin A, Glazer J et al: Report of the Subcommittee on Disease-Related Pain in Childhood Cancer. Pediatrics 1990;86:818.

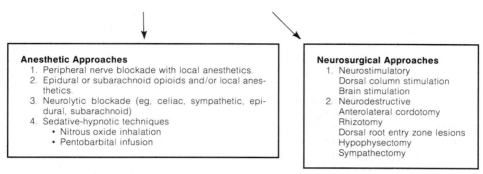

Anesthetic Approaches
1. Peripheral nerve blockade with local anesthetics.
2. Epidural or subarachnoid opioids and/or local anesthetics.
3. Neurolytic blockade (eg, celiac, sympathetic, epidural, subarachnoid)
4. Sedative-hypnotic techniques
   - Nitrous oxide inhalation
   - Pentobarbital infusion

Neurosurgical Approaches
1. Neurostimulatory
   Dorsal column stimulation
   Brain stimulation
2. Neurodestructive
   Anterolateral cordotomy
   Rhizotomy
   Dorsal root entry zone lesions
   Hypophysectomy
   Sympathectomy

Figure 28–1.   (Continued)

ing analgesic and anti-infective preparations. Several widely used oral preparations are indicated in Table 28–4.[60] If local control is insufficient and the patient still is able to swallow, oral systemic analgesics are appropriate. Although the nonsteroidal anti-inflammatory drugs offer excellent anti-inflammatory potential in these lesions, the antiplatelet effects usually prohibit their use in these patients. This is particularly true since mucositis is seen most commonly in the pancytopenic, postchemotherapy patient. Therefore, if oral acetaminophen (preferably alcohol-free to avoid irritation) is not adequate, stronger oral opi-

oids are indicated. If the patient is unable to swallow, then parenterally administered opioids may be necessary. Hill and colleagues[61] have reported on the success of patient-controlled analgesia in adults with mucositis.

Peripheral Neuropathy/Plexopathy

Vincristine or the other related vinca alkaloids almost invariably induce a diffuse, symmetric polyneuropathy.[5] Children typically will develop gnawing jaw pain that goes on to include dysesthesias in the hands and feet. Occasionally, cranial nerves can become in-

Table 28–4.
Topical Oral Anesthetics

Agent	Composition	Comments
Viscous lidocaine	2% lidocaine	Swish and spit; lidocaine can be swallowed by young children
Dyclonine hydrochloride	0.5% dyclonine	Topical anesthetic; possibly more suitable for young children
Antacids	Various	Soothing, coating
Peridex*	0.12% chlorhexidine	Microbicidal; may stain teeth
"Magic Mouthwash"	1 part viscous lidocaine 1 part diphenhydramine elixir 2 parts antacid (Maalox†) 2 parts water ± flavor	Swish and spit; coating and pleasant-tasting; caution in young children

* Proctor and Gamble, Cincinnati, OH
† Rorer Consumer Pharmaceuticals, Fort Washington, PA

volved, although such involvement usually is painless. The peripherally acting analgesics, as well as the opioids, often have only limited effect on this pain. The tricyclic antidepressants may prove useful; however, the periods of intense vinca treatment are often completed by the time these drugs become effective. More commonly, if the neuropathy results in unacceptable pain, the antineoplastic doses are adjusted downward in an attempt to avoid pain.

Herpes zoster infection and its associated postherpetic neuralgia can occur in children who are immunocompromised from therapy. It can initially present with localized severe pain that precedes the typical cutaneous lesions. Aggressive analgesic therapy, including the potent opioids, should be offered to these children until the acute infection is controlled. However, pain may be treated best by initiating antiviral therapy. Acyclovir has been shown not only to prevent dissemination and shorten the time of the rash, but also to reduce the pain of the infection.[62] Tricyclic antidepressants, and, if necessary, local neural blockade also may be of benefit.[63]

Irradiation of various tumors often may include neurologic structures such as the brachial or lumbosacral plexus. This can lead to local fibrosis and nerve entrapment syndromes. Systemic tricyclic antidepressants or local therapy may prove helpful. Transcutaneous electrical nerve stimulation or regional anesthesia may be required as well. When the spinal cord is included in the radiation field, postradiation myelopathy can develop. These pain syndromes can be localized or may include more distal dysesthetic complaints. They can be transient and self-limiting, or can develop into a progressive syndrome that may even result in complete transverse myelopathy. Treatment usually involves the use of the neuroleptic drugs.

SUMMARY

The management of pain is a vital aspect of the comprehensive care of a child with cancer. For parents, the notion of cancer is inextricably linked with the notion of pain and suffering, and it is therefore vital that pain assessment and management be integrated into cancer treatment.

A few key aspects of cancer pain treatment in children are essential. Assessment for pain should be a routine part of the medical care. The pain associated with diagnostic procedures should be managed aggressively. Poor management of this aspect of the child's care sets in motion a cycle of fear and dread that often generalizes to the child's caregivers. Behavioral approaches are vital, and should be taught early on after diagnosis and used throughout the child's illness. Pharmacologic approaches can be simple and geared to the traditional World Health Organization ladder. As much as possible, medication should be administered via non-noxious routes and in a scheduled manner. Parents have a vital role to play as advocates for their child, and should be involved as much as possible in the child's treatment. Available technology allows us to eliminate the overwhelming majority of pain associated with cancer in childhood. To ignore this important issue is to violate the fundamental right of the child to appropriate and humane medical care.

REFERENCES

1. Miser AW, Dothage JA, Wesley RA et al: The prevalence of pain in a pediatric and young adult cancer population. Pain 1987;29:73.
2. McGrath PJ, Hsu E, Cappelli M et al: Pain from pediatric cancer: A survey of an outpatient oncology clinic. Journal of Psychosocial Oncology 1990;8:109.
3. Miser AW, Miser JS: The treatment of cancer pain in children. Pediatr Clin North Am 1989;36:979.
4. Schechter NL: Pain in children with cancer. In Foley KM, Bonica JJ, Ventafridda V (eds): Advances in Pain Research and Therapy, vol 16, p 57. New York, Raven Press, 1990.
5. Allen JC: The effects of cancer therapy on the nervous system. J Pediatr 1978;93:903.
6. Weiss HD, Walker MD, Wiernik PH: Neurotoxicity of commonly used antineoplastic agents. N Engl J Med 1974;37:127.
7. Phillips T, Fu K: Quantification of combined radiation therapy and chemotherapy effects on critical normal tissues. Cancer 1976;37:1186.
8. McGrath PA: Pain in Children. New York, Guilford Press, 1990.

9. Cornaglia C, Massimo L, Haupt R et al: Incidence of pain in children with neoplastic disease. Pain 1984;2 (Suppl):S28.

10. Mohide EA, Royle JA, Montemuro M et al: Assessing the quality of cancer pain management. Journal of Palliative Care 1988;4:9.

11. World Health Organization: Cancer Pain Relief. Geneva, WHO, 1986.

12. Cronin C, Edmiston K, Griffin T: Hematologic safety of choline magnesium trisalicylate: A non-opioid analgesic. Journal of Pain and Symptom Management 1991;6:158.

13. Maunuksela EL, Olkkola KT, Kokki H: Pharmacokinetics of intravenous ketorolac and its efficacy in relieving postoperative pain in children. Journal of Pain and Symptom Management 1991;6:142.

14. Berde C, Ablin A, Glazer J et al: Report of the Subcommittee on Disease-Related Pain in Childhood Cancer. Pediatrics 1990;86:818.

15. Atchison N, Syzfelbein SK, Osgood PF et al: MS-Contin: Time released pain relief for burn patients. Journal of Pain and Symptom Management 1991; 6:156.

16. Payne R, Max M, Sunshine A et al: Principles of Analgesic Use in the Treatment of Acute Pain and Chronic Cancer Pain. Skokie, IL, American Pain Society, 1989.

17. Miser AW, Miser JS: The use of oral methadone to control severe pain in children and young adults with malignancy. Clinical Journal of Pain 1986;1:243.

18. Shannon M, Berde C: Pharmacologic management of pain in children and adolescents. Pediatr Clin North Am 1989;36:855.

19. Kaiko RF, Foley KM, Grabinsky P et al: Central nervous system excitatory effects of meperidine in cancer patients. Ann Neurol 1983;13:180.

20. Miser AW, Miser JS, Clark BS: Continuous intravenous infusion of morphine sulfate for control of severe pain in children with terminal malignancy. J Pediatr 1980;96:930.

21. Miser AW, Davis DM, Hughes CS et al: Continuous subcutaneous infusion of morphine in children with cancer. Am J Dis Child 1983;137:383.

22. Berde CB, Lehn BM, Yee JD et al: Patient-controlled analgesia in children and adolescents: A randomized prospective comparison with intramuscular morphine. J Pediatr 1991;118:460.

23. Schechter NL, Berrien FB, Katz SM: The use of patient controlled analgesia in patients with sickle cell disease: A preliminary report. Journal of Pain and Symptom Management 1988;3:109.

24. Schechter NL, Weisman SJ, Rosenblum M et al: Sedation for painful procedures in children with cancer using the fentanyl lollipop: A preliminary report. In Tyler DC, Krane EJ (eds): Advances in Pain Research and Therapy, vol 15, p 209. New York, Raven Press, 1990.

25. Ashburn MA, Olson L, Fine P et al: Oral transmucosal fentanyl citrate for the treatment of breakthrough cancer pain. Anesthesiology 1989;71:615.

26. Miser AW, Narang PK, Dothage JA et al: Transdermal fentanyl for pain control in patients with cancer. Pain 1989;37:15.

27. Massimo L, Haupt R, Zamorani ME: Control of pain with sublingual buprenorphine in children with cancer. European Paediatric Haematology and Oncology 1985;2:224.

28. Forrest W, Brown B, Brown C et al: Dextroamphetamine with morphine for treatment of postoperative pain. N Engl J Med 1977;296:712.

29. Yee JD, Berde CB: Methylphenidate or dextroamphetamine as adjuvants in opioid analgesia. Journal of Pain and Symptom Management 1991;6:162.

30. Walsh TD: Adjuvant analgesic therapy in cancer pain. In Foley KM, Bonica JJ, Ventafridda V (eds): Advances in Pain Research and Therapy, vol 16, p 155. New York, Raven Press, 1990.

31. Shaw E, Routh D: Effect of mother presence on children's reaction to aversive procedures. J Pediatr Psychol 1982;7:33.

32. Bauchner H, Waring C, Vinca R: Parental presence during proceduring in an emergency room: Results from 50 observations. Pediatrics 1991;87:544.

33. Kuttner L: Psychological treatment of distress, pain, and anxiety for young children with cancer. J Dev Behav Pediatr 1988;9:374.

34. Kuttner L: "No tears, no fears.' Canadian Cancer Society, 1987.

35. Kavanagh C: Psychological intervention with the severely burned child: Report of an experimental comparison of two approaches and their effects on psychological sequelae. J Am Acad Child Psychiatry 1983;22:145.

36. Kavanagh C, Lasoff E, Eide E et al: Learned helplessness and the pediatric burn patient. Journal of Pain and Symptom Management 1991;6:177.

37. Manne SL, Redd WH, Jacobsen PB et al: Behavioral intervention to reduce child and parent distress during venipuncture. J Consult Clin Psychol 1990;58:565.

38. Kolko DJ, Rickard-Figueroa JL: Effects of video games on the adverse corollaries of chemotherapy in pediatric oncology patients: A single case analysis. J Consult Clin Psychol 1985;53:223.

39. McCaffery M: Nursing Management of the Patient With Pain. Philadelphia, JB Lippincott, 1979.

40. Olness K: Hypnotherapy: A cyberphysiologic strategy in pain management. Pediatr Clin North Am 1989;36:873.

41. Zeltzer LK, Kellerman J, Ellenberg L et al: Hypnosis for reduction of vomiting associated with chemother-

apy and disease in adolescents with cancer. J Adolesc Health Care 1983;4:77.

42. Zeltzer LK, LeBaron S: The hypnotic treatment of children in pain. In Routh D, Wolraich M (eds): Advances in Developmental and Behavioral Pediatrics, vol 7, p 197. Greenwich, CT, JAI Press, 1986.

43. Scholtes JL, Veyckemans F, Ninane J: Cervical epidural analgesia for a cancer child at home. Journal of Pain and Symptom Management 1991;6:155.

44. Jay SM, Elliot C, Katz E: Cognitive, behavioral, and pharmacologic intervention for children's distress during painful medical procedures. J Consult Clin Psychol 1987;55:860.

45. Bernstein B, Schechter NL, Hickman T et al: Premedication for painful procedures in children: A national survey. Journal of Pain and Symptom Management 1991;6:190.

46. Schechter NL, Altman A, Weisman SJ: Report of the Consensus Conference on the Management of Pain in Childhood Cancer. Pediatrics 1990;85:813.

47. Zeltzer LK, Altman A, Cohen D et al: Report of the subcommittee on the management of pain associated with procedures in children with cancer. Pediatrics 1990;86:826.

48. Kapelushnik J, Koren G, Sohl H: Evaluating the efficacy of EMLA in alleviating pain associated with lumbar puncture. Pain 1990;42:31.

49. Zeltzer L, Lebaron S: Hypnosis and non-hypnotic techniques for reduction of pain and anxiety during painful procedures in children and adolescents with cancer. J Pediatr 1982;101:1032.

50. Maunuksela EL, Rajantie J, Siimes MA: Flunitrazepam-fentanyl induced sedation and analgesia for bone marrow aspiration and needle biopsy in children. Acta Anaesthesiol Scand 1986;30:409.

51. Schechter NL, Weisman SJ, Rosenblum M: Oral transmucosal fentanyl citrate for pediatric procedures: A randomized clinical trial. Journal of Pain and Symptom Management 1991;6:178.

52. Hendrickson M, Myre L, Johnson DG: Postoperative analgesia in children: A prospective study of intermittent intramuscular injection versus continuous intravenous infusion of morphine. J Pediatr Surg 1990; 25:185.

53. Bray RJ: Postoperative analgesia provided by morphine infusions in children. Anaesthesia 1983;38: 1075.

54. Sethna N, Strafford M, Berde CB: Experience with 852 epidural infusions in a children's hospital. Journal of Pain and Symptom Management 1991;6:164.

55. Bach S, Nirebg MF, Tjellden NU: Phantom limb pain in amputees during the first 12 months following limb amputation after preoperative lumbar epidural. Pain 1988;33:297.

56. Heiligenstein E, Jacobson PB: Differentiating depression in medically ill children and adolescents. J Am Acad Child Adolesc Psychiatry 1988;27:716.

57. Foley KM: The treatment of cancer pain. N Engl J Med 1985;313:84.

58. Watson CP, Evans RJ, Merskey H et al: Amitriptyline versus placebo in postherpetic neuralgia. Neurology 1982;32:671.

59. Spiegel K, Kalb R, Pasternak GB: Analgesic activity of tricyclic antidepressants. Ann Neurol 1981;54:451.

60. Ferretti GA, Ash RC, Brown AT et al: Chlorhexidine for prophylaxis against oral infections and associated complications in patients receiving bone marrow transplants. J Am Dent Assoc 1987;114:461.

61. Hill HF, Mackie AM, Coda BA: Patient-controlled analgesic administration. Cancer 1991;67:873.

62. Shepp DH, Dandliker PS, Myers JD: Treatment of varicella zoster virus infection in severely immunocompromised patients: A randomized comparison of acyclovir and vidarabine. N Engl J Med 1986;314: 208.

63. Watson CPN: Therapeutic window for amitriptyline. Can Med Assoc J 1984;130:105.

Chapter *29*

Oncologic Emergencies

Julia Ladd Smith

INTRODUCTION

Fortunately, oncologic emergencies are relatively uncommon occurrences. Recognition of the early signs, as well as maintaining a familiarity with the risk factors that characterize this relatively small group of disorders, are, however, important in order to reduce morbidity and mortality in cancer patients. This is particularly true for health care providers whose major activity is symptom control, since, in their early stages, many oncologic emergencies may mimic the signs and symptoms of slowly progressive neoplastic disease.

Some emergency situations, such as cardiac tamponade, spinal cord compression, and hypercalcemia characteristically are related to tumor growth and invasion. In contrast, the hematologic emergencies, such as neutropenic fever, thrombocytopenia, and tumor cell lysis syndrome, tend to be induced by cancer treatment. Some of the situations described in this chapter, such as pleural effusion, bowel obstruction, and ureteral obstruction, by no means are unique to the cancer population, but are encountered with sufficient frequency in cancer patients to warrant specific comments.

CARDIAC TAMPONADE

Cardiac tamponade occurs when fluid accumulates in the pericardial space and restricts the normal filling of the heart's chambers. Pericardial metastases may result in pericardial effusion as a result of increased fluid production and/or decreased fluid resorption. Whereas large volumes of fluid, even up to 1 liter, can be accommodated when sequestration is a gradual consequence of chronic disease, the rapid accumulation of even a few hundred milliliters of fluid results in mechanical dysfunction of the heart and acute symptomatology.[1] Symptomatic pericardial effusion may mimic pulmonary disease, pleural effusion, congestive heart failure, or progressive systemic cancer. It is important to distinguish among these entities, as their subsequent treatment and potential outcomes differ.

The most common cancers associated with cardiac tamponade are lung (36%), breast (22%), lymphoma, leukemia, and melanoma.[2] Primary tumors of the pericardium, such as mesothelioma, are quite rare.[3] In addition, more indolent tamponade may develop even years after mediastinal radiation due to radiation pericarditis with fibrosis and/or effusion, particularly after radiation doses in excess of 4,000 rad.[4] Nonmalignant effusions also can develop in cancer patients from a variety of causes, including infection, uremia, trauma, rheumatic disease, and postsurgical syndromes.

DIAGNOSIS

The signs and symptoms of tamponade are primarily those of acute right-sided heart failure, and are related directly to the hemodynamic changes that result from reduced filling volumes: cardiac output decreases and retrograde pressure in the venous system increases. Characteristic complaints are of shortness of breath, exercise intolerance, diaphoresis, and chest pain, often accompanied by a vague sense of apprehension. Classic physical signs include the presence of tachycardia, jugular venous distention, which may increase with inspiration (Kussmaul's sign), hepatic engorgement, distant heart sounds, and pulsus paradoxus. The latter is confirmed by observations of reductions in systolic blood pressure of greater than 10 mm Hg during inspiration. When extreme, pulsus paradoxus can be detected by attenuation or elimination of a palpable radial pulse on deep inspiration. Systemic hypotension and peripheral edema may be present. Electrocardiographic changes include tachycardia, reduced voltage, and electrical alternans, an abnormality characterized by an alternating amplitude of the QRS

complex (Fig. 29–1). Electrocardiographic evidence of coexisting myocardial ischemia and paroxysmal atrial fibrillation or flutter may be present as well. Chest radiographic findings usually demonstrate an enlarged cardiac silhouette.

Ultrasonography is the preferred means for diagnosing pericardial effusion, because it is both highly accurate and noninvasive. Using two-dimensional echocardiography, both the presence of pathologic accumulations of pericardial fluid and alterations in chamber filling can be identified. When findings are equivocal, the diagnosis can be confirmed with right-heart catheterization, which demonstrates a tendency toward equalization of the right atrial and ventricular diastolic pressures, and of the pulmonary wedge and arterial diastolic pressure.[5] Pericardiocentesis, when indicated (see below), is both therapeutic and further aids in confirming a diagnosis.

TREATMENT

Urgent pericardiocentesis may be life-sustaining, as the removal of even 50 ml of fluid characteristically improves cardiac output and usually results in dramatic, if transient, symptomatic relief. Aspirated fluid is sent for cytologic examination and yields a specific diagnosis in about 75% of cases.[2]

Definitive treatment depends on the underlying tumor type. Untreated patients with highly chemosensitive tumors (eg, lymphoma, small-cell lung cancer) may benefit from chemotherapy; radiotherapy can be instituted for patients with radiosensitive disease, such as recurrences of small-cell lung cancer or breast cancer. As a rule, however, surgery or instillation of a sclerosing agent is indicated to mechanically prevent recurrent cardiovascular compromise. Surgical treatment consists of either subxyphoid pericardotomy, which requires only a small incision and generally can be performed under local anesthesia, or, by means of a more extensive thoracic incision, creation of a pleuropericardial window to allow drainage into the larger pleural space.[2] An alternative, increasingly

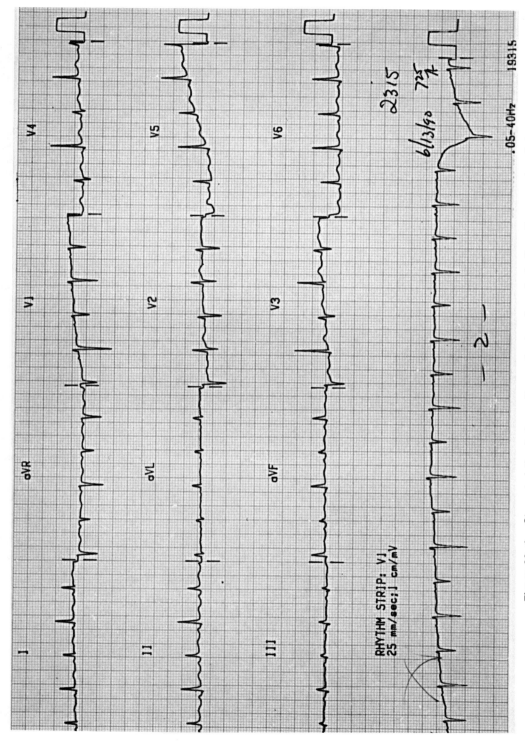

Figure 29–1. Characteristic electrocardiogram tracing of a patient with malignant pericardial tamponade.

well accepted form of management is sclerotherapy, which involves placement of the tip of a flexible catheter within the pericardial space. Pericardial fluid is drained, and tetracycline subsequently is instilled to cause scarring of the pericardial sac and obliteration of the space.[6] Effusions recur in up to 20% of patients after surgery.[5] Pericardiectomy, a major surgical procedure that sometimes requires cardiopulmonary bypass, may be required when symptomatic pericardial compromise is caused by radiation fibrosis.[7]

PROGNOSIS

The prognosis of the patient with malignant pericardial effusion and tamponade depends on the nature of the underlying malignancy, the timing of the diagnosis and prompt intervention, and ultimately on the ability to offer effective antineoplastic treatment. Thus, if effusion or tamponade is the first clinical manifestation of a highly treatment-responsive tumor such as lymphoma or breast cancer, after treatment the patient may do well for months or years. If the patient has received extensive prior treatment and the effusion is part of a pattern of disease recurrence or progression, then life expectancy is likely to be short, and depends on other systemic factors.

HYPERCALCEMIA

Hypercalcemia, when severe, is a metabolic emergency associated with direct central nervous system and cardiac effects that can lead to coma and death, and indirect effects on organs such as the kidney and bowel. The onset of symptoms is often insidious, and as a result may be mistaken for that of diabetes mellitus, hepatic metastases, opioid-induced constipation, or central nervous system invasion.

DIAGNOSIS

Hypercalcemia should be particularly suspected in symptomatic patients with osseous metastases or tumors that characteristically elaborate parathormone-like substances. Lung cancer meets both these criteria, and is the most common cause of hypercalcemia. Breast cancer is the next most common cause of hypercalcemia. Other patients at increased risk for its development include those with multiple myeloma, hypernephroma, and, to a lesser extent, lymphoma and tumors of the prostate, thyroid, ovary, colon, head, and neck. Immobilization and bed rest result in increased resorption of bony calcium, and further predispose to elevations in serum calcium.

Generally, hypercalcemia is an underdiagnosed disorder, particularly when symptoms are mild or only moderately severe. The onset of symptoms is often insidious, and as a result may be mistakenly attributed to other systemic abnormalities. Patients with advanced cancer who are not involved in active antitumor therapy are probably at greatest risk for a missed diagnosis because of a tendency for reduced exposure to routine laboratory testing.

Symptomatic hypercalcemia may be present at the time of the initial diagnosis of malignancy, or may complicate progressive disease. A myriad of often vague symptoms can occur. Polyuria and polydipsia are common, and may be confused with symptoms of diabetes mellitus. Calcium is one of the major cations involved in the activation of muscle and electrical conduction, and in hypercalcemia muscle and nerve activity are dampened. Skeletal and smooth muscle tone both are reduced, causing weakness, hyporeflexia, constipation, nausea, and anorexia. These symptoms may be mistaken for opioid-induced side effects in patients being treated for pain, or may be regarded as nonspecific signs of advancing disease. As serum calcium increases, progressive lethargy, confusion, and eventually coma and death result. Hypercalcemia should be suspected when evaluating any confused or comatose cancer patient. Finally, altered electrical conduction predisposes to the development of cardiac arrhythmias. Characteristic alterations in cardiac conduction include prolongation of the P-R interval, widening of the QRS complex, and shortening of the Q-T interval. Hypercalcemia potentiates the effects of digoxin, and may result in toxicity in the presence of therapeutic digoxin levels.

When hypercalcemia is suspected, the diagnosis should be confirmed or excluded by assessing a serum calcium level. Simultaneously, serum levels of other electrolytes, blood urea nitrogen, and creatinine should be obtained to evaluate fluid and electrolyte status and the presence of renal abnormalities before initiating therapy. Calcium is a largely protein-bound ion, so reductions in circulating albumin may result in symptoms at lower levels of measured calcium then ordinarily would be expected. Since a high incidence of hypoalbuminemia occurs in cancer patients secondary to nutritional deficiencies and hepatic disease, measurement of serum albumin should be considered as part of the assessment of the patient with suspected hypercalcemia. Normal levels of serum calcium range between 9.5–10.5 mg/dl. Elevations to levels of up to 12 mg/dl are often well tolerated, but calcium levels of 14 mg/dl produce symptoms in most patients.

TREATMENT

Hypercalcemia that is severe (>13 mg/dl) or markedly symptomatic requires urgent treatment. The management of hypercalcemia involves two major steps: hydration and pharmacologic intervention. The therapeutic mainstay is intravascular volume expansion. Hypercalcemic patients are dehydrated; intravenous fluid administration reduces serum calcium by a dilutional effect. Normal saline is administered preferentially, because sodium inhibits renal reabsorption of calcium.

Fluid therapy must be individualized to tolerance, but often volumes of 250 ml/hour are administered. Once normovolemia or moderate hypervolemia have been established, furosemide should be administered intravenously every 6–8 hours to reduce the risks of overhydration and further to enhance calciuria. Patients should be observed for clinical signs of congestive heart failure, and con-

sideration should be given to monitoring of cardiac filling pressures in patients with underlying cardiac disease.[8] Serial measurements of urinary output and serum electrolytes should be carried out. Potassium replacement may become necessary as forced diuresis continues. Dialysis occasionally is required if renal dysfunction prevents the establishment of adequate diuresis.

If, after 24 hours of treatment, the serum calcium level has fallen only slowly or not at all, a decision about further management needs to be made. If the underlying malignancy is responsive to chemotherapy, specific antineoplastic therapy should be considered, especially when a rapid response can be expected, as in the case of multiple myeloma. Calcium levels begin to normalize as the tumor responds to the chemotherapy. In situations where a less dramatic response is anticipated, treatment with other agents is considered, such as prednisone, phosphates, plicamycin (formerly called mithramycin), calcitonin, and diphosphonates (see below).

The selection of drug therapy for hypercalcemia that has not responded to conservative treatment is complex, and is based on multiple factors, including the nature of other planned treatment, ease of administration, safety, and cost (Table 29–1). Glucocorticoids (40–100 mg prednisone/day) act to lower serum calcium by multiple mechanisms. Their hypocalcemic effect takes several days to develop, and whereas efficacy is good for patients with hematologic malignancies (including multiple myeloma) and breast cancer, effectiveness is unpredictable for other solid tumors.[9]

For years, plicamycin, a cytotoxic antibiotic, was the only potent parenteral anticalcemic agent available. Plicamycin is a tissue irritant, and careful intravenous administration is required to avoid extravasation injuries. Its most common side effect is gastrointestinal upset, but of greater concern is the potential for myelosuppression (particularly thrombocytopenia), hepatic injury (with the potential for coagulation abnormalities), and renal toxicity. Dosage should be reduced in the presence of elevated levels of serum creatinine. The onset of effect usually occurs within

Table 29–1.
Treatment of Hypercalcemia

Drug	Route	Dose	Onset	Duration	Side Effects
Saline and lasix	IV	150 cc/hr 20–40 mg q 8h	12–24h	While in use	K^+, Mg^{2+} deficits, volume shifts
Plicamycin (Mithramycin)	IV	25 μg/kg	24–48h	96h–1 wk	Thrombocytopenia, clotting abnormalities, hepatocellular damage, nephrotoxicity
Calcitonin	IM	4–8 units q 6–12h	2–3h	4–5 days	Development of refractoriness
Phosphates	PO	Titrate to mild diarrhea	24h	While in use	Diarrhea
Glucocorticoids	PO	40–100 mg prednisone	48–96h	While in use	Usual steroid effects
Biphosphonates (Etidronate)	IV	7.5 mg/kg/d over 2 hrs × 3 days	24–48h	Up to 10 days	Cannot be given if creatinine $\geq$2.5, metallic taste
Pamidronate Dialysis	IV	60 or 90 mg/24h	24h	7–14 days	Fever, local skin reaction
Gallium nitrate	IV	200 mg/m²/d continuous infusion		11 days	Nephrotoxicity

24 to 48 hours of administration, and the duration of effect persists for variable periods.[9]

More recently, calcitonin has become available. Its probable mechanism of action involves suppression of osteoclast activity and bone resorption, and enhanced calciuresis.[9] It can be administered intramuscularly or subcutaneously, and often is effective within hours, frequently inducing a rapid decline in serum calcium by 1–4 mg/dl. It has a rapid onset of action and is not associated with marrow or renal toxicity. The major limitation in the use of calcitonin is the development of resistance due to antibody formation. Resistance may be delayed but not prevented by concomitant use of prednisone.[10]

Intravenous diphosphonate (Didronel; Norwich Eaton Pharmaceuticals, Norwich, NY) also inhibits osteoclast activity. It is administered intravenously over 2 to 4 hours for 3 to 5 days. Renal insufficiency represents a relative contraindication to its use. Also new in this class of drugs is pamidronate (Aredia; Ciba-Geigy, Summit, NJ), which requires a single 24-hour infusion. The diphosphonates may be a good therapeutic choice if antineoplastic agents are likely to be used in the near future.

The newest drug in the armamentarium against hypercalcemia is gallium nitrate, an investigational chemotherapeutic agent that was serendipitously observed to be associated with the potentially beneficial side effect of reducing serum calcium. It recently became available for use in the setting of hypercalcemia.[11]

PROGNOSIS

Untreated, progressive hypercalcemia leads inevitably to death. Once an acute episode has been resolved, maintenance therapy can be instituted with oral phosphates, prednisone, and/or oral diphosphonates. The effects of these oral drugs are significantly less potent than those of parenteral therapy. Ultimately, the ability to treat the underlying malignancy and prevent subsequent rises in calcium determines the longevity of affected patients. If reasonable options for treatment of the underlying disease have been exhausted, and the transitory correction of hypercalcemia promises only to return a patient to chronic symptomatic illness and recurring hypercalcemia, it may be appropriate to discuss the option of not treating the hypercalcemia at all. Death from hypercalcemia can be a humane release from the suffering of long-standing illness.

SPINAL CORD COMPRESSION

Spinal cord compression is in some respects the most challenging of the oncologic emergencies. Over 90% of the patients who develop cord compression from metastatic cancer have antecedent back pain,[12,13] (see Chapter 1) yet back pain is an exceedingly common symptom in the general population, especially in cancer patients, and on this basis is often disregarded. Additionally, the onset of progressive neurologic symptoms is often insidious and may go unrecognized, particularly in patients who already are multisymptomatic, until late signs are already established.

In most instances, mechanical compression of the spinal cord is caused by the growth of bony metastatic deposits in a vertebral body. As the lesion grows posteriorly, it extends into the epidural space, and pressure is transmitted across the dura to the cord and its vascular supply, which, if unchecked, leads to mechanical injury, ischemia, venous stasis, and infarction. Extradural tumor growth is responsible for about 95% of cases of cord compression, with intramedullary metastases and paraspinal extension of soft tissue tumors accounting for the remainder of cases.[14] The thoracic spinal cord is involved in about 70% of cases, the cervical cord in 15%, and the lumbosacral cord in the remainder of cases.[14] Since the spinal cord is the common pathway for the transmission of sensory and motor impulses to and from the periphery, compression leads to progressive loss of sensation and muscle strength and autonomic deregulation

below the site of the lesion. If symptom progression goes unrecognized and intervention consequently is delayed, paraplegia, numbness, and bowel and bladder dysfunction result. These symptoms add inestimable hardship to patients and families already struggling with the difficulties of cancer and its concomitant symptoms. With cord compression in the cervical or high thoracic region, patients are at further risk for quadriplegia and respiratory death.

Breast cancer and lung cancer are the most common primary malignancies associated with the development of spinal cord compression, followed by prostate cancer, lymphoma, and multiple myeloma.[15] Actually, any cancer that metastasizes to bone may be causal, including renal, melanoma, unknown primary, and more rarely gynecologic and gastrointestinal malignancies. Although there usually is initial involvement of the vertebral bodies, lymphoma can give rise to paraspinal nodal masses that infiltrate through the vertebral column's neural foramina to compress the cord.

DIAGNOSIS

The key to the diagnosis of epidural cord compression rests on the maintenance of a high degree of clinical suspicion, and the performance of careful serial neurologic examinations coupled with appropriate diagnostic imaging. Simple back strain and degenerative disc disease must be considered as part of the differential diagnosis of back pain, and in a patient without known cancer and an absence of neurologic abnormalities, observation and conservative management are warranted. In the patient with underlying cancer, a complaint of back pain should prompt more thorough investigation and concern about a metastatic cause. Localized paraspinal, radicular, or referred pain usually is the first sign of metastases to the bony vertebral column. Pain tends to be dull, steady, and aching, and increases gradually over time. Pain may be elicited by palpation or percussion of the spinous processes of the involved segments, may be

Table 29–2.
Physical Exam in Suspected Spinal Cord Compression

Motor Exam	Sensory Exam	Other
Ambulatory status	Look for dermatomal loss of sensation below affected level—	Palpation for enlarged bladder
Heel and toe walking		Consider straight catheterization for residual urine volume
Direct testing of muscle groups	Pin-prick	
Deep tendon reflexes (may be increased or absent)	Light touch	Decreased sweating below affected level
	Anal sphincter sensation	
Plantar response	Vibration and position sense	
Abdominal reflexes (T8–10 and T10–12)		
Cremasteric reflexes (L-1,2)		
Anal spincter tone		

exacerbated when lying down, and partially relieved by sitting or standing.

The clinical neurologic evaluation should include inquiry about symptoms of weakness, radicular pain, alterations in gait, numbness, urine retention or incontinence, and constipation. The examination should include testing of reflexes, muscle strength, sensation to light touch and pinprick, and the Babinski response. When practical, the patient's gait and ability to heel-walk and toe-walk should be observed. A rectal examination is performed to assess sphincter tone and sensation, and the abdomen is palpated to determine if the bladder is enlarged. A review of some of the recommended features of the neurologic examination is provided in Table 29–2.

Patients often present with localized back pain and a level of sensory deficit that serve to direct attention to a specific level of cord involvement, but regardless, neurologic integrity of the entire cord should be evaluated since pathology can be occult and multifocal. Plain films of the spine provide a rapid means to assess the presence of gross metastatic involvement. Scintigraphy (radionuclide bone scan) is more sensitive for osseous metastases but is not specific for cord involvement, and is too time-consuming if neurologic symptoms or findings are present. When it can be arranged, a multidisciplinary assess-

ment involving the oncologist, neurologist or neurosurgeon, and radiologist is most efficient of time. If spinal cord compression is suspected, urgent radiologic evaluation is undertaken. The choice of the most appropriate investigation is somewhat controversial.[14] Although the traditional "gold standard" radiologic study still is a myelogram, computed tomography (CT) and magnetic resonance imaging scanning are becoming increasingly well accepted in many communities. Myelography permits rapid visualization of all of the contents of the intrathecal sac, and, in addition, cerebrospinal fluid can be obtained for chemical and cytologic analysis. It is, however, invasive and uncomfortable, and in the presence of a high-grade block to the flow of contrast material, a second puncture may be required to visualize the entire cord. In addition, a small but actual risk of inducing herniation of the spinal cord exists if the pressure within the dural space is high. Computed tomography scans, with or without contrast, are readily obtainable, but require that the clinician estimate the location of the block so that the scan can be performed at the appropriate site. Scanning the entire cord in a detailed fashion is prohibitively time-consuming. Magnetic resonance imaging has become more readily available in recent years. Images in the axial and sagittal planes can be obtained, and are extremely sensitive to changes in tissue composition of bone and nervous tissue. Requirements include that the patient remain immobile in an enclosed space for about 2 hours, and an absence of surgical hardware or metallic prostheses.

TREATMENT

Once a diagnosis has been established, high-dose corticosteroids usually are administered to reduce peritumoral edema. Standard treatment is with dexamethasone 4–6 mg, administered intravenously every 6 hours, although some authorities advocate higher initial and maintenance doses.[13] Bed rest is indicated to prevent further displacement of unstable pathologic fractures. As noted, early detection and prompt intervention are the keys to successful treatment. Consequently, interdisciplinary consultation is advisable during the diagnostic phase so that therapeutic decisions can be made with a minimum of delay. Involvement of a medical oncologist, radiation oncologist, and neurosurgeon is ideal.

Emergency high-dose radiotherapy (3,000–4,000 rad delivered over 2–4 weeks) is considered in the presence of highly radiosensitive tumors, multiple or extensive lesions, and when patients otherwise are not fit for surgery. Factors favoring surgical intervention (emergency decompressive laminectomy) are: absence of a histologic diagnosis, progression of symptoms during or after radiotherapy, poor tumor radiosensitivity, and continued pain and instability after radiation.[13] When surgery is to be performed, spinal cord compression represents a true surgical emergency, since the presence of dermatomal sensory loss and frank muscle and bladder paresis usually precedes irreversible paraplegia or quadriplegia by only 12–24 hours.[16] In the absence of prior radiation to the involved area, postoperative irradiation commonly is used.

ANESTHESIA

If surgery is contemplated, there are many important anesthesiologic considerations. Since the patient and family members may be markedly anxious, contemplating the prospect of paralysis, major surgery, and further disability, a thorough, compassionate explanation of anesthesia, and, when the medical condition is sufficiently stable, generous premedication are indicated. Radiologic findings are reviewed and discussed with the surgeon to determine if instability of the cervical spine is present that may require consideration of special airway management, such as fiber-optic, nasal, and/or conscious intubation to minimize further neurologic injury. If conscious intubation is elected, topical anesthesia and sedation should be used to reduce coughing. Dehydration may be present as a consequence of chronic illness and steroid administration. In patients with advanced lesions, sympathetic nervous system dysfunction may result in impaired cardiovascular compensation for alterations in posture and blood loss. Preoperative hydration with a balanced salt solution and prompt replacement of blood loss are indicated to attenuate intraoperative reductions in blood pressure. Measurements of cardiac filling pressures are a useful guide to fluid therapy. Patients may become poikilothermic below the level of injury, and normothermia should be maintained aggressively. Patients with high lesions should be assessed for weakness of respiratory muscles, and should be observed carefully once sedatives have been administered. The risk of succinylcholine-induced hyperkalemia increases over the first few days after neurologic injury. Since the time of initial neurologic insult often is indeterminable, when possible, a nondepolarizing agent should be selected to facilitate tracheal intubation. Hypertension and bradycardia associated with autonomic hyperreflexia are of concern only when denervation is chronic.

PROGNOSIS

Although the radiosensitivity of the cancer and the overall condition of the patient are important indicators, the outcome in these patients depends primarily on the extent of disability established at the time treatment is started. Patients who are ambulatory at the time of presentation have a high probability of maintaining that ability, whereas patients who already are paretic or paraplegic are unlikely to regain ambulatory status.[17]

SUPERIOR VENA CAVA SYNDROME

Superior vena cava (SVC) syndrome is caused by tumor growth in the apex of the right lung or superior mediastinum. The mass of tumor grows around or against the compressible superior vena cava, resulting in a reduced flow of venous blood back to the heart from the head, neck, and upper extremities. Obstruction often develops slowly, in which case collateral veins gradually enlarge to facilitate venous return. However, in cases of rapid tumor growth, the onset of obstruction may be sufficiently acute to warrant immediate diagnosis and therapy. Thus, the syndrome may not represent a true emergency but rather an urgent problem of diagnostic and therapeutic importance.

Cancer now accounts for an estimated 97% of all cases of SVC syndrome.[5] The syndrome is most common in patients with carcinoma of the lung and malignant lymphoma. In an analysis of 84 cancer patients diagnosed with SVC syndrome, 75% of cases were due to bronchogenic carcinoma, 15% to lymphomas, and 7% from metastatic infiltration of the mediastinum.[18]

DIAGNOSIS

Signs and symptoms of SVC syndrome are relatively uniform, and usually permit a diagnosis to be made on clinical grounds alone (Table 29–3). Direct observation may reveal facial plethora, facial edema, and swelling of the upper extremities. Swelling typically is most severe in the morning and improves after hours spent upright. Other symptoms include hoarseness due to vocal cord edema,

headache from cerebral edema, cough, and shortness of breath. Key physical findings include dilated collateral veins over the chest wall, and distention of the arm veins that is unrelieved when the arms are raised above the level of the heart. Dyspnea and stridor indicate the need for urgent intervention.

Chest radiography is the single most useful confirmatory investigation. A right upper lobe mass adjacent to the SVC and mediastinal widening are the two most common findings. The indications for further testing are controversial, and depend on numerous factors, including the patient's overall physical status and whether the primary is known. Chest CT with contrast frequently will reveal the site of obstruction, and further delineates other intrathoracic disease. If CT is unavailable or the patient is unable to tolerate recumbency, nuclear or contrast bilateral upper extremity venograms can be performed, although raised intraluminal pressure introduces the risk of persistent hemorrhage from venipuncture sites.

Superior vena cava syndrome may be the initial manifestation of undiagnosed malignancy, in which case a definitive tissue diagnosis and analysis of the extent of disease need to be obtained. Methods include bronchoscopy, esophagoscopy, mediastinoscopy, scalene node biopsy, and exploratory thoracotomy. All are associated with increased risk of morbidity when symptoms are severe, and may be deferred until clinical improvement has been achieved.

TREATMENT

Initial symptomatic management consists simply of elevation of the head and avoidance of venipuncture in the upper extremities for blood samples and intravenous access. The role of diuretics and dexamethasone is controversial, but their administration may provide prompt, if transient relief of symptoms, especially dyspnea.[5] Anticoagulation and fibrinolysis are favored by some authorities,[19]

Table 29–3.
Signs and Symptoms of Superior Vena Cava Obstruction

Symptoms	Physical Signs
Swelling of face and arms	Edema of face and arms
Cough	Plethora
Headache	Arms veins distended even with arm above heart level
Hoarseness	
Dyspnea	Dilated chest wall veins

based on autopsy findings of intraluminal thrombosis in one-third to one-half of patients with SVC syndrome,[20] but the role of these interventions remains unclear.[21] Definitive therapy depends on the histology of the tumor, and involves complex decision-making. In newly diagnosed lymphoma or small-cell lung cancers, aggressive chemotherapy alone or combined with radiotherapy is as a rule associated with rapid regression of both tumor bulk and symptoms. The primary therapeutic modality usually is radiation therapy, which generally produces prompt and often complete symptomatic improvement.[5]

PROGNOSIS

Prognosis varies depending on the histologic diagnosis and extent of disease. The syndrome is not in itself a poor prognostic sign, and thus, for example, patients with indolent lymphoma tend ultimately to do well, whereas individuals with small-cell lung cancer do well initially but are subject to a high rate of relapse.

HEMATOLOGIC EMERGENCIES

The most common hematologic emergencies, thrombocytopenia and neutropenia, usually are induced iatrogenically by antineoplastic treatment. In addition, these conditions can occur as direct effects, usually in the course of

hematologic malignancies, or as a consequence of bone marrow replacement late in the course of patients with solid tumors. Although rarely a true emergency, anemia is discussed because of its potential to contribute to the progression of symptoms of terminal illness.

ANEMIA

Anemia is common and often multifactorial. Causes include occult or acute hemorrhage, tumor infiltration of bone marrow, nutritional deficiencies, hemolysis, the effects of chronic disease, hypersplenism, and chemotherapy or radiation therapy. Anemia often is chronic and well tolerated, particularly in the setting of a sedentary lifestyle. It may, however, contribute to dyspnea, fatigue, and indirectly to malnutrition if low energy levels interfere with a patient's ability and interest in the preparation of food. When correctable deficiencies such as iron, folate, or B12 are present, treatment is straightforward. Indications for transfusion are controversial,[22] especially in patients with chronic, irremediable conditions, but clinicians often will provide symptomatic patients with transfusions to achieve a hematocrit of 20%–30%.

THROMBOCYTOPENIA

Many of the same factors noted as potentially contributing to anemia also may cause thrombocytopenia. Patients with platelet counts below 20,000–30,000 are at increased risk for spontaneous hemorrhage, in which case petechiae, ecchymosis, and hematuria may be noted by the patient. Platelet counts below 50,000 are associated with increased risks of hemorrhage during invasive procedures. Prophylactic platelet transfusions are recommended for patients at risk for spontaneous hemorrhage, and immediately before a planned procedure when there is an increased risk of bleeding.

NEUTROPENIA

Absolute neutrophil counts (ANC) below 500 are associated with a high risk of spontaneous infection, especially by gastrointestinal flora, including *Pseudomonas*.[23] Patients with fever and an ANC below 500 should be evaluated by a physical examination that should include a gentle inspection of the skin and perirectal area. Complete cultures and a chest radiograph should be performed, followed by the institution of broad spectrum antibiotics to cover gram-positive and gram-negative organisms, including *Pseudomonas*. Antibiotic coverage should be adjusted according to culture results. In the setting of prolonged neutropenia and fever, consideration should be given to initiating antifungal therapy empirically.

LEUKOSTASIS

This phenomenon is seen almost exclusively in patients with acute myelogenic leukemia and high circulating volumes (>100,000) of blast cells. Because of the large diameter of the blasts, they can obstruct capillary beds and cause multiple cerebral and pulmonary microinfarctions and hemorrhage. If unrecognized, this syndrome is often fatal. Diagnosis depends on history, physical examination, and analysis of a peripheral blood smear. Immediate treatment with high doses of hydoxyurea and/or leukapheresis can provide temporary relief until definitive antileukemic therapy can be started.

DISSEMINATED INTRAVASCULAR COAGULATION

Disseminated intravascular coagulation (DIC) is more likely to be a subacute finding than a true emergency. This problem involves diffuse microthrombi within the vascular system. Due to consumption of clotting factors, including platelets, it paradoxically can precipitate clinical bleeding. It is associated with acute promyelocytic leukemia, metastatic prostate cancer, massive hepatic metastases, and, rarely, other solid tumors. Many types of tumor cells (promyelocytic leukemia, adenocarcinoma of the prostate) are rich in thromboplastin-like materials that can trigger the coagulation cascade.

As with most disorders of coagulation, a careful history and physical examination is the most useful screening procedure. Clinically there may be cutaneous manifestations and bleeding from phlebotomy sites. Prothrombin time, partial thromboplastin time test, and laboratory studies of platelets and bleeding time can be performed initially. In the presence of abnormalities of these tests, a more exact diagnosis often is suggested by analysis of levels of fibrinogen and fibrin split products, as well as with an examination of a peripheral blood smear, which may reveal abnormal red cells and red cell fragments. Ultimately, control of DIC depends on control of the underlying cancer, but temporizing measures may be necessary in fulminant cases. Transfusion of cryoprecipitate, platelets, plasma, and whole blood or packed cells may be required. In refractory cases, intravenous heparin potentially will interrupt the cycle of intravascular microcoagulation and the consumption of clotting factors, but is associated with risks of increased bleeding.[24]

RENAL EMERGENCIES

URETERAL OBSTRUCTION

Tumor growth within the pelvis or retroperitoneum can lead to obstruction of the ureters, hydronephrosis, and consequent renal failure. The cancers most associated with this complication are rectal, cervical, prostate, bladder, and lymphoma. The presenting symptoms are those of renal failure: oliguria or anuria, nausea, anorexia, mental status changes, and even coma. Associated electrolyte abnormalities are common. Renal ultrasound is a safe and direct way to evaluate for hydronephrosis. Treatment involves immediate drainage either via ureteral stents, or, more commonly, nephrostomy. In the presence of severe electrolyte or mental status changes, dialysis may be necessary on an urgent basis. Radiation therapy often will relieve obstruction, and should be strongly considered. It may be appropriate to elect not to treat ureteral obstruction in patients with prior pelvic irradiation or advanced systemic cancer in whom life expectancy is otherwise short, and other refractory symptoms are present. Death by uremia may be more humane than prolonging life when no other therapeutic options exist.

TUMOR LYSIS SYNDROME AND URIC ACID NEPHROPATHY

Tumor lysis syndrome is an emergency best treated by prevention. Some malignancies respond so robustly to chemotherapy that, in the presence of bulky disease, rapid cell death and subsequent high metabolic turnover can lead to clinical problems. Patients with lymphoma (especially American Burkitt's) and leukemia are predisposed to developing clinically significant disturbances.

The destruction of large numbers of malignant cells releases large quantities of nucleic acids with accumulation of uric acid, the major product of purine catabolism. Precipitation of uric acid crystals is associated with gouty arthritis and a variety of renal insults, the most important of which is acute hyperuricemic nephropathy.

Sudden onset of oliguric or anuric renal failure is characteristic, and is due to obstruction at the level of the distal nephron. Clumping of crystals within the ureters may occur, and is associated with flank pain. Hyperuri-

cemia is a common feature of renal failure, regardless of its etiology, but crystalluria and a disproportionate elevation in serum uric acid levels in susceptible patients suggest that it is causative. Excessive liberation of intracellular potassium also may precipitate life-threatening acidosis and cardiac arrhythmias.

Before cytotoxic therapy, susceptible patients should be identified and prophylaxis should be instituted, namely: pretreatment with allopurinol (an inhibitor of the enzyme xanthine oxidase) and high-dose hydration with forced diuresis, accompanied by frequent serum electrolyte testing. In the presence of preexisting renal dysfunction, additional caution is warranted. Treatment of established acute renal failure involves vigorous intravenous hydration, careful alkalinization of the urine with intravenously administered sodium bicarbonate, and the administration of allopurinol. Mannitol has been used successfully to reestablish urinary flow, and, in otherwise unresponsive cases, treatment with dialysis is indicated.

INTESTINAL OBSTRUCTION

When possible, true obstruction should be differentiated from simple advanced constipation with adynamic ileus, because management differs. Although constipation and its causative factors may contribute to true obstruction, most often other, often multiple, factors are present, including intraluminal obstruction, extramural mass compression, transluminal infiltration of the muscular wall, surgical or malignant adhesions, and radiation fibrosis. Onset is usually insidious, and is characterized by the presence of nausea, vomiting, colic, alternating diarrhea and constipation, and abdominal distention. Obstruction may occur in any setting, but most frequently accompanies colorectal or ovarian carcinoma, or occurs subsequent to abdominal or pelvic irradiation.

Palliative surgery should be considered in the otherwise fit patient with a simple, single lesion. These conditions often are unsatisfied in the patient with advanced carcinoma. The utility and appropriateness of the traditional hospital-based measures of intravenous hydration and nasogastric suction are controversial and generally are not favored in the hospice environment.[25] Although they are useful presurgically, and transiently on an emergency basis, applied chronically they contribute to patient discomfort and generally presuppose hospitalization.

Using alternative therapy, chronic nausea and colic can nearly be eliminated in most patients, even in the presence of severe obstruction, and symptoms can be limited to once- or twice-daily vomiting, which is not nearly as distressing as it sounds.[25] The conservative management of intestinal obstruction is summarized in Table 29-4.

PLEURAL EFFUSION

In most cases, pleural effusions progress gradually and do not require true emergency treatment. If unrecognized, however, they may contribute significantly to dyspnea and fatigue, conditions that often respond dramatically when the effusion is removed.

Any cancer within the thoracic cavity can lead to an effusion, either directly when the pleura is involved, or indirectly when lymphatic channels are obstructed. Cancers of the lung, breast, ovary, and lymphomas account for the majority of pleural effusions. Symptoms include shortness of breath, cough, and fatigue. Physical examination and chest radiography are the diagnostic interventions of choice. As with pericardial effusion, the initial treatment is with thoracentesis. If active chemotherapy or radiotherapy of a primary mediastinal mass is anticipated to reduce the effusion, then the chest radiograph can be used to follow the status of the effusion. If the effusion reaccumulates quickly, or the likelihood of systemic control of the cancer is low, then pleurodesis is indicated. Pleurodesis involves removal of the maximum amount of fluid possible by chest tube drainage, followed by the introduction of a chemical sclerosing agent (tetracycline, bleomycin) to adhere the parietal and visceral pleura. Although loculation

Table 29-4.
Principles of the Conservative Management of Malignant Intestinal Obstruction

1. Eliminate stimulant laxatives and properistaltic agents (metoclopramide).
2. If obstruction is subtotal, the regular oral administration of stool softeners (docusate sodium 100 mg bid or docusate calcium 240 mg/day) may help decrease intraluminal bulk.
3. Administer antiperistaltic–antidiarrheal agents to control colicky pain (diphenoxylate with atropine 1–2 tablets q 4 hr or loperamide 1–2 capsules q 4–6 hr).
4. Consider the introduction of nonopioid analgesics, but, if needed, administer opioid analgesics (morphine, hydromorphone) regularly to help control colic and coexisting abdominal pain.
5. Administer antiemetics, as needed.
6. Consider relatively high-dose steroids (dexamethasone 8 mg bid) to reduce inflammation secondary to tumor bulk, particularly in the presence of peritoneal carcinomatosis.
7. When possible, maintain the oral route for medication administration. If absorption is questionable, consider rectal suppositories and/or bolus or continuous subcutaneous administration. One formula recommended by St. Christopher's Hospice includes morphine 40 mg, atropine 0.8 mg, and haloperidol 5 mg administered continuously over 24 hr.
8. Reassure, and encourage maintenance of hydration. Intravenous hydration usually is not needed. Maintain mouth care when dehydration is present. Encourage regular vomiting, preferably once every morning. Once improvement of symptoms has been effected, patients often choose to eat and drink low-fiber foods liberally between episodes of vomiting.

of fluid may preclude full lung reexpansion, it usually is possible to improve pulmonary capacity.

REFERENCES

1. Fowler NO: Pericardial disease. In Hurst JW, Logue RB (eds): The Heart, 2nd ed, p 1254. New York, McGraw Hill, 1970.
2. Press OW, Livingston R: Management of malignant

pericardial effusion and tamponade. JAMA 1987; 257:1088.

3. Recant L, Lacy PE, eds. Clinicopathologic Conference: Pericardial disease with effusion, systemic involvement and pulmonary edema. Am J Med 1962;33:442.

4. Arsenau JC, Rubin P: Oncologic emergencies. In Rubin P (ed): Clinical Oncology: A Multidisciplinary Approach, 6th ed, p 516. Rochester, NY, American Cancer Society, 1983.

5. Helms SR, Carlson MD: Cardiovascular emergencies. Semin Oncol 1989;16:463.

6. Davis S, Rambotti P, Grignani F: Intrapericardial tetracycline sclerosis in the treatment of malignant pericardial effusion. J Clin Oncol 1984;2:631.

7. Appelfield MM, Slawson RG, Hall-Craigs M et al: Delayed pericardial disease after radiotherapy. Am J Cardiol 1981;47:210.

8. Mazzaferri EL, O'Dorisiao TM, Cobuglio AF: Treatment of hypercalcemia associated with malignancy. Semin Oncol 1978;5:141.

9. Ritch P: Treatment of cancer related hypercalcemia. Semin Oncol 1990;17 (Suppl 5):26.

10. Binstock ML, Mundy GR: Effect of calcitonin and glucocorticoids in combination in the hypercalcemia of malignancy. Ann Intern Med 1980;93:269.

11. Warrell RP Jr, Skelos A, Alcock NW et al: Gallium nitrate for acute treatment of cancer-related hypercalcemia: Clinicopharmacological and dose response analysis. Cancer Res 1986;46:4208.

12. Rodiochock LD, Harper GR, Ruckdeschel JC et al: Early diagnosis of spinal epidural metastases. Am J Med 1981;70:1181.

13. Posner JB: Back pain and epidural spinal cord compression. Med Clin North Am 1987;71:200.

14. Willson JKV, Masaryk TJ: Neurologic emergencies in the cancer patient. Semin Oncol 1989;16:494.

15. Gilbert RW, Kim JH, Posner JB: Epidural spinal cord compression from metastatic tumor: Diagnosis and treatment. Ann Neurol 1978;3:183.

16. Arsenau J, Rubin P: Oncologic emergencies. In Rubin P (ed): Clinical Oncology: A Multidisciplinary Approach, 6th ed, p 517. Rochester, NY, American Cancer Society, 1983.

17. Sorenson PS, Borgeson SE, Rohde K et al: Metastatic epidural spinal cord compression: Results of treatment and survival. Cancer 1990;65:1502.

18. Perez CA, Presant CA, Amburg AL: Management of the superior vena cava syndrome. Semin Oncol 1978;5:123.

19. Green J, Rubin P, Holzwasser G: The experimental production of superior vena cava syndrome. Radiology 1973;73:400.

20. Lokich JJ, Goodman RL: Superior vena cava syndrome. JAMA 1975;231:58.

21. Adelstein DJ, Hines JD, Carter SG et al: Thromboembolic events in patients with malignant superior vena cava syndrome and the role of anticoagulation. Cancer 1988;62:2258.

22. National Institutes of Health: Transfusion alert: Indications for the use of red blood cells, platelets, and fresh frozen plasma. Washington, DC, NIH Publication No. 89-2974 U.S. Department of Health and Human Services, Public Health Service, 1989.

23. Pizzo P, Young R: Infections in the cancer patient. In Devita V, Hellman S, Rosenberg S (eds): Cancer: Principles and Practice of Oncology, 3rd ed, p 2094. Philadelphia, JB Lippincott, 1989.

24. Ratnoff OD: Hemostatic emergencies in malignancy. Semin Oncol 1989;6:562.

25. Twycross R, Lack S: Therapeutics in Terminal Cancer Care, p 65. Edinburgh, Churchill Livingstone, 1990.

Chapter 30

Care of People Who Are Dying: The Hospice Approach

Julia Ladd Smith

PROLOGUE

The following has been reprinted with permission from Ajemian I, Mount B: The McGill University palliative care service. In Davidson GW (ed): The Hospice: Development and Administration, pp 47–49. New York, Hemisphere Publishing, 1985.

It had been a long day.

As we walked across the parking lot at Ross Pavilion, there was one last exchange before we went our separate ways, heading home for a late supper: "So, in the morning if you'll write the prescriptions and get reports from the nurses on the ward, I'll go over to the 'Neuro' and see that patient of Dr. Gauthier's. She's deteriorating and we've set up a meeting with the family and the resident on the floor."

The end of another day for the "Vic" PCS! As I nosed the car out into the traffic my mind wandered back over the events of the day. A collage of faces and situations. Problems and solutions. Stresses and reconciliations. Frustrations and achievements.

There had been two deaths on the ward. For the Bastorelli family it was the end of an era. The passing of their matriarch. Long denied, yet finally an unbelievable fact, she was gone. There had been moments of important mutual support in the softly-lit small lounge. An uncertain number of family members of all ages and shapes quietly consoling each other and sharing their new reality. For all concerned—patients, family members, caregivers—there was a sense of closure. For all the sadness there was a feeling of things coming together. The reassurance of knowing that a lot of people had come a very long way in a very short time. Much had been achieved there.

How different it had been for all of us that same morning as we watched Jacob Edmonds-Whyte drawing his last breaths. The dyspnea of pulmonary lymphangitic spread; the boring pain of pelvic nerve involvement; the anguish of fears and feelings unexpressed; the controlled tautness of the bowstring tension as husband and wife played out this final scene in a long and troubled marriage. Oh, there had been attention to detail in adjusting the doses of medication all right: the morphine, the dexamethasone, the amitryptiline, the dilantin—the lorazepam at bedtime. We had listened attentively. We had been very careful to give every possible inch of autonomy. We had struggled with the minutiae of details in considering how best to support the complex psychological, social and spiritual needs of this suffering couple. As far as we were concerned, we had failed. "I guess you don't always succeed," I thought to myself as the traffic light turned red.

There had been four new consults that morning, bringing the total number of patients being followed by Jeanne, Marcel, Charlie and their colleagues on the consultation team to twenty-eight. My mind went back to the events of the morning. Pressure on the beds in both the medical and surgical pavilions had led to the urgent transfer of two patients to the PCS. Jeanne had done everything she could to smooth the way but the timing was terrible. Jacob was dying, Mr. Kerry in status epilepticus, the ward was short-staffed, the Perrault family angry and, as one of the nurses pointed out, "Eleven of our sixteen patients require total care. There simply isn't going to be time this morning to give sufficient attention to the needs of the new patients being admitted!"

The traffic light turned green and the driver behind me leaned on his horn and something reminded me of the way the morning had started! Friday morning, 8:00 A.M.—Pathology Rounds. Command performance! Two cases from the Palliative Care Unit to be presented. One had been straightforward enough, but the other had been an elderly lady with ascites, renal failure and presumed pancreatic carcinoma. Autopsy had revealed chronic pancreatitis. Accountability! Peer review. Suddenly there it was. The heads of all departments, eight pairs of eyes, eight quick minds sifting over the facts and the decision-making processes, through the retrospectoscope and as we all know "hindsight is always 20/20." It had

been concluded that the actions of the Palliative Care team and the referring oncologist had been appropriate, but the issues were certainly reviewed!

The traffic was thinning out now and my mind drifted to the home care service. There had been two deaths that day—one at home that had gone well and one in the emergency department that would have been at home had the family only called the home care nurse rather than the ambulance when they panicked. Sue had touched base with them only the night before and everything had seemed under control. There was concern among the home care nurses about the family during their bereavement and the decision was made to have Sue continue her contact along with a volunteer from the bereavement team.

Quite a day. There had, however, been some real high points. Probably countless ones I didn't know about but the ones that came to mind as I pulled into the driveway included the highly animated interservice teaching session on Ross 4 that Jeanne had held in the early afternoon around the problems confronting old Mrs. Chiswick and her family; the minor triumph as Eugene, the music therapist, played his flute and used relaxation techniques in the "Cat Lab" to calm the anxious brittle, young woman as she underwent cardiac catheterization. And, there was the profitable session (the fourth in a series of consultations) with the group from Drummondville who are about to open their own program. Finally, there was the data presented by Stephanie at the four o'clock research meeting concerning the Meaning of Life Index project. Even Walter was pleased.

As the car door slammed and I headed for the front door, I had to smile as I recalled a conversation that had occurred on the way home yesterday evening. "You know, I really enjoy this work," I had commented absent-mindedly. "Why?" she asked. Without much thought, I responded "Because you can make such a difference." We had both laughed at the irony. These were the patients for "whom nothing more can be done."

INTRODUCTION

The care of dying persons has undergone major changes over the past 50 years. Formerly, medical technology provided only limited options to prolong life. As recently as the 1950s, the only ventilators available were "iron lungs." Today a vast array of lifesaving interventions are readily available. This phenomenon forces physicians, patients, and families consciously to choose the appropriate time to cease relying on technologic efforts intended to prolong life, a choice that necessitates confronting the equally challenging task of achieving comfort and a satisfying closure to life. The hospice movement focuses on people who are at this stage of terminal illness, and strives to balance the need to relieve physical suffering with the intense emotional needs of the patient and those around him or her. Although over 90% of patients on most hospice programs have cancer, people with AIDS, end-stage heart and lung disease, and progressive neurologic disorders are all appropriate hospice patients.

Hospice care has been called "a blend of clinical pharmacology and applied compassionate psychology."[1,1a] As such, it is a philosophy of providing intensive symptom control combined with psychosocial and spiritual support to dying people and their families. In many locales there is a formal hospice program certified to provide interdisciplinary care to patients and families at home, and, when needed, inpatient care is available either in a local hospital or in a free-standing hospice unit. In either type of inpatient setting, the hospice team remains actively involved with the patient's care and in providing support for the family.

DEFINING THE TERMINAL STATE

For hospice purposes, the definition of the terminal period is less than 6 months of life. For this reason, the majority of patients served by hospice programs are individuals with cancer, because that disease has a relatively predictable course once antineoplastic treatments are stopped. However, patients with AIDS, end-stage heart disease, pulmonary disease, and degenerative neurologic illness who are likely to live less than 6 months, or renal failure patients who elect to forgo dialysis, all can benefit from hospice care. Thus it is not the

diagnosis but the terminal status and the desire for comfort care that makes hospice an appropriate intervention.

The ability to estimate life expectancy is inexact at best. Even experienced oncologists and hospice workers tend to overestimate the prognosis by an average of 3.4 weeks.[2,2a] Reuben and colleagues[1] identified a low Karnofsky performance status (below 40) as the single most useful predictor of life expectancy. Included in this group are individuals who are sufficiently disabled to require help with activities of daily living, and those who are moribund (see Table 30–1). In addition, physical complaints of dry mouth, shortness of breath, problems with eating, weight loss within 2 weeks, and difficulty swallowing were identified as useful predictors of life expectancy.

DEFINING COMFORT CARE

The boundary between aggressive management of a disease such as cancer and comfort-oriented care of the patient is not always clear-cut. In fact, palliation of symptoms is part of good medical treatment from the moment that a chronic illness is diagnosed. The transition from the provision of aggressive treatment intended to arrest the underlying disease and prolong life to comfort-oriented treatment intended to optimize the quality of the remaining weeks or months of life is difficult for physicians as well as the patients and families they serve. Good hospice practice decries the belief that there is ever a point at which "nothing can be done" for the patient, advocating instead refocusing priorities on attention to comfort. The provision of an aggressive, proactive, and systematic approach to comfort care is the key to achieving symptom control and emotional peace, elements that equate with "quality of life." Hospice does not advocate hastening death, nor does it advocate prolonging the dying process.

Comfort-oriented care specifically focuses on alleviating symptoms, and often is not di-

Table 30–1.
Performance Scale (Karnofsky and ECOG)

Grade	ECOG	Karnofsky	
0	Fully active, able to carry on all predisease performance without restriction	100	Normal, no complaints, no evidence of disease
		90	Able to carry on normal activity; minor signs or symptoms of disease
1	Restricted in physically strenuous activity but ambulatory and able to carry out work of a light or sedentary nature (eg, light house work, office work)	80	Normal activity with effort; some signs or symptoms of disease
		70	Cares for self; unable to carry on normal activity or to do active work
2	Ambulatory and capable of all self-care but unable to carry out any work activities. Up and about more than 50% of waking hours	60	Requires occasional assistance, but is able to care for most of his or her needs
		50	Requires considerable assistance and frequent medical care
3	Capable of only limited self-care, confined to bed or chair more than 50% of waking hours	40	Disabled, requires special care and assistance
		30	Severely disabled, hospitalization indicated; death not imminent
4	Completely disabled. Cannot carry on any self-care. Totally confined to bed or chair	20	Very sick, hospitalization necessary, active supportive treatment necessary
		10	Moribund, fatal processes, progressing rapidly
5	Dead	0	Dead

rected at their underlying cause(s) (see Chapter 13). As a result, the need for laboratory investigations, from interventions as minor as blood tests to more sophisticated tests like computed tomography (CT) scans, is limited. The decision to perform any investigation should be subjected to a simple but key inquiry: will the results of the test alter symptom management and provide information that will help improve the patient's well-being? A repeat CT scan to determine whether brain metastases have increased in size does not lead to further treatment alternatives once maximal whole brain radiation has been ad-

ministered. Some additional guidelines to help determine whether an intervention is appropriate follow. These are not intended to be exhaustive, but to help provide guidance for practitioners.

• The human cost of an intervention must not outweigh the anticipated benefit. These costs include the effort involved in transportation or added side effects and discomfort likely to be associated with treatment. For example, a patient with limited energy may prefer to conserve his or her limited resources to participate in a family visit rather than choosing an ambulance ride to undergo additional radiography. Transfusions may not be appropriate, particularly in a bed-bound patient who is unlikely to benefit symptomatically, when weighed against the potential discomfort involved in transportation and obtaining intravenous access, as well as the risk of fluid overload. In this circumstance, the provision of nasal oxygen and attention to conserving energy may be a reasonable substitute for transfusion.

- The traditional medical approach sometimes is appropriate. Despite a preterminal status, under some circumstances, treatment directed at relieving the underlying source of symptoms does not merely prolong the dying process, but may lead to improved comfort, and therefore is elected. Treatment of the oncologic emergencies described in Chapter 29 is appropriate when further antineoplastic therapy offers significant promise of tumor response and meaningful relief of symptoms. On the other hand, medical resolution of an episode of hypercalcemia is not compassionate when it can be predicted to be followed by recurrent episodes of hypercalcemia or the prolongation of an uncomfortable bed-ridden existence. Likewise, palliative radiation for impending spinal cord compression, which sometimes produces dramatic resolution of symptoms, is likely to be burdensome and possibly counterproductive if the course of treatment is 3 weeks and the patient is likely to live only 3 or 4 weeks.

- The patient must desire to undergo the test or treatment. At times, well-meaning or uninformed family members may urge a patient to continue with interventions that are neither helpful nor desired by the patient. The physician, too, must be clear why he or she is ordering a test or treatment; the physician's own need to avoid uncertainty or to do "something" does not justify an order.

GOAL-ORIENTED CARE

The alternative to aggressive testing and treatment is goal-oriented symptom management

Table 30–2.
Setting Realistic Goals

1. Identify the problems as well as patient's strengths and abilities and resources. How has he or she dealt with them in the past?
2. Help the patient identify desired change.
3. Help patient prioritize desired changes.
4. Identify goals and order of approach. Goals will address what the patient will be doing that is different and better as a result of his care.
5. Break down long-term goals into manageable short-term segments.
6. Plan and carry out the treatment program.
7. Assess the progress of the patient related to the goals. Change treatment as needed.
8. Review goals often, especially in relation to changes in the patient's abilities as he or she physically deteriorates due to the illness.

Modified from Hillier ER, Lunt B: Goal setting in terminal cancer. In Twycross RG, Ventafridda V (eds): The Continuing Care of Terminal Cancer Patients, p 271. Oxford, Pergamon Press, 1979.[2]

(Table 30–2). Goal-oriented care requires a dialogue between the physician and patient, and, when appropriate, the family. The health care team must provide information in a gentle way (Table 30–3) and elicit the patient's desires. At times, realistic choices must be separated delicately from unrealistic and wishful thinking.

There are three guidelines that are useful to invoke in the discussion of any specific proposed treatment: 1) the treatment must be directed at controlling symptoms and optimizing comfort; 2) the treatment must not involve increased discomfort; and 3) the treatment uses the least invasive measure to accomplish the goal. One must carefully consider invasive measures if required for comfort. Comfort care most commonly is "low-tech and high-touch." When these guidelines are applied, sometimes seemingly innocuous measures such as blood transfusions become burdensome for the patient,

Table 30–3.
Treating the Patient as a Person

Nonverbal communication
- Greet the patient by name
- Introduce self by name
- Shake patient's hand
- Sit down, if possible
- Make eye contact
- Visit regularly
- Include family/visitors in greeting

Attention to detail
- Ask about specific known symptoms
- Ask about sleep, comfort, diet, mouth, and elimination

Verbal communication
- Provide opportunity to ask questions about patient's condition
- Avoid promises to relatives about nondisclosure of information to the patient
- Gentle truth is preferred by patients
- The doctor–patient relationship is founded on trust; it is fostered by honesty but poisoned by deceit
- The doctor's responsibility is to "nudge" the patient in the direction of reality, but never to force him or her

Modified from Twycross RG: Hospice care: Redressing the balance in medicine. J R Soc Med 1980;73:475.[3]

and simple interventions like conversation are therapeutic.

SPECIFIC ISSUES

PAIN

Most of the chapters in this book are related to various aspects of pain control. Nevertheless, a few comments relating to pain in the terminal stages of illness are appropriate here. When life expectancy is limited to a matter of weeks, the oral route should be used as long as feasible, the analgesic regimen should be simplified as much as possible, and alternate routes for administering analgesics should be made available when needed (see Chapters 6–12). "High-tech" delivery systems are

costly, and because the machinery may become the focus of attention rather than the person, these interventions actually may detract from the personal care provided to the patient. When used, these systems require a competent and capable person in the home to change the needle site, tubing, and medication cassettes, and to troubleshoot for problems, as well as professional support for this individual. Caregivers often are elderly, and may be overwhelmed by the machinery or may lack the manual dexterity or visual acuity required for safe operation. Continuous infusion pumps have the greatest application when the enteral route cannot be used, but are also useful in selected individuals who require large volumes of oral medication or in whom unwanted side effects might be resolved with continuous delivery. Infusion pumps are best used when there is a life expectancy of at least several weeks, due to the need for education and their relatively high initial costs. There usually are other options available that are equally effective and simpler to institute for patients with shorter life expectancies. With the recent availability of formulations of controlled-release morphine in tablets up to 100 mg and transdermal fentanyl delivery systems (see Chapter 11), continuous subcutaneous administration is now a less needed option. Controlled-release morphine tablets easily can be administered rectally (or vaginally) with nearly equivalent potency as when used orally.[4,5] This alternative may enable family members to feel more successful in their role as caregivers. The epidural administration of analgesics (see Chapter 18) is most appropriate for patients with a prognosis of several months. The application of sophisticated pain management techniques requires the same scrutiny of goal-oriented care as do other interventions.

Advance preparation for changes in the patient's ability to swallow helps families face new problems more calmly. Early education in the use of sustained-release tablets as suppositories, and the advance provision of short-acting opioids in suppository or concentrated liquid form avoids escalation of pain and panic both for family and patient. If repet-

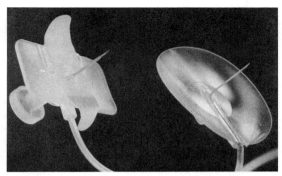

Figure 30–1. Two innovative devices intended to simplify the institution and administration of subcutaneous infusions of opioids and adjuvants. Both devices eliminate the need for repeated injections, facilitate sterile placement, and reduce the likelihood of injury to caregiver. The housing and needle of the device on the left detaches, leaving a small plastic cannula in the subcutaneous tissue. The disk on the right is applied flush to the patient's skin, and attaches with an adhesive backing.

itive doses of injectable medications are needed temporarily, either at home or in a hospital or hospice unit, the use of a subcutaneous disk (Fig. 30–1) left in place avoids the discomfort associated with repeated injections. The disk is a small-bore subcutaneous needle attached to an adhesive-backed disk and connected to tubing like a butterfly needle. The tubing must be primed with medication to avoid underdosing on the first occasion of use due to dead space within the tubing. The disk can be left in place for several days if skin irritation is absent. The site can be changed by either the family or a professional nurse. This technique helps family members overcome reluctance to participate in hands-on care by avoiding the necessity to puncture the skin for each dose of medication.

NAUSEA

Nausea is highly prevalent among patients with advanced terminal illness (see Chapters 12 and 13). Frequently multifactorial, its causes include the effects of analgesics and other medications, liver metastases, intra-abdominal tumor, bowel obstruction, brain metastases, hypercalcemia, and uremia. In patients who are otherwise reasonably fit, limited investigations may be undertaken to determine the exact cause of nausea and vomiting, but only insofar as the results of testing may recommend specific therapy that is both available and desirable. In other words, determination of a digoxin level potentially would be useful since a dosage reduction can be instituted, but findings of elevated levels of calcium or creatinine would be unlikely to result in other than symptomatic treatment (antiemetics, reassurance).

Multiple antiemetics are available and of potential clinical use, and, as with analgesics, it may be necessary to rotate or combine agents when symptoms persists. The oral route is preferred when possible, due to ease of administration. Suppositories, transdermal, and continuous subcutaneous administration are important alternatives when the oral route is ineffective. Beside the usual prochlorperazine and thiethylperazine, haloperidol and chlorpromazine have special usefulness in the terminal patient.

Haloperidol has the advantage of serving more than one use. It has excellent antiemetic properties, is useful to control agitation and hallucinations, and is an anxiolytic. It is available in tablet, concentrated liquid, and parenteral form. There are anecdotal reports of using haloperidol by continuous subcutaneous infusion.[6]

Chlorpromazine has the same multiple indications as haloperidol, is available in suppository form, and also is useful for hiccups.

Metoclopramide is beneficial in the presence of delayed gastric emptying, and has the advantage of being useful for continuous subcutaneous administration when other treatments have failed to relieve the nausea.[7]

Prednisone 10–20 mg/day reduces nausea and stimulates appetite in selected patients.

Transdermal scopolamine can reduce nausea, especially if there is associated vertigo. If side effects such as sedation or excessively dry mouth occur, the dose should be reduced carefully, in which case it is necessary to remove the hexagonal plastic cover. Cut the cover in half and discard half, replacing the remainder over the patch so only half is exposed. The patch with cover piece is adhered to the patient's skin, usually behind an ear. If the disk itself is cut, the controlled delivery system may be disrupted.[8]

NUTRITION AND HYDRATION

One of the most difficult situations for patients and especially their families occurs when the terminally ill person can no longer eat or drink (see Chapter 13), an event that can be regarded as tangible evidence of impending death. Food and love are interconnected in our society, and the healthy may unconsciously feel rejected by the ill person's failure to thrive. Family members also may feel helpless and that they are not doing enough for the patient. Gentle explanation that these events are expected, combined with instruction about mouth care, usually ease the anxiety of this transition. Frequent mouth care (see Chapter 13) is critical to patient comfort,[9] and engages the family in an active role, generally obviating the feeling that they must feed the patient. If the family remains uncomfortable, it usually is helpful to return to discussions of the goal-oriented approach to care. Interventions such as feeding tubes and intravenous hydration generally are not favored in hospice care, but are common subjects of families' interest. It is useful to consider these options in light of the trade-offs they represent. The maintenance of peripheral venous access often is difficult, and requires multiple restarts. Placement and maintenance of a nasogastric tube usually is regarded as uncomfortable, and introduces risks of aspiration. A restless or confused patient is likely to pull out tubes or lines, adding further discomfort to the patient and anxiety for the family. Conversely, as oral intake declines, production of urine and stool and resorption of third-

space fluids also decline, often with greater consequent comfort. Explanation of these trade-offs should be provided to the family, and to the patient if he or she still is capable of making decisions for himself or herself.

Since many coanalgesics are available only in oral formulations, both the patient and family need permission to eliminate them from the regimen as the patient becomes more debilitated and cannot swallow readily. The same applies to other oral medications such as chronic cardiac or diabetic medication. Decreased oral intake makes diabetic medications unnecessary, and decreased activity reduces the need for antianginal agents.

CHANGES IN MENTAL STATUS/ TERMINAL RESTLESSNESS

As death approaches, some patients become agitated and/or restless. A variety of conditions can contribute to this state, including unrelieved pain and medications such as opioid analgesics. This is another distressing symptom for family and care providers to witness. It is important to attempt to distinguish restlessness that is uncomfortable to the patient from restlessness that merely is distressful for those around him. The former requires urgent intervention, usually with an agent such as haloperidol or chlorpromazine. In the latter case, explanations and continued open communication and support may be of great benefit. If a restless patient is not eating and has no coherent wakeful periods, or has wakeful periods that are dominated by pain, nausea, or anxiety, sedation may be the most compassionate alternative. This should be implemented after discussing the goal of sedation with the patient, if possible, and with the family.

DYSPNEA

Dyspnea (see Chapter 13) is distressing to the patient and to caregivers. When further physical measures, such as repositioning or the use of fans, fail to provide relief or are too cumbersome, it often is necessary to provide low-dose morphine or an alternative opioid to ease air hunger. Bruera[10] has shown that although there are no significant changes in pO_2, pCO_2, or the respiratory rate, patients' subjective sense of well-being improves, and the family is more at ease. A related problem is the so-called death rattle, associated with inability to clear oral secretions. Although explanation helps the family, it is useful to employ transdermal scopolamine to dry the secretions and decrease sonorous breathing sounds. Suctioning often is ineffective and frightening, and should not be implemented if avoidable.

CONSTIPATION

An effective prophylactic bowel regimen (see Chapters 12 and 13) should be prescribed for all patients taking opioid analgesics chronically. Constipation increases nausea and is inherently uncomfortable. In the relatively fit individual, the first lines of defense against constipation are increased activity and fluids coupled with dietary measures to increase roughage. Standard agents include docusate with or without senna, lactulose, milk of magnesia, and bisacodyl tablets or suppositories. Enemas and digital disimpaction may be required, particularly when cord compression or other neurologic involvement prevents the patient from being aware of the urge to defecate. Education for both patient and caregivers is vital for prevention and treatment of constipation.

There are several excellent handbooks with additional suggestions for specific symptom management.[9,11–13]

INTERDISCIPLINARY CARE

The prospect of providing good symptom relief as well as psychological and spiritual support for dying people and their loved ones would be daunting if it were not shared among a team of caregivers. Ideally, a team consisting of a registered hospice nurse, social worker, pastoral care counselor, coordinator of volunteer services, and hospice medical director monitors the ongoing care of each patient. Generally, the patient's own physician continues to have direct patient responsibility, along with a designated hospice nurse. Continued involvement of a physician, either in the office or on home visits, is immensely comforting to patients and their families. Other services often available through hospice programs are dietary and financial counseling, physical and occupational therapy, and involvement of a clinical pharmacist.

The medical director is available as a teacher and advisor to the team and as a resource to the attending physician. The hospice nurse visits the patient frequently at home, and communicates physical changes to the attending physician, implementing treatment ordered by the attending physician. The pastoral counselor provides nondenominational support to the patient and family regarding the search for meaning and connectedness during the dying process. He or she also acts as liaison to individual churches as required by patients. The social worker provides emotional counseling, and offers both the patient and family the opportunity to address, communicate, and, if possible, resolve emotional concerns. This interdisciplinary approach permits each team member to better identify issues of all types, and to have ready access to the skills of other professionals.

Although not usually considered formally as team members, the family plays a central role in direct support for the patient. In this context, family encompasses any significant person in the life of the dying person. Hospice programs in the United States developed as home care programs, and continue both philosophically and by regulation to promote care at home. The professional staff provides expert supervision and instruction; the volunteer staff provides personal attention or errand running; and, when required, home health aides assist in personal care. These individuals are facilitators for the family rather than substitutes. There are times when 24-

hour care in an inpatient setting becomes necessary. These times would include rapidly changing symptoms, overwhelming family stress, respite for the family, family teaching, and for some, the terminal period may require inpatient management.

Care of the hospice family does not end with the death of the patient. Formal bereavement programs are an important component of the hospice concept. Immediate help at the time of death is followed with continuing contact at intervals over the first year. If a family is identified as having extra difficulty, referral to community agencies or private counseling is advised and facilitated.

SUMMARY

Caring for people in the final stages of a terminal illness can be both challenging and rewarding. The necessary skills include a compassionate nature, knowledge of medications and other measures to relieve an array of symptoms, as well as the ability to be flexible. Symptoms such as pain, nausea, dyspnea, and restlessness must be resolved to permit emotional and spiritual issues to be addressed. The work involves communication with the patient, the family, and a team of caregivers. It is important to define goals at each step of treatment and at each phase of the patient's physical decline. Hospice seeks neither to prolong dying nor to hasten death, but rather to ease the path and to comfort the bereaved.

REFERENCES

1. Reuben DB, Mor V, Hiris J: Clinical symptoms and length of survival in patients with terminal cancer. Arch Intern Med 1988;148:1586.

1a. Doyle D: Education and training in palliative care. J Pall Care 1987;2:5.

2. Hillier ER, Lunt B: Goal setting in terminal cancer. In Twycross RG, Ventafridda V (eds): The Continuing Care of Terminal Cancer Patients, p 271. Oxford, Pergamon Press, 1979.

2a. Forster LE, Lynn J: Predicting life span for applicants to inpatient hospice. Arch Intern Med 1988;148:2540.

3. Twycross RG: Hospice care: Redressing the balance in medicine. J R Soc Med 1980;73:475.

4. Kaiko RF, Healy N, Pav GB et al: The comparative bioavailability of MS Contin tablets (controlled release oral morphine) following rectal and oral administration. In Twycross RG (ed): The Edinburgh Symposium on Pain Control and Medical Education, p 235. London, Society of Medical Services Ltd., 1989.

5. Maloney CM, Kesner K, Klein G et al: The rectal administration of MS Contin: Clinical implications of use in end stage cancer. American Journal of Hospice Care, 1989;6:34.

6. Storey P, Hill H, St Louis R et al: Subcutaneous infusions for control of cancer symptoms. Journal of Pain and Symptom Management 1990;5:33.

7. Bruera E, Michaud M, Partington J et al: Continuous subcutaneous (sc) infusion of metoclopramide (MCP) using a plastic disposable infusor for the treatment of chemotherapy-induced emesis. Journal of Pain and Symptom Management 1988;3:105.

8. Osier C: Communication to the New York State Hospice Association, April, 1990.

9. Twycross RG, Lack S; Therapeutics in Terminal Cancer. New York, Churchill Livingstone, 1990.

10. Bruera E, Macmillan K, Pither J et al: Effects of morphine on the dyspnea of terminal cancer patients. Journal of Pain and Symptom Management 1990;5:341.

11. Billings JA: Outpatient Management of Advanced Cancer. Philadelphia, JB Lippincott, 1985.

12. Saunders C, Baines M: Living with Dying: The Management of Terminal Disease. New York, Oxford University Press, 1989.

13. Walsh TD (ed): Symptom Control. Blackwell Scientific Pub, 1989.

Appendix A

Pain Assessment Tools

Figure A-1. Brief Pain Inventory. A reliable means for assessing patients with cancer pain. Requires about 15 minutes to complete. May be self-administered or administered by interviewer. See text for details. (Reprinted with permission of the Pain Research Group, Department of Neurology, University of Wisconsin-Madison Medical School.)

DO NOT WRITE ABOVE THIS LINE

Brief Pain Inventory

Date: __ / __ / __

Name: _____ _____ _____
                     Last   First   Middle Initial

Phone: (__) _____   Sex: ☐ Female   ☐ Male

Date of Birth: __ / __ / __

1) Marital Status (at present)

    1. ☐ Single   3. ☐ Widowed

    2. ☐ Married   4. ☐ Separated/Divorced

2) Education (Circle only the highest grade or degree completed)

Grade   0   1   2   3   4   5   6   7   8   9

           10 11 12 13 14 15 16 M.A./M.S.

Professional degree (please specify)

3) Current occupation _____
(specify titles; if you are not working, tell us your previous occupation)

4) Spouse's Occupation _____

5) Which of the following best describes your current job status?

    ☐ 1. Employed outside the home, full-time
    ☐ 2. Employed outside the home, part-time
    ☐ 3. Homemaker
    ☐ 4. Retired
    ☐ 5. Unemployed
    ☐ 6. Other

6) How long has it been since you first learned your diagnosis ? [_____] months

7) Have you ever had pain due to your present disease?

    1. ☐ Yes   2. ☐ No   3. ☐ Uncertain

Figure A-1. (*Continued*)

8) When you first received your diagnosis, was pain one of your symptoms?

      1. ☐ Yes   2. ☐ No   3. ☐ Uncertain

9) Have you had surgery in the past month?   1. ☐ Yes   2. ☐ No

10) Throughout our lives, most of us have had pain from time to time (such as minor headaches, sprains, and toothaches). Have you had pain other than these everyday kinds of pain during the last week?

      1. ☐ Yes   2. ☐ No

IF YOU ANSWERED YES TO THE LAST QUESTION, PLEASE GO ON TO QUESTION 11 AND FINISH THIS QUESTIONNAIRE. IF NO, YOU ARE FINISHED WITH THE QUESTIONNAIRE. THANK YOU.

11) On the diagram, shade in the areas where you feel pain. Put an X on the area that hurts the most.

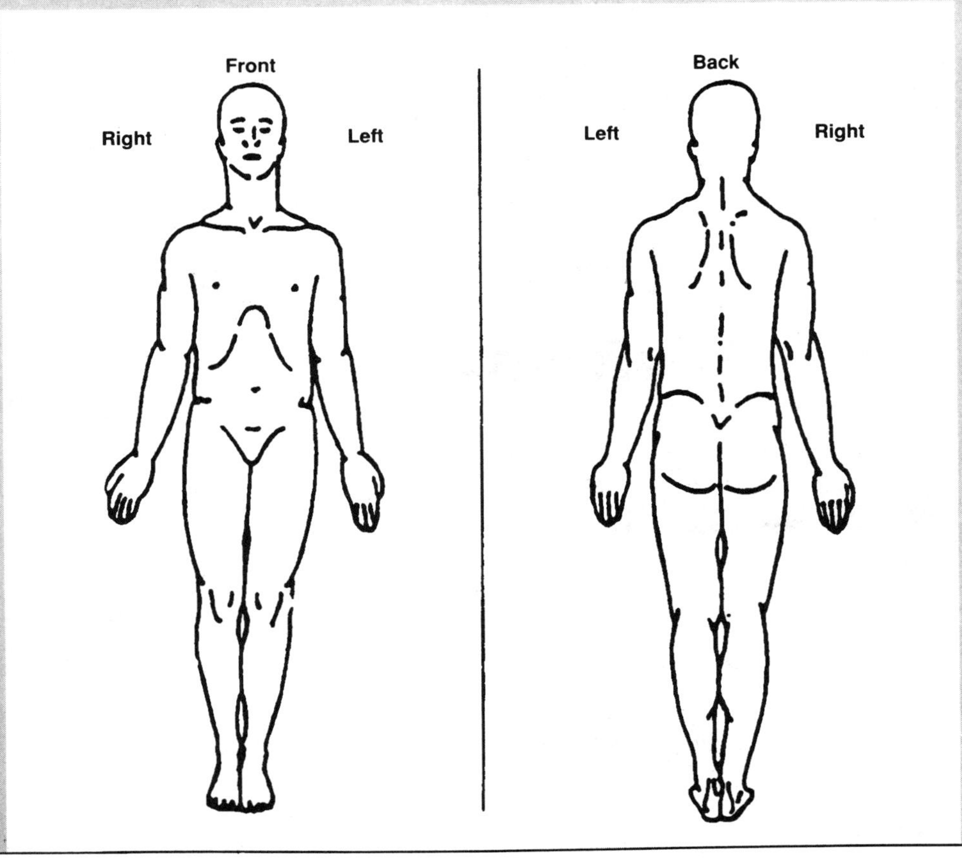

Figure A-1. (*Continued*)

556

12) Please rate your pain by circling the one number that best describes your pain at its `worst` in the last week.

0	1	2	3	4	5	6	7	8	9	10
No Pain										Pain as bad as you can imagine

13) Please rate your pain by circling the one number that best describes your pain at its `least` in the last week.

0	1	2	3	4	5	6	7	8	9	10
No Pain										Pain as bad as you can imagine

14) Please rate your pain by circling the one number that best describes your pain on the `average`.

0	1	2	3	4	5	6	7	8	9	10
No Pain										Pain as bad as you can imagine

15) Please rate your pain by circling the one number that tells how much pain you have `right now.`

0	1	2	3	4	5	6	7	8	9	10
No Pain										Pain as bad as you can imagine

16) What kinds of things make your pain feel better (for example, heat, medicine, rest?)

_____

_____

17) What kinds of things make your pain worse (for example, walking, standing, lifting?)

_____

_____

18) What treatments or medications are you receiving for your pain?

_____

_____

19) In the last week, how much relief have pain treatments or medications provided? Please circle the one percentage that most shows how much relief you have received.

0%	10%	20%	30%	40%	50%	60%	70%	80%	90%	100%
No Relief										Complete Relief

Figure A-1. (*Continued*)

20) If you take pain medication, how many hours does it take before the pain returns?

□ 1. Pain medication doesn't help at all.   □ 5. Four hours.

□ 2. One hour.   □ 6. Five to twelve hours.

□ 3. Two hours.   □ 7. More than twelve hours.

□ 4. Three hours.   □ 8. I do not take pain medication.

21) Circle the appropriate answer for each item.
I believe my pain is due to:

Yes □ No □ 1. The effects of treatment (for example, medication, surgery, radiation, prosthetic device).

Yes □ No □ 2. My primary disease (meaning the disease currently being treated and evaluated).

Yes □ No □ 3. A medical condition unrelated to primary disease (for example, arthritis)

22) For each of the following words, check yes or no if that adjective applies to your pain.

Aching	□ Yes	□ No
Throbbing	□ Yes	□ No
Shooting	□ Yes	□ No
Stabbing	□ Yes	□ No
Gnawing	□ Yes	□ No
Sharp	□ Yes	□ No
Tender	□ Yes	□ No
Burning	□ Yes	□ No
Exhausting	□ Yes	□ No
Tiring	□ Yes	□ No
Penetrating	□ Yes	□ No
Nagging	□ Yes	□ No
Numb	□ Yes	□ No
Miserable	□ Yes	□ No
Unbearable	□ Yes	□ No

Figure A-1. *(Continued)*

23) Circle the one number that describes how, during the past week, pain has interfered with your:

A. General Activity

0	1	2	3	4	5	6	7	8	9	10

Does not interfere

Completely interferes

B. Mood

0	1	2	3	4	5	6	7	8	9	10

Does not interfere

Completely interferes

C. Walking ability

0	1	2	3	4	5	6	7	8	9	10

Does not interfere

Completely interferes

D. Normal work (includes both work outside the home and housework)

0	1	2	3	4	5	6	7	8	9	10

Does not interfere

Completely interferes

E. Relations with other people

0	1	2	3	4	5	6	7	8	9	10

Does not interfere

Completely interferes

F. Sleep

0	1	2	3	4	5	6	7	8	9	10

Does not interfere

Completely interferes

G. Enjoyment of life

0	1	2	3	4	5	6	7	8	9	10

Does not interfere

Completely interferes

Pain Research Group
Department of Neurology
University of Wisconsin-Madison

Figure A-1. (*Continued*)

DO NOT WRITE ABOVE THIS LINE

Brief Pain Inventory (Short Form)

Date: ___/___/___   Time: _____

Name: _____
         Last   First   Middle Initial

1) Throughout our lives, most of us have had pain from time to time (such as minor headaches, sprains, and toothaches). Have you had pain other than these everyday kinds of pain today?

   1.   Yes   2.   No

2) On the diagram, shade in the areas where you feel pain. Put an X on the area that hurts the most.

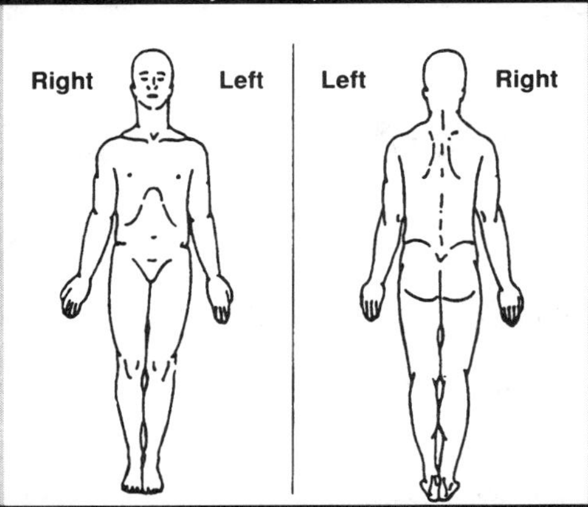

Right [face] Left   Left   Right

3) Please rate your pain by circling the one number that best describes your pain at its **worst** in the last 24 hours.

0	1	2	3	4	5	6	7	8	9	10
No Pain										Pain as bad as you can imagine

4) Please rate your pain by circling the one number that best describes your pain at its **least** in the last 24 hours.

0	1	2	3	4	5	6	7	8	9	10
No Pain										Pain as bad as you can imagine

5) Please rate your pain by circling the one number that best describes your pain on the **average.**

0	1	2	3	4	5	6	7	8	9	10
No Pain										Pain as bad as you can imagine

6) Please rate your pain by circling the one number that tells how much pain you have **right now.**

0	1	2	3	4	5	6	7	8	9	10
No Pain										Pain as bad as you can imagine

Figure A-2. Brief Pain Inventory (short form). See text for details. (Reprinted with permission of the Pain Research Group, Department of Neurology, University of Wisconsin-Madison Medical School.)

7) What treatments or medications are you receiving for your pain?

_____

8) In the last 24 hours, how much relief have pain treatments or medications provided? Please circle the one percentage that most shows how much relief you have received.

| 0% | 10% | 20% | 30% | 40% | 50% | 60% | 70% | 80% | 90% | 100% |
| No Relief | | | | | | | | | | Complete Relief |

9) Circle the one number that describes how, during the past 24 hours, pain has interfered with your:

A. General Activity

| 0 | 1 | 2 | 3 | 4 | 5 | 6 | 7 | 8 | 9 | 10 |
| Does not interfere | | | | | | | | | | Completely interferes |

B. Mood

| 0 | 1 | 2 | 3 | 4 | 5 | 6 | 7 | 8 | 9 | 10 |
| Does not interfere | | | | | | | | | | Completely interferes |

C. Walking ability

| 0 | 1 | 2 | 3 | 4 | 5 | 6 | 7 | 8 | 9 | 10 |
| Does not interfere | | | | | | | | | | Completely interferes |

D. Normal work (includes both work outside the home and housework)

| 0 | 1 | 2 | 3 | 4 | 5 | 6 | 7 | 8 | 9 | 10 |
| Does not interfere | | | | | | | | | | Completely interferes |

E. Relations with other people

| 0 | 1 | 2 | 3 | 4 | 5 | 6 | 7 | 8 | 9 | 10 |
| Does not interfere | | | | | | | | | | Completely interferes |

F. Sleep

| 0 | 1 | 2 | 3 | 4 | 5 | 6 | 7 | 8 | 9 | 10 |
| Does not interfere | | | | | | | | | | Completely interferes |

G. Enjoyment of life

| 0 | 1 | 2 | 3 | 4 | 5 | 6 | 7 | 8 | 9 | 10 |
| Does not interfere | | | | | | | | | | Completely interferes |

Pain Research Group
Department of Neurology
University of Wisconsin-Madison

Figure A-2. (*Continued*)

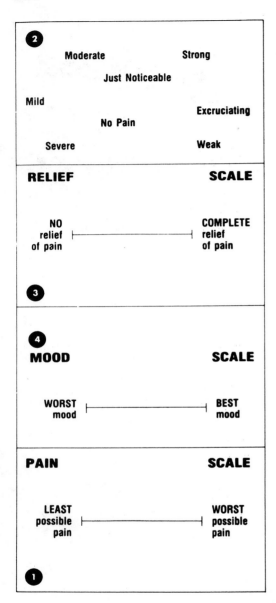

Figure A-3. Memorial Pain Assessment Card. A simple, efficient, and valid assessment instrument that provides rapid evaluation, in clinical settings, of the major aspects of pain experienced by cancer patients. It is easy to understand and use, and can be completed by experienced patients in less than 20 seconds. It consists of a two-sided 8 1/2″ × 11″ card that is folded so that four separate measures are created. See text for details. (Reprinted with permission of the Department of Neurology, Memorial Sloan Kettering Cancer Center.)

Appendix B

Where to Obtain Instruments Used in Assessing Pediatric Pain

The Oucher

Judith E. Beyer, RN, PhD, Associate Professor, University of Colorado Health Sciences Center, School of Nursing, Campus Box C-288, 4200 East Ninth Avenue, Denver, CO 80262. (303) 270-4317

Eland's Color Tool

JoAnn Eland, RN, PhD, Associate Professor, School of Nursing, University of Iowa, 316 Nursing Building, Iowa City, IA 52242. (319) 351-7146

Poker Chip Tool

Nancy O. Hester, RN, PhD, Associate Professor, University of Colorado Health Sciences Center, School of Nursing, Campus Box C-288, 4200 East Ninth Avenue, Denver, CO 80262. (303) 270-8664

Varni/Thompson

James Varni, PhD, Behavioral Pediatrics Program, Orthopaedic Hospital, 2400 S. Flower Street, Los Angeles, CA 90007.

McGrath Faces

Patricia A. McGrath, PhD, Director, Pain Programme, Child Health Research Institute, Children's Hospital of Western Ontario, London, Ontario, Canada N6C 2V5.

Gustave-Roussy Child Pain Scale

Annie Gauvain-Piquard, MD, Psychiatry and Psycho-Oncology Unit, Gustave-Roussy Institute, Rue Camille Desmoulins, 94805 Villejuif, France.

CHEOPS

Patrick J. McGrath, PhD, Department of Psychology, Dalhousie University, Halifax, Nova Scotia, Canada B3H 4J1.

OSBD-Revised

Susan M. Jay, PhD, Psychosocial Program, Division of Hematology-Oncology, Children's Hospital of Los Angeles, 4650 Sunset Boulevard, Los Angeles, CA 90027.

Modified Frankl Behavior Rating Scale

Marion E. Broome, PhD, Maternal-Child Nursing, Rush Presbyterian, St. Luke's Medical Center, Chicago, IL 60612.

The Faces Pain Scale: Bieri, et al

Dr. G. David Champion, MB, BS, FRACP, St. Vincent's Clinic, Level 9, Suite 903, 438 Victoria Street, Darlinghurst, NW 2010, Australia.

Maunuksela Scales

Eeva-Liisa Maunuksela, MD, The Children's Hospital, University of Helsinki, Stenbäckinkatu 11, SF-00290, Helsinki, Finland.

Appendix C

Pharmacotherapeutic Guidelines

Richard B. Patt
James E. Szalados
Christopher L. Wu

Table C-1.
Guidelines for the Use of Opioid Analgesics in Patients with Chronic Cancer Pain (Moderate to Severe)*

Pure (morphine-like) Agonists			Equian-algesic Dose§	Recommended Schedule**	Form-ulations†	Comments, Toxicity††
Generic Name	Trade Name†	Route‡				
Immediate release morphine	MSIR Roxanol	oral	30–60 mg***	2–4 hr	15,30 mg 2 mg/ml 4 mg/ml 20 mg/ml	1,2
Controlled release morphine	MS Contin Oromorph	oral	30–60 mg	12–8 hr	15,30,60, 100 mg	2,3
Morphine		I.M.	10 mg	2–4 hr	various	2,4
Morphine	RMS	rectal	5 mg		5,10,20	—
Hydromorphone	Dilaudid	oral	7.5 mg	2–4 hr	1,2,3,4 mg	5
Hydromorphone	Dilaudid	I.M.	1.5 mg	2–4 hr	1,2,4,10 mg/ml	5
Hydromorphone	Dilaudid	rectal	7.5 mg	3–6 hr	3 mg	5
Meperidine	Demerol Pethedine	P.O.	300 mg	2–4 hr	50,100 50 mg/5 ml	6
Meperidine	Demerol Pethedine	I.M.	75 mg	2–4 hr	various	6
Diamorphine	Heroin	oral	60 mg	—	—	7
Diamorphine	Heroin	I.M.	5 mg	—	—	7
Methadone	Dolophine	oral	20 mg	4–12 hr	5,10,40 mg 1,2,10 mg/ml	8
Methadone	Dolophine	I.M.	10 mg	4–12 hr	10 mg/ml	8
Levorphanol	Levodromoran	oral	4 mg	4–8 hr	2 mg	9
Levorphanol	Levodromoran	I.M.	2 mg	4–8 hr	2 mg/ml	9
Oxymorphone	Numorphan	I.M.	1 mg	3–6 hr	1 or 1.5 mg/ml	10
Oxymorphone	Numorphan	rectal	5–10 mg	3–6 hr	5 mg	
	Brompton's Cocktail	oral	—	—	—	11
Propoxyphene	Darvon See Table C-2	oral	65–130 mg	4–6 hr	Table C-2	12
Codeine	See Table C-2	oral	200 mg	3–6 hr	15,30,60 mg Table C-2	13,14
Codeine		I.M.	130 mg	same	30 mg/ml	13,14
Oxycodone	Roxycodone See Table C-2	oral	20–30 mg	3–6 hr	5 mg 1,20 mg/ml	15
Hydrocodone	See Table C-2	oral	—	4–6 hr	—	13
Dihydrocodeine	See Table C-2		—	—	—	13
Fentanyl	Sublimaze	I.V.	0.1 mg	continuous	50 μg/ml	16
Fentanyl	Duragesic	T.D.	0.1 mg	72–48 hr	25,50,75 & 100 μg/hr	17
Sufentanil	Sufenta	I.V.	.15 mg	—	50 μg/ml	16
Alfentanil	Alfenta	I.V.	.75 mg	—	500 μg/ml	16

(continued)

Table C-1.
(*Continued*)

Generic Name	Trade Name†	Route‡	Equian-algesic Dose§	Recommended Schedule**	Form-ulations†	Comments, Toxicity††
Partial Agonists						
Buprenorphine	Buprenex	I.M.	0.4 mg	4–6 hr	0.3 mg/ml	18,19
Buprenorphine	Temgesic	S.L.	0.8 mg	6 hr		18,19
Dezocine	Dalgan	I.M.	10 mg	3–4 hr	5–15 mg/ml	20,21
Mixed Agonists/Antagonists						
Butorphanol	Stadol	I.M.	2–2.5 mg	3–4 hr	1 mg/ml	18,21
Pentazocine	Talwin	oral	180 mg	3–4 hr	50 mg	18,22
Pentazocine	Talwin	I.M.	60 mg	3–4 hr	30 mg/ml	18
Nalbuphine	Nubain	I.M.	10 mg	3–6 hr	10 mg/ml	18,21

* See text for complete explanation.

† Listing is partial, comprised primarily of formulations available in the United States. In mg unless stated otherwise.

‡ For parenteral routes, only the most commonly used route is listed, although most agents can be administered either intramuscularly, subcutaneously, or intravenously.

§ Dose that provides analgesia equivalent to 10 mg intramuscular morphine. Equianalgesic doses are based on values most frequently cited in the literature and on clinical findings, although these sometimes conflict. They are approximate and are intended to serve as guidelines only.

** This is intended as a rough guide only. It is hoped that this characterization will be maximally useful to the clinician. Discussions of half-life, peak, and duration appear in the text and in recommended readings.

†† Potential toxicity for all agents includes constipation, sedation, dysphoria, confusion, hallucinations, nausea, vomiting, respiratory depression (rare in tolerant patients), urinary retention, itching. Toxicity profile varies from patient-to-patient and from agent-to-agent, often even in the same patient (incomplete cross tolerance).

*** See comment 3, below.

1. Usually recommended as the first drug of choice for moderate to severe cancer pain. Best oral to parenteral conversion ratio is controversial. Single dose studies suggest a 6:1 ratio (6 mg oral morphine = 1 mg parenteral morphine), but clinical experience has shown that, administered chronically, a 2 or 3:1 ratio is more applicable.

2. Despite single-dose studies that suggest an IM:PO conversion ratio of 1:6, clinical experience that suggests a ratio of 2–3:1 with chronic use are generally considered more applicable.

3. Timed release mechanism is employed to provide slow absorption and consequently, long dosing interval. May result in more consistent blood levels and hence more consistent analgesia with fewer episodes of "breakthrough pain." Extremely useful as basal analgesic; good compliance because of convenient dosing schedule. Usually supplemented with "rescue doses" of shorter acting agents for breakthrough pain. Cannot be broken, crushed, or chewed. Anecdotal reports of good, consistent analgesia with rectal, vaginal, and stomal use.

4. Prototypical pure agonist opioid; standard against which other agents are compared.

5. Relatively rapid in onset, short in duration, particularly effective for breakthrough pain. Due to its high solubility, parenteral form is often used in high concentrations to limit the administered volume in patients needing high dose subcutaneous opioid therapy.

6. Useful for acute pain, not recommended for chronic use (especially in patients with renal failure) due to short duration of effect, poor oral bioavailability and potential for CNS toxicity (myoclonus, seizures) due to accumulation of metabolite,normeperidine.

7. Unavailable in the United States; analgesic action due primarily to action of metabolites. Due to its high solubility, parenteral form is sometimes used in high concentrations to limit the administered volume in selected patients needing high dose subcutaneous opioid therapy. A controlled study found no differences in analgesia between parenteral hydromorphone and parenteral heroin.

(continued)

Table C-1.
(*Continued*)

8. As a result of long half life (15–57 hrs) has the potential to accumulate and produce sedation, and respiratory depression, particularly in the elderly and in individuals with decreased renal function. Should be administered initially prn.
9. See comments on methadone.
10. No oral formulation available.
11. Conceived of at Brompton's Hospital in U.K. Usually consists of morphine hydrochloride (15 mg), cocaine hydrochloride (15 mg), 90% alcohol (2 ml), syrup (4 ml), chlorophorm water (15 ml). Studies show no benefits over oral opioids alone; use should therefore be discouraged.
12. Traditionally used for mild pain, often combined with aspirin or acetaminophen (see Table 2). Available as propoxyphene hydrochloride or napsylate. Although toxic metabolite may accumulate with high doses used chronically, this is rarely a problem with doses used clinically.
13. For mild to moderate pain, traditionally administered as combined product with aspirin or acetaminophen (see Table C-2).
14. Despite probable equianalgesia at this dose, single doses of this magnitude are undesirable because of the likelihood of toxicity.
15. For mild to moderate pain, traditionally marketed as combined product with aspirin or acetaminophen (see Table C-2). Recently made available without coanalgesic.
16. Not available orally; used primarily as a component of anesthesia or in intensive care setting. Chest wall rigidity may occur when large doses are administered rapidly. May be used by the intraspinal route.
17. Once steady state is achieved, characteristics of delivery system result in even blood levels of analgesic for about 72 hr. After first administration or dose increment, plasma concentration slowly rises to steady state levels, which are usually achieved by 24 hours. Depending on the minimal effective concentration for a given individual, hours or days may be required to achieve analgesia. Adverse effects may persist for 8–12 hr after system is removed due to formation of a skin depot. Extremely useful as a long acting basal analgesic, particularly in noncompliant patients, in individuals with difficulty swallowing, and in patients for whom frequent requirements to take analgesics represent a discouraging reminder of the status of their illness.
18. Same potential toxicities as pure opioid agonists with the addition of potential for withdrawal/abstinence syndrome in opioid dependent patients, and greater propensity for psychomimetic side effects. Probable ceiling dose for analgesia. In general, the use of the partial agonist and mixed agonist/antagonist agents are not preferred in patients with cancer pain.
19. Sublingual form not currently available in U.S. Probable ceiling effect for analgesia. Unlike other similar agents, may have role in management of cancer pain.
20. Recently introduced, clinical experience limited. Probably a partial agonist.
21. No oral formulation.
22. Psychomimetic side effects prominent. Marketed in the U.S. combined with naloxone to reduce potential abuse.

Table C-2.
Commonly Available Formulations of Combined Analgesics

Codeine Combinations

Empirin with codeine
  aspirin 325 mg plus codeine phosphate
    #2—15 mg, #3—30 mg, #4—60 mg
Empracet with codeine
  acetaminophen 300 mg plus codeine phosphate
    #2—15 mg, #3—30 mg, #4—60 mg
Phenaphen with codeine/Phenaphen-650 with
  codeine
  acetaminophen 300 or 650 mg plus codeine
  phosphate
    #2—15 mg, #3—30 mg, #4—60 mg
Tylenol with codeine (also available as elixir)
  acetaminophen 300 mg plus codeine phosphate
    #1—7.5 mg, #2—15 mg, #3—30 mg,
    #4—60 mg

Hydrocodone Combinations

Vicodin
  acetaminophen 500 mg, hydrocodone bitartrate
  5 mg
Vicodin ES
  acetaminophen 750 mg, hydrocodone bitartrate
  7.5 mg
Bancap HC, Hydrocet, Hy-phen
  acetaminophen 500 mg, hydrocodone bitartrate
  5 mg
Co-gesic
  acetaminophen 500 mg, hydrocodone bitartrate
  5 mg

Oxycodone Combinations

Roxicet
  acetaminophen 325 mg, oxycodone 5 mg
  acetaminophen 325 mg, oxycodone 5 mg per 5 ml
Percodan
  aspirin 325 mg
  oxycodone hydrochloride 4.5 mg, oxycodone
  terepthalate—0.38 mg
Percodan-demi
  aspirin 325 mg
  oxycodone hydrochloride 2.25 mg, oxycodone
  terepthalate—0.19 mg
Tylox
  acetaminophen 500 mg, oxycodone hydrochloride
  5 mg
Percocet
  acetaminophen 325 mg, oxycodone hydrochloride
  5 mg

Propoxyphene Combinations

Darvon with ASA
  aspirin 325 mg, propoxyphene hydrochloride
  65 mg
Darvon-N with ASA
  aspirin 325 mg, propoxyphene napsylate 100 mg
Darvon Compound/Darvon Compound-65
  aspirin 389 mg, caffeine 32.4 mg
  propoxyphene hydrochloride 32/65 mg
Darvocet-N 50/Darvocet-N 100
  acetaminophen 325 mg/650 mg, propoxyphene
  napsylate 50 mg/100 mg
Wygesic
  acetaminophen 650 mg, propoxyphene
  hydrochloride 65 mg

Meperidine Combinations

Mepergan Fortis
  promethazine hydrochloride 25 mg, meperidine
  hydrochloride 50 mg

Pentazocine Compounds

Talwin Compound
  aspirin 325 mg, pentazocine hydrochloride
  12.5 mg
Talacen
  acetaminophen 650 mg, pentazocine
  hydrochloride 25 mg
Talwin Nx
  pentazocine hydrochloride 25 mg, naloxone
  hydrochloride 0.5 mg

Dihydrocodeine Combinations

Synalgos-DC
  aspirin 356.4 mg, caffeine 30 mg, dihydrocodeine
  bitartrate 16 mg

Table C-3.
Nonsteroidal Anti-inflammatory Drugs

Generic Name and Class*	Trade Name†	Approx. Half Life (hr)	Dosing Schedule	Recommended Starting Dose (mg/day)‡	Maximum Recommended Dose (mg/day)	Comments, Toxicity§**
Para-aminophenol Derivatives						
Acetaminophen	Tylenol, Datril, Panadol	2–4	q 4–6 hr	2600	6000	1
Salicylates						
Acetylsalicylic acid	Aspirin, etc	3–12	q 4–6 hr	2600	6000	2
Choline magnesium trisalicylate	Trilisate	8–12	q 8–12 hr	1500 × 1 then 500 q 12	4000	3
Salsalate	Disalcid	8–12	q 8–12 hr	1500 × 1 then 500 q 12	4000	3
Diflunisal	Dolobid, Dolobis	8–12	q 12 hr	1000 × 1 then 500 q 12	1500	4
Pyrazolon Derivatives						
Phenylbutazone	Butazoladin, Antadol, Phebuzine	50–100	q 6–8 hr	300	400	5
Oxyphenbutazone	Tandearil, Rapostan, Rheumapax, Oxalid	50–100	q 6–8 hr	300	400	6
Acetic Acid Derivatives						
Indomethacin	Indocin, Indocid, Indomethine	4–5	q 8–12 hr	75	200	7
Sulindac	Clinoril, Arthrobid	14	q 12 hr	300	400	8
Tolmetin	Tolectin	1	q 6–8 hr	600	2000	
Ketorolac	Toradol	4–7	q 4–6 hr	120	240	
Suprofen		2–4	q 6 hr	600	800	9
Fenamates						
Mefenamic acid	Ponstel, Ponstan, Ponstil, Namphen	2	q 6 hr	4	1000	10
Meclofenamate sodium	Meclomen	2–4	q 6–8 hr	150	400	11
Proprionic Acid Derivatives						
Ibuprofen	Motrin, Advil, Nuprin, Rufen	3–4	q 4–8 hr	1200	4200	12
Naproxen	Naprosyn, Naprosine, Proxen	13	q 12 hr	500	1000	13
Fenoprofen	Nalfon, Fenopran, Nalgesic, Progesic	2–3	q 6 hr	800	3200	
Ketoprofen	Orudis, Alrheumat	2–3	q 6–8 hr	150	300	
Flurbiprofen	Ansaid	5–6	q 8–12 hr	100	300	
Diclofenac	Voltaren	2	q 6 hr	75	200	
Oxicams						
Piroxicam	Feldene	45	q 24 hr	20	40	14

(continued)

Table C-3.
(Continued)

Pyranocarboxylic Acids						
Etodolac	Lodine	7.3	q 6–8 hr	800	1200	15
Naphthylalkanones						
Nabumetone	Relafen	22–30	q 12–24 hr	1000	2000	15

* Various schema of chemical classification have been advanced.

† Predominantly U.S. trade names.

‡ It is recommended to reduce the normal starting dose by 1/2 to 2/3 in patients who are elderly, on multiple medications or in the presence of renal impairment. If clinical effects are inadequate, initial doses should be titrated upwards as tolerated, usually on a weekly basis. Studies of the NSAIDs in cancer patients are meager and as a result, dosing guidelines are empiric.

§ All agents (except in some cases acetaminophen) are associated with a variety of potential toxicities, the most prominent of which is gastrointestinal. Other potential adverse effects include hemorrhage, confusion, renal impairment, hepatic dysfunction, bronchospasm, rash and allergy. See text for greater detail.

** At high doses, prudence dictates that stool should be checked every two weeks for blood; liver function tests, BUN, creatinine, and urinalysis should be performed every 1–2 months.

1. Available over-the-counter in various preparations. Possesses weak anti-inflammatory activity, and is therefore not recommended as a drug of first-choice for bone pain or pain that is accompanied by inflammation. Lack of gastropathy and antiplatelet activity makes this drug an excellent choice in patients predisposed to such complications. Acute overdosage produces dose-dependent, potentially fatal hepatic toxicity. When used chronically at high doses, renal, hepatic, and bone marrow function should be monitored periodically.

2. Standard to which other agents are compared, available over-the-counter in various preparations. May not be as well tolerated as newer alternative agents.

3. May be particularly useful in some cancer patients due to minimal effects on platelets and gastrointestinal tract. Available in liquid formulation.

4. Less gastrointestinal toxicity than aspirin.

5. Not recommended as a first-line drug in the treatment of cancer pain due to relatively greater risk of bone marrow toxicity. Periodic monitoring of CBC indicated in addition to other monitoring.

6. May cause less gastric irritation than phenylbutazone, otherwise, see above.

7. Available in sustained release and rectal formulations. Potent anti-inflammatory, but is associated with relatively greater incidence of toxicity, especially to GI tract and CNS than some alternative agents.

8. Appears to be responsible for less renal toxicity than other NSAIDs.

9. Parenteral formulation available. Appears to be equianalgesic to morphine in low dose ranges, but like other NSAIDs, has ceiling dose above which further analgesia is not achieved.

10. Considerable incidence of gastrointestinal toxicity has resulted in recommendations that therapy persist no longer than one week, making it an inappropriate choice for patients with cancer pain.

11. Relatively short latency of onset (30 minutes), relatively high incidence of gastrointestinal toxicity.

12. Available over-the-counter in low dose formulations, relatively economical. Relatively well-tolerated for long term use.

13. Relatively well-tolerated and rapidly absorbed. Has been reported anecdotally to be effective in its parenteral form for relatively severe pain. Has also been anecdotally reported to be particularly effective in the management of neoplastic fever.

14. Convenient once-daily dosing is an advantage for many patients with cancer. Higher doses (>20 mg) are associated with increased risks of ulceration, particularly in the elderly. May take 5–7 days to reach steady state and may accumulate in the presence of significantly altered renal or hepatic function.

15. Recently released in U.S. Relatively low G.I.blood loss and endoscopy scores, findings not necessarily correlated with incidence of G.I. upset.

Table C-4.
Guidelines for the Use of the Heterocyclic Antidepressants in Patients with Chronic Cancer Pain† # ††

Generic Name	Trade Name§	Dose Range**	Anti-chol-inergic	Sedative Effects	Ortho-stasis	Recep-tors	Comments, Toxicity‡ ††
Amitriptyline*	Elavil Endep	10–300	+++	+++	++	S(NE)	1,2,3,4
Imipramine*	Tofranil	20–300	+++	++	+++	NE(S)	1,4
Doxepin*	Sinequan Adapin	30–300	+++	+++	+++	S/NE	1,5
Desipramine*	Norpramin Pertofrane	75–300	+	+	+	NE(S)	1
Nortriptyline*	Pamelor Aventyl	50–100	++	+	+	NE(S)	1,5,6
Trimiptramine†††	Surmontil	50–225	+++	+++	+++	S(NE)	—
Protriptyline	Vivactil	15–40	+++	+	++	NE(S)	—
Amoxapine†††	Asendin	200–300	+	+	++	S/NE/D	7
Fluoxetine†††	Prozac	20–60	0	+	0	S	8
Second Generation/Atypical Heterocyclics							
Trazadone†††	Desyrel	50–600	0	+++	+++	S	9
Maprotiline†††	Ludiomil	75–300	+	+++	+	NE	10

* Drugs for which evidence for analgesic effects independent of antidepressant effects has been demonstrated in controlled studies are marked with an asterisk.

† Doses and quantification of anticholinergic effects, sedation and activity at receptor sites are estimated based on surveys of the literature. Intended as a rough guide only.

The prescription of the heterocyclic antidepressants specifically for the management of pain is most often considered for neuropathic pain, i.e. pain that is characteristically of a burning or dysesthetic quality due to injury to the nervous system (brachial or lumbosacral plexopathy due to tumor invasion or radiation injury, myelopathy, chemotherapy-induced polyneuropathy, herpes zoster, nerve invasion, nerve impingement).

‡ As a class, the heterocyclic antidepressants are generally associated with a range of side effects, most of which are due to their anticholinergic effects. These may include dry mouth, constipation, urinary retention, cardiac dysrhythmias, orthostatic hypotension, drowsiness and delerium. More infrequent events include hypertension, rash, bone marrow depression, visual impairment, sexual dysfunction, gynecomastia, jaundice and alopecia. Only especially noteworthy side effects are listed.

§ In U.S.A.

** The values listed reflect the range between minimum and maximum recommended doses. In general, the higher range of doses are intended to treat clinical depression, and even then it is recommended that dosage be reduced for maintenance therapy. In general, when antidepressants are prescribed to treat neuropathic pain, they are prescribed in the low range of the dose spectrum, often initially at the lowest possible dose.

†† The heterocyclic antidepressants are purported to produce analgesia independent of their effect on mood. In support of a distinction between modulation of pain and affect, treatment for pain is generally with low doses, usually considered inadequate to combat depression. Initial treatment is usually with low night time doses (amitriptyline 10–25 mg hs or its equivalent). Relief of pain, when it occurs, is often not established until one to three weeks of treatment have elapsed, although restoration of more normal nighttime sleep occurs more rapidly. Dosage may be titrated upwards as tolerated, particularly when there is coexisting depression. See text for details.

††† Analgesic activity independent of antidepressant effects has not been demonstrated in controlled studies.

  1. Preferred for the management of neuropathic pain due to relatively greater clinical experience.

(continued)

Table C-4.
(*Continued*)

2. Best studied drug of this class for the relief of neuropathic pain, and therefore thought to be most reliable. This must be balanced against the relatively greater potential for (anticholinergic) toxicity.
3. Available for I.M. use.
4. Use may be associated with weight gain.
5. Available as elixir.
6. Is a metabolite of amitriptyline. Some authorities feel that this factor combined with its relatively favorable side effect profile may favor its use.
7. Occasionally associated with extrapyramidal side effects.
8. In contrast to other heterocyclic antidepressants, is relatively nonsedating and may even produce increased activation. Use may be associated with weight loss.
9. Use is occasionally associated with priapism.
10. Most eleptogenic.

Table C-5.
Guidelines for the Use of Anticonvulsants in Patients with Chronic Cancer Pain*

Generic Name	Trade Name	Dose Range		Toxicity, Comments†
		Usual Starting Dose	Usual Dose Range	
Carbamezapine	Tegretol	100 mg bid	200 mg TID–400 mg qid	1
Clonazepam	Klonopin Rivotril	0.5 mg bid	2–8 mg/day	2
Phenytoin	Dilantin Epanutine	300 mg/day	300–400 mg/day	3
Valproic Acid Divalproex	Depakene Depakote	125 mg TID	500 mg tid–1000 mg tid	4

* Useful primarily as either first line drugs for neuropathic pain with a predominant shooting or lancinating component or as a second line therapeutic agent for neuropathic pain, independent of character. See text for details.

† All are associated with a relatively high incidence of dose-related toxicity. Most prominent adverse effects are loss of mental acuity and sedation. Less common are slurred speech, ataxia, nystagmus, confusion, dizziness, and nausea. Rarely serious hepatic or hematopoietic disturbances may occur. Drugs with a predeliction for specific adverse effects are noted below.

1. Often selected first because of clinical experience and efficacy. Dose-related dizziness, ataxia, sedation, diplopia, nausea and vomiting relatively prominent. Bone marrow depression is relatively common but serious marrow toxicity and liver dysfunction are rare. Nonetheless, periodic monitoring is indicated and other drugs should be used if marrow integrity is of concern (eg, patients receiving chemotherapy or hemibody radiation). Induces metabolism of phenytoin, valproic acid, theophylline, warfarin and thyroxine, lowering their blood levels.
2. Dizziness, sedation and fatigue are relatively prominent. Like other benzodiazepines, after chronic use a true abstinence syndrome may follow abrupt withdrawal.
3. Gingival hyperplasia may occur, but can often be prevented or managed with the institution of meticulous oral hygienic measures. Other adverse effects include acne and hirsutism. Rapid hydroxylation of coadministered steroids, which takes several weeks to develop, may reduce the effectiveness of oral contraceptives, thyroxine and corticosteroids (manage with dose escalations of the latter drugs). Rare effects include macrocystosis, vitamin D dependent rickets, osteoporosis, folate-responsive megaloblastic anemia, exfoliative dermatitis, Stevens-Johnson syndrome, hepatitis, nephritis, peripheral neuropathy and pseudolymphoma. Highly bound to plasma proteins (90%). Chlorpromazine, cimetidine, isoniazid and disulfiram increase phenytoin levels.
4. Adverse effects include liver dysfunction (either hepatocellular toxicity or hyperammonemia syndrome which may occur with normal LFT's), pancreatitis, nausea and vomiting, blood dyscrasias, insomnia, headache, tremor, alopecia, and weight gain. Rarely interferes with hemostasis due to dose-related thrombocytopenia and platelet dysfunction. Highly bound to plasma proteins (80%), so may cause displacement drug reactions (see phenytoin).

Table C-6.
Miscellaneous Drugs with Analgesic Potential

Generic Name	Trade Name	Dose Range	Comments
Oral Local Anesthetics/Sodium Channel Blockers			
Mexilitene	Mexitil	600–900 mg/day	1
Tocainide	Tonocard	200–400 mg tid	2
Psychostimulants			
Dextroamphetamine	Dexedrine	5–20 mg q 6–12 hr	3
Methylphenidate	Ritalin	5–20 mg bid	3
Major Tranquilizers			
Methotrimeprazine	Levoprome	10–50 mg/4–8 hr	4
Phenothiazines	—	—	5
Anxiolytics/Antihistamines			
Hydroxyzine	Vistaril, Atarax	50–100 mg/4–6 hr	6
Antihistamines			7
Benzodiazepines			8
Miscellaneous			
Baclofen	Lioresal	20–120 mg/day	9
Nifedipine	Procardia	10–60 mg/day	10
Phenoxybenzamine	Dibenzyline	10–120 mg/day	11
Clonidine	Catapres		12
Tetrahydrocannibinol	Marinol	5–15 mg/m^2	13

1. Frequently considered for management of neuropathic pain in patients who have failed trials of antidepressants and/or anticonvulsants. Potential adverse effects include cardiac arrhythmia, confusion, dysarthria, nystagmus, tremor, nausea, vomiting, constipation.
2. Considered as a third line drug for neuropathic pain for patients who have failed trials of antidepressants, anticonvulsants and mexiletine. Side effect profile similar to but more severe than that of mexiletine. In addition, administration has been associated with rare incidences of pneumonitis, hepatitis, immunologic, allergic and psychotic reactions.
3. Primary indication is as a psychostimulant, to enhance alertness in patients with opioid-induced sedation. Analgesic effect has been demonstrated with some reliability, although pain per se is not a primary indication. Although not indicated as an analgesic, this effect together with its rapid antidepressant activity are beneficial side effects.
4. Phenothiazine. Available only in parenteral (I.M.) form, although there is anecdotal support for safe I.V. use. Equianalgesic with morphine (15 mg methotrimeprazine = 10 mg MSO4). Use is associated with sedation, making it a good choice in anxious patients with advanced illness who have not responded to more conventional analgesics or who are unable to take opioids. Potent antiemetic. Use may be associated with the appearance of extrapyramidal signs. See text for details.
5. With the exception of methotrimeprazine, generally regarded as not possessing intrinsic analgesic activity although sedative and antiemetic properties make these agents useful in the treatment of agitation, nausea and vomiting.
6. Antihistamine. Only drug of this class with demonstrated analgesic activity. Often coadministered with an opioid for acute pain and anxiety. I.M. injection may be painful. Not recommended in the management of chronic cancer pain.
7. With the exception of hydroxyzine, generally regarded as not possessing intrinsic analgesic activity although sedative and antipruritic actions may be useful.

(continued)

Table C-6.
(*Continued*)

8. Direct analgesic/coanalgesic activity have not been demonstrated. Well-established role in treatment of insomnia and anxiety. May have an indirect role in managing pain when complaints are presumed to stem in large part from anxiety or sleep deprivation. Should not be used as a substitute for analgesics.

9. Antispasmodic agent (gamma-amino butyric acid analogue). Has not been studied in cancer patients, but may be useful as an adjunctive pharmacologic agent in the treatment of neuropathic pain.

10. Calcium channel blocker. Has not been studied in patients with cancer pain. Anecdotal support for use as a systemic vasodilator in the presence of sympathetically maintained pain. Common adverse effects include orthostatic hypotension, headache and peripheral edema.

11. Alpha-adrenergic antagonist. Has not been studied in patients with cancer pain. Anecdotal support for use as a systemic vasodilator in the presence of sympathetically maintained pain. Common adverse effects include orthostatic hypotension, headache and peripheral edema.

12. Centrally acting antihypertensive. Has not been studied in cancer pain. Indications for use still unclear. Analgesic by intraspinal routes, available as transdermal patch, used as an adjunct in the management of opioid and nicotine withdrawal.

13. Cannabinoid/psychotropic. Capacity to relieve pain is controversial. Use is associated with psychomimetic effects that many patients find undesirable. Indication is mainly as an antiemetic and more recently, appetite stimulant.

Table C-7.
Comparison of Selected Corticosteroids*

Generic Name	Approximate Duration	Equivalent Dose	Relative Anti-inflammatory Potency	Relative Mineralocorticoid Potency
Short Duration	12 hr			
Cortisone		25	0.8	2
Hydrocortisone		20	1	2
Intermediate Duration	12–36 hr			
Prednisone		5	4	1
Prednisolone		5	4	1
Methylprednisolone		4	5	0.5
Triamcinalone		4	5	0
Long Duration	48 hr			
Paramethasone		2	10	0
Dexamethasone		0.75	25	0
Betamethasone		0.6	25	0

* Based on oral administration

Appendix D

Anatomic Charts

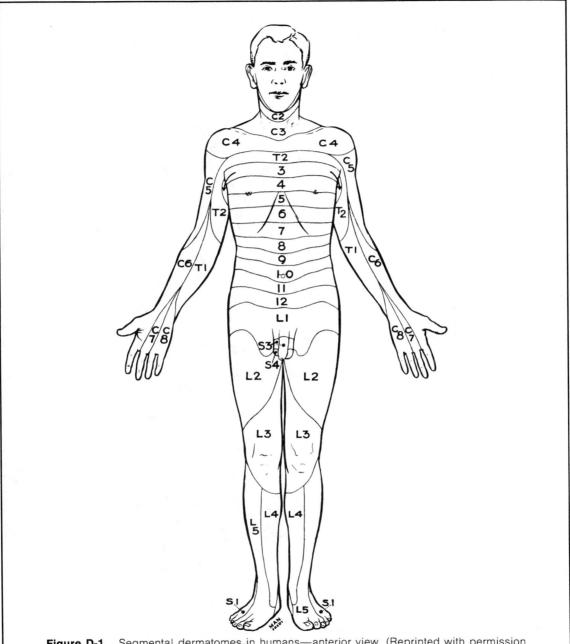

Figure D-1. Segmental dermatomes in humans—anterior view. (Reprinted with permission from Haymaker W, Woodhall B: Peripheral Nerve Injuries, 2nd ed. Philadelphia: WB Saunders, 1953.)

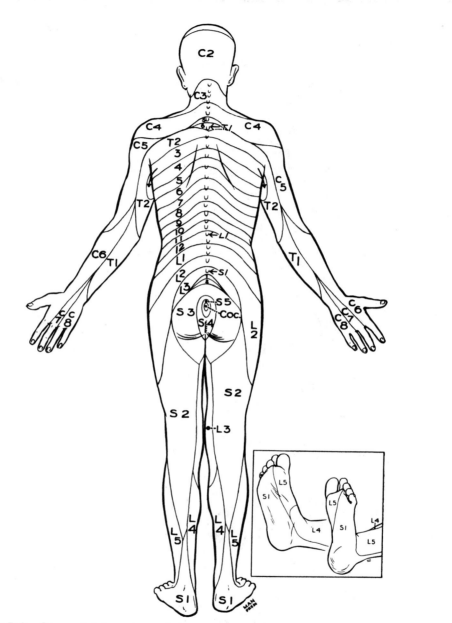

Figure D-2.   Segmental dermatomes in humans—posterior view. (Reprinted with permission from Haymaker W, Woodhall B: Peripheral Nerve Injuries, 2nd ed. Philadelphia: WB Saunders, 1953.)

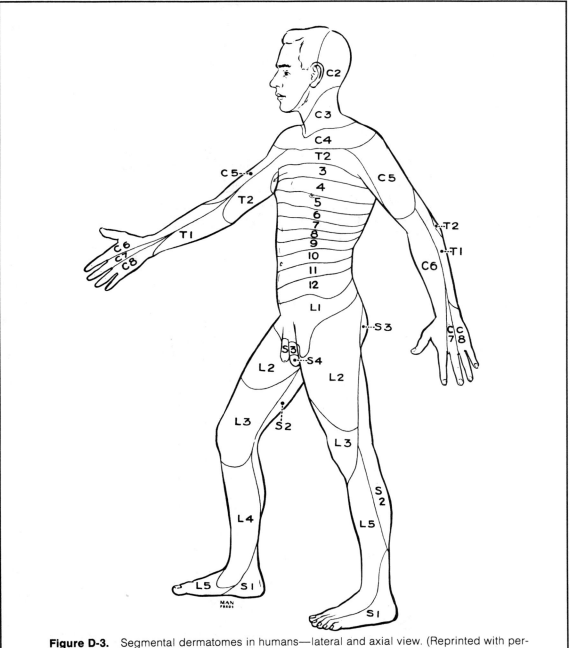

Figure D-3.   Segmental dermatomes in humans—lateral and axial view. (Reprinted with permission from Haymaker W, Woodhall B: Peripheral Nerve Injuries, 2nd ed. Philadelphia: WB Saunders, 1953.)

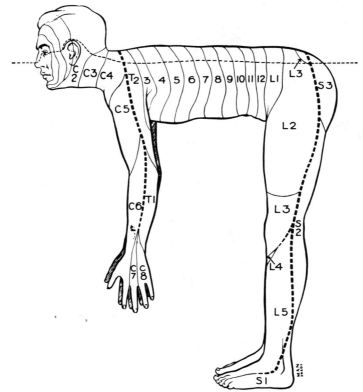

Figure D-4. Segmental dermatomes in humans—lateral and axial view. (Reprinted with permission from Haymaker W, Woodhall B: Peripheral Nerve Injuries, 2nd ed. Philadelphia: WB Saunders, 1953.)

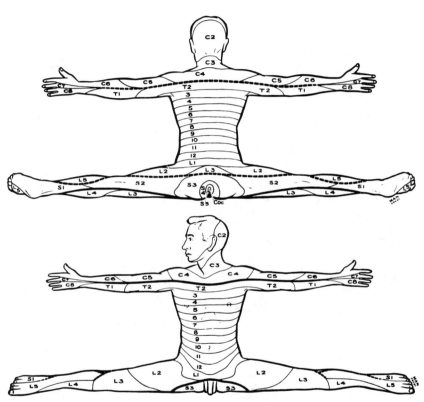

Figure D-5. Segmental dermatomes in humans—axial and anterior/posterior views. (Reprinted with permission from Haymaker W, Woodhall B: Peripheral Nerve Injuries, 2nd ed. Philadelphia: WB Saunders, 1953.)

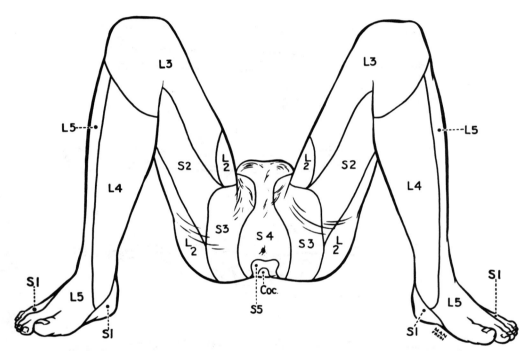

Figure D-6. Segmental dermatomes in humans—perineal view. (Reprinted with permission from Haymaker W, Woodhall B: Peripheral Nerve Injuries, 2nd ed. Philadelphia: WB Saunders, 1953.)

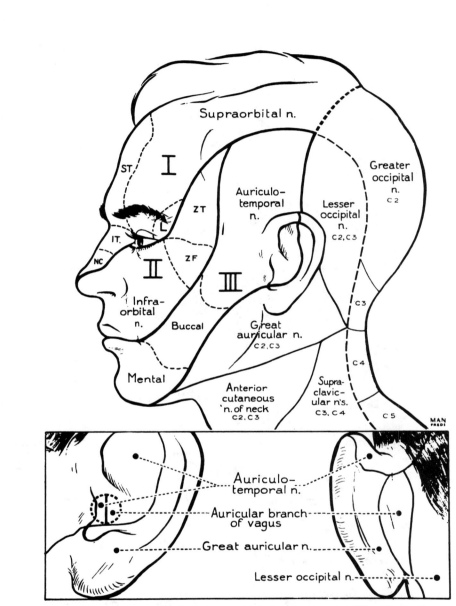

Figure D-7.   Peripheral distribution of trigeminal nerve in humans. (Reprinted with permission from Haymaker W, Woodhall B: Peripheral Nerve Injuries, 2nd ed. Philadelphia: WB Saunders, 1953.)

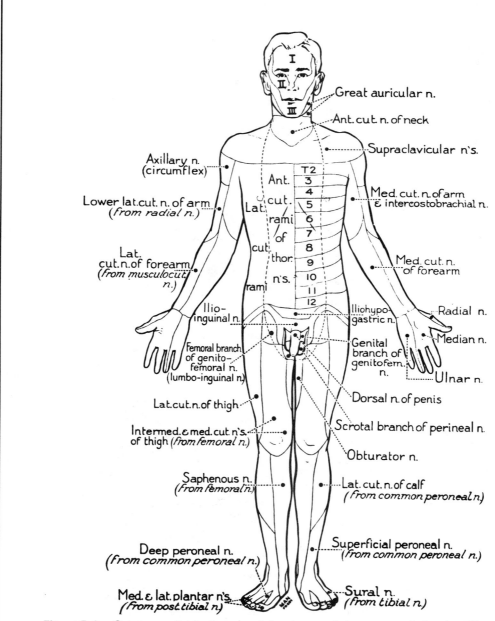

Figure D-8.   Cutaneous distribution of peripheral nerves in humans—anterior view. (Reprinted with permission from Haymaker W, Woodhall B: Peripheral Nerve Injuries, 2nd ed. Philadelphia: WB Saunders, 1953.)

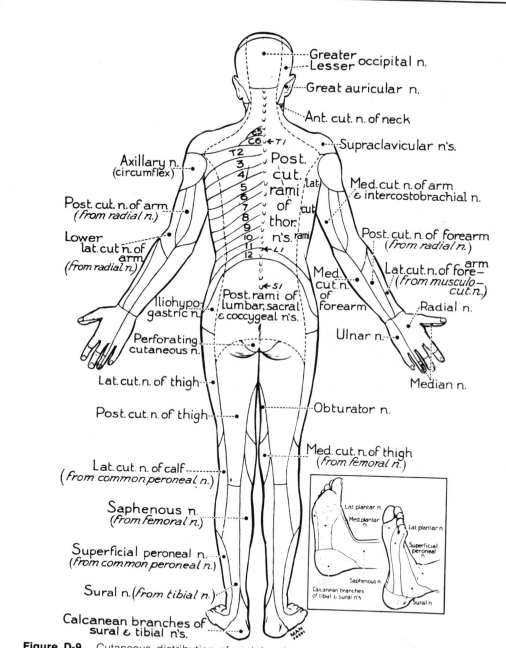

Figure D-9. Cutaneous distribution of peripheral nerves in humans—posterior view. (Reprinted with permission from Haymaker W, Woodhall B: Peripheral Nerve Injuries, 2nd ed. Philadelphia: WB Saunders, 1953.)

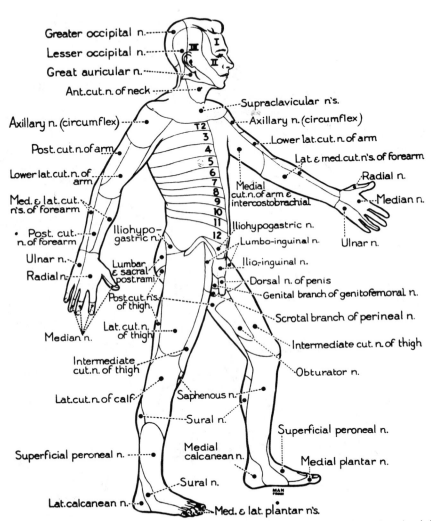

Figure D-10. Cutaneous distribution of peripheral nerves in humans—lateral and axial view. (Reprinted with permission from Haymaker W, Woodhall B: Peripheral Nerve Injuries, 2nd ed. Philadelphia: WB Saunders, 1953.)

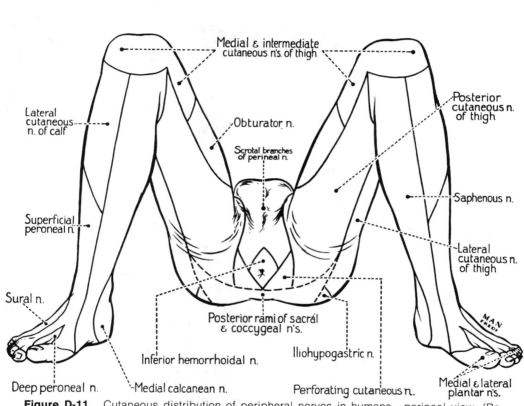

Figure D-11. Cutaneous distribution of peripheral nerves in humans—perineal view. (Reprinted with permission from Haymaker W, Woodhall B: Peripheral Nerve Injuries, 2nd ed. Philadelphia: WB Saunders, 1953.)

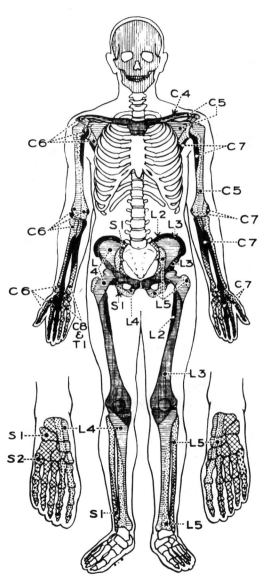

Figure D-12. Segmental osteotomes in humans—anterior view. (Reprinted with permission from Haymaker W, Woodhall B: Peripheral Nerve Injuries, 2nd ed. Philadelphia: WB Saunders, 1953.)

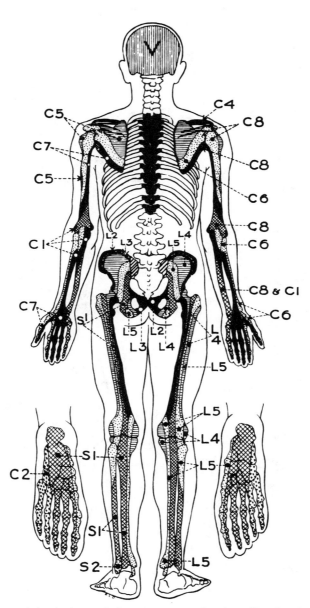

Figure D-13. Segmental osteotomes in humans—posterior view. (Reprinted with permission from Haymaker W, Woodhall B: Peripheral Nerve Injuries, 2nd ed. Philadelphia: WB Saunders, 1953.)

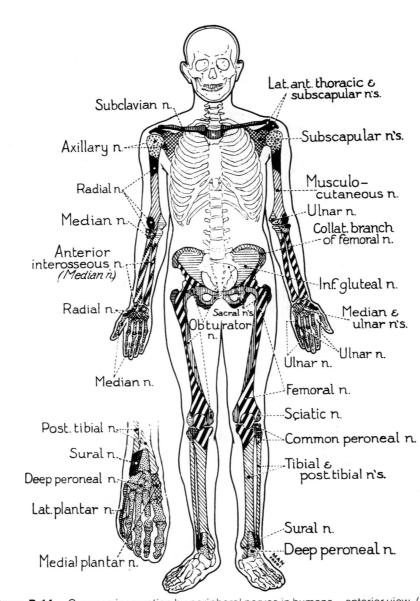

Figure D-14.   Osseous innervation by peripheral nerves in humans—anterior view. (Reprinted with permission from Haymaker W, Woodhall B: Peripheral Nerve Injuries, 2nd ed. Philadelphia: WB Saunders, 1953.)

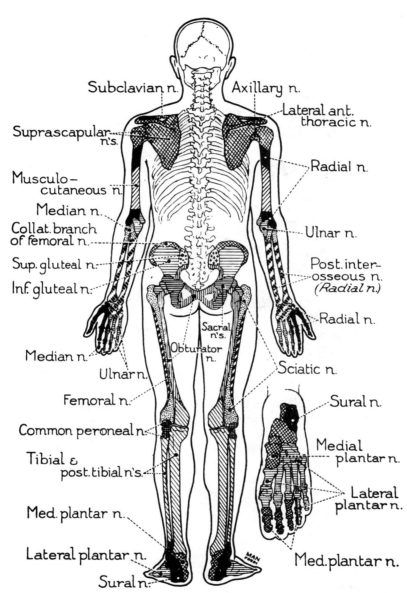

Figure D-15. Osseous innervation by peripheral nerves in man—posterior view. (Reprinted with permission from Haymaker W, Woodhall B: Peripheral Nerve Injuries, 2nd ed. Philadelphia: WB Saunders, 1953.)

Appendix E
_____

Needles, Catheters, and Syringes: Design, Development, and Selection

John R. Roschuck

NEEDLES

The design and selection of needles for use in pain management procedures involves the consideration of a variety of attributes, some of which are discussed below.

BEVEL DESIGN

The use of a sharp needle facilitates penetration of the skin but may increase the risk of nerve injury[1] or of unintentionally piercing an adjacent biologic membrane such as the pleura, the dura, or a vessel wall. Virtually all disposable and reusable needles have a bevel cut on three planes (Figure E-1), a design intended to minimize tissue laceration and coring.[2] The term "A" bevel has been used to refer to the configuration of the conventional "cutting" needle (17 degrees). The tip of a true short beveled or "Chiba-type" needle is 45 degrees, while a so-called "B" bevel needle is configured somewhere between these two extremes.[3] The use of a short beveled needle confers enhanced tactile recognition of the needle's anatomic location during its passage by helping to distinguish among different tissue planes. In experienced hands this may be manifest by (1) perception of variable degrees of resistance to the needles's passage through tissue of varying compliance and (2) the sensation of a "pop" or "click" that corresponds to passage through a fascial or vascular barrier.[2] In addition, with a shorter beveled needle it is more likely that the needle's entire orifice will be located within a single tissue plane,[4] thus facilitating passage of a catheter and potentially reducing the likelihood of (1) failure due to incomplete deposition of the injected solution in the proper space and (2) complications due to partial intravascular, epidural, or intrathecal injection. Penetration of the skin with a sharper needle may be required to facil-

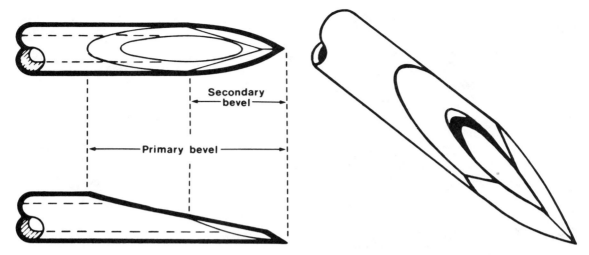

Figure E-1. Basic design of hypodermic needle point demonstrating standard practice of design with a bevel cut on three planes. Reprinted with permission: McMahon D: Managing regional anesthesia equipment. In Brown DL (ed): Problems in Anesthesia: 1987;1:592.

itate the subsequent introduction of a blunter needle. Excessively blunt needles should be avoided. Too blunt a needle tip may impede the optimal gradual and steady passage of the needle through soft tissue and may encourage rapid uncontrolled advances due to requirements for excessive pressure.

A variety of specific modifications have been introduced and have enjoyed varying popularity for specific uses. Further, unless specific patent and licensing agreements exist, manufacturers often slightly alter their version of similar needle types.[5] The Quincke-Babcock needle (Figure E-2), usually referred to as the "standard" spinal needle, is equipped with a sharp point and medium-length cutting bevel. It differs from the standard (Diamond) hypodermic needle in that in the former the secondary bevel is at an acute (30 degree) angle to the primary bevel, as opposed to the perpendicular (90 degree) junction in the latter. The Pitkin spinal needle has a sharp point and a short bevel with cutting edges and a rounded heel, and despite claims of a reduced incidence of headache is generally regarded to have no specific advantages. The Greene spinal needle has a sharp rounded

point and a rounded, noncutting bevel of medium length.[6] The so-called "pencil-point" spinal needles (see Figure E-2) include the Greene, Whitacre, and Sprotte varieties. The Whitacre needle has a completely rounded, noncutting bevel with a solid tip, the opening of the needle being on the side, 2 mm proximal to its tip.[7] The Sprotte needle is only significantly different in that the orifice is somewhat further from the tip and is wider than the inner diameter of the cannula to promote an axial flow rather than a jet effect. The noncutting bevel of the Greene, Whitacre, and Sprotte needles are intended to part rather than cut the longitudinal fibers of the dura and to reduce the incidence of postdural puncture headache.[4] The Huber tip epidural needle, with its rounded, blunt, gently curved tip and slightly laterally disposed orifice may be less likely to puncture the dura than other types. The Tuohy needle,[8] preferred by most for epidural puncture, differs only in that its edges are sharper than those of the Huber needle. The curve of both devices facilitates smooth cephalad passage of an epidural catheter. The R-K needle[9] is designed to be used with the Racz epidural catheter (see Chapter

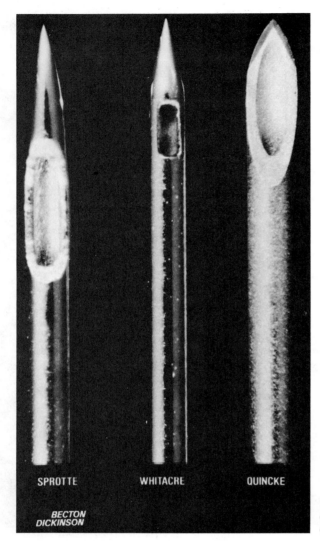

SPROTTE   WHITACRE   QUINCKE

BECTON
DICKINSON

Figure E-2. Comparison of tips of three commonly employed regional anesthesia needles (see text for details). Courtesy Becton Dickson Corp.

17) and is similar in design to the standard Touhy needle except that the back end of its orifice is blunted in place of the standard (sharp) V-shape (Figure E-3). This design is intended to eliminate the risk of shearing an epidural catheter and permits multiple passes without the need for removal of the catheter and needle simultaneously. The thin-walled Crawford needle is preferred by some for a paramedian or lateral approach to the epidural space. Its relatively short bevel and blunt tip make smooth advancement somewhat difficult, especially at the skin. The shaft of the Scott needle protrudes slightly from its hub, making advancement of a catheter somewhat easier. Contemporary kits now usually include a small disposable plastic device for this purpose. The Weiss needle refers to the

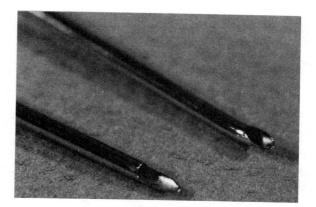

Figure E-3. Comparison of standard Tuohy needle (above) and R-K needle (below). Note blunt back end of orifice intended to reduce risk of catheter shearing, especially when used with the Racz epidural catheter. Courtesy Gabor Racz, M.D., Lubbock, Texas.

most popular of a variety of needles with a winged hub, a modification that facilitates location of the epidural space by the "hanging drop" technique of Gutierrez.

NEEDLE CALIBER

Intuitively, the use of thin needles would be expected to be associated with less tissue trauma and pain incidental to insertion.[10] For these reasons the use of finer gauge (25–27 G) needles is preferred for initial, preliminary local infiltration. In contrast, however, a larger caliber needle (18–22 G) is usually preferred for the definitive placement of the needle for nerve block. The use of such a needle helps to more precisely identify its anatomic location by permitting a greater appreciation of tissue compliance.[11] This is manifest by fine variations in feel that may be discerned during passage through tissue,[12] *eg*, the grittiness of the ligamentum flavum, the leatheriness of an intervertebral disc, a fascial or vascular "pop" or "click,"[2] the smooth, marblelike hardness of the rib or transverse process and rough, gritty, yielding feel of the vertebral body.[13] In addition the use of a larger bore needle ensures that the degree of resistance encountered to the injection of air or solution through a large bore needle is influenced less by the needle's caliber and as a result more accu-

rately reflects tissue compliance.[14] A larger needle permits more reliable aspiration of blood and cerebrospinal fluid. Finally, problems with a finer needle breaking or, more commonly, bending are avoided. Long thin needles must be supported along their shafts during insertion, but even so may bend in response to the resistance offered by deeper tissues.

NEEDLE LENGTH

The length of the needle that is selected will depend on the patient's body habitus, the procedure that is to be undertaken and the anatomic approach that is to be utilized. Most regional block procedures, especially in the periphery can be accomplished with a 2.5–8.75 cm (1–3.5 inch) needle. For procedures that require deeper penetration, especially truncal sympathetic blocks, needles of 12.5–20 cm (5–8 inch) are utilized.

REUSABLE VERSUS DISPOSABLE DEVICES

"With careful cleansing needles can be used repeatedly and when slightly damaged may be restored by polishing on emery cloth and sharpening on a small stone. For operating on his friends the operator will do well invariably to use a new needle."[15] The above passage from a text published in 1916 demonstrates the degree to which the practice of regional anesthesia has changed with the passage of time.

The tradition of the exclusive use of reusable needles (Figure E-4) has given way to the predominant use of disposable devices. The apparent economy of reusing needles may be offset by other factors. Repeated use of needles (especially after contact with periosteum) will eventually result in blunting of their tips and the potential for the development of barbs (Figure E-5), both of which may inhibit needle passage and increase iatrogenic trauma. Early proponents of regional anesthesia recommended regular inspection of needles and hand-sharpening[16], arts that have become relatively obscure in the context of contemporary practice and that introduce risks of human error. When reusing needles it is also important to inspect for barely perceptible bowing that may cause the needle to deviate from its expected course, and to dispose of such needles since manual correction may predispose to breakage. A final concern relates to the means of sterilization that is used and the potential for contamination by bacteria, viruses and detergents. In the 1950s, reports of permanent paraplegia after routine spinal anesthesia were determined to have resulted from contamination of ampules of local anesthetic immersed in phenol that had been used as a disinfectant and presumably gained entry by means of minute cracks in the glass ampules.[17] The acceptance of spinal anesthesia in the United Kingdom was dramatically reduced for years following this highly publicized event (Wooley and Rowe). The reader is referred to an in-depth account of the various means of maintaining and sterilizing reusable equipment that is of primarily historical interest.[12]

SECURITY NEEDLES, DEPTH MARKERS

Traditionally, authorities have advocated the use of so-called "security" needles which are fitted with a metal bead 4–6 mm distal to the junction of the needle shaft and hub.[18] The bead is intended to prevent insertion of the entire length of the needle so that, if it were to break at its weakest point, the junction of the shaft and hub, the needle could be readily removed with a forceps. Improvements in the materials used for manufacture and less reliance on reusable needles have reduced the necessity for security type needles.

Historically, sterile pieces of cork or rubber were threaded over the shaft of the needle,[3] and were then advanced flush to the patient's skin as a measure of depth of a preliminary insertion and referred to as a guide during subsequent insertions. Many needles now come from the manufacturer with prefitted latex depth markers. Alternatively, more experienced operators may prefer to simply pinch the substance of the shaft of the needle between their thumb and forefinger as a guide to depth.

MATERIAL

Needles are traditionally composed entirely of metal, although nonmetallic needles have recently been developed for use with magnetic resonance imaging. In the past, a variety of materials were used in manufacture including platino-iridium, platinum, tempered gold, nickeloid, and steel. Today most needles are composed of the American Iron and Steel Institute type 304 stainless steel, often referred to as "18-8" steel, by virtue of the 18% chromium and 8% nickel that impart its qualities.[2,19] A microscopic layer of chromium oxide protects against most corrosives, while the nickel lends the alloy its workability. In the case of disposable devices a metal cannula is usually combined with a plastic hub and, often, a plastic stylet. If disposable needles are utilized, one with a transparent hub is preferred to facilitate the observation of aspirated blood or cerebrospinal fluid.

A most important factor to be considered in the selection of the material that comprises the hub and cannula is that it is resistant to local anesthetics, opioids and organic solvents (alcohol, phenol) that might be used to pro-

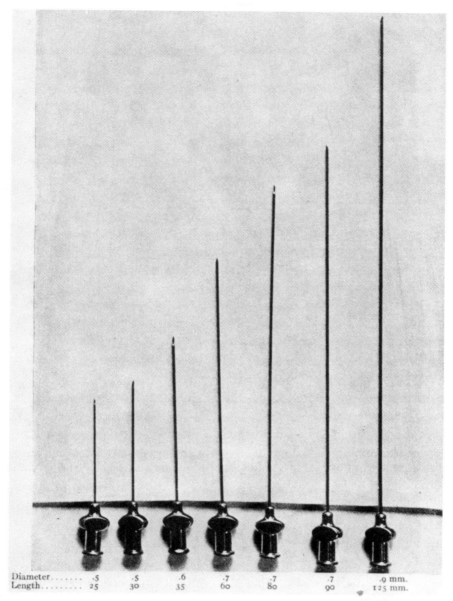

Diameter	.5	.5	.6	.7	.7	.7	.9 mm.
Length	25	30	35	60	80	90	125 mm.

Figure E-4. Assortment of reusable regional anesthesia needles. Of primary historic interest.

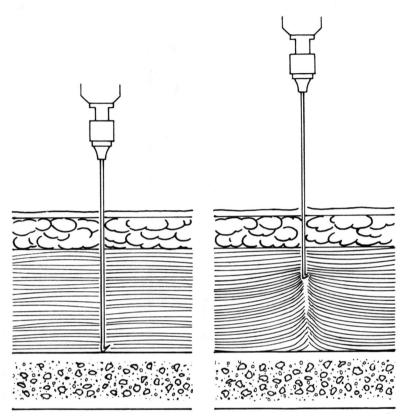

Figure E-5. Demonstrates suggested mechanism by which the tips of reused needles may become blunted and barbed by repeated contact with periosteum resulting in potential injury to adjacent soft tissue.

duce regional anesthesia or neurolytic blockade. Many plastics are susceptible to degradation by the latter substances and it is therefore important that all plastic parts be composed of resistant materials such as polypropylene or polyethylene rather than acrylic or polycarbonate. We have recently reported a case of the acute degradation of a needle hub of the latter type during alcohol celiac plexus block (Figure E-6).[20] The 302 stainless steel that is generally used for a needle's metal component parts is resistant to the above substances.

When a nerve stimulator is utilized, it is preferable that the shaft of the needle be coated with Teflon.[21,22] Such insulation aids in accurately positioning the needle's tip beside the nerve that is to be blocked by eliminating artifact that may be introduced by transmission of electrical current through the needle shaft. An alternative approach involves the use of an over-the-needle catheter which also provides effective insulation. A non-insulated needle can be used,[10,11] but requires greater expertise.

CATHETERS

Malleable needles[23] and ureteral catheters[24] were the first devices utilized to administer anesthetics in serial doses, usually in the caudal epidural space. Catheter design has since undergone numerous modifications that have helped to make possible investigators' efforts to place catheters in various other regions including the celiac plexus,[25] lumbar plexus,[26] stellate ganglion,[27] and near peripheral nerves.[28,29,30] The Racz epidural catheter[31] is a specially designed radio-opaque device that incorporates a spring wire in its design with

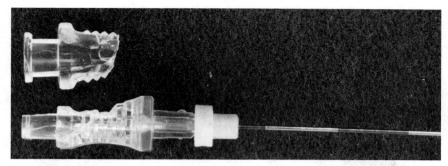

Figure E-6. Hub of needle composed of polycarbonate material that underwent acute degeneration at the bedside during alcohol celiac plexus block, interfering with completion of the procedure.

the intention of increasing durability and, when used with the R-K needle (see above), reducing the risk of shearing.

The selection and design of catheters intended for use in chronic pain management must take into account numerous factors including whether the catheter is to be introduced over or from within a needle, intended location and duration of use, radio-opacity, volume/flow requirements and properties that discourage kinking and migration in ambulatory patients. Ideal catheter characteristics are incompletely understood. The routine incorporation of radio-opaque materials and use of an external marking system are desirable to facilitate accurate placement and subsequent verification. While stiffer catheters may be easier to insert, their introduction may be more likely to result in trauma and once placed they may be prone to migration. The use of a soft thermal-conductive material, such as polyurethane may be desirable because once introduced the more pliable catheter is less likely to become displaced. When styletted, such catheters can be readily positioned. Over-the-needle systems are necessarily larger and therefore potentially more traumatic and in addition, catheters may buckle and tear tissue during their passage. Through-the-needle catheters introduce a theoretical potential for leakage around the catheter once the needle has been removed, although this has not emerged as a practical problem in clinical practice. Early experience

with the flow properties of 24 gauge catheters positioned with external 20 gauge needles is quite encouraging (Patt R, Jain S: Unpublished data; see Figs. E-8 and E-9). Before any catheter is used for the introduction of a neurolytic substance, it should be determined that it is manufactured of a specifically chemical resistant material. Finally, catheters that are intended for greater than thirty days of use are considered by the FDA as implanted devices (FDA Class III devices) and are subject to more rigorous testing and controls than the typical catheter used in acute settings (FDA Class II device).

SYRINGES

Once composed of metal and combinations of metal and glass, syringes (see Figure E-7) are now routinely composed of plastic. Glass syringes are preferred when it is important to distinguish among tissues of varying compliance because of the reduced friction that results from contact between the syringe's plunger and the internal walls of its barrel. The use of a so-called "control" syringe, fitted with three rings configured to be occupied by the thumb, index, and middle finger is desirable for better control, particularly when assistance is lacking. When sufficient manpower is available, the use of sterile extension tubing permits even greater control.

Independent of whether a luer slip or luer lock syringe is used, the act of connecting or

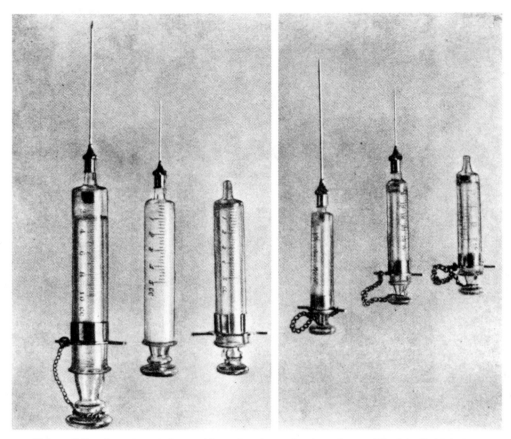

Figure E-7.   Assortment of reusable regional anesthesia syringes. Of primarily historic interest.

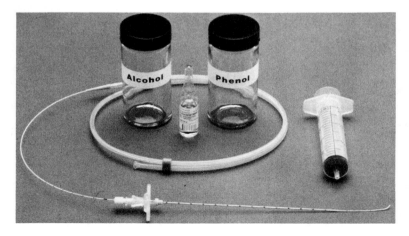

Figure E-8.   Specialized equipment suitable for continuous local anesthetic or neurolytic celiac plexus block. Consists of a 20 gauge, eight inch graduated needle with sliding depth indicator, removable wings and Chiba point designed to transmit a 24 gauge radio-opaque, styletted catheter, manufactured to be resistant to degradation by alcohol and phenol. Courtesy, Preferred Medical Products, Lewiston, NY

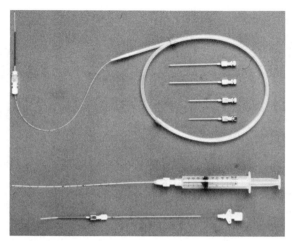

Figure E-9. A variety of needles and catheters designed for continuous peripheral, sympathetic and epidural blockade. Uppermost is a 24 gauge 8-inch styletted, chemically resistant catheter advanced through a 20 gauge 1½ inch insulated needle for continuous peripheral nerve, stellate ganglion or epidural block. A variety of needles suitable for transmitting such a catheter are arranged within its sheath including 20 gauge 1½ and 2½ inch needles with Touhy and Crawford tips. The lower portion of the figure depicts this catheter attached to a 10 ml syringe and introduced through 20 gauge 1½ inch insulated needle. Courtesy, Preferred Medical Products, Lewiston, NY

disconnecting the syringe from the needle during a nerve block is one of the procedure's most critical moments since it is at this time that the sharp needle may accidentally migrate. When using a luer slip syringe to inject hyperbaric phenol, extreme caution should be taken that the pressure required does not separate the syringe and needle unexpectedly, splashing the patient and physician with solution. Eye protection is recommended. The use of a small syringe permits increased force to be generated and a 1–3 ml syringe is recommended to facilitate the instillation of phenol and glycerine through a 20 or 22 gauge needle/catheter. Small caliber syringes and glass syringes are also often used preferentially so that differences in the

magnitude of resistance to injection can be more readily appreciated.

STATUS OF THE INDUSTRY AND FUTURE TRENDS

The overall market for devices specifically designed for the management of pain has until recently been relatively small, and as a result, activity in the area of product development has been relatively meager. Equipment is designed and manufactured predominantly by large multinational institutions that traditionally engage in very careful scrutiny of the demand and market for devices before investing in development. As a result of these shortcomings, anesthesiologists have used existing devices for alternate innovative purposes (eg, intravenous cannulae for brachial plexus blockade, epidural catheters for lumbar sympathetic blockade), a practice that would in general be expected to limit success. Increased interest in the management of chronic pain has led to the development of new implantable products (silastic intraspinal catheters and pumps; see Chapter 17), and there are signs that this increased commitment on the part of industry is beginning to be mirrored in other areas as well. Small innovative specialty manufacturers have recently begun designing and developing devices specific to the needs of the emerging chronic pain management market. As a result, a variety of new devices have recently become available and it is anticipated that their use will become more widespread. These devices include pediatric caudal sets, micro-bore spinal needle-catheter sets, and catheters intended by design to be placed near the lumbar sympathetic chain, celiac plexus, stellate ganglion, and peripheral nerves. (See Figures E-8 and E-9.)

REFERENCES

1. Selander D, Dhuner KG, Lundberg G: Peripheral nerve injury due to injection needles used for regional

anesthesia. Acta Anaesthesiol Scand 1977;21:182.

2. McMahon D: Managing regional anesthesia equipment. In Brown DL (ed): Problems in Anesthesia: 1987;1:592.

3. Winnie AP: Plexus Anesthesia, p 126. Philadelphia, WB Saunders, 1983.

4. Carron H, Korbon GA, Rowlingson JC: Regional Anesthesia, p 167. Orlando, Grune and Stratton, 1984.

5. Dixon CL: The Sprotte, Whitacre, and Quincke spinal needles. Anesth Review 1991;18:42.

6. Greene HM: Lumbar puncture and the prevention of postpuncture headache. JAMA 1926;86:391.

7. Hart JR, Whitacre RJ: Pencil-point needle in prevention of postspinal headache. JAMA 1951;147:657.

8. Tuohy EB: Continuous spinal anesthesia: A new method of utilizing a ureteral catheter. Surg Clin NA 1945:845.

9. Racz GB, Kline WM: Technical advance: New epidural adaptor and needle. In Racz GB (ed): Techniques of Neurolysis, p 95. Boston, Kluwer, 1989.

10. Labat G: Regional Anesthesia. Philadelphia, WB Saunders, 1922.

11. Bromage PR: Spinal Epidural Analgesia, p 52. Baltimore, Williams and Wilkins, 1954.

12. Sherwood-Dunn B: Regional Anesthesia, p 30. Philadelphia, FA Davis, 1922.

13. Lofstrom JB, Cousins MJ: Sympathetic neural blockade of the upper and lower extremity. In Cousins MJ, Bridenbaugh PO: Neural Blockade, 2nd ed., p 482. Philadelphia, JB Lippincott, 1988.

14. Thompson GE, Moore DC: Celiac plexus, intercostal and minor peripheral blockade. In Cousins MJ, Bridenbaugh PO: Neural Blockade, 2nd ed., p 519. Philadelphia, JB Lippincott, 1988.

15. Hertzler AE: Surgical Operations with Local Anesthesia, 2nd ed. New York, Surgery Pub, 1916.

16. Smith AE: Block Anesthesia and Allied Subjects. St. Louis, CV Mosby, 1920.

17. Cope RW: The Wooley and Rowe case: Wooley and Rowe v the Ministry of Health and others. Anaesthesia 1954;9:249.

18. Bonica JJ: Sympathetic Nerve Blocks for Pain Diagnosis and Therapy, vol. I, p 21. Seattle, Breon, 1980.

19. Brown J, Jacobs J, Stark L: Biomedical engineering, p 308. Philadelphia, FA Davis, 1978.

20. Catania J, Patt R, Voisine R: Acute deterioration of a needle hub during alcohol celiac plexus block. In press.

21. Pither CE, Raj PP, Ford DJ: Peripheral nerve stimulation with insulated and uninsulated needles: Efficacy of characteristics. Reg Anesth 1984;9:9.

22. Bashein G, Ready LB, Haschke RH: Electrolocation: Insulated versus noninsulated needles. Reg Anesth 1984;9:31.

23. Lemmon WT: A method for continuous spinal anesthesia. Ann Surg 1940;111:141.

24. Tuohy EB: Continuous spinal anesthesia: Its usefulness and technique involved. Anesthesiology 1944;5:142.

25. Humbles FH, Mahaffey JE: Teflon epidural catheter placement for intermittent celiac plexus blockade and celiac plexus neurolytic blockade. Reg Anesth 1990;15:103.

26. Schultz P, Anker-Moller E, Dahl JB et al: Postoperative pain treatment after open knee surgery: Continuous lumbar plexus block with bupivacaine versus epidural morphine. Reg Anesth 1991;16:34.

27. Linson MA, Leffert R, Todd DP: The treatment of upper extremity reflex sympathetic dystrophy with prolonged stellate ganglion blockade. J Hand Surg 1983;8:153.

28. Safran D, Kuhlman G, Orhant EE et al: Continuous intercostal blockade with lidocaine after thoracic surgery. Anesth Analg 1990;70:345.

29. Borzecki M, Hilgier M: Treatment of chronic pain by continuous blockade of peripheral nervous system. Reg Anesth 1979;4:16.

30. Fisher A: Continuous postoperative regional analgesia by nerve sheath block for amputation surgery: A pilot study. Anesth Analg 1991;72:300.

31. Racz GB, Sabonghy M, Gintautas J et al: Intractable pain therapy using a new epidural catheter. JAMA 1982;238:646.

Long-Term Epidural Catheter Implantation for Cancer Pain

EPIDURAL HOME CARE SUPPLY LIST

Daily Supplies

12-ml syringes (one per injection time)
Monoject 19- or 20-gauge 1.5-inch needle with
5-μm filter [Monoject #250] (one per injection)
Duramorph PF

Weekly Supplies

Tegaderm dressing [3M #1626] (two or three
per week)
0.22 μm filter [Concord MP-094 or Millex
#SLGS0250S] (one per week)

Miscellaneous Supplies

Betadine swabs or swabsticks
Acetone/alcohol swabsticks or alcohol wipes
4" × 4" gauze
Porous tape (*eg*, Dermacel)

Note: This appendix originally appeared in The Pain Clinic
Manual, *Abram SE, Haddox JD, Kettler RE, eds. Philadelphia:
JB Lippincott, 1990, pp 321–331.*

INDIVIDUAL DOSAGE SCHEDULE

For _____ *(patient's name)* _____

1. Use only preservative-free morphine
   (Duramorph PF), in a strength of _____
   mg/10 ml. Inject _____ ml every _____
   hours.
2. Change dressing every three days or more
   often if required (see Dressing Change
   Technique).
3. Change filter once a week (see Filter
   Change Technique).

   Note that some syringes are labeled in
   "ml" and some are in "cc." For our
   purposes, they are the same, so that
   10 ml = 10 cc.

Note

You are to call us at the pain clinic and/or your
physician if any of the following happen:

1. You have an unexplained fever or an
   extremely sore and tender back.
2. You have inadequate pain relief or the
   pain returns before the next dose.
3. You require Narcan (naloxone). You
   should be given Narcan 0.4 mg (one vial)
   into the thigh or arm muscle if you

603

become *very* drowsy (or unarousable), if you have *severe* nausea and vomiting, or if you have *severe* itching. If you require Narcan you should be taken to an emergency room after receiving it.

INJECTION TECHNIQUE FOR EPIDURAL CATHETER

1. *Wash hands before starting procedure.*
2. Avoid contaminating the filter port, filter cap, needle (including the hub), and the tip of the syringe (Fig. F-1). If any of these contact anything that is not sterile (such as the table top, fingers, or an area outside of the drug vial) they must be discarded.

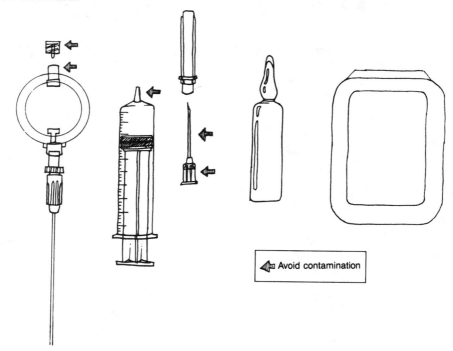

☐ Avoid contamination

Figure F-1.

3. Assemble the following equipment
   a. 4" × 4" gauze
   b. the Duramorph vial
   c. one needle
   d. one syringe
4. Take the catheter out of the carrying pouch and place the filter where it can be worked with easily.
5. Open the syringe by twisting the cover and its end cap in different directions. Remove the syringe from the cover and lay it down, taking care not to touch the tip.
6. Open the needle by twisting the two parts of its cover in opposite directions. *Do not touch the hub.* Keep a grasp on the needle by holding onto the long part of the cover.

7. Place the tip of the syringe firmly into the hub of the needle: do not twist (Fig. F-2). Draw 1 ml of air into the syringe through the covered needle to break the plunger seal and then push the air back out.

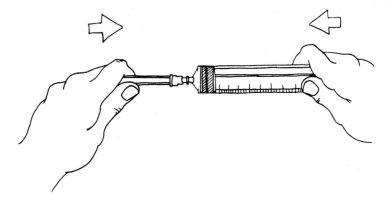

Figure F-2.

8. Set the syringe and attached needle down.
9. Using gauze to protect your hands, break the top of the Duramorph vial off by snapping it away from you sharply (Fig. F-3). Beware of glass fragments.

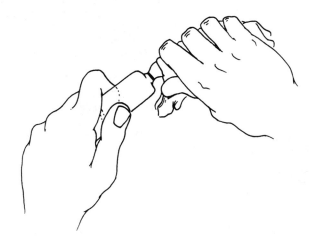

Figure F-3.

10. Remove the needle cover by pulling it straight off (do not twist) and set the cover down. Carefully insert the needle into the vial and draw up all of the Duramorph (Fig. F-4).

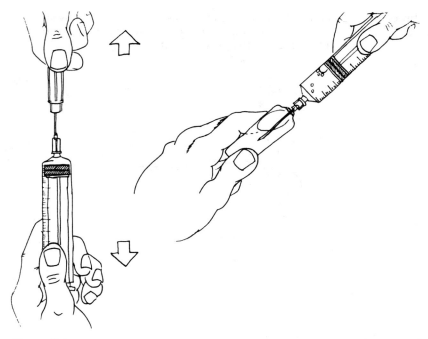

Figure F-4.

11. With the needle pointing up, tap the side of the syringe to get all the air bubbles to the top and then expel the air slowly by gently pushing up on the plunger of the syringe (Fig. F-5). Point the needle at a receptacle (sink, trash can) and watch the top edge of the plunger while pushing gently until the top of the plunger is at the dose indicated on your "Individual Dosage Schedule" (Fig. F-5).
12. Replace the cover over the needle.
13. With the filter held firmly between the thumb and first two fingers of the left hand, place the needle cover into the left palm and grasp it with the ring and little fingers (Fig. F-6).
14. Twist the syringe out of the needle and place the syringe down on a clean flat surface, taking care not to contaminate the tip (Fig. F-7).
15. With the right hand twist the cap off of the filter and place it on the needle hub, giving it a slight twist to secure it (Fig. F-8).
16. Place the tip of the syringe into the filter port snugly without twisting (Fig. F-9).
17. Now hold the syringe in the left hand and pull back on the plunger with the right hand to cause some suction (move the plunger about 1 ml) and hold it there for several seconds (Fig. F-10). Watch for blood filling up the catheter or for clear fluid filling up the syringe. A few bubbles are to be expected in the syringe. If either blood or clear fluid appear, recap the filter, and call the pain clinic.

(text continues on page 609)

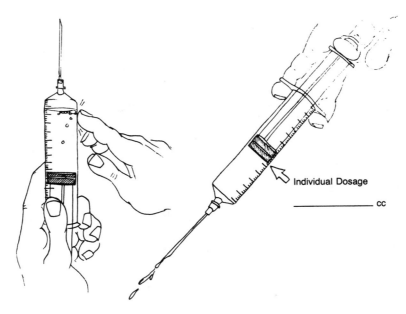

Individual Dosage

_____ cc

Figure F-5.

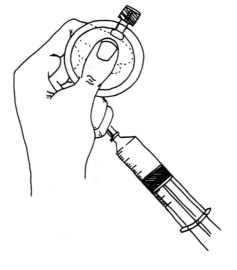

Figure F-6.

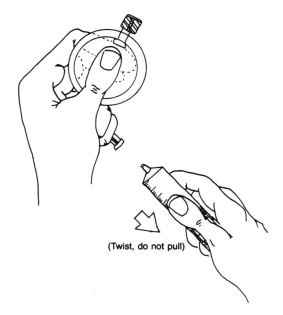

(Twist, do not pull)

Figure F-7.

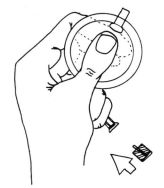

Figure F-8.

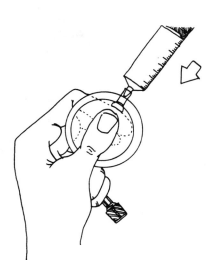

Figure F-9.

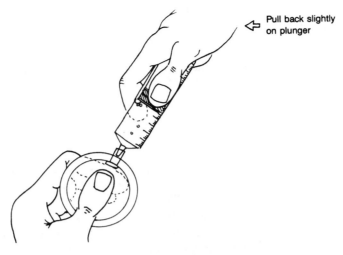

Pull back slightly
on plunger

Figure F-10.

18. Push the Duramorph into the filter by gentle steady pressure on the plunger (Fig. F-11). If the drug requires excessive pressure to push in or will not go in, call the pain clinic.
19. When injection is complete, grasp the filter and needle (with the filter cap still attached) in the left hand as before. Remove the syringe and lay it down.

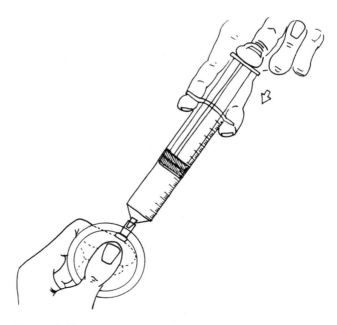

Figure F-11.

20. Remove the filter cap from the needle hub and place it securely on the filter port, giving it a slight twist.
21. Check to make sure all connections are secure (catheter adapter to catheter, filter to catheter, cap to filter).
22. Discard the needle and all parts of the vial in a container with a lid, such as a plastic milk carton, before placing the container in the garbage.

DRESSING CHANGE TECHNIQUE

1. *Wash hands before starting procedure.*
2. Assemble the following items:
   a. 3 Betadine swabs or swabsticks
   b. 3 alcohol wipes or acetone/alcohol swabsticks
   c. Gauze
   d. Tegaderm dressing
3. Holding the catheter with one hand, carefully peel the dressing off skin going from front to back. *Be careful not to pull on catheter* (Fig. F-12).

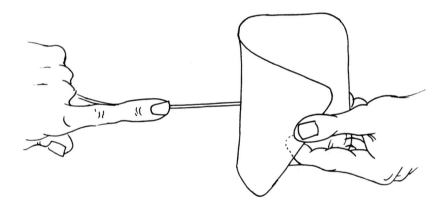

Figure F-12.

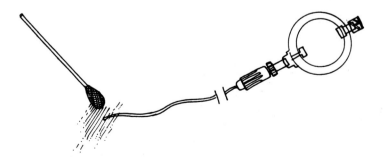

Figure F-13.

4. Wipe the catheter exit site with a Betadine swab starting at the center of the site and wiping outward in an ever-widening circular spiral motion (Fig. F-13). Do not wipe over the same area twice with the same swab. Repeat with the remaining swabs. Allow the area to dry.
5. Wipe the area in a similar manner with the three acetone/alcohol swabs.
6. Pat the area gently with gauze, touching skin and catheter only with the gauze, not the fingers.
7. Apply the dressing according to the instructions on the package. Remember that the sticky side is also the sterile side, so be careful not to touch it, except at the edges.

FILTER CHANGE TECHNIQUE

1. *Wash hands before starting procedure.*
2. Open a new filter and leave it in the package.
3. Hold the catheter adapter in your left hand, taking care not to pull on the catheter.
4. Grasp the old filter with your right hand and twist it counterclockwise to disengage the filter from the adapter. Take care not to loosen the adapter from the catheter. Set the old filter down.
5. Pick up the new filter, being careful not to touch the uncapped end.
6. Place the uncapped end into the catheter adapter and twist it clockwise until it is snug.
7. Check to make sure the cap is secure on the filter port.

Manufacturing Processes

Chad Swenson

Richard B. Patt

APPENDIX G-1

Phenol in Glycerin—10%
Phenol in Glycerin 3%, 6%, 12%*

MATERIALS AND INGREDIENTS
3 ml luer lock plastic syringe and needle
10 ml luer lock plastic syringe and needle
gloves
protective eyewear

disposable plastic medicine cups
Millex-FG 0.2 micron filter
ethyl alcohol
89% liquefied phenol U.S.P.
glycerin U.S.P.
10 ml sterile empty vial

METHOD OF PREPARATION

1. Under aseptic conditions, using protective eyewear and gloves and a Class 100 laminar flow hood, draw up approximately 2 ml of absolute ethanol into a 3 ml luer lock syringe. Remove the needle and attach a 0.2 micron FG filter (Millex®-FG, Millipore Corp., Product no. SLFG025LS). Wet the filter by gently pushing the alcohol through and into a disposable medicine cup. Set the filter aside maintaining its sterility. Clear the filter unit of any residual ethanol by drawing up approximately 2 ml of liquefied phenol into a 3 ml luer lock syringe pushing it slowly through the filter and into the disposable medicine cup.

2. Filter 1.1 ml of 89% liquefied phenol into a 10 ml sterile empty vial (Solopak or Lyphomed) utilizing the previously

---

* Alternatively, phenol and glycerin can be compounded in various other proportions by following the same procedure but altering the volumes as follows:

** 3% phenol in glycerin	.33 ml of 89% liquefied phenol
	9.66 ml of glycerin U.S.P.
** 6% phenol in glycerin	.65 ml of 89% liquefied phenol
	9.35 ml of glycerin U.S.P.
12% phenol in glycerin	1.3 ml of 89% liquefied phenol
	8.7 ml of glycerin U.S.P.

** If small syringes of adequate accuracy are not readily available, larger total volumes (*eg*, 30 ml) may be compounded, in which case the volumes of each ingredient are increased proportionately.

primed 0.2 micron FG filter. Add 8.9 ml of glycerin U.S.P. to the vial by filtration through a large volume 5 micron conical filter (Burron Medical Inc., Product Code LV-5000). Mix thoroughly by shaking. The resulting solution is 10% W/V (weight/volume) phenol in glycerin.*

3. Subject the vial containing the phenol and glycerin mixture to dry heat sterilization by exposing them to 150°C for 1 hour.
4. Confirm sterilization by aseptically adding the contents of one vial to a liter of sterile water for injection. Filter the resulting solution through a bacterial retentive filter unit (QC testers, Health-Tek) and then culture using tryptic soy broth at 39°C. The cultures are examined at 48 hours and 14 days for microbiologic growth.
5. Endotoxin test utilizing limulus amebocyte lysate (Pyrotell®, Associates of Cape Cod).
6. Protect from light, 1 year expiration.

APPENDIX G-2
*Aqueous Phenol**

A. 12% AQUEOUS PHENOL (IN 20% GLYCERIN)

MATERIALS AND INGREDIENTS
3 ml luer lock plastic syringe and needles
10 ml luer lock plastic syringe and needles
gloves
protective eyewear
disposable plastic medicine cups
Millex-FG 0.2 micron filter
Millex-GS 0.2 micron filter
ethyl alcohol
89% liquefied phenol USP
glycerin USP
sterile water for injection USP
10 ml sterile empty vial

* Phenol's maximum solubility in water at room temperature is 6.7%. One means of compounding higher concentrations of aqueous phenol involves the utilization of a solution of 20% glycerin in water. This results in a solution that is only minimally more viscous than plain aqueous phenol.

METHOD OF PREPARATION

1. Under aseptic conditions, using protective eyewear and gloves and a Class 100 laminar flow hood, draw up approximately 2 ml of absolute ethanol into a 3 ml luer lock syringe. Remove the needle and attach a 0.2 micron FG filter (Millex®-FG, Millipore Corp., Product no. SLFG025LS). Wet the filter by gently pushing the alcohol through and into a disposable medicine cup. Set the filter aside maintaining its sterility. Clear the filter unit of any residual ethanol by drawing up approximately 2 ml of liquefied phenol into a 3 ml luer lock syringe pushing it slowly through the filter and into the disposable medicine cup.
2. Filter 1.3 ml of 89% liquefied phenol into a 10 ml sterile empty vial utilizing the previously primed 0.2 micron FG filter. Mix 1.6 ml of anhydrous glycerin USP with 7.1 ml of sterile water for injection USP in a 10 ml syringe. Filter the resulting solution into the vial using a 0.2 micron GS filter (Millex®-GS, Millipore Corp., Product no. SLGS020S). Mix thoroughly. The resulting solution is a 12% W/V phenol and 20% W/V glycerin in water.
3. Autoclave the preparation at 121°C for 30 minutes.
4. Confirm sterilization by aseptically adding the contents of one vial to a liter of sterile water for injection. Filter the resulting solution through a bacterial retentive filter unit (QC Testers, Health-Tek) and then culture using tryptic soy broth at 39°C. Examine the cultures at 48 hours and 14 days for microbiologic growth.
5. Endotoxin test utilizing Limulus Amebocyte Lysate (Pyrotell®, Associates of Cape Cod).
6. Protect from light, 1 year expiration.

B. 6% AQUEOUS PHENOL

Follow the above procedure with the exception of the following changes in step #2:
a. Use .65 ml 89% liquefied phenol.
b. Use 9.35 ml sterile water.
c. Omit anhydrous glycerin.

C. PHENOL IN CONTRAST MEDIUM

Boas et al[1,2] have recommended the use of a preparation of phenol and contrast medium as the preferred solution for neurolysis. The obvious exception would be for intrathecal neurolysis which requires the use of a hyperbaric solution of phenol. Boas has demonstrated that the iodinated contrast solution Conray 420 may be used for this purpose and that its phenol solubility exceeds that of water. Using ultraviolet spectrophotometry his group has demonstrated that each compound remains chemically stable when mixed (ie, no release of free iodine, no degradation of, phenol) and that the resulting compound remains stable for a minimum of three months. Boas has also advocated the use of Renografin-76,[1] another ionic compound, and Raj[3] has described the use of Amipaque, a nonionic, low osmolar contrast agent.

In order to compound phenol with such contrast agents, the procedures outlined above are followed, using the contrast agent as a diluent.

APPENDIX G-3

Preservative Free Morphine Sulfate in Sterile Water for Injection 50 mg/ml Solution (18 ml)*

MATERIALS AND INGREDIENTS
20 gauge needles
20 ml plastic luer lock syringes (2)
Millex-GS 0.2 micron filter
disposable plastic medicine cup
sterile syringe cap
Morphine Sulfate U.S.P. powder
Sterile Water for Injection U.S.P.

METHOD OF PREPARATION

1. Weigh out 900 mg of morphine sulfate U.S.P. powder on a Class A prescription balance and place into a disposable plastic medicine cup.
2. In a Class 100 laminar flow hood dissolve the powder in 18 ml of preservative free sterile water for injection to yield a 50 mg/ml solution.
3. Draw the morphine sulfate solution with a few milliliters of air into a 20 ml plastic luer lock syringe. This will allow for the expressing of residual solution from the filter during the filtration process.
4. Take a second 20 ml plastic luer lock syringe and draw the plunger back to the 20 ml graduation mark. Place a 0.2 micron GS filter with a 20 gauge needle on the syringe containing the morphine sulfate solution. Insert the needle into the lumen of the empty syringe and slowly filter and solution into it. Expel any air present in the filled syringe and then place a syringe cap on it.
5. Place a label on the barrel of the syringe that describes the contents.

---

* Morphine can technically be concentrated to 64.52 mg/ml in an aqueous solution at room temperature before crystalization occurs, but clinically, concentrations of 50 mg/ml are rarely exceeded. Various lesser concentrations of preservative free morphine sulfate can be prepared by following the above procedure and modifying the quantities of morphine in the sterile water, eg: 18 ml of a 25 mg/ml solution can be prepared by utilizing 440 mg instead of 900 mg morphine sulfate USP powder in 18 ml sterile water.

** The morphine sulfate powder may be endotoxin tested with Limulus Amebocyte Lysate (Pyrotell®, Associates of Cape Cod) to determine its pyrogenicity potential prior to employing it. The injection is ideally prepared on the day of pump fill.

*** Alternatively, a commercial preparation of preservative free morphine (Infumorph® 25 mg/ml morphine sulfate solution manufactured by Wyeth, Duramorph® .5 or 1 mg/ml morphine sulfate solution manufactured by Elkins-Sinn, or Astramorph .5 or 1 mg/ml morphine sulfate solution manufactured by Astra®) may be used. The decision to use extemporaneously prepared versus commercially prepared morphine sulfate solution depends on a variety of factors including cost, clinical requirements and access to a skilled pharmacist and manufacturing facility.

APPENDIX G-4
*Preservative Free Hydromorphone
in Sterile Water for Injection*

Hydromorphone solutions can be prepared using the above procedure except that hydromorphone U.S.P. powder is substituted for morphine sulfate U.S.P. powder. Hydromorphone can technically be concentrated to a 333 mg/ml aqueous solution, although concentrations above 100–200 mg/ml are rarely exceeded in clinical practice. The greater solubility of hydromorphone compared to that of morphine combined with the former's greater potency dramatically increases both the amount of analgesic and analgesia that can be delivered in a given volume for hydromorphone compared to morphine.

REFERENCES

1. Boas RA: The sympathetic nervous system and pain relief. In Swerdlow M, Charlton JE (eds): Relief of Intractable Pain. New York, Elsevier, 1989, p 259.
2. Boas RA, Hatangdi VS, Richards EG: Lumbar sympathectomy: A percutaneous chemical technique. Adv Pain Res Ther 1976;1:685.
3. Meissner W: Formulas. In Raj PP (ed): Practical Management of Pain. Chicago, Yearbook Medical Publishers, 1986, p 858.

Radiologic Guidance, Contrast Medium, and Untoward Reactions

Joseph A. Catania

Richard B. Patt

RADIOLOGIC GUIDANCE

The use of radiologic guidance as an adjunct to neural blockade has in recent years become not only more commonplace and well-accepted, but has come to be regarded by some authorities as essential in some settings (*eg*, neurolytic celiac plexus block, gasserian ganglion injection).[1,2] Indeed, in such settings the old argument of "guidance versus no guidance" has in some quarters been superceded by "traditional radiography versus CT scanning,"[3,4] and with the advent of nonferromagnetic needles[5] it may be a matter of time before magnetic resonance imaging is advocated. Specific indications for various types of radiologic guidance in neural blockade are described in Chapters 18–24.

PLAIN RADIOGRAPHY

Plain radiography is simple to use, readily available, and generally produces sharp images of bony and gaseous structures. Plain radiography is not however generally preferred because it is time consuming and, because most cameras are mounted in a fixed position, obtaining multiple views is awkward.

FLUOROSCOPY

Despite its higher cost, greater technical complexity, lesser availability, and a tendency toward inferior imaging capability, fluoroscopy is by far the most widely used radiographic adjunct to neural blockade. Of its advantages over plain radiography, perhaps most important is the ability to view serial images without pausing to develop film. This can be accomplished either in "real time," the effect of which is like that of a movie camera, or by obtaining serial "snapshots" during a procedure. More sophisticated units permit storage of a variable number of images for later reproduction for documentation and to assist in teaching. Another advantage is that when c-arm or biplanar units are employed, multiple tangential images can be obtained to assist in localization. Modern c-arm units, though costly, are portable and many do not require the presence of lead-lined walls. Units can be operated safely and effectively by a variety of medical personnel, including anesthesiologists.

COMPUTED TOMOGRAPHY

Computed tomography (CT) scanning has enjoyed increasing but more limited use. Its drawbacks include cost, limited availability, greater technical complexity, the need for a specially trained staff, and the requirement for patients to remain immobile for more prolonged periods. The advantages of CT scanning include better visualization of soft tissue, especially vasculature, tumor, nerves, solid and hollow organs, as well as better overall resolution.

CONTRAST MEDIUM

The use of contrast medium for nerve blocks represents a tiny fraction of its global use for diagnostic and interventional radiology. As a result, the overwhelming bulk of literature on contrast agents applies to neural blockade only by inference. Many of the comments that follow include references to the administration of contrast by intravenous and even oral routes. Inclusion is nevertheless deemed pertinent since perineural injections of contrast medium may be accidentally injected intravenously, are ultimately absorbed into the bloodstream, and in the case of CT guidance, contrast medium is often administered intravenously or orally to enhance imaging.

Independent of the type of imaging that is selected, the use of radiologic contrast medium is essential. Contrast medium is used to better determine that the needle(s) are properly localized and that the material injected

through them spreads as expected. As a corollary, the judicious use of contrast medium helps exclude aberrant spread of the injectate into areas where an intended therapeutic injection could produce harm, *eg*, vasculature, neuraxis, and organs. Further, during CT scanning, the intravascular and/or oral administration of contrast material enhances the imaging quality of the vasculature, gut, and certain end organs, further facilitating needle localization.

HISTORICAL

The potential benefit of enhancing radiologic visualization by employing radio-opaque contrast agents has long been recognized. In the mid-1920s, Swick[6] developed the first water-soluble iodinated contrast medium for use in urography. His intention was to develop a stable, water-soluble compound that could be administered intravenously and which would enhance diagnostic imaging while minimizing patient risk. Swick worked with Lichtwitz, Binz, Rath, and von Lichtenberg to develop Iopax (Uroselectan), a N-pyridone monoiodinated compound, as well as a diiodinated compound, neoiopax (Uroselectan-B). These agents provided adequate imaging qualities for excretory urography, but were accompanied by a high incidence of untoward side effects, most notably nausea and vomiting. Swick's perseverance led to the development of a monoiodinated benzoic acid derivative, iodohippurate sodium (Hippuran, Mallinkrodt Medical Inc., St Louis, MO) which continues to be used for renal scintigraphy. Diodrast (Winthrop Labs, New York, NY), a diiodinated N-pyridone compound eventually replaced neoiopax as the agent of choice for urography. When it became known that attaching an acetylated amide side chain to the structure's benzene ring resulted in reduced toxicity, Wallingford introduced sodium acetriozoate (Urokon) as an additional alternative.

Technological advances occurred at a rapid rate. Diatrizoic acid and iothalamic acid (Conray, Mallinckrodt Medical, St Louis, MO) were introduced in 1956 and 1962, respectively and soon replaced earlier agents.[7] Their triiodinated, fully substituted benzene structure produced less chemotoxicity while further improving imaging capabilities.

The quest for further improvement, especially with regard to reducing the incidence of adverse effects, prompted Almen in the late 1960s, to begin focusing on the development of lower osmolar compounds.[8] It was at this time that a correlation between toxicity, ionicity, and osmolality was first established. The development and acceptance of modern agents resulted in the near-elimination of pain associated with intravascular injection, improved intravenous tolerance, and reduced neurotoxicity.

In the 1960s, metrizamide (Amipaque, Winthrop-Breon, New York, NY) came to be regarded as the agent of choice for myelography.[8] More recently, even newer nonionic, low osmolar compounds have been introduced and are preferred in many settings. These include iohexol (Omnipaque, Winthrop Breon, New York, NY), iopamidol (Isovue, Squibb Diagnostics, New Brunswick, NJ), and ioversol (Optiray, Mallinkrodt Medical, St. Louis, MO). Ioxaglate (Hexabrix, Guerbet, Aulnay-sous-Bois, France) is also a low osmolar agent, but as opposed to the former agents, is an ionic substance. These changes in clinical practice are based on a recognition that reduced osmo- and chemotoxicity are associated with a decreased incidence of side effects with preservation of imaging quality. These agents are, however, considerably more expensive, costing in many cases 10–20 times the price of previously used agents.

CHEMISTRY AND CLINICAL CORRELATES

The array of different agents available for clinical use and the distinctions among their chemical makeup create the potential for confusion for the nonspecialist, but are nevertheless important. The chemical structure of contrast agents determines their physiobiologic behavior, and as such, to a large extent, their clinical effects.

There are four general types of contrast media: ionic monomers, ionic monoacidic dimers, nonionic monomers, and nonionic dimers.[7] The important differences between agents in these groups include the presence of a carboxyl group and the absence of a carbonyl group in nonionic agents. Monomers are characterized by the presence of an iodinated benzene ring, while dimers possess two iodinated benzene rings. The presence of hydroxyl groups in nonionic monomers confers water solubility. Ionic contrast agents typically have no hydroxyl group, with the exception of ioxithalamate and ioxaglate which each possess one hydroxyl group. Nonionic agents are generally more water-soluble (hydrophilic) than their ionic counterparts. Although ionic agents are relatively less hydrophilic, the presence of carboxyl groups confer modest degrees of water solubility. The greater hydrophilicity of the newer nonionic agents contributes to their lower intravenous and subarachnoid toxicity.[9]

Ionic agents derive their name from the presence of two ions, a negatively charged entity (anion) and a positively charged entity (cation). The anion generally contains three iodine atoms for attenuation or absorption of radiation and one carbonyl group.

OSMOLALITY AND OSMOTOXICITY

Osmotoxicity refers to a spectrum of adverse effects related to the net movement of water across cell membranes induced by the administration of a relatively hyperosmolar agent. The osmolality of agents in current clincial use may exceed that of plasma by as much as seven times for high osmolar and as little as two times for low osmolar compounds.[10] Effects attributed to high osmotic loads include sensations of warmth during arteriography, vasodilation, hypotension, changes in red blood cell plasticity, and alterations in the blood–brain barrier.

As a means to quantitate and characterize osmotoxicity, a ratio between the imaging ef-

Table H-1.
Currently Available Low Osmolar Contrast Agents*

Type	Generic Name	Trade Name
Ionic	Ioxaglate	Hexabrix
Nonionic	Iohexol	Omnipaque
	Iopamidol	Isovue
	Ioversol	Optiray

* Low osmolar agents are associated with reduced neurotoxicity and are therefore preferred for use near the spinal axis and major nerve plexi. In addition, the lower incidence of associated anaphylactoid reactions has increased their popularity in a variety of settings.

fect and osmotic effect of contrast medium is used. The imaging effect corresponds to the number of iodine atoms present, while the osmotic effect relates to the number of particles in an ideal solution.[9] The higher this ratio, the lower the osmotoxicity. For example, ionic monomers with three iodine atoms dissociating into two particles yield a ratio of 1.5. Such an agent is referred to as a ratio 3 contrast substance and has twice the number of iodine atoms and half the osmotic effect of a ratio 1.5 contrast agent.

All ionic monomeric compounds are 1.5 ratio agents and are referred to as **high osmolar** contrast media. **Low osmolar** agents have ratios of 3 and 6 and include nonionic monomers and dimers, and ionic monoacidic dimers (Table H–1).

In summary, nonionic compounds are relatively water-soluble (hydrophilic) based on the absence of charged groups and the presence of numerous hydroxyl groups. This further decreases their protein-binding and tissue-binding properties and renders these compounds more biologically inert.[7] Consequently, nonionic agents are less osmotoxic and are better tolerated when administered intravenously and intrathecally.

ADVERSE EFFECTS

The purpose of contrast medium is to enhance imaging capabilities during radiologic studies.

All other effects are unnecessary and often problematic. Pain, hemodynamic alterations, organ toxicity, and interference with clotting have all been observed. In general, the more newly synthesized low osmolar agents are associated with a lower incidence and reduced severity of adverse effects than are the older high osmolar agents. All high osmolar contrast media are ionic structures, while low osmolar media may be nonionic or ionic compounds.

CARDIOVASCULAR EFFECTS

The administration of contrast media is associated with a variety of hemodynamic sequelae. Regardless of type, administration may be associated with pain on injection, a subjective sensation of warmth, vasodilation, and hemodilution, all of which are in part related to shifts of extravascular fluid into the intravascular compartment. These effects are markedly reduced when low osmolar agents, including all nonionic compounds, are utilized.

Hyperosmolality has also been implicated in alterations in red blood cell plasticity and morphology, an effect that may precipitate erythrocyte aggregation.[8] Damage to vascular endothelium may also result, with consequent release of endogenous vasoactive substances such as histamine, serotonin, bradykinin, kallikreins, fibrinolysins, and prostaglandins.[8]

Cardiac output may decrease due to reductions in preload and/or myocardial contractility. Clinically significant changes in pulmonary artery pressure and plasma volume may occur.[11] Acute alterations in cardiac conduction including delayed atrioventricular conduction and other dysrhythmias have also been observed.[7] The likelihood and degree of these effects is significantly less both with the use of low osmolar agents and in patients with an absence of preexisting cardiac disease.

RENAL EFFECTS

The administration of contrast agents may be associated with acute renal dysfunction. This is particularly true for the high osmolar, ionized agents and with intravenous administration. Reductions in glomerular filtration rate by up to 27% have been demonstrated after angiography.[7] The frequency of renal disturbances tends to be somewhat higher in patients with pre-existing azotemia, diabetes mellitus, or documented elevations in serum creatinine.[7] Elderly patients (over age 65) and/or patients with multiple myeloma, hypertension, or hyperuricemia may also be at increased risk for developing contrast-induced nephrotoxicity.

Mechanisms of renal injury are complex and incompletely understood. Fortunately, disruptions in renal function tend to be self-limited and many mild reactions may not even be detected clinically. Proposed mechanisms include alterations in renal blood flow related to vascular damage and the release of chemical markers of tissue injury and direct tubular damage.[7] The utility of pretreatment creatinine levels to predict the likelihood of renal toxicity is controversial.[10]

COAGULATION EFFECTS

Controversy over the so-called "clotting issue" persists, in part due to conflicting evidence that supports effects that may potentially both enhance and hinder the coagulation process. Hypercoagulability is suggested by reports of thrombi observed either at or within intravascular catheters and syringes during angiographic procedures performed with nonionic contrast media.[12] While hypercoagulability is a concern for procedures that demand an anticoagulated state like angiography, there is considerably less relevance in the case of nerve blocks, where normal hemostasis is essential to avoid complications.

Thrombin contributes to coagulation by two routes: it acts specifically to convert fibrinogen to fibrin and stimulates platelet aggregation. Ionic contrast agents have been shown to interfere with clot formation by disturbing fibrin polymerization, an effect that seems to be absent with nonionic agents, which have also been observed to affect clot

formation to a lesser degree.[12] Platelet aggregation is adversely affected by the administration of contrast media, an effect that is exaggerated as osmolality and/or ionic strength is increased.[12] Even nonionic compounds are considered by some authorities as weak inhibitors of coagulation.[8]

RATIONALE FOR THE SELECTION OF CONTRAST MEDIUM

An understanding of the chemical structures of these agents leads to better selection. There is debate however, as to the actual clinical significance of some of the theoretical distinctions between agents noted above. In addition to clinical concerns, the controversy between low osmolar and high osmolar contrast medium is also one of expense, because a cost differential of up to 10–20 times exists between low osmolar and high osmolar compounds.

Guidelines for predicting toxicity and clinical suitability have been addressed by Almen[9] and summarized into three rules. Rule I states that the use of agents that are ratio 3 or higher minimizes pain during arteriography. Rule II relates to intravenous tolerance and patient safety and concludes that compounds that are low in osmolality and whose structure is characterized by high ratios of hydroxyl groups to iodine atoms are better tolerated. Rule III states that neurotoxicity is reduced, particularly in the subarachnoid space, with agents that possess fewer carboxyl groups and more evenly distributed hydroxyl groups. Thus, the radiologic literature states that all myelography and many intravascular injections in and around the central nervous system are optimally performed with nonionic agents.[7]

CONTRAST REACTIONS

The overall incidence of reactions attributed to the intravenous use of high osmolar contrast material is 5%–8%.[8] The incidence of reactions to contrast medium is greatest in the third and fourth decade, although reactions tend to be more severe in patients over age 50. Although reactions are relatively rare in children, patients less than age 1 are considered to be at relatively high risk for experiencing such reactions.[10]

Patients with a history of previous untoward reactions to contrast agents are at particular risk as are those with a history of significant allergies.[10] Patients with reactive airway disease and documented bronchospasm are predisposed to reactions, as are individuals with compromised cardiovascular status (angina, congestive heart failure, pulmonary edema, or hypertension).[7] Minor risk factors include renal insufficiency, diabetes mellitus, dehydration, dysproteinemia, and anxiety.

Both minor and severe reactions are less common with low osmolar agents, although severe reactions (epiglottic edema, hypotension, severe skin reactions) still may occur.[13] The incidence of adverse effects in patients with a history of prior reactions is lower (2.7%) with low osmolar contrast material then with high osmolar contrast material (16%–20%).[10] The overall rate of all reactions with nonionic agents has been reported as ranging from 0.6%–3.1%.[7] Nausea, vomiting, sensations of heat and pain are uncommon with low osmolar agents. If cost were not a concern, safety factors would certainly dictate that low osmolar agents be used exclusively, a trend that is evidenced in many contemporary practices.

Serious systemic reactions related to contrast media, (ionic and nonionic) can be considered either anaphylactoid-type or vasovagal in origin. Anaphylactoid-type reactions stem from the close association of these reactions with true allergy while vaso-vagal episodes are typically associated with a symptom complex consisting of bradycardia, hypotension, and alterations in mental status or loss of consciousness. Identification of the type of reaction is critical to implementing treatment (Table H–2).

ANAPHYLACTOID REACTIONS

Anaphylactoid reactions vary in severity and may be simply manifest as flushing, erythema, and/or urticaria. Manifestations of more severe reactions include airway edema, bronchospasm, and hemodynamic instability. Coughing or vomiting are frequent precursors to serious reactions.[13]

The etiology of anaphylactoid reactions is unclear and although these events clinically resemble true allergic reactions, a true antibody reaction is difficult to confirm. Release of histamine, activation of the complement and coagulation cascades, prekallikrein transformation, and generation of bradykinin have all been implicated as initiators of severe reactions.[14] In addition, patients with a strong history of atopy have a slightly higher incidence of developing a contrast medium reaction, especially if the allergy is to shellfish.[13]

Treatment of an anaphylactoid reaction begins with recognition and assessment of its severity (Table H–3). Mild reactions without evidence of airway compromise or cardiovascular dysfunction may require only careful observation, reassurance, and the administration of antihistamines. An H-1 receptor antagonist such as diphenhydramine (25–50 mg IV or IM) or hydroxyzine (50 mg IM) is usually considered effective.[13] H-2 receptor antagonists are particularly effective in minimizing cutaneous manifestations.[13] Options include cimetidine (300 mg PO or IV), ranitidine (50 mg IV) or Pepcid (20 mg IV). Although effective in mild reactions, antihistamines do not sufficiently block receptor sites to blunt the massive histamine release associated with severe reactions.

Outcome from severe reactions is dependent on prompt recognition and intervention as fatal reactions may occur within 15 minutes of injection.[13] Initial therapy includes the provision of supplemental oxygen and maintenance of the airway if it is jeopardized. Intravenous access is required to administer resuscitation medications. Vital signs and level of consciousness should be continually assessed.

Table H-2.
Management of Adverse Reactions to Contrast Media

Type	Symptoms	Recommended Treatment
Anaphylactoid	Urticaria	Antihistamines
		H-1 receptor antagonists (diphenhydramine 25–50 mg IV or hydroxyzine 50 mg IM); may add H-2 receptor antagonists (cimetidine 300 mg IVSS or ranitidine 50 mg IVSS)
	Bronchospasm	Inhaled beta adrenergics (albuterol, metaproterenol, or terbutaline) q 4–6 hr, prn
	Hypotension	Intravenous isotonic fluids (up to three liters)
		Intravenous epinephrine (dose depends on severity, see text for details)
Vaso-vagal		Trendelenberg position
	Mental clouding	Verbal and manual stimulation
	Bradycardia	IV atropine (0.8–1.0 mg)
	Hypotension	IV isotonic fluids
		Ephedrine (5–20 mg IV)

Hypotension and tachycardia frequently accompany severe reactions, and are usually most effectively treated with the rapid infusion of isotonic intravenous fluids such as sodium chloride. Volumes of up to three liters are commonly required.[13] Histamine receptor blocking agents, although insufficient as sole therapy, should be included in the treatment regimen.

Refractory hypotension or symptoms strongly suggestive of respiratory and cardiovascular compromise may be best treated with the administration of adrenergic agents.[13] Epinephrine is the preferred drug as its alpha- and beta-stimulating properties act on the heart, peripheral vasculature, and the airway. Arteriolar and venous constriction are produced by alpha agonist effects, intropy and chronotropy are augmented by beta-1 stimulation, and smooth muscle relaxation in both the vascular tree and the bronchioles is achieved by beta-2 adrenergic agonism. On a cellular level, beta-1 stimulation increases cyclic AMP, thereby restricting the release of vasoactive mediators like histamine and leukotrienes. A recommended initial intravenous dose in adults is 10–100 μg/min depending upon the severity of symptoms and signs. This may be followed by the initiation of an infusion of a preparation of 1 ml of 1:000 epinephrine in 250 ml of normal saline that is then titrated to a rate of 1–4 mcg/min. The recommended rate of infusion in children is 0.1 mcg/kg/min.[13]

Epinephrine must be administered cautiously in elderly patients, especially in the presence of known ischemic heart disease. Caution is also advised in patients chronically receiving beta-antagonist and alpha-blocking drugs. Pre-existing beta-blockade may prevent increases in the levels of AMP and may actually decrease AMP because of unopposed alpha-agonism. Alpha-blockade may reverse the expected vasopressor effect of epinephrine with subsequent falls in blood pressure due to unopposed vasodilation.

Corticosteroids may be helpful in the treatment of anaphylactoid-type reactions and some authorities recommend their use prophylactically.[14] The mechanism of action is somewhat unclear but appears to relate to their cell membrane stabilizing properties. This tends to prevent the generation and release of potent chemical mediators such as arachidonic acid, leukotrienes, prostaglandins, and platelet-activating factor.[15] Dose ranges of 200–1000 mg of hydrocortisone have been used intravenously.[13] A proposed pro-

Table H-3.
Standardized Prophylactic Treatment Regimen to Avoid Anaphylactoid Reaction in Patients at Increased Risk*

1. Document necessity of study.
2. Explain potential risks and obtain consent.
3. Pretreatment:
   a. Diphenhydramine 50 mg IM one hour beforehand;
   b. Prednisone 50 mg orally 13, 7 and 1 hr beforehand;
   c. Ephedrine 25 mg orally beforehand (if not contraindicated)
4. Employ a low osmolar agent (see Table H-1).

Also:

May add an H-2 antagonist (orally three hours before or intravenously one hour before the procedure);
Consider discontinuing beta adrenergic blockers if feasible;
For urgent procedures, may substitute 200 mg intravenous hydrocortisone immediately and every four hours until the procedure is performed.

---

* Modified from: Lieberman P: Anaphylactoid reactions to radiocontrast material. Annals of Allergy 1991;67:91.

---

phylactic regimen includes prednisone 50 mg orally thirteen hours, seven hours, and one hour before the procedure.[14]

Bronchospasm may occur alone or in combination with hemodynamic alterations. Inhaled bronchodilators such as albuterol, metaproterenol, and terbutaline may be administered for their selective beta-2 agonist effects.[13] The inhaled route of administration affords maximum local effect at airway tissue while minimizing systemic effects. A standard adult dose is typically used and may be repeated at 4- to 6-hour intervals.

VASO-VAGAL REACTIONS

Vaso-vagal reactions are an entirely different phenomena from those of an anaphylactoid type. They may result from a variety of stressful events but nevertheless remain incompletely understood. Clouding of consciousness typically results in a confused, apprehensive, and diaphoretic patient. A combination of hypotension and sinus bradycardia may develop which if untreated may progress to loss of consciousness and cardiac arrest. Vagotonicity is manifested by depression of sinoatrial and atrioventricular node activity and inhibition of the atrioventricular conduction system. In addition, peripheral vasodilation may occur as a result of increased vagal tone.

If detected early, severe reactions may be averted by manual and verbal stimulation, the application of a cool washcloth, and the Trendelenberg position. Treatment of severe vagal reactions requires correction of sinus bradycardia and hypotension, which may be aggravated by a relative fluid deficit. Atropine may be administered intravenously in a dose range of 0.8–1.0 mg. Smaller doses have been associated with worsening bradycardia and the emergence of other arrhythmias. The administration of atropine may be repeated if needed after allowing for adequate circulation time of the first dose. Intravenous administration of isotonic saline may be required to fully restore hemodynamic stability, because atropine affects cardiac slowing but not peripheral vasodilation. Ephedrine, an indirect-acting combined alpha and beta agonist agent, may be useful by augmenting cardiac intropy and chronotropy while inducing peripheral vasoconstriction. Initially, 5–10 mg should be administered intravenously. Repeated dosing may be necessary, although tachyphylaxis has been observed.

REFERENCES

1. Abram SE, Boas RA: Sympathetic and visceral nerve block. In Benumof JL: Clinical Procedures in Anesthesia and Intensive Care. Philadelphia, JB Lippincott, 1992, p 787.
2. Scott DB: Techniques of Regional Anaesthesia. Norwalk, CT, Appleton & Lange, 1989, pp 56, 210.
3. Singler RC: An improved technique for alcohol neu-

rolysis of the celiac plexus. Anesthesiology 1982; 56:137.

4. Jain S, Alagesan R, Harris A, Chiang J: Elective neurolysis of carnial nerve using computerized tomography. Anesthesiology 1991;75(suppl):A-748.

5. Mueller P, Stark D, Simeone JF: Clinical use of a nonferromagnetic needle for magnetic resonance guided biopsy. Gastrointestinal Rad 1989;14:61.

6. Swick M: Radiographic media in urology: The discovery of excretion urography: Historical and developmental aspects of the organically bound urographic media and their role in the varied diagnostic angiographic areas. Surg Clin NA 1978;58:977.

7. McClennan BL, Stolberg HO: Intravascular contrast media: Ionic versus nonionic: Current status. Radiologic Clinics of North America 1991;155:225.

8. McClennan BL: Ionic and nonionic iodinated contrast media: Evolution and strategies for use. Am J Roentgenology 1990;155:225.

9. Almen T: Contrast media: The relationship of chemical structure, animal toxicity and adverse clinical effects. Am J Cardiology 1990;66:1F.

10. King BF, Hartman GW, Williamson Jr B, LeRoy Jr A, Hattery RR: Low-osmolality contrast media: A current perspective. Mayo Clinic Proceedings 1989;6: 976.

11. Hirshfeld JW: Cardiovascular effects of iodinated contrast. Am J Cardiology 1990;66:9F.

12. Stormorken HV: Effects of contrast media on the hemostatic and thrombotic mechanisms. Investigative Radiology 1988;23(suppl):S-318.

13. Bush WH: Treatment of systemic reactions to contrast media. Urology 1990;35:145.

14. Lieberman P: Anaphylactoid reactions to radiocontrast material. Annals of Allergy 1991;67:91.

15. Zipser RD, Laffi CT: Prostaglandins, thromboxanes, and leukotrienes in clinical medicine. West J Med 1985;143:485.

Index

Page numbers followed by f *indicate figures; those followed by* t *indicate tabular material.*